Daniel Oertli · Robert Udelsman (Eds.)

Surgery of the Thyroid and Parathyroid Glands

With 235 Figures and 52 Tables

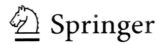

Springer

Editors

Daniel Oertli
Division of General Surgery,
University Hospital Basel,
Vice-Dean of the Medical Faculty,
University of Basel
4031 Basel
Switzerland

Robert Udelsman
Lampman Professor of Surgery and Oncology,
Chairman, Department of Surgery,
Surgeon-in-Chief – Yale-New Haven Hospital
Yale University School of Medicine
PO Box 208062
New Haven, CT 06520-8062
USA

ISBN-13 978-3-642-06713-6   e-ISBN-13 978-3-540-68043-7

Springer is a part of Springer Science + Business Media
springer.com
© Springer-Verlag Berlin Heidelberg 2010

Editor: Gabriele M. Schröder, Heidelberg, Germany
Desk Editor: Stephanie Benko, Heidelberg, Germany

Cover Design: estudio calamar, Spain
Printed on acid-free paper 24/3100/YL - 5 4 3 2 1 0

Acknowledgement

The Editors are deeply indebted to all authors and coauthors who have contributed to *Surgery of the Thyroid and Parathyroid Glands*. The Editors believe that this textbook is among the most comprehensive international references on surgical diseases of the thyroid and parathyroid glands. The diligent efforts of the contributors, who have provided insightful state-of-the art presentations, are gratefully acknowledged.

The Editors also wish to pay tribute to the diligent work of the Springer-Verlag staff members, who enabled the realization of this first edition. Particularly appreciated were the efforts of Gabriele M. Schroeder, Executive Editor, and Stephanie Benko, Desk Editor, who provided strong encouragement and ongoing support during the creation of this textbook. Furthermore, the Editors are most appreciative of the principal artist, Mr. Jörg Kühn, who provided us with excellent drawings.

We also express our gratitude to the valuable coordinative work of our editorial assistants in Basel and New Haven: special thanks are addressed to Susan Demou, Madeleine Moser, and Dotty Franco.

Finally, our profound gratitude goes to all who were involved in the development of this text, including our immediate families, who expressed interest and encouragement in the completion of this textbook. We greatly appreciate their support, which stimulated us to pursue the ambitious goal of preparing what we consider to be a concise, comprehensive textbook.

DANIEL OERTLI and ROBERT UDELSMAN

Preface

Thyroid and parathyroid disorders are frequently encountered by the endocrine surgeon in daily practice. The Editors therefore have designed this comprehensive textbook focusing on surgically relevant thyroid and parathyroid diseases. The Editors intend this book to become an important reference presenting the latest information regarding the management of both common and rare thyroid and parathyroid disorders. Internationally renowned physicians and surgeons have provided detailed outlines and discussions on operative techniques and treatments accompanied by rationales for particular approaches advocated by the authors. The topics cover all surgically relevant thyroid and parathyroid pathologies, the preoperative surgical evaluation, decision making, and operative strategies including high quality step-by-step illustrations of the current surgical techniques. Furthermore, experts are presenting the molecular basis for thyroid neoplasia and the current understanding of the genetics of inherited thyroid and parathyroid diseases. Moreover, evolving modern operative techniques like the minimally invasive videoscopic approach to the thyroid and parathyroid glands are discussed in this textbook.

The current edition has been designed primarily to meet the requirements of young surgeons who wish to acquire profound knowledge of basic, clinical, and laboratory concepts as well as surgical techniques regarding the thyroid and parathyroid glands, thus complementing the surgeons' training. These principles are presented together with advancements in technologic, molecular, cellular, and biologic sciences, thus meeting the criteria of the 21st century definition of each subspecialty involving care of patients with thyroid and parathyroid disease. The preparation of the text material has been a labor of love and represents an honest attempt to provide information that we believe is not only of clinical importance to surgeons, but also to endocrinologists, radiologists, and pathologists dealing with patients with thyroid and parathyroid disorders.

It is hoped that the reader will find the material in our textbook as helpful and exciting as we do.

Daniel Oertli and Robert Udelsman

Table of Contents

List of Contributors

Michel Adamina
Division of General Surgery,
University Hospital Basel,
Spitalstrasse 21,
4031 Basel,
Switzerland

Reza Asari
Division of Endocrine Surgery,
Department of Surgery,
Vienna University Hospital,
Vienna,
Austria

Zubair W. Baloch
Department of Pathology and Laboratory Medicine,
University of Pennsylvania Medical Center,
Philadelphia, PA,
USA

Detlef K. Bartsch
Department of Surgery,
Philipps-University, Marburg,
Germany

Prabhat K. Bhama
Division of Endocrine Surgery,
University of Michigan Medical School,
Ann Arbor, MI,
USA

Leon D. Boudourakis
Yale University School of Medicine,
New Haven, CT,
USA

Anne E. Busseniers
Metropolitan FNA Service,
Washington, DC; Bethesda, MD,
USA
and
Department of Pathology,
Vrije Universiteit Brussels,
Brussels,
Belgium

Tobias Carling
Department of Surgery,
Yale University School of Medicine,
New Haven, CT,
USA

Nadine Caron
Department of Surgery,
University of California San Francisco and
UCSF Comprehensive Cancer Center at Mt Zion
Medical Center,
San Francisco, CA,
USA

Herbert Chen
Department of Surgery,
University of Wisconsin,
H4/750 Clinical Science Center, 600 Highland
Avenue,
Madison, WI,
USA

David W. Cheng
Department of Diagnostic Radiology,
Yale University School of Medicine,
New Haven, CT,
USA

Mirjam Christ-Crain
Department of Endocrinology,
John Vane Science Centre,
Barts and the London Medical School,
Charterhouse Square,
London,
UK

Gerard M. Doherty
Division of Endocrine Surgery,
University of Michigan Medical School,
Ann Arbor, MI; 2920B Taubman Health Care Center,
Box 0331, 1500 E. Medical Center Drive,
Ann Arbor, MI,
USA

Quan-Yang Duh
Department of Surgery,
University of California San Francisco and
Veterans Affairs Medical Center,
San Francisco, CA,
USA

Hermann Engel
Institute of Radiology and Nuclear Medicine,
Hospital Waid,
Zürich,
Switzerland

Andrea Frilling
Department of General Surgery,
Visceral surgery and Transplantation,
University Hospital Essen,
Essen,
Germany

Oliver Gimm
Department of General,
Visceral and Vascular Surgery, University of Halle,
Ernst-Grube-Strasse 40,
06097 Halle,
Germany

Peter E. Goretzki
Department of Surgery,
Lukaskrankenhaus of the Heinrich-Heine University
Düsseldorf,
Neuss,
Germany

Ulrich Güller
Department of Surgery,
Divisions of General Surgery and Surgical Research,
University of Basel,
Basel,
Switzerland

Elizabeth H. Holt
Section of Endocrinology,
Yale University School of Medicine,
New Haven, CT,
USA

Silvio E. Inzucchi
Section of Endocrinology,
Yale University School of Medicine,
New Haven, CT,
USA

Ludwig A. Jacob
Section of Interventional Radiology,
Department of Radiology,
University Hospital Basel,
Basel,
Switzerland

Moosa Khalil
University of Calgary,
Pathologist, Calgary Laboratory Services,
Calgary, Alberta,
Canada

Bernhard J. Lammers
Department of Surgery,
Lukaskrankenhaus of the Heinrich-Heine University
Düsseldorf,
Neuss,
Germany

Peter Langer
Department of Surgery,
Philipps-University Hospital, Baldingerstrasse,
D-35043 Marburg,
Germany

Virginia A. LiVolsi
Department of Pathology and Laboratory Medicine,
University of Pennsylvania Medical Center,
Philadelphia, PA,
USA

Gabriele Materazzi
Department of Surgery,
Azienda Ospedale Università di Pisa,
Pisa,
Italy

Michael Mayr
Division of Transplantation Immunology and
Nephrology, Department of Internal Medicine,
University of Basel, Basel,
Switzerland

Christoph A. Meier
Endocrine Unit, Division of Endocrinology,
Diabetes and Nutrition,
Department of Internal Medicine, University
Hospital Geneva,
CH-1211 Geneva 14,
Switzerland

Paolo Miccoli
Department of Surgery,
Azienda Ospedale Università di Pisa,
Pisa,
Italy

Nils G. Morgenthaler
Institut für Experimentelle Endokrinologie,
Charité Campus Mitte,
Universitätsmedizin Berlin,
Berlin,
Germany

Jan Mueller-Brand
University of Basel,
School of Medicine, Basel;
Division of Nuclear Medicine and PET Center,
University Hospital Basel,
Basel,
Switzerland

Beat Müller
Dept. of Endocrinology,
Diabetology and Clinical Nutrition,
University Hospital,
Petersgraben 4,
Basel,
Switzerland

Bruno Niederle
Division of Endocrine Surgery,
Department of Surgery,
Medical University of Vienna,
Währingergürtel 18–20,
A-1090 Vienna,
Austria

Egbert U. Nitzsche
University of Basel,
School of Medicine,
Basel;
Division of Nuclear Medicine and PET Center,
Aarau General (Cantonal) Hospital, Aarau,
Switzerland

Daniel Oertli
Division of General Surgery,
University Hospital Basel,
Vice-Dean of the Medical Faculty,
University of Basel,
Basel,
Switzerland

Janice L. Pasieka
Division of General Surgery,
Department of Surgery,
Faculty of Medicine, University of Calgary,
Calgary, Alberta,
Canada

Christian Passler
Division of Endocrine Surgery,
Department of Surgery,
Vienny University Hospital,
Vienna,
Austria

Michel Procopiou
Division of Endocrinology, Diabetes and Nutrition,
Department of Internal Medicine,
University Hospital Geneva,
CH-1211 Geneva 14,
Switzerland

Lawrence J. Rizzolo
Section of Anatomy,
Department of Surgery,
Yale University School of Medicine,
PO Box 208062,
New Haven, CT 06520-8062,
USA

Hans-Dietrich Röher
Klinik für Allgemein und Unfallchirurgie,
Universitätsklinikum Duesseldorf,
Moorenstrasse 5,
40225 Düsseldorf,
Germany

Sanziana Alina Roman
Section of Endocrine Surgery,
Department of Surgery,
Yale University School of Medicine,
PO Box 208062,
New Haven, CT 06520,
USA

Rachel Rosenthal
Division of General Surgery,
Department of Surgery,
University Hospital Basel,
Spitalstrasse 21,
CH-4031 Basel,
Switzerland

Matthias Rothmund
Department of Surgery,
Philipps-University,
Marburg,
Germany

Christian Scheuba
Division of Endocrine Surgery,
Department of Surgery,
Vienny University Hospital,
Vienna,
Austria

Klaus-Martin Schulte
Department of Endocrine and General Surgery,
King's College Hospital,
Denmark Hill,
London SE5 9RS,
UK

Leslie M. Scoutt
Department of Diagnostic Radiology,
Yale University School of Medicine,
New Haven, Connecticut
USA

Susan A. Silver
Metropolitan FNA Service,
Bethesda, Washington, DC,
USA

Rebecca S. Sippel
Department of Surgery,
University of Wisconsin,
H4/710 Clinical Science Center,
600 Highland Avenue,
Madison, WI,
USA

Julie Ann Sosa
Sections of Oncologic,
Endocrine, and General Surgery,
Yale University School of Medicine,
330 Cedar Street,
New Haven, CT 06520-8062,
USA

Wolfgang Steinbrich
Institute of Diagnostic Radiology,
University Hospital Basel,
Petersgraben 4, 4031 Basel,
Basel,
Switzerland

William B. Stewart
Department of Surgery,
Yale University School of Medicine,
PO Box 208062,
New Haven, CT 06520-8062,
USA

Cord Sturgeon
Department of Surgery,
Northwestern University Feinberg School of
Medicine,
Division of Gastrointestinal and Endocrine Surgery,
Chicago, IL,
USA

Robert Udelsman
Department of Surgery,
Yale University School of Medicine,
PO Box 208062,
New Haven, CT 06520-8062,
USA

Ana Paola Uranga
Department of Surgery,
Yale University School of Medicine,
330 Cedar Street FMB 102,
New Haven, CT 06520, USA

Kate V. Viola
Sections of Oncologic,
Endocrine, and General Surgery,
Yale University School of Medicine,
330 Cedar Street,
New Haven, CT 06520-8062,
USA

Frank Weber
Department of General Surgery,
Visceral Surgery and Transplantation,
University Hospital Essen,
Essen,
Germany

Walter Wiesner
Medical Radiology Center,
Klinik Stephanshorn,
Brauerstrasse 95,
9016 St. Gallen,
Switzerland

Heather Yeo
Department of Surgery,
Yale University School of Medicine,
330 Cedar Street FMB 102,
New Haven, CT 06520-8062,
USA

1 History of Thyroid and Parathyroid Surgery

Hans-Dietrich Röher and Klaus-Martin Schulte

CONTENTS

1.1 Introduction

Endocrine surgery is the concept and practice of surgically applied human physiology. This concept has deep historical roots and has been nourished by many thoughts, ideas, and discoveries. Several individuals influenced this interesting field primarily providing answers to human physiology and secondarily to questions on surgical technique. Indeed, the proper function of the thyroid as an endocrine gland was discovered by a surgeon. Moreover, surgeons pioneered the recognition of parathyroid disease. Unlike in any other field, operative principles in endocrine surgery have been developed after recognition of the homeostatic regulations of different endocrine organ systems. Hence interest in molecular biology resulted in a profound understanding of the endocrine control of cellular homeostasis. This resulted in the first entirely gene-directed surgical procedure in man, the prophylactic thyroidectomy in multiple endocrine syndrome 2A. Historically, endocrine surgery represents a major pathway for the import and export of ideas, a trafficking place, where anatomy, physiology, biological and analytical chemistry, imaging, and surgical technique have ideally met and influenced each other.

1.2 Recognition of Goitrous Disease

In the first and second centuries, Celsus and Galen described cervical masses such as cysts, tuberculous lymph nodes (scrofula), and goiters. In the eleventh century, the Arabic scientist Abulkasim, working in Cordoba, Spain, differentiated natural, endemic goiter from non-natural goiter [17]. Between the eleventh and the mid-thirteenth century, the renowned medical school of Salerno near Naples, Italy, gave advice for conservative treatment of goiter disease using sea products such as burned sponge. On the other hand, the school recommended cauterization or seton implants in order to induce necrotizing inflammation and tissue destruction for selected cases [9]. In these times, nothing was really known about the organic source of goiter formation.

1.3 Anatomy of the Thyroid Gland

In 1543, the anatomist Andrea Vesalius (1514–1564; Fig. 1.1) originally described "glandulae laryngis" in his inauguration of modern anatomy *De Humani Corporis Fabrica* published in Basel, Switzerland. The first distinct image of the thyroid gland with the typical horseshoe shape dates back to the work of Julius Casserius (1545–1616) [23]. Casserius was a servant of Hieronymus Fabricius of Aquapendente, Professor and Chairman of Anatomy and Surgery at the University of Padua between 1609 and 1616. The first utilization of the term "glandula thyreoidea" was made by Thomas Wharton, London, UK (1656) and by Albrecht von Haller, Göttingen, Germany. They attributed endocrine secretory properties to this ductless gland.

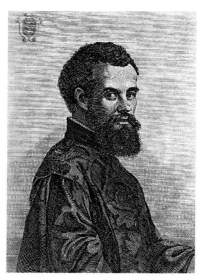

Fig. 1.1 Andreas Vesalius (1514–1564) was a Belgian anatomist and physician whose dissections of the human body and descriptions of his findings helped to correct misconceptions prevailing since ancient times. As Professor of Anatomy in Padua (Italy) Vesalius wrote the revolutionary texts *De Humani Corporis Fabrica*, seven illustrated volumes on the structure of the human body

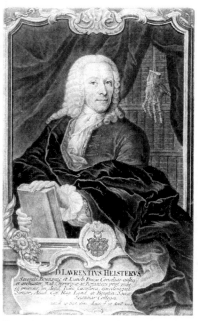

Fig. 1.2 Lorenz Heister (1683–1758) served as an army surgeon in several German campaigns before becoming Professor of Anatomy and Surgery at Altdorf. Distressed at the inferior state of surgery he published his *Chirurgie* (Nuremberg, 1718)

1.4   Early Attempts at Surgery

Over several following centuries, written sources documented that attempts were undertaken for surgical removal of goiters. The indication for surgery was primarily given by extensive cervical masses or severe tracheal obstruction resulting in dyspnea. However, the operative results were disastrous with extremely high mortality because of fatal bleeding or infection.

In 1742, Lorenz Heister (1683–1758; Fig. 1.2), who had founded scientific surgery in Germany, first described the surgical removal of a thyroid gland. While describing thyroid colloid substance in 1754, he was among the first who acknowledged the practical value of the understanding of endocrine substances. Heister already knew that goiters can turn malignant, as he thought, after they had been treated with acid substances. He also recognized the erosion of neck vessels by malignant goiters and gave attention to thyroid cancer. In 1792, the French surgeon Pierre Joseph Desault (1744–1795) demonstrated that a partial thyroid resection may be feasible and thereby opened the proper way into thyroid surgery at a time when hormone replacement was not even theoretically known [10].

Following this, Johann August Wilhelm Hedenus (1760–1836) operated on six patients who had suffered from airway obstruction by giant goiters [24].

Thyroid surgery remained a life-threatening procedure during these times even in the hands of the most skilled surgeons. The mainly fatal outcome after goiter surgery motivated the leading German surgeon Johann Dieffenbach from Berlin to make the statement in 1848 that "goiter surgery is one of the most thankless, most perilous undertakings." Also the French Academy of Medicine criticized any thyroid operation in 1850, and Bernhard Rudolph Conrad Langenbeck (1810–1887) vehemently warned to avoid it.

1.5   Thyroid Physiology

Surgeons provided the first substantial evidence of endocrine secretion by the thyroid gland. Thomas Wilkinson King (1809–1847) from London wrote in his observations on the thyroid gland:

The most important novel fact concerning the thyroid gland is doubtless this, that its absorbent vessels carry its peculiar secretion to the great veins of the body and the most simple and satisfactory method of demonstrating this fact is to expel the contents of the healthy gland by repeated and gentle compressions, into the lymphatics of the surface and then to coagulate the fluid on the surface... Whilst the nourishment of a part is indispensable to its existence, the influence which it exerts upon the circulating fluids may be more or less needful for the healthful subsistence of the entire animal [27].

In the same volume, Sir Astley Cooper (1768–1841) had included a report on his experimental thyroidectomies in dogs. In 1827 he observed how slowly the dogs recovered after a period of stupor and tiredness. In 1859 the German physiologist Moritz Schiff (1823–1896) published his experiences of total thyroidectomy and showed that all thyroidectomized dogs and guinea pigs eventually died postoperatively. Some simultaneously appearing treatises on the coincidence of goiter and cretinism should have rendered obvious the nature of an "endocrine organ," but these observations remained without general practical consequences. Because this seemed so ridiculous to his contemporaries, Sir Felix Semon (1849–1921) was unable to publish his hypothesis in 1883 that myxedema and cretinism were caused by the loss of thyroid function.

1.6   Morbidity of Thyroid Surgery During the Nineteenth Century

Intra- and postoperative bleeding was the major problem in thyroid surgery of those days and surgeons had just learned how to tackle it. William Blizzard (1743–1835) tried to cure thyroid overfunction by ligation of the upper pole arteries. Luigi Porta (1800–1875) contributed in two major respects. First he performed a targeted adenoma excision in 1849. Second, his attempt to cure thyroid hyperfunction by unilateral arterial ligation failed and therefore Porta concluded that bilateral ligations would be necessary. Edmund Rose (1836–1914) followed up this idea. After succeeding Theodor Billroth as the Surgical Chairman in Zurich, Switzerland, Rose published his treaty on *Der Kropftod und die Radikalkur der Kröpfe* (death by goiter and radical cure of goiters). He stated that goitrous recurrence could only be prevented by a complete removal of the gland. For this he described meticulous ligation of every single vessel feeding the gland whilst respecting the recurrent laryngeal nerves, the vagal nerves, as well as the hypoglossal nerves.

The main problems during the nineteenth century were bleeding and infection. Being among the leading surgical experts in Europe, Theodor Billroth (1829–1894; Fig. 1.3) reported an intraoperative mortality of 36% for thyroid surgery. During the second half of the nineteenth century, three key factors largely contributed to the development and progress of thyroid surgery. First, William Morton from Boston, USA, invented inhalation anesthesia in 1846. Second, in 1867, Lord Joseph Lister from Glasgow, UK, introduced the

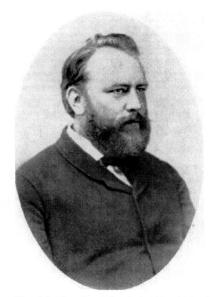

Fig. 1.3 Theodor Billroth (1829–1894) obtained his medical degree from the University in Berlin in 1852 and became assistant to Bernhard von Langenbeck in 1854. He was appointed Professor of Clinical Surgery in Zurich in 1860 and Professor of Surgery at the University of Vienna in 1867. Courtesy of Prof. U. Boschung, Institute of Medicine History, University of Berne, Switzerland

principles of antisepsis [30]. Third, in 1874, Thomas Spencer Welles developed "hemostatic forceps" for surgery. These new developments enabled surgeons to substantially refine their operating technique.

This pioneering era in thyroid surgery was dominated by Theodor Billroth, who worked in Zurich, Switzerland, between 1860 and 1867 and later on in Vienna, Austria, and by his disciple Anton Wölfler (1850–1917). Their efforts targeted at complete removal of the thyroid gland in order to facilitate intraoperative hemostasis after describing techniques using ligation of the arteries [57].

In 1879, Claude Bernard stated that "We do not know anything about the use of these organs (i.e. thyroid, thymus), we don't even have an idea about their utility and importance..." Of note, this statement coincides with the first thyroidectomy for a goiter associated with exophthalmus performed by Ludwig Rehn (1849–1930).

1.7   Relevance of Postoperative Loss of Thyroid Function

The discovery of the importance of human thyroid function dates back to 1882 and should be attributed to the surgeon Jacques-Louis Reverdin (1842–1929;

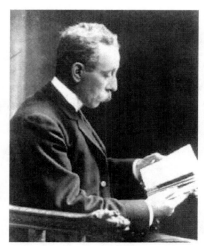

Fig. 1.4 Jacques-Louis Reverdin (1842–1929), Professor of Surgery, Geneva, Switzerland. Courtesy of Prof. U. Boschung, Institute of Medicine History, University of Berne, Switzerland

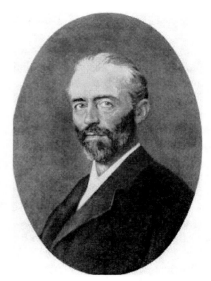

Fig. 1.5 Theodor Kocher (1841–1917), Professor of Surgery. In 1872, he became Chairman at the University Hospital in Berne and remained in this post in spite of several invitations to foreign universities. Courtesy of Prof. U. Boschung, Institute of Medicine History, University of Berne, Switzerland

Fig. 1.4), and to his cousin Auguste Reverdin (1848–1908). They called this postoperative state "myxoedeme opératoire." A letter of J.-L. Reverdin to Theodor Kocher in 1882 described a case of cretinism following thyroidectomy. In 1883, Reverdin published on the thyroprivic consequences of 22 thyroidectomies. Thereafter, he vehemently advocated to avoid thyroidectomy and omitted this operation [47]. Theodor Kocher (1841–1917; Fig. 1.5), however, resolutely pursued the issue that had been raised by the Reverdins. This culminated in his historic manuscript *Ueber Kropfexstirpation und ihre Folgen* (on the removal of goiter and its consequences) [28]. For his work, Kocher was later awarded the Nobel prize for physiology or medicine in 1909.

Starting from the personal case of the eleven-year-old Maria Bichsel in 1874, Kocher developed the concept of "kachexia thyreopriva" that summarizes the various consequences for the entire body due to the lack of thyroid hormone function. After 1883, Kocher strongly promoted the use of the unilateral operation to avoid the thyroprivic state. This concept found worldwide acceptance and was transferred to the United States by Charles Mayo, the pioneer of endocrine surgery in the new world [36–38].

In parallel one of Billroth's disciples Johann v. Mikulicz-Radecki (1850–1905) recognized the problems of too extensive thyroid surgery. He replaced the complete thyroidectomy by a bilateral partial resection in order to reduce the potential local harm to the parathyroids (whose function was only partially understood) and to the laryngeal nerves. The remnant would take over the thyroid function. Whereas the understanding of the consequence of complete loss of thyroid function can be attributed to the Reverdins and to Kocher, the recognition of postoperative tetany was made by Billroth and his pupils Wölfler and von Eiselsberg. They recognized the association between parathyroprivic symptoms and the loss of the parathyroid glands.

1.8   Surgery for Hyperthyroidism

Thyroid operations were initially performed to solve mechanical airway obstruction. Attention to hyperthyroidism was paid much later in time. Caleb Hillier Parry first described an "exophthalmic goiter" [43]. In the English and the German literature, the clinical complex of autoimmune hyperthyroidism was described by Robert James Graves (Fig. 1.6) and by Carl Adolf von Basedow (Fig. 1.7), respectively [1,15]. In 1884, Ludwig Rehn (1849–1930) from Frankfurt, Germany, opened the way for surgical cure of Graves' disease [46]. Mikulicz expanded the indication for surgery by "exophthalmic goitre." Initially, many of these patients were treated with a unilateral approach, resulting in recurrences.

During the first two decades of the twentieth century, the unilateral operation for thyroid toxicosis was still the mainstay in the United States. In many instances a multistage procedure was performed. After

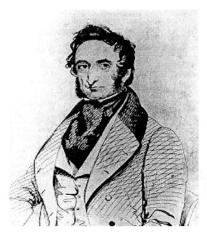

Fig. 1.6 Robert James Graves (1796–1853)

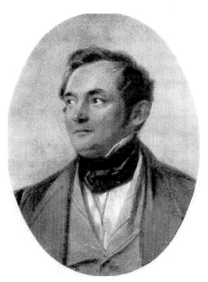

Fig. 1.7 Carl Adolf von Basedow (1799–1854)

initial occlusion of the thyroid arteries, a lobectomy was done in a second operation. A third intervention was often indicated if the disease persisted or recurred. F. Hartley (New York, USA, 1905) and Thomas Dunhill (Melbourne, Australia, 1907) changed this paradigm [11,22]. They showed that hyperthyroidism can be cured by unilateral lobectomy and contralateral subtotal resection. Dunhill also surmounted the contraindications for surgery in the presence of cardiac symptoms. He demonstrated that surgery may be successful even in patients with tachyarrhythmia and cardiac failure. The reports on his successes were first doubted and ignored, and Dunhill decided to travel from Australia to the United Kingdom and the United States. In the United States, his technique and his indications were well accepted, although without being quoted by the leading surgeons. This may be the reason why both Dunhill and Hartley were ignored until their preferred operation was elevated to the standard surgical technique for hyperthyroidism. Another milestone was made by Charles Mayo, Henry Plummer, and Walter Boothby from the Mayo Clinic in the 1920s. They showed that the risks and severity of perioperative thyroid storm were greatly reduced by preoperative peroral administration of large doses of iodine using the Wolff-Chaikoff effect [44,45,55]. Perioperative mortality in 600 patients was reduced from 5% to less than 1%. The introduction of radioiodine ablation therapy in 1942 and of thyrostatic drugs in 1943 dramatically changed the treatment patterns in hyperthyroidism and almost replaced surgery for a while.

During the 1950s the repertoire of diagnostic tools expanded. By detection of stimulating antibodies, the immunogenic nature of hyperthyroidism can now be proven and classified. The preoperative therapy using high-dose iodine according to Plummer has been replaced by thyrostatic drug therapy that allows for a fine hormonal tuning and for timing of surgery. Modern surgical treatment of hyperthyroidism consists of a differentiated approach with either near-total or total thyroidectomy for immunogenic hyperthyroidism and with lobectomy for toxic adenomas.

1.9   Thyroid Cancer Surgery

Histopathology has emerged as the preeminent tool for the classification of thyroid cancers. This led to the recognition of the biologically different behavior of different cancer subtypes and to the introduction of differentiated surgical strategies. Another major step is the, still incomplete, acceptance of prognostic scoring systems including tumor, node, metastases (TNM), European Organization for Research and Treatment of Cancer (EORTC), Age, Grade, Extent, Size (AGES), Age, Metastases, Extent, Size (AMES), and the Metastases, Age, Completeness of resection, Invasion, Size (MACIS). All these classifications allow the comparison of treatment results in cohorts from different continents treated with a broad range of regimens.

1.10   Thyroid Surgery in Modern Times

Since 1980 molecular medicine has provided major insights into the impact of genetic mutations eventually leading to thyroid tumors. This has not only yielded a further possibility of tumor classification according to their specific genetic changes, but it has also opened the path to the recognition of specific cancer predispositions in individual family members. Since mutations of the RET protooncogene can be detected in peripheral blood lymphocytes, prophylactic thyroidectomy can be cancer preventive. Presymptomatic thyroidectomy in individuals with the mutated RET protooncogene represents the first indication in the history of surgery which is fully and solely based on the genetic proof of a malignant trait, i.e., medullary thyroid cancer. Genetic research has also proven the unifying causative changes in familiar syndromes, such as multiple endocrine neoplasia type I and II [53,54] and diseases caused by changes in the succinate dehydrogenase complex. The lively interchange between basic molecular research and clinical practice has revolutionized endocrine surgical practice.

The recent years represent an industrious period of relentless technical research and improvement in endocrine surgery. This has reduced the operative risks with regard to all forms of complications. Bleeding is now rare, and most thyroid surgery can safely be performed without the need of drainage. Infection has virtually disappeared. Due to vigorous protection of the anatomical structures and consequent identification of the recurrent laryngeal nerve, permanent nerve palsies occur in less than 1% of cases. Hypoparathyroidism has been reduced to frequencies below 1% due to meticulous preparation techniques and the generous use of parathyroid autotransplantation. Mortality is almost nil.

The most recent enrichments of the surgical repertoire are the targeted, minimally invasive, and endoscopic approaches. The evolutionary progress of techniques and indications is underway. A more secure estimation of the safety of these techniques needs further consolidation of data and experiences.

1.11 Discovery of the Parathyroid Glands

Small things often go unnoticed. It is no surprise that this holds true for the parathyroid glands that even today may sometimes be difficult to retrieve. Although Thomas Wharton gave a detailed report on the "glandulae thyroideae" in 1656, he did not mention the parathyroid glands.

The first description of the parathyroid glands was by the London anatomist and curator of the Natural History Museum, Sir Richard Owen, in 1850

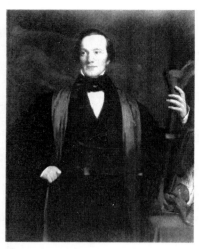

Fig. 1.8 Sir Richard Owen (1804–1892) was a pioneering British comparative anatomist who coined the term dinosauria

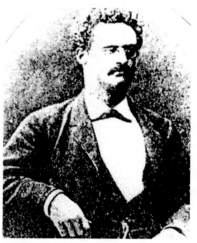

Fig. 1.9 Ivar Sandström. Reprinted with permission from Organ CH (2000) J Am Coll Surg 191:284

(Fig. 1.8). He discovered them when he was dissecting a rhinoceros that had died in the London Zoo. The respective paper was eventually published in the Zoological Proceedings of London [41]. He was not given credit for his observation because he never performed histological confirmation. This state of affairs lasted until 1887 when the medical student Ivar Sandström (Fig. 1.9) described tiny glandular elements in 50 dissected human bodies. He gave a comprehensive description of their appearance, position, size, and blood supply. His publication contains various issues of far-reaching importance, such as the finding that the blood supply derives from the inferior thyroid artery and may be multiple. His work *On a New Gland in Man and Several Animals* was rejected by German editors and eventually published in Swedish in the Uppsala Medical Journal [48]. This may have contributed to the lack of recognition of this brilliant young man who later committed suicide.

1.12   Parathyroid Preservation

Sandström's detailed dissection of the parathyroids and their blood supply were consolidated by the meticulous work of Herbert M. Evans, Johns Hopkins, Baltimore, who identified the variations of blood vessels and thereby heralded the protection of glandular function by maintenance of their blood supply. His mentor, William Halsted (Fig. 1.10) immediately derived the correct instinctive conclusion, that the thyroid artery should be ligated proximal to the thyroid gland while sparing the parathyroid end arteries [20].

Kocher and Billroth were the two exponents of thyroid surgery at the end of the nineteenth century. Each had founded a surgical school—Kocher in Bern and Billroth in Vienna—and the respective postoperative outcomes reflected the particular techniques utilized in each school. Kocher experienced the symptoms associated with radical removal of the thyroid, leading to postoperative hypothyroidism "cachexia strumipriva." Billroth's patients experienced tetany. Halsted gives another example of his surgical instinct when he associated these differences to the characters of operating surgeons:

Kocher, neat and precise, operating in a relatively bloodless manner, scrupulously removed the entire thyroid gland, doing little damage outside the capsule. Billroth, operating more rapidly, and as I recall his manner, with less regard for tissues and less concern for hemorrhage, might easily have removed the parathyroids or at least interfered with their blood supply, and have left remnants of the thyroid [19].

This description still is of enormous value since it teaches us about some of the virtues needed for successful endocrine surgery.

Billroth's pupils discovered the symptom complex of postoperative hypocalcaemia. Anton Wölfler gave a full and detailed account of tetany in the first patient who had undergone a total thyroidectomy by Theodor Billroth [56]. The patient recovered after having experienced the full range of symptoms over a period of three weeks. Nathan Weiss collected more data from patients with postoperative tetany [51]. These experiences stimulated Mikulicz to develop his technique of protection of the posterior thyroid capsule. Surgical knowledge about the parathyroids emerged from sur-

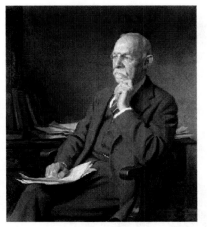

Fig. 1.10 William Stewart Halsted (1852–1922) was a true surgical innovator. Halsted revolutionized surgery by insisting on skill and technique rather than brute strength. Using an experimental approach, he developed new operations for intestinal and stomach surgery, gallstone removal, hernia repair, and disorders of the thyroid gland. He first practiced in New York and in 1886 became the first Professor of Surgery at Johns Hopkins

gical complications and preceded the discovery of the parathyroid function.

1.13   Tetany and Hypoparathyroidism

In 1891 the French physiologist Eugene Gley clarified the relation between parathyroid gland function and tetany [14]. He described tetany in rats and rabbits as a consequence of the removal of the thyroid and parathyroid glands. Moreover, he could show that removal of the parathyroids alone would have the same effect. The concept of parathyroid transplantation was born.

The first parathyroid autotransplantation was performed in 1892 by Anton von Eiselsberg (Fig. 1.11), Vienna, Austria. He transplanted thyroid and parathyroid tissue into the preperitoneal space of cats and showed that tetany was absent and new vessels had formed at the transplants. In contrast, tetany occurred after these transplant were removed [12].

Also William J. MacCallum at Johns Hopkins, Baltimore, described the use of parathyroid extracts to cure tetany in experimental animals [31,32]. He transferred upcoming knowledge about the role of calcium in nerve conduction and muscle action and formed a hypothesis that the parathyroid glands may play a role in calcium metabolism. This ingenious conclusion was later proven in experiments by Carl Voegtlin and it was shown that tetany caused by parathyroid-

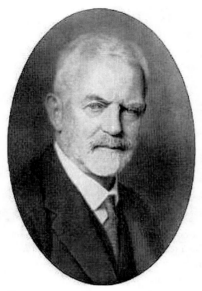

Fig. 1.11 Baron Anton von Eiselsberg was Professor and Chairman at the Allgemeines Krankenhaus in Vienna, Austria

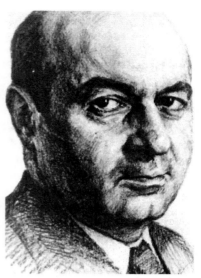

Fig. 1.12 Felix Mandl (1892–1957) was Professor of Surgery and Chairman of the Department of Surgery at the Franz-Joseph-Spital, Vienna, Austria. Reprinted with permission from Organ CH (2000) J Am Coll Surg 191:284

ectomy could be corrected with parathyroid extract or by injections of calcium [33]. This was a major advance, although MacCallum remained uncertain about the value of his own discoveries for another decade. In 1907, William Halsted at Johns Hopkins used parathyroid extract and calcium chloride to treat postoperative tetany [18]. He reported on the cure of "hypoparathyrosis" by parathyroid transplantation. However, the problems with parathyroid extracts were the difficulty of their production, the lack of stability, and the variability of biological activity. Adolf Hansen developed a method for hormone extraction from bovine parathyroid glands. In animal experiments, these extracts were able to cure tetany and raise the serum calcium of parathyroprivic dogs. They also induced osteoporosis after administration over a prolonged period [21]. These findings were substantiated with detailed experiments conducted by James P. Collip [6,7]. An immunoassay for parathyroid hormone detection in peripheral blood was developed by Yalow and Berson [4,58]. In 1977 the DNA sequence of the gene for parathyroid hormone was identified [3] and the respective cDNA was cloned in 1981 [25]. Today, human recombinant parathyroid hormone is available for treatment of hypoparathyroidism.

1.14   Hyperparathyroidism and Parathyroidectomy

After parathormone (PTH) deficiency was recognized and could be treated during the first decade of the twentieth century, the problems of hyperparathyroidism still remained unrecognized. Both physiologists and surgeons investigated parathyroid action and regulation of calcium metabolism. In 1906 Jacob Erdheim reported that the enlarged parathyroid glands were associated with bone diseases like osteitis fibrosa cystica and osteomalacia. His false conclusion was that the glands were enlarged as a consequence of bone disease [13]. Although no evidence was produced to support this assumption, it was generally accepted. With this background of medical error, we can understand how Felix Mandl (1892–1957; Fig. 1.12) treated his patient Albert Gahne. The patient suffered from bone pain and from a fracture of the femur. Radiographs demonstrated numerous bone cysts and the patient's blood and urinary calcium levels were elevated. Mandl first administered parathyroid extract which failed. He concluded that the dose was too low and obtained fresh parathyroid tissue from a trauma victim; this was grafted into the patient without success. Mandl received sharp criticism from his colleagues at the annual meeting of the Vienna Surgical Society just because he had failed to prove that he really had transplanted parathyroid tissue and not something else. Somehow his mind turned around and in 1925 he explored the neck of his patient and removed a parathyroid tumor. This was now followed by a clinical success and it inverted the paradigm [34,35]. However, the patient later died from a recurrence. Mandl might have operated on the first case of parathyroid cancer.

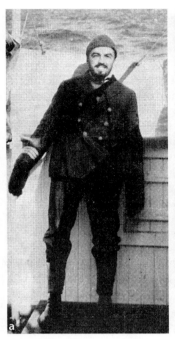
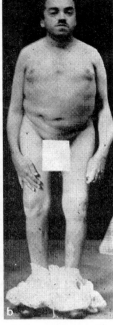

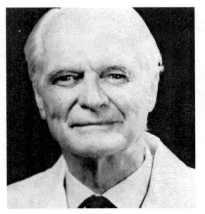

Fig. 1.14 Oliver Cope. Reprinted with permission from Organ CH (2000) J Am Coll Surg 191:284

Fig. 1.13a,b Charles Martell, Captain of US merchant marine. Reprinted with permission from Bauer E, Federman DD (1962) Metabolism 11:22

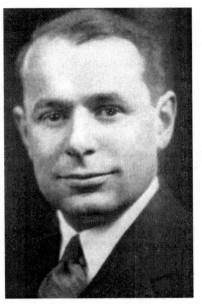

Fig. 1.15 Edward Churchill. Reprinted with permission from Organ CH (2000) J Am Coll Surg 191:284

In the United States E.J. Lewis at Cook County Hospital, Chicago, performed the first excision of a parathyroid tumor, again likely to be a carcinoma, in 1926 [16]. Unfortunately, the patient suffered from recurrences.

The case of Captain Charles Martell (Fig. 1.13) illustrates the problems of ectopic parathyroid adenoma [2]. The patient was a master mariner of the U.S. merchant marine with transport duties in the North Atlantic. In 1918, he was 22 years of age, about 1.85 m tall, and obviously in fine physical condition (Fig. 1.13a). A year later, Captain Martell's disease became manifest with severe osteopathy and nephrolithiasis. In 1926 when Martell entered the Massachusetts General Hospital (MGH) for surgery, the patient had shrunk by about 18 cm (Fig. 1.13b). By this time he had experienced eight fractures and suffered from marked kyphosis and bone deformities. The two first cervical explorations done by Dr. E.P. Richardson were unsuccessful. A third operation was performed in 1932 by Dr. Russell Patterson in New York City, with no tumor being discovered, and Martell returned to the MGH. Dr. Oliver Cope (Fig. 1.14) and Dr. Edward D. Churchill (Fig. 1.15) performed three subsequent cervical reinterventions without finding an adenoma.

The captain, who was often found in his room reading anatomy texts, was now convinced that the tumor was to be sought in the chest, and he urged a mediastinotomy. The seventh operation was performed by Churchill, with Cope's assistance, and a mediastinal encapsulated brown tumor of 3 cm in diameter was found. The two surgeons excised only 90% of the adenoma, attaching the remnant with its vascular pedicle to the region of the sternal notch. Despite this, tetany developed three days after surgery. Six weeks postoperatively a kidney stone became impacted in the ureter and Captain Martell died from larnygospasm shortly after a surgical intervention to relieve his ureteral obstruction. After 1932, Cope and Churchill performed a number of successful parathyroidectomies.

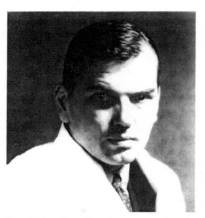

Fig. 1.16 Fuller Albright. Reprinted with permission from Organ CH (2000) J Am Coll Surg 191:284

Isaac Y. Olch performed the first successful operation of a parathyroid gland in the United States. In 1928, he removed a 3×3 cm adenoma from the left inferior thyroid pole from a patient at Barnes Hospital of the Washington University School of Medicine in St. Louis, Missouri. The definitive breakthrough of parathyroid surgery occurred in the late 1920s and early 1930s and can be ascribed to the group around Fuller Albright (Fig. 1.16) who studied in detail the pathophysiology of parathyroid bone disease and recognized hyperparathyroidism as a distinct clinical syndrome.

1.15 Different Forms of Hyperparathyroidism

One of the major issues was the discovery that parathyroid surgery may well be unsuccessful despite removal of one adenoma. Double adenomas and multiglandular hyperplasia became recognized disease entities of primary hyperparathyroidism. This led Paloyan and many others to the recommendation of subtotal parathyroidectomy in all cases. The dominant adenoma and at least two further glands would have to be resected to prevent recurrence [42]. With the more widespread availability of calcium and PTH assays the disease was considered to be due to hormone excess rather than adenoma formation. Early unsuccessful operations in cases of multiple diseased glands shifted the entire field of parathyroid surgery toward a principal bilateral exploration of all glands. In 1982, this paradigm was challenged when Tibblin advocated unilateral surgery for single adenomas [49].

In the late 1960s and 1970s surgery for secondary hyperparathyroidism due to chronic renal failure became popular [26]. The general recommendation was that of total or subtotal parathyroidectomy with or without autotransplantation and cryopreservation of tissue [52].

For both situations, the difficult adenoma in primary hyperparathyroidism and for retrieval of supernumerary glands in secondary hyperparathyroidism, attempts were made to improve preoperative localization by selective catheter angiography and venous sampling and computed tomography. Both did not offer satisfactory results. Rather they led to the quotation: "The most convincing localisation is to locate an experienced endocrine surgeon."

Further technical innovations significantly influenced parathyroid surgery. In 1989, A.J. Coakely noticed that technetium sestamibi is rapidly taken up by the parathyroids [5]. This has provided surgery with a potent tool for preoperative imaging, useful both in primary and redo situations. A focused surgical access is possible thanks to preoperative scintigraphy and cervical ultrasonography. Quick methods for assessment of PTH emerged. In 1988, Nussbaum provided evidence that PTH measures can be produced during the operation and thereby identify success [39]. This has rendered intraoperative frozen section much less important. Various combinations of imaging techniques and intraoperative hormone assessments are actually under consideration with regard to success rates and cost efficiency.

Uniglandular disease may well be approached by minimally invasive techniques, such as focused mini-incisions or endoscopy.

Today, the diagnosis of hyperparathyroidism can readily be made. The association between elevated PTH and bone disease is well understood, whereas the effects of elevated PTH on the central nervous system needs further investigation. Parathyroid surgery for primary hyperparathyroidism has nowadays a success rate close to 99%, operative complications are below 1%, and mortality is virtually nil.

References

1. Basedow CA von (1840) Exopthalmos durch Hypertrophie des Zellgewebes in der Augenhöhle. Wochenschr Gesamte Heilkunde 6:197
2. Bauer W, Federman DD (1962) Hyperparathyroidism epitomized: the case of Captain Charles E. Martell. Metabolism 11:21–29
3. Baxter JD, Seeburg PH, Shine J, Martial JA, Goodmann HM (1977) DNA sequence of a human coding for a polypeptide hormone. Clin Res 25:514A

4. Berson SA, Yalow RS, Aurbach GD, Potts JT Jr (1963) Immunoassay of bovine and human parathyroid hormone. Proc Natl Acad Sci USA 49:613–617

5. Coakley AJ, Kettle AG, Wells CP, et al (1989) ^{99m}Tc sestamibi a new agent for parathyroid imaging. Nucl Med Commun 10:791–794

6. Collip JP (1925a) A case of tetany treated with parathyrin. Can Med Assoc 15:59–60

7. Collip JP (1925b) Extraction of a parathyroid hormone which will prevent or control parathyroid tetany and which regulates the levels of blood calcium. J Biol Chem 63:395–438

8. Cope O (1966) The story of hyperparathyroidism at the Massachusetts General Hospital. N Engl J Med 274:1174–1182

9. Corner A (1931) Rise of medicine at Salerno in the twelfth century. Am Med Hist New Series 3:1–16

10. Desault PJ (1792) Giraud. J Chir (Paris) iii:3

11. Dunhill T (1909) Remarks on partial thyroidectomy, with special reference to exophthalmic goitre, and observations on 113 operations under local anaesthesia. BMJ 1:1222

12. Eiselsberg A von (1892) Ueber erfolgreiche Einheilung der Katzenschilddrüse in die Bauchdecke und Auftreten von Tetanie nach deren Extirpation. Wien Klin Wochenschr 5:81–85

13. Erdheim J (1906) Tetania parathyreopriva. Mitt Grenzgeb Med Chir 16:632–744

14. Gley ME (1891) Sur les functions du corps thyroide. CR Soc Biol 43:841–843

15. Graves RJ (1835) Clinical lectures (part II). London Med Surg J 7:516

16. Guy CC (1929) Tumors of the parathyroid glands. Surg Gynaecol Obstet 48:557–565

17. Haddad FS (1968) Albucasin. Abbotempo 3:22

18. Halsted WS (1907) Hypoparathyreosis, status parathyreoprivus, and transplantation of the parathyroid glands. Am J Med Sci 134:1–12

19. Halsted WS (1920) The operative story of goiter. The author's operation. John Hopkins Hosp Rep 19:71–257

20. Halsted WS, Evans HM (1907) The parathyroid glandules: their blood supply and their preservation in operations upon the thyroid gland. Ann Surg 46:489

21. Hanson AM (1923) An elementary chemical study of the parathyroid glands of cattle. Mil Surg 52:280–284

22. Hartley F (1905) Thyroidectomy for exophthalmic goiter. Ann Surg 42:33

23. Hast M (1970). The anatomy of the larynx: an aspect of renaissance anatomy by Julius Casserius. Proc Inst Med Chic 28:64

24. Heidel G, Wundrich B, Dehne A (1986) Our surgical heritage. The Dresden surgeon Johann August Wilhelm Hedenus (1760–1836). Zentralbl Chir 111:1551–1558

25. Hendy GN, Kronenberg HM, Potts JT Jr, Rich A (1981) Nucleotide sequence of cloned cDNAs encoding human preproparathyroid hormone. Proc Natl Acad Sci U S A 78:7365–7369

26. Katz AI, Hampers CL, Wilson RE, Bernstein DS, Wachman A, Merrill JP (1968) The place of subtotal parathyroidectomy in the management of patients with chronic renal failure. Trans Am Soc Artif Intern Organs 14:376–384

27. King TW (1836) Guy's Hospital Reports 1:429–446

28. Kocher T (1883) Über Kropfextirpation und ihre Folgen. Arch Klin Chir 29:254

29. Kocher T (1910) Ueber Jodbasedow. Arch Klin Chir 92:1166–1193

30. Lister J (1909) The collected papers of Joseph Baron Lister. Clarendon, London

31. MacCallum WJ (1905) The physiology and the pathology of the parathyroid glands. Bull Johns Hopkins Hosp 86:625–633

32. MacCallum WG (1912) The function of the parathyroid glands. JAMA 59:319

33. MacCallum WJ, Voegtlin C (1908) On the relation of the parathyroid to calcium metabolism and the nature of tetany. Bull Johns Hopkins Hosp 19:91–92

34. Mandl F (1925) Therapeutischer Versuch bei Ostitis fibrosa generalisata mittels Exstirpation eine Epithelkörperchens. Wien Klin Wochenschr 38:1343–1344

35. Mandl F (1926) Attempt to treat generalized fibrous osteitis by extirpation of parathyroid tumor. Zentralbl Chir 53:260–264

36. Mayo CH (1909) Ligation of the thyroid vessels in certain cases of hyperthyroidism. Ann Surg 50:1018–1024

37. Mayo CH (1910) Ligation and partial thyroidectomy for hyperthyroidism. In: Mellish MH (ed) Collected papers by the staff of St. Mary's Hospital, Mayo Clinic. Mayo Clinic, Rochester, MN, p 476

38. Mayo CH (1913) Surgery of the thyroid. Observations on 5,000 operations. JAMA 61:10

39. Nussbaum SR, Thompson AR, Hutcheson KA, et al (1988) Intraoperative measurement of parathyroid hormone in the surgical management of hyperparathyroidism. Surgery 104:1121–1127

40. Organ CH (2000) The history of parathyroid surgery, 1850–1996: the Excelsior Surgical Society 1998 Edward D. Churchill lecture. J Am Coll Surg 191:284–299

41. Owen R (1862) On the anatomy of the Indian rhinoceros (*Rh. Unicornis*, L). Trans Zool Soc London 4:31–58

42. Paloyan E, Lawrence AM, Baker WH, Straus FH II (1969) Near-total parathyroidectomy. Surg Clin North Am 49:43–48

43. Parry CH (1825) Collections from the unpublished papers of the late Caleb Hilliel Parry, vol 2. Underwood, Fleetstreet Press, London

44. Plummer HS (1923a) The value of iodine in exophthalmic goitre. Collect Pap Mayo Clin 15:565–576

45. Plummer HS (1923b) Results of administering iodine to patients having exopthalmic goiter. JAMA 80:1955

46. Rehn L (1884) Ueber die Exstirpation des Kropfs bei Morbus Basedowii. Berl Klin Wochenschr 163–166

47. Reverdin J, Reverdin A (1883) Note sur vingt-deux opérations de goitre, avec 3 pl. photographiques. Rev Med Suisse Romande 3:169–198

48. Sandström I (1880) On a new gland in man and several mammals (in Swedish). Upsala Laekarefoeren Foerh 15:441–471

49. Tibblin SA, Bondeson AG, Ljungberg O (1982) Unilateral parathyroidectomy in hyperparathyroidism due to single adenoma. Ann Surg 195:245–252

50. Vassale G, Generali F (1896) Sugli effeti dell'estirpazione delle ghiandole paratiroide. Riv Patol Nerv Ment 1:95–99

51. Weiss N (1881) Ueber Tetanie. Sammlung Klinischer Vorträge 189. Innere Medizin 63:1675–1704

52. Wells SA, Christiansen C (1974) The transplanted parathyroid gland: evaluation of cryopreservation and other environmental factors which affect its function. Surgery 75:49–55

53. Wells SA, Chi D, Toshima K (1994) Predictive DNA testing and prophylactic thyroidectomy in patients at risk for multiple endocrine neoplasia type 2A. Ann Surg 220:237–250

54. Wermer P (1954) Genetic aspects of adenomatosis of endocrine glands. Am J Med 16:363

55. Wolff J. Chaikoff I (1948) Plasma inorganic iodide as a homeostatic regulator of thyroid function. J Biol Chem 174:555–564

56. Wölfler A (1882) Die Kropfextirpationen an Hofr. Billroth's Klinik von 1877 bis 1881. Wien Med Wochenschr 32:5

57. Wölfler A (1886) Die operative Behandlung des Kropfes durch Unterbindung der zuführenden Arterien. Wien Med Wochenschr 36:1013–1017

58. Yalow RS, Berson SA (1953) Assay of plasma insulin in human subjects by immunologic methods. Nature 184:1648

2   Embryology and Surgical Anatomy of the Thyroid and Parathyroid Glands

William B. Stewart and Lawrence J. Rizzolo

2.1   Embryology of the Thyroid

The primordial thyroid gland is first identifiable during the fourth week of gestation, beginning as an endodermal invagination of the tongue at the site of the foramen cecum (Fig. 2.1a). The foramen cecum lies where the midline intersects the sulcus terminalis, which divides the tongue into anterior two thirds (oral part) and posterior one third (pharyngeal part). The thyroid diverticulum begins its descent through the tongue carrying with it the thyroglossal duct. The path of descent carries the developing gland anterior to the hyoid bone and the larynx. During the descent in the fifth week, the superior part of the duct degenerates. By this time, the gland has achieved its rudimentary shape with two lobes connected by an isthmus. It continues to descend until it reaches the level of the cricoid cartilage at about the seventh week. By the twelfth week of development, thyroid hormone is secreted. The distal part of the thyroglossal duct degenerates but may remain as a pyramidal lobe [8].

There is also a contribution to the thyroid from the fifth pharyngeal pouch (ultimobranchial body). These cells are believed to be neural crest in origin. They migrate into the thyroid and differentiate into the calcitonin-producing C cells (Fig. 2.1a) [4].

A number of developmental errors can affect thyroid development. The thyroid may fail to descend.

In this case, a lingual thyroid is located at the junction of the oral and pharyngeal parts of the tongue (Fig. 2.1b). Ectopic thyroid tissue may occur at any point along the pathway of the descent of the thyroid. In rare conditions, the thyroid may descend into the thorax. There may also be remnants of the thyroglossal duct that hypertrophy and become cystic (Fig. 2.1c). Ectopic thyroid tissue may also be encountered laterally in the neck [9]. Evaluation of the patient should consider whether the ectopic tissue is the sole active thyroid tissue. In very rare circumstances thyroid tissue may be encountered inferior to the diaphragm in association with the gastrointestinal tract. This thyroid tissue, a struma ovarii, is derived from an ovarian germ cell tumor [5].

2.2   Embryology of the Parathyroid Glands

The parathyroid glands develop from the third and fourth pharyngeal (branchial) pouches (Fig. 2.1a). These pharyngeal pouches develop in association with the aortic arches that encircle the developing foregut. The pharyngeal arches have a mesodermal core, covered on their superficial surface by ectoderm and on their deep surface by endoderm. The pharyngeal pouches lie between successive pharyngeal arches and are endodermal evaginations of the foregut. The inferior parathyroid glands (parathyroid III) come from the third pharyngeal pouch and the superior parathyroid glands (parathyroid IV) come from the fourth pharyngeal pouch. During the fifth week of development, the developing glands detach from the pouches and descend to join the thyroid gland during the seventh week. It should be noted that the inferior parathyroid glands actually arise from a more superior pharyngeal location (pouch III) than the superior thyroids (pouch IV). This relationship may be explained by the relationship of the developing inferior parathyroid gland with the thymus. The thymus arises from the caudal portion of the third pharyngeal pouch. As the thymus descends into the thorax,

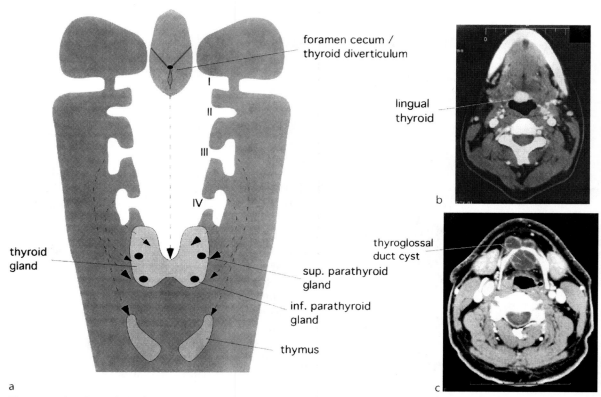

Fig. 2.1 Embryology of the thyroid and parathyroid. **a** Schematic view from behind with the vertebral column, esophagus, and trachea removed. The foramen cecum and emerging thyroglossal duct are indicated in the tongue. *Dashed arrow* shows migration of thyroid along the anterior wall of the neck. Laterally, the pharyngeal pouches are numbered. These are evaginations of the foregut into the mesoderm that contains the aortic arches. Each pouch lies inferior to the aortic arch of the same number. The parathyroid glands originate in the pharyngeal pouches and migrate into position as indicated by the *dashed arrows*. Note the co-migration of the inferior parathyroids with the thymus gland. **b** CAT scan with intravenous contrast demonstrates the concentration of iodine into an undescended (lingual) thyroid gland. The anterior two thirds of the tongue lies anteriorly to the gland. **c** CAT scan at the level of the hyoid bone exhibits a thyroglossal duct cyst. **b** and **c** courtesy of Dr. James Abrahams, Department of Diagnostic Imaging, Yale University School of Medicine

Table 2.1 Location of 54 ectopic parathyroid glands identified by Shen and co-workers [13]

Location	Number
High cervical	1
Aorticopulmonary window	2
Posterior mediastinum	3
Carotid sheath	5
Intrathyroid	6
Anterior mediastinum (non-thymic)	9
Intrathymic	13
Paraesophageal (neck)	15

it is accompanied by the inferior parathyroid glands. Normally the attachment to the thymus is lost and the inferior parathyroid glands take up their normal position posterior to the thyroid. Sometimes, however, the inferior parathyroid glands are carried into the thorax along with the thymus. The ectopic parathyroid gland may be found in a number of locations (Table 2.1). The most common locations were intrathymic or paraesophageal in the neck [13].

2.3   Anatomy of the Thyroid Gland

2.3.1   General Topography and Relations

The right and left lobes of the thyroid are connected at the midline by the isthmus of the gland. A pyramidal lobe may extend superiorly from the isthmus or from the medial portions of the left or right lobes. The thyroid extends from the level of the fifth cervical vertebra to the first thoracic vertebra. The gland weighs

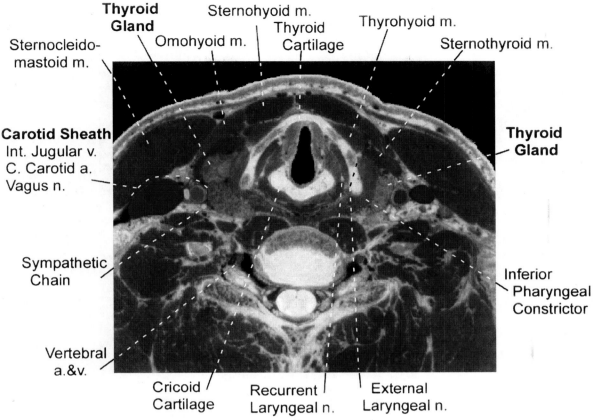

Fig. 2.2 Thyroid gland and its relations at the level of the thyroid cartilage. An unembalmed cadaver was frozen and sectioned (Visible Human Project, National Institutes of Health). The orientation is the same as for a CAT scan with patient's left on the right side of the image. Color enhancement demonstrates major arteries (*red*), veins (*blue*), and nerves (*yellow*). Note the close relationship of the superior pole of the thyroid gland with the carotid sheath and sympathetic chain

about 30 g, being somewhat heavier in females than in males [12]. The thyroid is surrounded by a sleeve of pretracheal fascia sometimes called the perithyroid sheath. Posteriorly, a thickening of this fascia attaches the gland to the cricoid cartilage. This fascia is the lateral ligament of the thyroid (ligament of Berry).

The anterior surface of the thyroid is related to the deep surface of the sternothyroid, sternohyoid, and omohyoid muscles (Figs. 2.2, 2.3). Where these muscles are absent in the midline, the isthmus of the gland is subcutaneous. Laterally the gland is related to the carotid sheath, which contains the common carotid artery, the internal jugular vein, and the vagus nerve. Posteriorly, the superior parts of the lobes of the thyroid are related to the longus colli and longus capitis muscles. Medially, the superior part of the thyroid is related to the larynx and laryngopharynx, which includes the cricothyroid and inferior pharyngeal constrictor muscles and the thyroid and cricoid cartilages. Medially, the inferior part of the thyroid is related to the trachea and the esophagus. The isthmus

of the thyroid lies anterior to the second and third tracheal rings. The description of relationships to important neural structures will be deferred to that section.

2.3.2 Blood Supply

As with other endocrine organs, the thyroid gland has a rich blood supply with abundant anastomoses. The arterial supply is bilateral from both the external carotid system, through the superior thyroid artery, and the subclavian system, through the inferior thyroid branch of the thyrocervical trunk (Fig. 2.4). There may be a single thyroid ima artery that arises from the brachiocephalic artery.

The superior thyroid artery is normally the first branch of the external carotid artery, though frequently it may arise more inferiorly from the common carotid artery. This vessel descends to the superior pole of the thyroid along with the external laryngeal

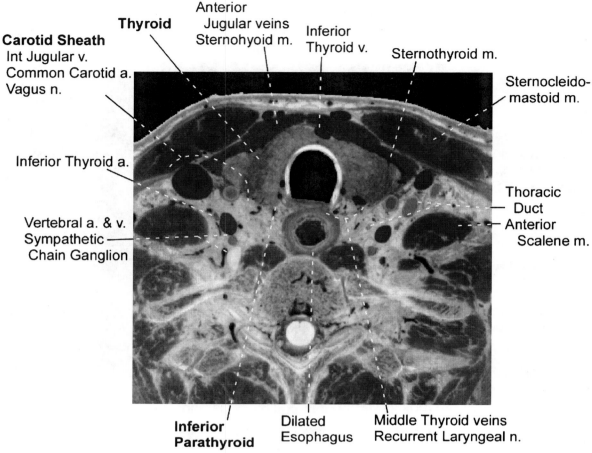

Fig. 2.3 Thyroid gland and its relations at the level of the third tracheal ring. Note the posteromedial relationships of the thyroid gland with the recurrent laryngeal nerve and middle thyroid veins. The thoracic duct (*green*) is atypically dilated close to where it joins the left internal jugular and subclavian veins. The inferior thyroid artery follows a looping course. In this image it is seen superior to its origin from the thyrocervical trunk of the subclavian artery. It will loop superiorly and medially before descending to join the thyroid gland near the recurrent laryngeal nerve. An inferior right parathyroid gland (*orange*) is evident near the recurrent laryngeal nerve and middle thyroid veins. Major nerves (*yellow*), arteries (*red*), and veins (*blue*) are indicated

nerve. As it reaches the thyroid, the artery divides into anterior and posterior branches (Fig. 2.5). The anterior branch parallels the medial border of the lobe and anastomoses in the midline with the anterior branch of the other side. The posterior branch anastomoses with branches of the inferior thyroid artery.

The inferior thyroid artery takes a looping course. It ascends along the anterior scalene muscle (Fig. 2.3). It turns medially to pass posteriorly to the carotid sheath and usually posteriorly to the sympathetic trunk as well. It descends along the longus colli to reach the inferior pole of the thyroid. There it passes to the thyroid either anteriorly or posteriorly to the recurrent laryngeal artery. At the thyroid, the artery branches into superior and inferior branches. The superior branch ascends on the posterior part of the gland to anastomose with the posterior branch of the superior thyroid artery. The inferior branch supplies the inferior part of the gland as well as the inferior parathyroid glands. The inferior thyroid artery may be absent on either side. There is evidence that there are anthropologic differences in the incidence of thyroid ima arteries, as well as in the symmetric origin of the superior thyroid arteries [17].

There are three main venous pathways from the thyroid: the superior, middle, and inferior thyroid veins (Fig. 2.6). The superior thyroid vein accompanies the superior thyroid artery and drains into the internal jugular vein. The middle thyroid vein is unaccompanied and drains directly into the internal jugular vein. Because of its posterior course, it is at risk when forward traction is applied to the gland, as

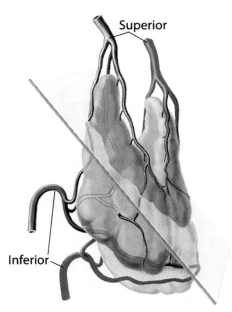

Fig. 2.4 Arterial supply of thyroid and parathyroid glands is divided into a superior and a inferior system. Superior and inferior thyroid arteries are indicated.

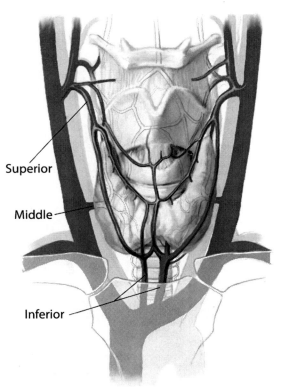

Fig. 2.6 Venous drainage of the thyroid and parathyroid glands. Superior, middle and inferior thyroid veins are indicated.

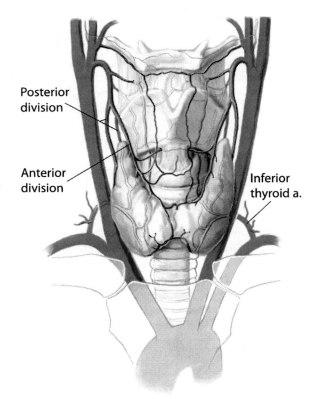

Fig. 2.5 Arterial supply of the thyroid derived from the four main vessels of the gland. Note the anterior and posterior divisions of the superior artery. The inferior thyroid artery comes from a posterolateral position to enter the thyroid gland close to the recurrent laryngeal nerve

in a thyroidectomy (Fig. 2.3). There are often a number of inferior thyroid veins that drain into the internal jugular or the brachiocephalic veins.

The lymphatic drainage of the lateral part of the thyroid follows the arterial supply. These lymphatic vessels either ascend with the superior thyroid artery or descend with the inferior thyroid artery to reach the jugular chain of nodes. Between these two arteries, lymphatic vessels may pass directly to the jugular nodes. The medial aspect of the gland drains superiorly to the digastric nodes and inferiorly to the pretracheal and brachiocephalic nodes [15].

2.4 Anatomy of the Parathyroid Glands

There are normally two pairs of parathyroid glands, located along the posterior aspect of the thyroid gland (Fig. 2.7). The superior parathyroid glands normally lie at the level of the middle third of the thyroid, while the inferior parathyroid glands lie at the level of the inferior third. Generally, the superior parathyroid glands are supplied by the inferior thyroid artery, the

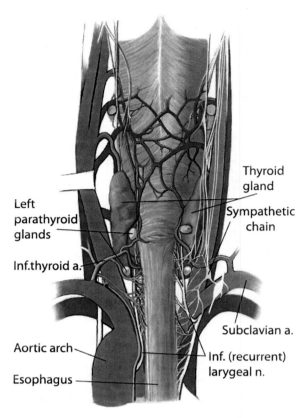

Left parathyroid glands

Thyroid gland

Sympathetic chain

Inf. thyroid a.

Subclavian a.

Aortic arch

Inf. (recurrent) larygeal n.

Esophagus

Fig. 2.7 Schematic dorsal view shows the course of the inferior laryngeal nerve in relation to the inferior thyroid artery, the thyroid gland, and the parathyroid glands

superior thyroid artery, or both. Anastomotic connections within the thyroid allow both vessels to contribute, especially to the superior parathyroid glands. A number of methods have been advocated for localizing the glands. These include ultrasonography [6], intraoperative methylene blue [7], and technetium sestamibi scans [18].

2.5 Nearby Relations of the Thyroid and Parathyroid at Risk During Surgery

2.5.1 External Laryngeal Nerve

The external laryngeal is a division of the superior laryngeal nerve, a branch of the vagus. This nerve supplies the cricothyroid muscle. Since this muscle is involved in movements of the vocal apparatus, damage to the nerve will impair phonation. The nerve may run near the superior pole of the thyroid on the way

to its target. The external laryngeal nerve is frequently entrapped in the vascular pedicle that transmits the superior thyroid vessels. Consequently the nerve may be injured during the ligation of these vessels [2,3].

2.5.2 Recurrent Laryngeal Nerve

The recurrent laryngeal nerve, a branch of the vagus, supplies the remainder of the laryngeal musculature as well as sensation on and inferior to the vocal folds (Figs. 2.2, 2.3). On the right side, the nerve loops posteriorly to the subclavian artery to ascend obliquely until it reaches the tracheoesophageal groove near the inferior extent of the thyroid (Fig. 2.7). On the left side the nerve loops posteriorly to the arch of the aorta and ascends to the larynx in the tracheoesophageal groove. The nerve may divide into a number of branches that also supply the trachea and esophagus [10]. The nerve has a very close relationship with the inferior thyroid artery, where it might lie either anteriorly or posteriorly to the vessel (Fig. 2.7). Because the left inferior thyroid artery may be absent in 6% of individuals, the identification of the recurrent laryngeal nerve may be more complicated [14]. The nerve may also be closely related to or within the ligament of Berry. Care must be taken in both retraction and division of the ligament to ensure that the nerve is preserved. There are some cases where the nerve may run through the substance of the gland [11,16].

In a small number of individuals (approximately 1%) the right subclavian artery arises distally from the arch of the aorta [1]. As a consequence the right recurrent laryngeal nerve is not pulled into the thorax by its relationship with the subclavian artery. This non-recurrent right laryngeal nerve passes directly to the larynx posterior to the common carotid artery. It runs parallel to the inferior thyroid artery and can ascend for a short distance in the tracheoesophageal groove [15]. It is, therefore, at risk for injury during surgery.

The vagus nerve and sympathetic trunk are within or closely related to the carotid sheath (Figs. 2.2, 2.3, 2.8). The vagus nerve may receive some of its blood supply from the inferior thyroid artery [15]. Consequently, the artery should not be ligated too close to its origin. Lymph node dissection along the carotid artery and near the vertebral artery or any manipulation near the superior pole of the thyroid gland should also be performed with care to ensure that the cervical sympathetic chain ganglia are not damaged or removed (Figs. 2.2, 2.3).

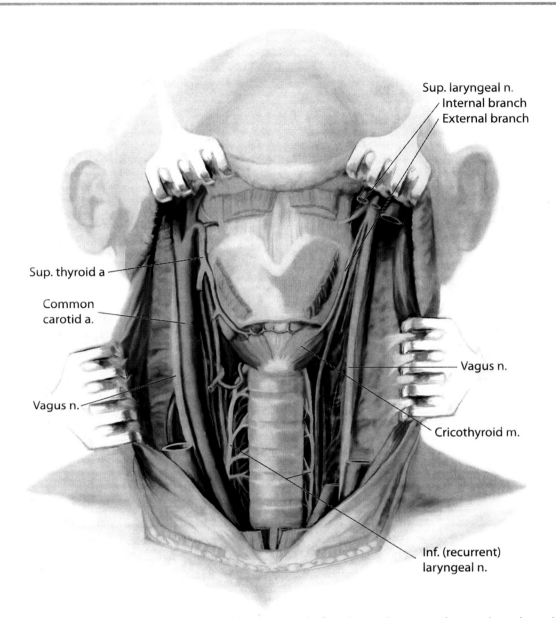

Sup. laryngeal n.
Internal branch
External branch

Sup. thyroid a

Common
carotid a.

Vagus n.

Vagus n.

Cricothyroid m.

Inf. (recurrent)
laryngeal n.

Fig. 2.8 Schematic anterior view depicts the courses of the superior and inferior laryngeal nerves in relation to the trachea and the larynx. Note also the course of the vagus nerve within the sheet of the common carotid artery and the internal jugular vein

Removal of large thyroid tumors may require division of the infrahyoid muscles. Care must be taken to identify the branches of the ansa cervicalis that supply these muscles. The course of the ansa as it descends from the hypoglossal nerve is highly variable. Normally, a superior division of the muscles will ensure the preservation of the nerve supply.

References

1. Abboud B, Aouad R (2004) Non-recurrent inferior laryngeal nerve in thyroid surgery: report of three cases and review of the literature. J Laryngol Otol 118:139–142
2. Bellantone R, Boscherini M, et al (2001) Is the identification of the external branch of the superior laryngeal nerve mandatory in thyroid operation? Results of a prospective randomized study. Surgery 130:1055–1059
3. Droulias C, Tzinas S, et al (1976) The superior laryngeal nerve. Am Surg 42:635–638

4. Dyson MD (1995) Endocrine system. In: Williams PL (ed) Gray's anatomy. Churchill Livingstone, New York, pp 1881–1906

5. Ghanem N, Bley T, et al (2003) Ectopic thyroid gland in the porta hepatis and lingua. Thyroid 13:503–507

6. Haber RS, Kim CK, et al (2002) Ultrasonography for preoperative localization of enlarged parathyroid glands in primary hyperparathyroidism: comparison with (99m)technetium sestamibi scintigraphy. Clin Endocrinol (Oxf) 57:241–249

7. Kuriloff DB, Sanborn KV (2004) Rapid intraoperative localization of parathyroid glands utilizing methylene blue infusion. Otolaryngol Head Neck Surg 131:616–622

8. Larsen WJ (2001) Human embryology. Churchill Livingstone, New York

9. Livolsi VA (1990) Surgical pathology of the thyroid. Saunders, Philadelphia

10. Mirilas P, Skandalakis JE (2002) Benign anatomical mistakes: the correct anatomical term for the recurrent laryngeal nerve. Am Surg 68:95–97

11. Page C, Foulon P, et al (2003) The inferior laryngeal nerve: surgical and anatomic considerations. Report of 251 thyroidectomies. Surg Radiol Anat 25:188–191

12. Shaheen OH (2003) Thyroid surgery. Parthenon Publishing, New York

13. Shen W, Duren M, et al (1996) Reoperation for persistent or recurrent primary hyperparathyroidism. Arch Surg 131:861–867; discussion 867–869

14. Sherman JH, Colborn GL (2003) Absence of the left inferior thyroid artery: clinical implications. Clin Anat 16:534–537

15. Skandalakis JE, Carlson GW, et al (2004) Neck. In: Skandalakis JE (ed) Surgical anatomy, vol 1. Paschalidis Medical, Athens, pp 3–116

16. Sturniolo G, D'Alia C, et al (1999) The recurrent laryngeal nerve related to thyroid surgery. Am J Surg 177:485–488

17. Toni R, Della Casa C, et al (2003) Anthropological variations in the anatomy of the human thyroid arteries. Thyroid 13:183–192

18. Udelsman R, Donovan PI (2004) Open minimally invasive parathyroid surgery. World J Surg 28:1224–1226

3 Evaluation of Hyperthyroidism and Hyperthyroid Goiter

Mirjam Christ-Crain, Nils G. Morgenthaler, and Beat Müller

CONTENTS

3.1 Introduction

The primary intention of this chapter is to focus on the diagnosis and treatment of the two most prevalent hyperthyroid states, i.e., Graves' disease and solitary and multinodular goiter. In addition, we aim to provide some concise information on thyroid physiology and thyroid function tests.

3.2 Thyroid Physiology

The thyroidal parenchyma consists of two major cell types, the thyrocytes releasing thyroid hormones and the C cells secreting mature calcitonin [1]. The two main thyroid hormones l-thyroxin (T_4) and to a much lesser extent l-triiodothyronin (T_3) are produced by the follicular epithelial cells of the thyroid gland. The synthesis requires the availability of iodine and is increased by thyroid-stimulating hormone (thyrotropin; TSH) from the anterior pituitary gland through a specific thyroidal TSH receptor. Thyroid hormones are almost entirely bound to plasma proteins and only a small percentage circulates in the free, bioavailable form.

The synthesis of T_4 and T_3 by the thyroid gland involves four major steps: (1) active transport of iodine into the thyroid cell; (2) oxidation of iodine and iodination of tyrosyl residues in thyroglobulin (Tg); (3) coupling of iodotyrosine molecules within thyroglobulin to form T_3 and T_4; (4) proteolysis of thyroglobulin, with release of free hormones into the circulation (Fig. 3.1).

After iodine is transported into the thyroid cell, it is oxidized and incorporated into tyrosyl residues in Tg. Tg is stored in the colloid space at the center of the thyroid follicles. The coupling of iodotyrosyl residues in Tg is catalyzed by the enzyme thyroperoxidase. Thereby, two molecules of diiodotyrosine (DIT) couple to form T_4, and one molecule of monoiodotyrosine (MIT) and a DIT couple to form T_3. Antithyroid drugs are potent inhibitors of thyroperoxidase and will block thyroid hormone synthesis. With the process of proteolysis through lysosomal enzymes hydrolysis of thyroglobulin occurs, releasing T_4, T_3, DIT, and MIT. T_4 and T_3 are released into the circulation, while DIT and MIT are deiodinated and the iodine is conserved within the thyroid. Iodide organification and Tg proteolysis are inhibited by excess iodide, called the Wolff-Chaikoff effect. As this is a transient effect, both normal and autonomous thyroid cells can escape from the inhibiting iodide effect within days to weeks with recurrence of euthyroidism or hyperthyroidism, respectively. Conversely, if the gland is unable to escape iodide-induced hypothyroidism will ensue, especially in the presence of autoimmune Hashimoto thyroiditis.

In the circulation, thyroid hormones are transported bound to carrier proteins. Only 0.04% of T_4 and 0.4% of T_3 are free, which represents the fraction that is indeed responsible for hormonal activity. There

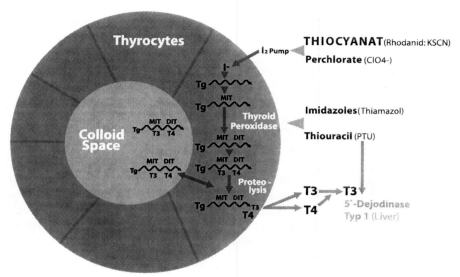

Fig. 3.1 Synthesis of thyroid hormones in the thyroid follicles

are three major thyroid binding hormones: thyroxin-binding globulin (TBG), transthyretin, and albumin.

The daily secretion of the normal thyroid gland is about 100 nmol of T_4 and about 5 nmol of T_3. The biologic activity of thyroid hormones is greatly dependent on the location of the iodine atoms. Deiodination of the outer ring of T_4 produces T_3, which is three to eight times more potent than T_4. On the other hand, deiodination of the inner ring of T_4 produces reverse T_3, which is metabolically inert. The deinodinase processes depend on specific deiodinating enzymes that differ in their local concentration and activity dependent on localization within the tissue and the organism. The most important, type 1 5′-deiodinase, is largely found in liver and kidney and in lesser quantities in the thyroid gland, skeletal muscle, and other tissues. The major function of type 1 5′-deiodinase is to provide T_3 to the plasma and hence the peripheral target tissues of thyroid hormone action. This activity of this enzyme is increased in hyperthyroidism and decreased in hypothyroidism. About 80% of T_4 is metabolized by deiodination, 35% to T_3, and 45% to reverse T_3. The remainder is inactivated in the liver and secreted into the bile. The metabolic clearance rate of T_4 is about 10% per day and the half-life of T_4 is about 7 days. The body pool of T_3 is much smaller and the turnover rate more rapid, with a plasma half-life of only 0.2 days. The rapid clearance of T_3 is due to lower binding affinity for thyroid binding proteins.

The growth and function of the thyroid gland and the peripheral effects of thyroid hormones are mainly controlled by the hypothalamic-pituitary-thyroid axis, where hypothalamic thyrotropin-releasing hormone (TRH) stimulates the synthesis and release of anterior pituitary TSH, which in turn stimulates growth and hormone secretion by the thyroid gland.

3.3   Thyroid Function Tests

Secretion of thyroid hormones T_4 and T_3 is regulated by pituitary thyrotropin (TSH). TSH secretion, in turn, is controlled through negative feedback by thyroid hormones. There is a negative log-linear relationship between serum-free T_4 and TSH concentrations [2]. This means that very small changes in serum-free T_4 concentrations induce very large reciprocal changes in serum TSH concentrations. As a result, thyroid function is best assessed by measuring serum TSH.

First- and second-generation TSH radioimmunoassay had detection limits of about 1 and 0.1 mU/l, respectively. Since this detection limit is just below the normal range for TSH, about 0.3–4.0 mU/l, these assays can be used as screening tests to distinguish hyperthyroidism from euthyroidism and hypothyroidism. However, since the range of subnormal TSH measurement is very limited in values near or at the detection limit, TRH testing was necessary to distinguish the degree of hyperthyroidism. With third-generation TSH chemoluminescent assays the detection limit is about 0.01 mU/l. They can therefore provide detectable TSH measurements even in mild, subclinical hyperthyroidism and make stimulation tests obsolete [3].

Serum total T_4 and T_3 are usually measured by radioimmunoassay, chemoluminometric assay, or a similar immunometric technique. Virtually all of serum T_4 and T_3 are bound to TBG or albumin. Serum total T_4 and T_3 measure both bound and unbound (free) T_4. Since drugs and illness can alter concentrations of binding proteins, the free and total hormone levels may not be concordant. It is therefore necessary to measure free hormone concentrations. Free T_4 concentrations are in the nanomolar range, in contrast to free T_3 levels which are present only in picomolar levels in the circulation. Therefore, the assays for free T_4 are considered more reliable.

3.4 Hyperthyroidism

Hyperthyroidism is the clinical syndrome that results when tissues are exposed to high levels of circulating thyroid hormones. In most instances, hyperthyroidism is due to hyperactivity of the thyroid gland. Occasionally, hyperthyroidism may be due to other causes such as excessive ingestion of thyroid hormones or excessive secretion of thyroid hormones from ectopic sites. Of the various forms of hyperthyroidism, the most common forms are Graves' disease, toxic adenoma, and toxic multinodular goiter.

3.4.1 Graves' Disease

Graves' disease is the most common form of hyperthyroidism. It may occur at any age, with a peak incidence in the 20- to 40-year age group. As with most autoimmune diseases, it is more commonly found in females than in males. The syndrome consists of one or more of the following features, which can occur together or independently: hyperthyroidism, ophthalmopathy, and dermopathy (pretibial myxedema). Graves' disease is an autoimmune disorder in which TSH receptor antibodies bind to and stimulate the thyroid gland, causing an excessive secretion of T_4 or T_3 or both, resulting in the clinical manifestation of hyperthyroidism.

3.4.1.1 Etiology of Graves' Disease

Graves' disease is an autoimmune disorder of unknown cause with a prevalence of 0.2%. There is a strong family predisposition in that about 15% of patients with Graves' disease have a close relative with the same disorder and about 50% of relatives of patients with Graves' disease have circulating thyroid antibodies. Females are affected five times more commonly than males and smoking is another risk factor for the development and severity of Graves' disease and especially ophthalmopathy [4].

3.4.1.2 Pathogenesis of Graves' Disease

T lymphocytes become sensitized to antigens within the thyroid gland and stimulate B lymphocytes to synthesize antibodies to these antigens. One group of autoantibodies is directed against the TSH receptor site on the thyroid cell membrane. These autoantibodies stimulate the TSH receptor independently of TSH, which leads to an increase in growth and activity of the thyroid cell. Rarely, a subgroup of these autoantibodies, although picked up by the assay, block the TSH receptor without intrinsic stimulation and thus are inhibitory to the thyroid function resulting in hypothyroidism. Conversely, in some patients with hyperthyroid autoimmune thyroiditis, TSH receptor antibodies are not found but thyroperoxidase autoantibodies are present, also referred to as "hashitoxicosis." This might suggest an overlap in the pathogenesis of hyperthyroid (i.e., Graves' disease) and hypothyroid (i.e., Hashimoto's disease) autoimmunity. Alternatively, transient hashitoxicosis could also be due to an initial and transient release of thyroid hormone as a result of the inflammatory destruction of thyroid follicles. In this context, a common pathogenesis might exist in patients suffering from "silent" thyroiditis, a lymphocytic thyroiditis that can occur during the postpartal period.

The presence of TSH receptor antibodies is positively correlated with activity and with relapse rate of the disease. There is an underlying genetic predisposition, but it is unclear what triggers the acute episode. Some factors are suggested to incite the immune response of Graves' disease, namely iodide excess, lithium therapy, viral or bacterial infections, and withdrawal of glucocorticoids. It has been suggested that stressful life events may trigger an episode of Graves' disease [5]. Conversely, during pregnancy the clinical manifestations of the autoimmune syndrome can be attenuated, with a common recurrence during the postpartal period. The pathogenesis of Graves' ophthalmopathy may involve cytotoxic lymphocytes and antibodies sensitized to a common antigen such as the TSH receptor found in orbital fibroblasts, orbital muscle, and thyroid tissue.

3.4.1.3 Clinical Manifestations of Graves' Disease

The clinical manifestations of Graves' disease can involve almost any organ system and can be divided into symptoms common to any form of hyperthyroidism and those specific to Graves' disease [6]. Usually there is a palpable, diffusely enlarged, smooth goiter that initially is soft but becomes progressively firmer. Because of the increased vascularity of the gland, there may be a systolic bruit heard with the stethoscope. Patients commonly report nervousness, malaise, irritability, inability to concentrate, easy fatigability, and intolerance to heat. There is often marked weight loss without loss of appetite. Other clinical symptoms are excessive sweating, hand tremor, and mild or moderate muscle weakness. In patients over 60 years of age, cardiovascular and myopathic manifestations may predominate with the most common presenting complaints of palpitations, dyspnea on exertion, tremor, nervousness, and weight loss. A clinical score may be used to quantify the clinical symptomatology and for follow-up examination [7]. In addition, vitiligo, pruritus, osteoporosis, and gynecomastia can also occur.

Graves' ophthalmopathy (GO) occurs together with hyperthyroidism in 46–60% of patients, in 30% of patients hyperthyroidism may occur several years before any eye symptoms are present, and only in about 10% of cases may the eye symptoms precede the thyroidal symptoms [8]. GO is most likely to occur between 40 and 50 years. Clinical signs are (in descending frequency) lid retraction, edema, exophthalmus, motility disorders, and visual impairments (Fig. 3.2). About 50% of all patients with Graves' disease develop visible eye symptoms, however, more

Table 3.1 Clinical activity score (CAS) for a standardized clinical assessment of Graves Ophthalmopathy

CAS item		Score
Pain	Painful, oppressive feeling on or behind the globe during the last 4 weeks	1
	Pain on attempted up, side, or down-gaze during the last 4 weeks	1
Redness	Redness of the eyelids	1
	Diffuse redness of the conjunctiva, covering at least one quadrant	1
Swelling	Swelling of the eyelids	1
	Chemosis	1
	Swollen caruncle	1
Impaired function	Increase of proptosis of ≥2 mm during a period of 1–3 months	1
	Decrease of eye movements in any direction ≥5° during a period of 1–3 months	1
	Decrease of visual acuity of ≥1 line(s) (using a pinhole) during a period of 1–3 months	1
Maximal CAS score		10

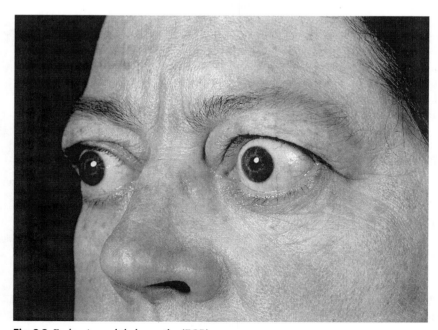

Fig. 3.2 Endocrine ophthalmopathy (EOP)

Table 3.2 NOSPECS classification of Graves Ophthalmopathy

NOSPECS score	0	1	2	3
Lid retraction	No	Yes		
Soft tissue inflammation[a]	0	1–4	5–8	>8
Proptosis	<17 mm	17–18 mm	19–22 mm	>22 mm
Site difference	<1 mm	1–2 mm	3–4 mm	>4 mm
Extraocular muscle involvement	No	Upgaze >20° Abduction >35°		Upgaze <20° Abduction <35°
Corneal defects	No	Yes		
Optic nerve compression	No			Yes

[a] Upper lid edema 0–2, lower lid edema 0–2, conjunctival injection 1, conjunctival chemosis 1

than two thirds of symptom-free Graves' disease patients show eye muscle enlargement in the magnetic resonance tomography (MRT) [9]. Most Graves' disease patients develop mild to moderate GO, but only 3–5% of patients develop very severe GO with opticus compression.

Standardized clinical assessment of the severity and activity of GO is mandatory for successful treatment. The most recent and widely accepted protocol for a standardized assessment of the clinical activity score (CAS) was proposed by Mourits and colleagues [10]. The severity of the disease can be assessed by a modified NOSPECS classification, which includes all disease manifestations (Tables 3.1, 3.2) [11].

Thyroid dermopathy consists of thickening of the skin, particularly over the lower tibia, due to accumulation of glycosaminoglycans. It is relatively rare, occurring in about 2–3% of patients with Graves' disease and is usually associated with ophthalmopathy with a very high serum titer of TSH receptor antibodies.

Symptoms specific for Graves' disease are diffuse goiter, ophthalmopathy, and dermopathy; all other symptoms are common to any form of hyperthyroidism.

3.4.1.4 Laboratory Assessment of Graves' Disease

The laboratory findings in Graves' disease are essentially the combination of a suppressed TSH and elevated free T_4 and T_3 levels. If eye signs are present, the diagnosis of Graves' disease is obvious. If eye signs are absent, TSH receptor autoantibodies confirm the diagnosis. Modern assays employing human recombinant TSH receptor have a greater than 95% sensitivity, and if they are positive, the diagnosis of Graves' disease is confirmed and no other diagnostic tests are

necessary [12,13]. If they are negative, a radioactive iodine uptake should be determined to differentiate Graves' disease from other causes of hyperthyroidism. A diffusely elevated uptake of radioiodine is diagnostic for Graves' disease, whereas a localized increased uptake is suggestive for toxic nodular disease. A low uptake is seen in patients with subacute thyroiditis or a flare-up of Hashimoto's thyroiditis. Low uptakes will also be found in patients who are iodine loaded or, rarely, in association with a *struma ovarii*.

3.4.1.5 Treatment of Graves' Disease

Although autoimmune mechanisms are responsible for the syndrome of Graves' disease, management has been largely directed toward controlling the hyperthyroidism. The initial therapeutic approach consists of both rapid amelioration of symptoms with a beta-blocker and measures aimed at decreasing thyroid hormone synthesis. For this purpose, three treatment options are available: antithyroid drug therapy, radioactive iodine, and surgery [14]. There is regional variation in their use. Initial radioiodine treatment is favored in North America and antithyroid drugs nearly everywhere else. The treatment options and advantages and disadvantages should be discussed with each patient. Whatever treatment is used, initial monitoring should consist of periodic clinical assessment and measurement of free T_4. Serum TSH concentration may remain low for several weeks after the patient becomes euthyroid.

Antithyroid Drug Therapy

Antithyroid drug therapy is most useful primarily in young patients with a first episode of Graves' disease.

In Europe and in Asian countries it is the preferred initial therapy for most patients. Either propylthiouracil (PTU) or methimazole (MMI) is considered a first-line agent in the treatment of Graves' disease. PTU and MMI inhibit iodination of Tg, iodotyrosine coupling, and Tg synthesis. In addition, PTU, but not MMI, inhibits conversion of T_4 to T_3 [15]. PTU should be administered 2–3 times daily because of a shorter half-life, whereas <20 mg MMI can be given once daily. The customary starting dose of PTU may be 300–450 mg/day in divided doses and of MMI 30–45 mg daily. PTU is preferred during pregnancy, since it may cross the placenta to a lesser degree than MMI. The aim of antithyroid drug treatment is to restore a euthyroid state within 1–2 months. When the patient becomes euthyroid, maintenance therapy may be achieved with a lower single morning dose, commonly 25–50 mg PTU or 2.5–5 mg MMI. Allergic reactions to antithyroid drugs involve either a rash (about 5% of patients) or agranulocytosis (about 0.5% of patients). The rash can be managed by simply administering antihistaminics, and unless it is severe it is not an indication for discontinuing the medication. Agranulocytosis requires immediate cessation of all antithyroid drugs, institution of appropriate antibiotic therapy, and shifting to an alternative therapy, usually radioactive iodine. Agranulocytosis is usually heralded by sore throat and fever. Thus, all patients receiving antithyroid drugs should be instructed that if sore throat or fever develops they should see a physician for a white blood cell and differential count. Cholestatic jaundice, angioneurotic edema, hepatocellular toxicity, and acute arthralgia are serious, but rare, side effects that also require cessation of therapy. A complete blood count and liver function tests should be obtained initially and perhaps every 3 months during treatment, although the side effects of agranulocytosis cannot be accurately predicted.

The duration of antithyroid drug therapy is quite variable, but should be at least 6 months [16]. At our center, the most common treatment duration is 18 months. After discontinuation of antithyroid drugs, the incidence of relapse is quite high and is 50–60% even in selected patients [6]. Predictors of persisting remission are a reduction of the size of the thyroid to normal after treatment, TSH receptor antibodies that are no longer detectable, and a low dose of antithyroid drugs to control the disease. Conversely, large goiter size, persisting high levels of TSH receptor autoantibodies, and severe hyperthyroidism initially (i.e., markedly elevated T_3 levels) are negative prognostic factors [17].

Radioactive Iodine

In the USA, treatment of Graves' disease with iodine-131 (^{131}I) is the preferred therapy for most patients over the age of 21 years. It has this popularity because of its efficacy and few side effects, the most frequent of which is treatable thyroid failure. Follow-up studies have not implicated ^{131}I treatment in a higher risk of carcinoma in general, leukemia, or lymphoma [18]. Therapy with ^{131}I does increase the gonadal radiation exposure, but a higher risk of fetal malformation in subsequent pregnancies has not been demonstrated, however this is based only from anecdotal experience. Thus, ^{131}I should be administered with caution to any female patient of childbearing age. Radioactive iodine is given in a dose of 5–15 mCi on the basis of assessment of the size of the thyroid [19]. This results in ablation of the thyroid within 6–18 weeks [20]. The main side effect of radioiodine treatment is development of hypothyroidism. Conversely, approximately 10% of patients fail the first radioiodine treatment and require a second dose. These are usually patients with severe hyperthyroidism or very large goiters. Pretreatment with antithyroid drugs before radioiodine treatment reduces its effectiveness, primarily due to a radioiodine-uptake independent effect [21]. This is particularly a problem with PTU which can have a radioprotective effect [22]. However, in patients with severe hyperthyroidism, especially in the presence of cardiac comorbidity, antithyroid drug pretreatment should be performed for 4–8 weeks before radioiodine administration, since the drugs reduce thyroid hormone secretion rapidly and thereby reduce the risk of development of thyrotoxic crisis soon after radioiodine treatment. An interruption of thyrostatic therapy for 3 days prior to radiotherapy will restore radioiodine uptake with stable thyroid hormone levels [23].

Radioiodine treatment can induce worsening of GO, particularly in smokers. The worsening of ophthalmopathy is often transient and can be prevented by glucocorticoid treatment (40 mg prednisone daily with tapering over a period of 3 months) [24].

Surgery

Subtotal thyroidectomy is the preferred treatment option in selected patients with Graves' hyperthyroidism, especially those with a large goiter, and those with a coexistent thyroid nodule whose oncologic nature is unclear. To minimize perioperative risk, the patient should be treated with an antithyroid drug until clinical euthyroidism is achieved. There is disagreement about how much thyroid should be removed. Total thyroidectomy is usually not necessary, unless maybe in patients with severe progressive ophthalmopathy to remove antigen stimulation. However, if too much tissue is left, the risk for relapse increases. Thus, most surgeons perform subtotal thyroidectomy and leave 2–3 g of thyroid tissue on either side of the neck. Thereafter, a significant fraction of patients require TSH-guided thyroid supplementation following thyroidectomy for Graves' disease. Hypoparathyroidism and recurrent laryngeal nerve injury occur as complications of surgery in about 1% of cases, depending on the experience of the surgeon.

3.4.1.6 Treatment of Graves' Ophthalmopathy

Mild-to-moderate ophthalmopathy often improves spontaneously. The only treatment modality shown to improve mild disease is smoking cessation. Other, symptomatic options for therapy are sleeping with head raised, use of artificial tears, and diuretic treatment. An important therapeutic aim is to obtain euthyroidism of the thyroid. Severe ophthalmopathy, in particular impaired vision, improves in about two thirds of patients who are treated with high-dose glucocorticoid treatment, orbital radiation, or both [25]. Due to the fluctuating nature of the disease, it is debated which fraction of this beneficial effect can be attributed to a side effect-prone steroid therapy. Orbital decompression is effective in patients with optic neuropathy and exophthalmus, either as initial therapy or after the failure of glucocorticoid treatment [26]. However, it has to be emphasized that there are no adequately powered, randomized, placebo-controlled studies available for the treatment of GO. In particular, the place of other medical treatments, for example, immunosuppressive drugs and octreotide, remains unclear.

3.4.2 Toxic Adenoma and Toxic Multinodular Goiter

Toxic adenoma and toxic multinodular goiter are common causes of hyperthyroidism, second in prevalence only to Graves' disease. They can appear at any age, although they most frequently occur in patients older than 40 years. Toxic nodular or multinodular goiters are not believed to have an autoimmune etiology since TSH receptor antibodies are absent.

3.4.2.1 Toxic Adenoma

Patients who have a solitary autonomous nodule as the cause of their hyperthyroidism generally have a palpable thyroid nodule. The prototypic patient is an older individual, usually over 40, who has noted recent growth of a long-standing thyroid nodule. These lesions slowly increase in size and gradually suppress the other lobe of the gland. Nodules more than 3 cm in diameter evolve to cause more frequently clinical hyperthyroidism than do smaller nodules. The diagnosis is made by a thyroid scan, where a localized increased uptake of radioiodine is seen with a decreased or completely absent uptake in the remaining thyroid gland. Clinical symptoms of a toxic adenoma are the classic symptoms of hyperthyroidism, indistinguishable from the symptoms in Graves' disease, except that ophthalmopathy and dermopathy do not occur. The differential diagnosis from other causes of hyperthyroidism usually poses no difficulty, with the distinction resting on the anatomy of the thyroid by physical and scan examination and the presence or absence of typical signs of Graves' disease or TSH receptor antibody. Toxic adenomas are almost always follicular adenomas and virtually never malignant. They are easily managed by administration of antithyroid drugs such as PTU or MMI, followed by treatment with radioactive iodine or unilateral lobectomy. ^{131}I doses of 20–30 mCi are usually required to destroy the benign neoplasm. Radioactive iodine is preferable for smaller toxic nodules but larger ones are best managed surgically.

3.4.2.2 Toxic Multinodular Goiter

Toxic multinodular goiters that cause hyperthyroidism are usually very large. They occur mostly in older patients, similar to toxic adenomas. Clinically, the patients present with typical symptoms of hyperthyroidism, and ophthalmopathy is extremely rare. Toxic multinodular goiters occur equally in men and women. On physical examination, the thyroid gland is multinodular and enlarged. The nodules usually are benign follicular adenomas.

Radioiodine scans reveal multiple functioning nodules in the gland or occasionally an irregular, patchy distribution of radioactive iodine.

Hyperthyroidism in patients with multinodular goiters can often be precipitated by the administration of iodide (iodide-induced hyperthyroidism). Thereby, some thyroid adenomas do not develop or escape the Wolff-Chaikoff effect and cannot adapt to an iodide load. Thus, they are driven to excess hormone production by a high level of circulating iodide.

The long-term management of toxic multinodular goiter using antithyroid drugs is cumbersome as, in contrast to thyroid autoimmunity, autonomy will persist. Control of the hyperthyroid state with antithyroid drugs followed by subtotal thyroidectomy is the therapy of choice, but often these patients are elderly and have other illnesses that make them poor candidates for surgery. In these cases, the toxic nodules can be destroyed with ^{131}I, but the multinodular goiter will remain, and other nodules may become toxic, requiring repeated doses of ^{131}I.

3.4.3   Complication of Hyperthyroidism: Thyrotoxic Crisis ("Thyroid Storm")

Thyrotoxic crisis is the acute exacerbation of all of the symptoms of hyperthyroidism, often presenting as a syndrome that may be of life-threatening severity. Hyperpyrexia, agitation, delirium, psychosis, stupor, or coma are common. Although thyrotoxic crisis may occur in patients with longstanding untreated hyperthyroidism without a known precipitating event, it is more often precipitated by thyroidal or non-thyroidal surgery, by the peripartum or postpartum period, by ^{131}I therapy, by administration of iodine-containing materials, or by infections.

3.4.3.1   Treatment of Complications of Hyperthyroidism

The therapeutic options for the treatment of thyrotoxic crisis are the same as those for uncomplicated hyperthyroidism, except that the drugs are given in higher doses and more frequently. In addition, full support of the patient in an intensive care unit is essential, since the mortality rate from thyroid storm is substantial. In addition to specific therapy directed against the thyroid gland, supportive therapy may be critical to the final outcome. Many patients require a substantial amount of fluid, while others may require diuresis because of congestive heart failure. Infections need to be identified and treated, and hyperpyrexia should be aggressively corrected. Acetaminophen is preferable to aspirin, which can increase serum-free T_4 and T_3 concentrations by interfering with protein binding.

The therapeutic regimen typically consists of multiple medications, each of which has a different mechanism of action: beta-blockers to control the symptoms induced by increased adrenergic tone, antithyroid drugs to block new hormone synthesis, an iodinated radiocontrast dye to inhibit the peripheral conversion of T_4 to T_3, an iodine solution to block the release of thyroid hormone, and glucocorticoids to reduce T_4-to-T_3 conversion.

References

1. Wartofsky L (2001) The thyroid gland. In: Becker KL (ed) Principles and practice of endocrinology and metabolism. Lippincott Williams & Wilkins, Philadelphia, pp 308–471

2. Spencer CA, et al (1990) Applications of a new chemi-luminometric thyrotropin assay to subnormal measurement. J Clin Endocrinol Metab 70:453–460

3. Christ-Crain M, et al (2002) Basal TSH levels compared with TRH-stimulated TSH levels to diagnose different degrees of TSH suppression: diagnostic and therapeutic impact of assay performance. Eur J Clin Invest 32:931–937

4. Utiger RD (1995) Cigarette smoking and the thyroid. N Engl J Med 333:1001–1002

5. Winsa B, et al (1991) Stressful life events and Graves' disease. Lancet 338:1475–1479

6. Weetman AP (2000) Graves' disease. N Engl J Med 343:1236–1248

7. Zulewski H, et al (1999) Evaluation of procollagen III peptide as a marker of tissue hyperthyroidism in long-term treated women with TSH suppressive doses of thyroxine. Exp Clin Endocrinol Diabetes 107:190–194

8. Bartley GB, et al (1996) Chronology of Graves' ophthalmopathy in an incidence cohort. Am J Ophthalmol 121:426–434

9. Kendall-Taylor P, et al (1998) Clinical presentation of thyroid associated orbitopathy. Thyroid 8:427–428

10. Mourits MP, et al (1997) Clinical activity score as a guide in the management of patients with Graves' ophthalmopathy. Clin Endocrinol (Oxf) 47:9–14

11. Gerding MN, et al (2000) Assessment of disease activity in Graves' ophthalmopathy by orbital ultrasonography and clinical parameters. Clin Endocrinol (Oxf) 52:641–646

12. Morgenthaler NG (1999) New assay systems for thyrotropin receptor antibodies. Curr Opin Endocrinol Diabetes 6:251–260

13. Schott M, et al (2005) TSH-receptor autoantibodies in Graves' disease: recent developments in the diagnosis and therapy monitoring. Trends Endocrinol Metab 16:243–248

14. Singer PA, et al (1995) Treatment guidelines for patients with hyperthyroidism and hypothyroidism. Standards of Care Committee, American Thyroid Association. JAMA 273:808–812

15. Cooper DS (1984) Antithyroid drugs. N Engl J Med 311:1353–1362

16. Maugendre D, et al (1999) Antithyroid drugs and Graves' disease: prospective randomized assessment of long-term treatment. Clin Endocrinol (Oxf) 50:127–132

17. Schott M, et al (2004) Levels of autoantibodies against human TSH receptor predict relapse of hyperthyroidism in Graves' disease. Horm Metab Res 36:92–96

18. Saenger EL, et al (1968) Incidence of leukemia following treatment of hyperthyroidism. Preliminary report of the Cooperative Thyrotoxicosis Therapy Follow-Up Study. JAMA 205:855–862

19. Farrar JJ, et al (1991) Iodine-131 treatment of hyperthyroidism: current issues. Clin Endocrinol (Oxf) 35:207–212

20. Franklyn JA (1994) The management of hyperthyroidism. N Engl J Med 330:1731–1738

21. Walter MA, et al (2004) Radioiodine therapy in hyperthyroidism: inverse correlation of pretherapeutic iodine uptake level and post-therapeutic outcome. Eur J Clin Invest 34:365–370

22. Imseis RE, et al (1998) Pretreatment with propylthiouracil but not methimazole reduces the therapeutic efficacy of iodine-131 in hyperthyroidism. J Clin Endocrinol Metab 83:685–687

23. Walter MA, et al (2005) Paired comparison of radioiodine uptakes and thyroid hormone levels on/off simultaneous carbimazole medication. A prospective paired comparison. Nuklearmedizin 44:33–36

24. Bartalena L, et al (1998) Relation between therapy for hyperthyroidism and the course of Graves' ophthalmopathy. N Engl J Med 338:73–78

25. Bartalena L, et al (1997) Treating severe Graves' ophthalmopathy. Baillieres Clin Endocrinol Metab 11:521–536

26. Garrity JA, et al (1993) Results of transantral orbital decompression in 428 patients with severe Graves' ophthalmopathy. Am J Ophthalmol 116:533–547

4 Diagnostic Imaging of the Thyroid and Radioiodine Therapy

4.1 Walter Wiesner, Hermann Engel, and Wolfgang Steinbrich
4.2 Egbert U. Nitzsche and Jan Mueller-Brand

CONTENTS

4.1 Sonography of the Thyroid

4.1.1 Basics and Technique

According to its superficial anatomic location, the thyroid gland may easily be assessed by sonography. Linear transducers with a width of 7.5–9 cm and frequencies of around 10 MHz are used. Sonography of the thyroid gland should also always be combined with a sonography of the surrounding soft tissues and of the cervical vessels. It allows the exact measurement of the thyroid volume and assessment of the parenchymal texture of the thyroid gland with identification of diffuse or focal abnormalities of the gland itself and of potential abnormalities within the surrounding structures [1–4].

Compared to other imaging modalities sonography of the thyroid gland offers the best spatial resolution. Lateral resolution is 0.5–1 mm and this is also valid for tiny calcifications. For solid or cystic lesions the detection levels are 3–4 mm and 2 mm, respectively. By using the combination with color Doppler sonography additional information may be achieved regarding the local perfusion in focal or diffuse abnormalities. Furthermore, exact fine-needle aspirations or biopsies may be performed under sonographic guidance. As an imaging modality sonography is particularly attractive due to its low cost and lack of toxicity.

4.1.2 Examination and Findings

For sonography of the thyroid the patient should be positioned supine. A pillow may be placed beyond the neck of the patient in order to achieve good dorsal flexion of the cervical spine. During a systematic analysis of the thyroid the gland should be first imaged entirely in axial planes including the isthmus, and then each lobe should be imaged in its axial and longitudinal plane separately. Every sonographic examination of the thyroid must include measurement of the thyroid volume.

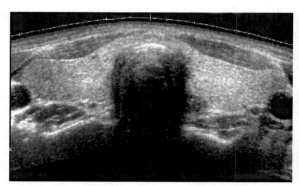

Fig. 4.1 Normal thyroid gland. Symmetric lobes with homogeneous parenchyma

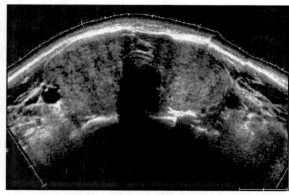

Fig. 4.2 Diffuse goiter. Symmetrically enlarged thyroid gland with mildly inhomogeneous and hypoechoic echotexture of its parenchyma

Regarding the description of sonographic findings the international terminology should be used: isoechoic, hypoechoic, hyperechoic, anechoic, diffuse or focal, homogeneous or heterogeneous, smooth or irregular, with dorsal echoenhancement or dorsal echoblock. Findings within the thyroid gland should be separated from findings outside the gland, and interpretation of findings should always be made at the end of the report and also be separated strictly from their initial description.

The volume of the thyroid gland may be achieved by using the formula: anteroposterior (AP) diameter × craniocaudal (CC) diameter × lateral diameter × 0.53 for each lobe (= volume in milliliters).

The normal thyroid has a smooth contour and shows a fine granular homogeneous, slightly hyperechoic sonographic pattern (Fig. 4.1). Its total volume may range up to 18 ml in women and up to 25 ml in men. The isthmus should not exceed 1 cm in its anteroposterior diameter and both lobes should perform a symmetric elevation during swallowing.

Regarding abnormalities of the thyroid gland that may be detected by sonography one has to differentiate between focal and diffuse findings, although these may of course also be found in combination. Diffuse and focal abnormalities of the thyroid gland and their sonographic appearances will be discussed separately.

4.1.3   Diffuse Abnormalities of the Thyroid

4.1.3.1   Diffuse Goiter

A diffuse enlargement of the thyroid gland with a normal echogenicity of its parenchyma is termed *struma diffusa*. In such cases both lobes of the thyroid gland are usually symmetrically enlarged especially in their craniocaudal and lateral diameters, while their anteroposterior diameter enlarges only relative to the total increase in size. The longer a struma diffusa persists, the more it happens that small regressive changes will be observed within the gland. These range from a mild irregularity of the parenchyma to anechoic, hypoechoic, or hyperechoic areas that represent small cystic degenerations, fibrosis, or calcification, respectively (Fig. 4.2) [1–4].

Attention: In any diffuse goiter one can find preexistent or new focal lesions that range from degenerative and regressive changes to benign or malignant neoplasias. However, independently from the presence of a struma diffusa the sonographic criteria for such focal lesions are always the same and correspond to those discussed in the following section.

4.1.3.2   Nodular Goiter

A thyroid with multiple nodules is termed struma nodosa or multinodosa. Usually the nodules represent colloidal, regressive and cystic, hemorrhagic or hyperplastic nodules, which may appear hyperechoic or hypoechoic on sonography. The function of a nodule can not be estimated by sonography; for this scintigraphy is needed. Furthermore, application of iodine should be avoided in nodular goiters because of the risk of inducing hyperthyrosis.

4.1.3.3   Graves' Disease

Graves' disease (morbus Basedow) represents an autoimmune disease that leads to a diffuse enlargement of the thyroid gland in combination with a hyperthyrosis and an endocrine ophthalmopathy. The thyroid gland is usually enlarged especially in its anteropos-

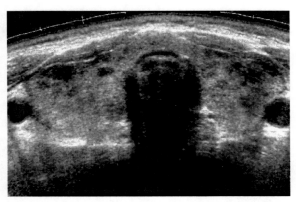

Fig. 4.3 Graves' disease (morbus Basedow). Slightly asymmetrically enlarged gland with inhomogeneous parenchyma, hypoechoic areas, and ball-shaped lobes

terior diameter (depth) which results in ball-shaped lobes (Fig. 4.3). The gland is typically hypoechogenic and this is caused by the microfollicular texture, the low content of colloid, as well as by the relative hyperperfusion of the gland [5].

However, in cases where Graves' disease involves an endemic goiter this hypoechoic pattern may be absent since it will be overlaid by the preexistent fibrotic and regressive changes within the gland. Regression of the anteroposterior diameter of the thyroid gland in Graves' disease and an increasing echogenicity of the parenchyma may be signs of remission, although hypoechogenicity of the gland may persist for months even after euthyrosis is reached in certain cases.

4.1.3.4 Acute Thyroiditis

Acute infectious thyroiditis is rare. It usually represents pyogenic infection in combination with focal or diffuse infections of the surrounding soft tissues and rarely an isolated viral infection. In such cases the parenchyma of the gland will appear homogeneously or inhomogeneously hypoechoic and enlarged. Especially in pyogenic cases local inflammatory changes such as edema, hyperthermia, and hyperemia will be present as well as tenderness of the gland and the surrounding tissues, depending on the degree of inflammation.

4.1.3.5 Subacute Thyroiditis de Quervain

Subacute thyroiditis de Quervain is a granulomatous inflammation of the thyroid gland, which is usually preceded by a simple infection of the upper airways. The thyroid gland is typically enlarged asymmetri-

cally and shows an inhomogeneous and hypoechoic pattern. Occasionally the hypoechoic regions may appear as quite well defined hypoechoic nodules that may be palpable and quite painful, although typically there is also pronounced tenderness of the entire organ in such cases [6]. Together with the typical clinical presentation of an ill patient presenting with fever and increased infectious parameters despite normal or even decreased WBC count, the clinical diagnosis is usually easy to make. Therefore, scintigraphy or a biopsy are not needed in these cases.

4.1.3.6 Hashimoto's Thyroiditis

Hashimoto's thyroiditis represents an autoimmune thyroiditis with diffuse infiltration of the thyroid gland by numerous lymphocytes and plasma cells. This disease usually affects middle-aged women and, apart from a certain genetic predisposition and a predisposing age and gender, mainly dysregulations in the cellular immune system and viral infections are discussed as etiologic factors.

In the initial stage the thyroid gland is usually of normal size or just slightly and asymmetrically enlarged and shows a mild inhomogeneous hypoechogenicity. However, the hypoechoic pattern of the thyroid parenchyma usually appears only after manifested hypothyrosis. Tenderness is absent and rarely hyperthyrosis may be present for a short time in the very initial phase of inflammation [7]. A variant of this acute or hypertrophic form of Hashimoto's thyroiditis is the so-called atrophic Hashimoto's thyroiditis that represents the chronic and late stage of the disease. Here, the gland is typically atrophic with areas or bands of hyperechoic, fibrotic parenchyma within (Fig. 4.4). Hashimoto's thyroiditis is associated

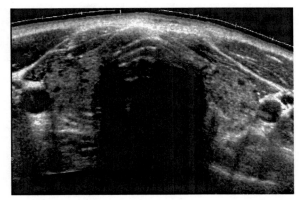

Fig. 4.4 Hashimoto's thyroiditis, chronic stage. Small gland with inhomogeneous hyperechoic echotexture of the parenchyma

with an increased risk of papillary carcinoma and of primary lymphoma of the thyroid (see following section on thyroiditis) and there is also an increased frequency of polyendocrinopathies.

4.1.3.7 Chronic Fibrosing Thyroiditis (Morbus Riedel)

Chronic fibrosing thyroiditis (morbus Riedel) represents an autoimmune thyroiditis as well, but here it is the fibrosing component with subsequent hypothyrosis that is dominating. The thyroid gland may be diffusely enlarged or already atrophic and it may be impossible to distinguish the organ sonographically from the surrounding fibroses [8]. The entire organ and the surrounding tissues may be very hard during palpation and the thyroid gland will typically show a significantly reduced mobility and elevation during swallowing. According to the increased amount of fibrotic tissue the gland will appear hyperechoic and in contrast to chronic Hashimoto's thyroiditis the sonographic distinction between the gland and the surrounding tissues may be extremely difficult.

4.1.3.8 Involvement of the Thyroid in Autoimmune Disorders

Hashimoto's thyroiditis may occur in combination with atrophic sialadenitis (Sjögren's syndrome), rheumatoid arthritis, lupus erythematodes, primary biliary cirrhosis, and other autoimmune endocrinopathies or even (cutaneous) autoimmune disorders [9]. Riedel's syndrome may also occur together with other fibrosing autoimmune disorders, such as idiopathic retroperitoneal fibrosis (Ormond's disease), pelvic fibrosis, mediastinal fibrosis, primary sclerosing cholangitis, or orbital pseudotumor [10]. In such cases the terms multifocal autoimmune syndrome or multifocal idiopathic fibrosclerosis (MIF) are used, respectively. However, the sonographic appearances in such cases are identical to those described above.

4.1.4 Focal Lesions

4.1.4.1 Cysts

Dysontogenetic cysts of the thyroid gland are rare and appear as round, well-defined anechoic lesions with dorsal echoenhancement. However, dorsal echoenhancement may be absent in small cysts or cysts with

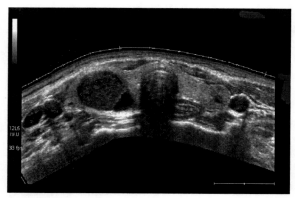

Fig. 4.5 Complicated (hemorrhagic) cysts. Well-defined cyst with multiple echoes

a viscous content and with high protein levels or in hemorrhagic cysts (Fig. 4.5) [1–4]. Most cysts in the thyroid gland represent cystic changes within primary solid lesions such as cystic degenerations in nodular hyperplasias, adenomas, or rarely even carcinomas. These so-called complicated cysts are usually irregularly shaped with tiny echoes, septations, lobulations, and diffuse or focally thickened walls and rarely even solid wall adherent papillary formations that protrude into the cyst lumen.

4.1.4.2 Calcifications

Calcifications are often found in a nodular goiter. Solid calcifications appear as bright reflexes with dorsal echoblock. However, rarely calcifications may also be limited to the walls of complicated cysts or be found as tiny stipulated calcifications within hyperplastic or regressive nodules [1–4]. These must be differentiated from so-called psammomatous microcalcifications that may be found in papillary carcinomas of thyroid.

4.1.4.3 Hyperplastic Nodules

Hyperplastic nodules that occur especially in endemic nodular goiters represent nodular hyperplasias but not true autonomous neoplasias and must therefore be strictly differentiated from true adenomas [1–4]. Sonographically hyperplastic nodules show an isoechoic to hyperechoic pattern in almost 90% of cases (Fig. 4.6). They often present with some small cysts and calcifications resulting from necroses and hemorrhage. However, if such secondary changes involve larger areas of a hyperplastic nod-

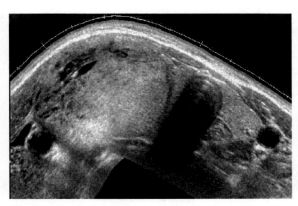

Fig. 4.6 Huge hyperplastic nodule. Solid, isoechoic, and homogeneous nodule

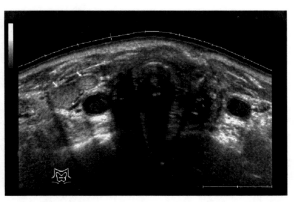

Fig. 4.7 Follicular carcinoma: two solid, hyperechoic nodules. Differentiation from hyperplastic nodules or adenomas is impossible by sonography alone

ule it may become more and more hypoechoic on sonography.

4.1.4.4   Adenoma

Adenoma represents a true epithelial neoplasia and it may have different microscopic subtypes, including, for example, oncocytic adenoma (oncocytoma). These lesions are usually hypoechoic and they often also show pronounced hypervascularization on Doppler sonography [11].

Attention: The term "autonomous adenoma" as used in scintigraphy does not always represent a true adenoma but it may also rarely represent an autonomous hyperplastic nodule and, therefore, the term focal autonomia should be used instead for the scintigraphic description of such lesions (see below).

4.1.4.5   Carcinoma

Carcinomas of the thyroid gland are hypoechoic in almost 80% of cases and in 20% of cases they appear as inhomogeneous lesions with solid hypoechoic and cystic changes [1–4]. However, 1% of all carcinomas may show a homogeneously hyperechoic echotexture (Fig. 4.7). Papillary carcinomas may appear with a distinct image due to microcalcifications and psammoma bodies and may be distinguished sonographically from other types of tumors. Papillary carcinomas have an increased incidence in patients with Hashimoto's thyroiditis and medullary carcinomas may occur in patients with multiple endocrine neoplasias (MEN2) or in association with the familial medullary thyroid carcinoma syndrome [12].

4.1.4.6   Metastases and Lymphomas

Rarely metastases from melanomas, lung carcinomas, breast carcinomas, renal carcinomas, and even adenocarcinomas of the gastrointestinal tract may be found in the thyroid gland [13]. Furthermore, lymphomas—with increased incidence in Hashimoto's thyroiditis—and leukemias may involve the thyroid gland. Most of these lesions are hypoechoic but apart from a potential bilaterality and multifocality they can not be differentiated from other neoplasias on the basis of their sonographic presentation. The diagnosis in such cases is usually based on the medical history of the patient and on the results of fine-needle aspirations and biopsies.

4.1.4.7   Cervical Lymph Nodes

Evaluation of cervical lymph nodes should be included during sonographic assessment of the thyroid gland. Low-level echogenicity of well-circumscribed masses is the classic sonographic appearance of enlarged lymph nodes (Fig. 4.8). However, in some cases the appearance is echo-free. Inflammatory processes may also exhibit a cystic nature. Differentiation of inflammatory from neoplastic processes is not always possible by sonographic criteria alone. To confirm a neoplastic process, biopsy is therefore recommended.

4.1.5   Analysis and Interpretation of Sonographic Findings

The points mentioned above make it clear that, apart from cysts, an isolated interpretation of the sonographic aspect of a focal lesion in the thyroid

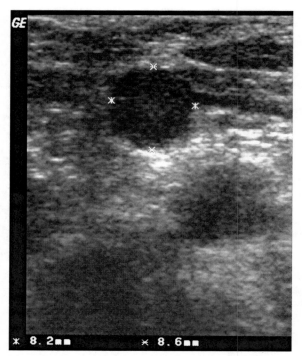

Fig. 4.8 Ultrasonographic appearance of an enlarged hypoechogenic cervical lymph node. The histology of the surgically removed specimen revealed a metastasis from a papillary thyroid carcinoma

gland will usually not allow its definite characterization. Here, the clinical constellation, laboratory findings, as well as scintigraphy must be included into the diagnostic workup in order to make the right decision for fine-needle aspirations, if needed.

In cases where a sonographically detected nodule shows focal autonomia on scintigraphy, the diagnosis is established and, disregarding if it is a hypoechoic nodule (probably autonomous adenoma) or a hyperechoic nodule (probably autonomous hyperplastic nodule), fine-needle aspiration biopsy is not generally recommended since the risk of a malignant autonomia (carcinoma) is only 1% in such cases.

Isoechoic or hyperechoic nodules in an endemic nodular goiter do not need to be biopsied, since the risk of malignancy is only about 1% in such cases even when the lesions appear as a cold nodules on scintigraphy. Nevertheless, sonographic follow-up examinations must be performed and fine-needle aspiration or biopsy are essential when the nodule grows over time.

In contrast, a scintigraphically cold nodule that appears hypoechoic on sonography must always be biopsied according to the statistically significantly increased risk of malignancy in such cases. Since false-

negative results from fine-needle aspirations or biopsies may occur in up to 10% of cases, surgery is often recommended for growing nodules.

Complicated cysts with solid, hypoechoic areas (wall thickening, papillary, or polypoid formations) should also be punctured or biopsied for diagnostic reasons. Simple cysts should be tapped only for therapeutic reasons to reduce their size.

4.1.6   Sonographic Follow-up of Patients with Thyroid Carcinoma

Ultrasonography is an accessible and non-invasive examination that is of great value in the determination of postsurgical remnants before ablative therapy and has proved to be highly sensitive in the monitoring of local recurrence and metastatic lymph nodes [14]. High-resolution ultrasonography also enables early detection of recurrent cancer in the thyroid bed or within the cervical lymphatic basin especially in patients with elevated serum thyroglobulin [15]. Moreover, sonography is useful in patients who have undergone partial thyroidectomy in whom follow-up with serum thyroglobulin measurements and radioiodine studies are not optimal.

When suspicious lymph nodes are detected, their possible metastatic nature may be ascertained by fine-needle aspiration cytology and by measurement of thyroglobulin in the aspirate.

High-resolution ultrasonography was positive in almost one third of 100 thyroid cancer patients studied by Simeone and coworkers and only seven were false-positive studies [16]. In 25 patients the diagnosis of recurrent cancer was confirmed with surgery or radioactive iodine scanning (sensitivity 96%, specificity 83%). In contrast, palpation was negative in 17 out of the 25 patients (sensitivity 32%, specificity 100%). In another study evaluating 89 subjects who underwent surgery for thyroid carcinoma, ultrasonography detected neoplastic disease with a sensitivity of 65%, specificity of 86%, and overall accuracy of 82%. The overall accuracy for scintigraphy was 88% and for thyroglobulin was 91% [15].

4.2 Nuclear Medicine Imaging of the Thyroid and Radioiodine Therapy

4.2.1 Radioisotopic Imaging of the Thyroid Gland

4.2.1.1 Introduction

Thyroid scintigraphy renders, at one point in time, information about the global and regional functional status of the thyroid. It is observer independent and reproducible with low inherent radiation exposure. In contrast, ultrasound (see above) is a sensitive means of detecting structural changes of the thyroid gland. Scintigraphic imaging of the thyroid includes determination whether either solitary or multiple nodules are functional (normal, hot, cold), whether cervical masses contain thyroid tissue, and it can demonstrate whether metastases from thyroid cancer concentrate iodine for the purpose of radioiodine therapy. In the majority of cases conclusive interpretation of ultrasonic and scintigraphic imaging findings is possible in combination with clinical, laboratory, and cytological findings.

The technique of thyroid scintigraphy is based on the principle that functional active thyroid cells incorporate iodine. Iodine uptake proceeds in two phases. First, iodine is actively taken up through the sodium/iodine symporter, a protein of the basal cell membrane (iodination). Second, iodine is quickly incorporated into organic iodine compounds (iodization). While the first of the two phases represents an unspecific process in which other ions such as pertechnetate may compete with iodine, the incorporation to organic compounds is a very specific process.

Quantitative thyroid scintigraphy enables assessment of the rate of thyroidal iodine uptake. Iodine uptake is self-controlled, in part by the iodine content of the thyroid cells and in part by stimulators such as thyroid-stimulating hormone (TSH). In case of autonomy, thyroid uptake may be increased despite these regulating mechanisms.

4.2.1.2 Radioactive Nuclides Commonly Used for a Thyroid Scan

For thyroid scintigraphy the following radionuclides are in use: ^{99m}Tc, ^{123}I, and ^{131}I.

^{99m}Tc is mainly used as a radionuclide in the form of ^{99m}Tc pertechnetate for thyroid scintigraphy. In contrast to ^{131}I, ^{99m}Tc has beneficial physical properties

such as pure gamma radiation, low energy of 140 keV, and short physical half-life of 6 hours. Since ^{99m}Tc is a generator-produced radionuclide, it is quickly available for routine use. Following intravenous injection, it takes about 15–20 minutes for maximum uptake, which is a factor of 10 lower compared to iodine. In this early phase the percent uptake of ^{99m}Tc pertechnetate reflects the iodination rate. Between 15 and 30 minutes a plateau is reached for ^{99m}Tc pertechnetate kinetics while, in contrast, uptake of iodine raises continuously. This difference in kinetics occurs because ^{99m}Tc pertechnetate is not incorporated into organic iodine compounds of the thyroid. It should be noted that the uptake of ^{99m}Tc pertechnetate is not specific for thyroid cells.

^{123}I has a physical half-life of 13 hours, pure gamma radiation, and low energy of 159 keV. It is taken up into thyroid cells and incorporated into organic iodine compounds. Because of the latter, imaging at later time points is enabled with the benefit of improved thyroid to background ratio. This defines its special use for the detection of dystopically situated lingual thyroid tissue, substernal mediastinal thyroid tissue, or rarely a struma ovarii.

Today the use of ^{131}I is limited to follow-up diagnostics in the case of thyroid cancer and in the course of radioiodine therapy. This is because of its unfavorable physical properties for scintigraphic imaging (i.e., physical half-life of 8.1 days, beta and gamma radiation, and high energy of 364 keV).

4.2.1.3 Quantitative Scintigraphy

This is the present method of choice for scintigraphic evaluation of the thyroid gland. The image is recorded using a specially designed "thyroid" collimator with a computer-linked gamma camera. Use of such a system enables high-quality images of the thyroid to be taken paralleled by calculation of global and regional thyroidal radiopharmaceutical uptake in percent of the administered amount of radioactivity. In this regard, ^{99m}Tc uptake is to be considered equivalent to thyroidal iodine clearance (Fig. 4.9), while ^{123}I uptake represents true iodine uptake.

^{99m}Tc uptake is dependent on endogenous TSH stimulation and, via autoregulation of the thyroid, on intrathyroidal iodine content. ^{99m}Tc uptake in a healthy thyroid gland amounts to between 0.5% and 2% of total body radioactivity. In geographic regions with iodine deficiency ^{99m}Tc uptake is between 2% and 8% in a euthyroid goiter.

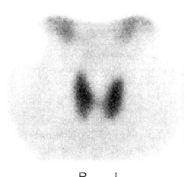

R   L

Fig. 4.9 ^{99m}Tc scintigraphy: normal thyroid scintigraphy, there is homogeneous uptake throughout the gland

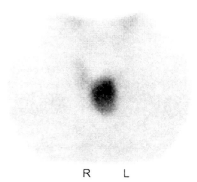

R   L

Fig. 4.11 ^{99m}Tc scintigraphy: high uptake throughout both lobes in Graves' disease

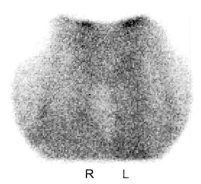

R   L

Fig. 4.10 ^{99m}Tc scintigraphy: virtually no uptake in a thyroid gland with autoimmune thyroiditis

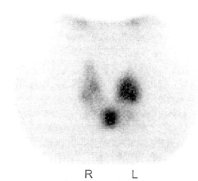

R   L

Fig. 4.12 ^{99m}Tc scintigraphy: high unifocal uptake in a case of unifocal autonomy (singular toxic nodule, toxic adenoma)

Low ^{99m}Tc uptake is observed after iodine exposition, such as application of iodine-containing contrast agents for radiodiagnostic imaging, iodine-containing drugs and beauty aids, disinfectants, following administration of perchlorate, during thyroid hormone therapy, as well as disease-related in cases of autoimmune thyroiditis, subacute thyroiditis de Quervain (Fig. 4.10), and secondary hypothyroidism. In contrast, high ^{99m}Tc uptake is observed for several causes of hyperthyroidism (Figs. 4.11–4.13), most frequently Graves' disease, iodine deficiency, during antithyroid drug and lithium therapy, and in cases of inherited enzymatic defects.

In addition to basal thyroid scintigraphy (in cases of normal TSH concentration) the suppression scintigram of the thyroid (rare but important) enables depiction of the global and regional regulation of thyroidal iodine uptake in cases of disseminated or focal (uninodular, e.g., unifocal or multinodular, e.g., multifocal) thyroidal autonomy. Following thyrosuppressive therapy based on thyroid hormone administration, ^{99m}Tc uptake declines to less than 0.5% in healthy thyroid glands or small diffuse goiters without auton-

R   L

Fig. 4.13 ^{99m}Tc scintigraphy: high multifocal uptake in multifocal autonomy (toxic multinodular goiter)

omy. In cases of functional relevant autonomy ^{99m}Tc uptake ranges from >1% up to 2%, because of slight if any depression of ^{99m}Tc uptake via TSH suppression. The extent of autonomy results from the amount of autonomic thyroid tissue and its functional activity. Today it is well known that under suppression a ^{99m}Tc uptake of >2.5% indicates increased risk of manifestation of hyperthyroidism in cases of increased iodine

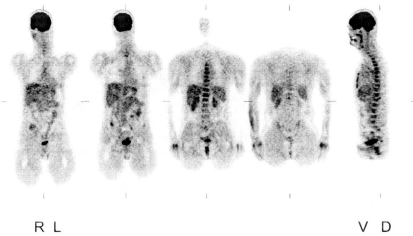

R L   V D

Fig. 4.14 A normal FDG PET scan. Coronal sections from ventral to dorsal at different depth levels of the body and a sagittal section at the slice level of the vertebral column. There is high uptake in the brain. The urinary bladder is illustrated because of renal elimination of FDG. There is moderate uptake in the skeletal muscles, liver, spleen, kidneys, and red bone marrow

intake. Therefore, the result of the suppression scintigram is an important parameter for a definitive therapeutic decision to eliminate autonomy as a cause of hyperthyroidism.

For positron emission tomography (PET) imaging of the thyroid, ^{124}I (physical half-life 4.15 days) and ^{94m}Tc (physical half-life 52 minutes) may be used in cases of benign disease. For evaluation of cancer disease of the thyroid, fluorine-18 (^{18}F; half-life 109.8 minutes)-labeled 2-deoxy-2-d-glucose (FDG) (Fig. 4.14) is used. It is indicated especially for the detection of recurrent and metastatic disease of differentiated (papillary or follicular) thyroid cancer. For medullary thyroid cancer, ^{18}F-labeled 3,4-dihydroxyphenylalanine (F-DOPA) is increasingly used in addition to established imaging techniques. Because of its broad availability, FDG PET is widely used for cancer imaging in almost all known PET sites throughout the world, while the other agents are available at selected PET sites.

Positron emission tomography enables an improved cancer lesion to background ratio resulting in higher sensitivity in cancer detection compared with other nuclear medicine imaging techniques. The use of FDG PET for detection of cancer is based on the observation of enhanced glycolysis in malignant transformed (cancer) cells. It is used as a glucose analog following the principle of competitive substrate kinetics until formation of ^{18}F-labeled FDG-6-phosphate via the hexokinase reaction in cancer cells. The latter means in practice, normal blood glucose levels are mandatory in order to have optimized conditions for cancer detection. It should be noted that a less-differentiated and fast-growing tumor is likely to take up an increased amount of FDG (means G3 is much better suited than G2, G1 is not suitable for FDG PET imaging), and a high mitotic rate permits better FDG PET imaging results. However, FDG is not a specific cancer imaging PET agent, and false-positive results may be observed because of inflammation. Today's state of the art examination is integrated PET/computed tomography (CT), a single, two-in-one approach to cancer imaging that permits both functional (PET) and morphologic (CT) examination at a single appointment rather than two separate PET and CT examinations and subsequent imperfect image fusion.

4.2.2   Radioiodine Therapy for Treatment of Hyperthyroidism and Benign Non-toxic Multinodular Goiter

Radioiodine therapy is safe and effective and is the most popular treatment option for hyperthyroidism in the United States. Elsewhere its use becomes increasingly popular. While the treatment of non-toxic nodular goiter was limited to thyroxine (T_4)-suppressive hormone therapy or thyroidectomy in the past, radioiodine therapy is now being considered as an alternative treatment option. Radioiodine is administered orally as sodium ^{131}I in a capsule. It is rapidly incorporated into the thyroid. Its beta emission causes extensive local thyroid tissue damage. The aim of the radioiodine therapy is elimination of the cause of hyperthyroidism, accepting hypothyroidism and lifetime thyroxine hormone replacement therapy, and/or decrease of goiter size. Apart from causing hypothyroidism, radioiodine therapy is quite safe and effective. Regarding the side effects of radioiodine therapy, in about 1% of treated patients radiation thyroiditis may be observed, which is usually adequately treated with non-steroidal antiinflammatory drugs for analgesia. Radioiodine therapy is a valid, safe, and effective treatment option, especially for elderly patients in whom surgery is contraindicated. A multicystic goiter with individual cystic lesions exceeding 2 cm in diameter is not well suited for radioiodine-mediated decrease of goiter size. Pregnancy is an absolute contraindication for radioiodine therapy.

4.2.3   Radioiodine Treatment of Differentiated Thyroid Cancer

For differentiated thyroid cancer, the aims of the radioiodine therapy are first, postsurgical thyroid remnant ablation, and with that elimination and cure of possible small thyroid cancer remnant(s), and second, therapy of radioiodine-concentrating metastases.

Three rationales exist for ablation of residual thyroid tissue with ^{131}I: (1) destruction of any microscopic foci of disease remaining after surgery, (2) increased specificity of ^{131}I scanning for detection of recurrent or metastatic disease based on elimination of uptake by residual normal thyroid tissue, and (3) improved value of measurements of serum thyroglobulin as a tumor marker.

Cancer of the thyroid is a rare tumor. Most patients suffering from thyroid cancer present with a thyroid nodule (Fig. 4.15), while a few patients present with cervical lymphadenopathy or lung, bone, liver, or brain metastases. Thyroid carcinomas are classified

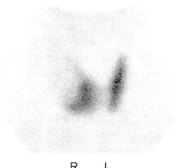

R   L

Fig. 4.15 An ^{123}I scan shows a cold nodule in the right lobe of the thyroid. Fine-needle aspiration revealed papillary thyroid cancer

into two varieties, carcinomas of the follicular epithelium and carcinoma of the parafollicular or C cells.

The most common thyroid cancer type is papillary carcinoma. Papillary cancer usually grows slowly and metastasizes typically into regional lymph nodes, where it may remain indolent for many years. However, acceleration of disease may occur at any time in the individual course of the disease. Overall, follicular carcinoma or follicular elements in papillary cancer account for those cases of thyroid carcinoma in which significant quantities of radioiodine are concentrated in situ or in metastases. Less common are the follicular tumors with three different variants that differ in their clinical course and abilities to take up radioiodine. Follicular carcinomas mimic histologically normal thyroid tissue and predominantly metastasize into lung and/or bone. Medullary thyroid cancer does not take up radioiodine and is discussed separately (see Chapter 11). Anaplastic carcinoma is histologically undifferentiated, highly malignant, fast growing, and usually afflicts the elderly. It is rapidly fatal because of extensive local invasion and it is refractory to radiation.

4.2.3.1   Indications for and Details of Radioiodine Therapy

Two indications are generally accepted for ^{131}I administration in patients with differentiated thyroid cancer: ablation of presumably normal thyroid tissue that may remain after thyroidectomy, and treatment and cure of known residual or metastatic disease. Radioiodine therapy in form of ^{131}I is the most effective non-surgical treatment for differentiated thyroid carcinoma. ^{131}I causes cytotoxicity by the emission of short path length (1–2 mm) beta radiation. ^{131}I uptake is dependent upon adequate stimulation by TSH, and is reduced in the presence of stable iodide. Therefore, whenever radioiodine imaging or treatment are planned, the patient should avoid all iodine-containing medications and dietary intake of iodine (foods allowed are fresh meat, poultry, potatoes, rice, wheat or rye bread, fresh or frozen vegetables, and fresh or frozen fruit).

For destruction of any microscopic foci of disease remaining after surgery, ablation of postoperative remnant thyroid tissue is recommended for almost all patients with differentiated thyroid carcinoma (exception: papillary cancer of 1.0 cm in diameter or less) and those with extrathyroidal tumor disease (i.e., direct invasion through the capsule of the gland or local and/or regional lymph node metastases). Thyroid remnant ablation destroys any remaining thyroid tissue in the neck, which may be present even after total thyroidectomy. Ablation after primary surgery is associated with a reduction of about 50% in local and regional recurrence. In addition, long-term disease-specific mortality appears to be reduced in patients with primary tumors 1.0–1.5 cm in diameter or greater, multicentric tumors, or soft tissue invasion at diagnosis [17–19].

The uptake of radioiodine by thyroid tissue is determined by imaging of the gamma radiation that is emitted by radioiodine. Thyroid remnant imaging and ablation are performed 4–6 weeks after surgery in the hypothyroid patient. The serum TSH concentration should be at least 25 mU/l before imaging is performed. As an alternative to thyroid hormone withdrawal, injection of recombinant human TSH (rhTSH) on l-thyroxine therapy is available as a useful method to stimulate radioiodine uptake and thyroglobulin secretion by neoplastic thyroid follicular cells. The use of rhTSH has the great advantage of avoiding the unpleasant side effects of hypothyroidism experienced by most patients undergoing the conventional follow-up strategy.

Treatment of known residual or recurrent and/or metastatic disease is performed following the same patient preparations as described for ablation. Regarding the extent of disease, 5,550–7,400 MBq are administered, dependent on the location of metastases and presence of soft tissue or skeletal metastatic disease. Higher doses may be given to patients presenting with recurrent disease after previous therapy. Post-therapy scanning is performed about 7 days after ^{131}I administration for documentation of therapeutic radioiodine concentration in the target (remnant and/or metastatic) thyroid tissue and for screening of further metastatic lesions.

All patients following surgery and radioiodine thyroid remnant ablation should receive thyroid hormone supplementation to prevent hypothyroidism and to minimize potential TSH stimulation of tumor growth. For the latter, the hypothesis is that reduction of serum TSH concentrations to below normal lower concentration decreases morbidity and mortality in patients with differentiated thyroid carcinoma. Although not proven, at least one study suggested improved relapse-free survival when serum TSH concentrations were undetectable during follow-up [20]. Results from a multicenter prospective tumor registry suggest that increasing TSH suppression is associated with improved progression-free survival in high-risk papillary carcinoma patients [21]. However, aggressive thyroxine therapy has some risks such as acceleration of bone loss, atrial fibrillation, and cardiac dysfunction [22–24]. Therefore, it seems reasonable to vary the dose of thyroxine according to the extent of disease and the likelihood of recurrence based on clinicopathologic staging for differentiated thyroid cancer. For low-risk and high-risk thyroid cancer patients, we recommend target basal TSH levels of 0.1–0.3 mU/l and 0.01–0.05 mU/l, respectively. If either risk factor of cardiac or skeletal disease are present, a lower level of TSH suppression is mandatory. In addition, in patients who remain disease free for more than 10 years after primary therapy the dose may be lowered.

External beam radiotherapy may be useful for patients with metastatic disease refractory to radioiodine or with tumors not concentrating iodine. Results of a recent multicenter study indicate a diminished acceptance of adjuvant external beam radiotherapy for differentiated thyroid carcinoma [25]. The discussion about the benefit of adjuvant radiation after surgical resection is controversial. It may be useful in selected individual cases as a result of interdisciplinary consent of involved specialty representatives. External radiotherapy after incomplete surgical resection may be helpful to control local residual tumor and it is used for palliation in patients with skeletal metastases, spinal cord compression from vertebral metastases, or intracranial metastases [26]. Recurrent tumor in the neck may be diagnosed based upon clinical examination and/or rising serum thyroglobulin concentrations and/or diagnostic imaging. The most sensitive technique for detection of local or regional cervical tumor recurrence is ultrasound. In addition, iodine scintigraphy (Fig. 4.16), ^{99m}Tc-labeled methoxy-isobutyl-isonitril (MIBI) scintigraphy (Fig. 4.17), or PET (Fig. 4.18) as a whole body tool for search of metastatic spread may be used. Recent study results indicate that uptake of FDG in a large volume of tissue correlated with poor survival. More lesions were detected if thyroxine therapy was discontinued and if the patient was hypothyroid before PET scanning or recombinant TSH was administered [27,28].

4.2.3.2   *Follow-up after Radioiodine Treatment*

Although most recurrences of differentiated thyroid cancer occur within the first 5 years after initial treatment, recurrences may occur many years or even decades later and long-term follow-up is warranted. For follow-up, the frequency of examinations for the individual patient depends on risk stratification, based on primary complete staging. A low-risk carcinoma means women aged 15–45 years, unifocal, highly differentiated papillary or follicular cancer, less than or equal to $T_2 N_0 M_0$ tumor stage, and target basal TSH level 0.1–0.3 mU/l [T1 (<1 cm) usually hemithyroidectomy only, no radioiodine therapy, thyroid hormone (T_4) suppression]. High-risk thyroid cancer includes any tumor stage higher than $T_2 N_0 M_0$ and

target basal TSH level 0.01–0.05 mU/l. Several follow-up schemes are recommended, but none of them is generally accepted.

At our institution we are practicing the following management:

- Completion of primary therapy and confirmation of successful thyroid remnant ablation (^{131}I scan, thyroglobulin, cervical ultrasound). Effectiveness of T_3 hormone medication is based on clinical and laboratory examination, and thyroid hormone therapy is later switched to T_4 hormone.
- Follow-up examinations include physical examination, thyroglobulin, chest X-ray, cervical ultrasound, and a ^{99m}Tc MIBI scan. In *high-risk patients*, this is done annually until 5 years, at 2-year intervals until 10 years, and thereafter at 3-years intervals. *Low-risk patients* are followed up annually until 2 years, at 2-year intervals until 6 years, and subsequently and finally after a 4-year interval.

A single negative ^{131}I scintigraphic study after complete ablation has a lower predictive value for relapse-

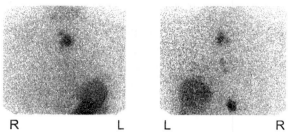

Fig. 4.16 An ^{131}I scan demonstrating metastatic spread of differentiated thyroid cancer and its ability to concentrate radioiodine for the purpose of radioiodine therapy. Depicted are anterior (*left*) and posterior (*right*) views of the body trunk of a patient with bony metastatic disease from follicular carcinoma. Note, there is normal depiction of the stomach

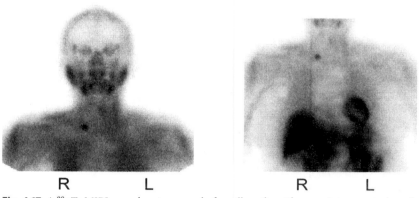

Fig. 4.17 A ^{99m}Tc MIBI scan showing spread of papillary thyroid cancer into a contralateral right cervical lymph node

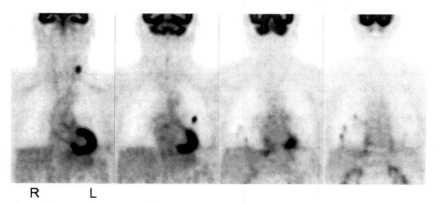

Fig. 4.18 An FDG PET scan of the body trunk for detection of metastatic spread of papillary thyroid cancer in a case of repeatedly measured rising serum thyroglobulin level but negative ^{131}I scan, indicating on coronal sections from ventral to dorsal at different depth levels of the body lymph node and bilateral lung metastatic disease

free survival than do two consecutive annual negative studies. Annual ^{131}I imaging is recommended by Grigsby et al. for surveillance until two consecutive annual negative studies are obtained, after which repeat imaging at 3–5 years appears to be satisfactory [29].

Side effects of radioiodine therapy are overall rarely observed. In the short term, radiation thyroiditis, painless neck edema, sialadenitis (promotion of salivary flow reduces such risk), nausea, tumor hemorrhage, or edema may occur, in particular when high doses are administered. Regarding chronic complications, secondary malignancies and infertility have been reported, primarily for high-dose radioiodine treatment. Maxon and Smith [30] have reviewed the literature on leukemia occurring after ^{131}I therapy and found 14 cases from a group of over 2,700 patients who received large activities of ^{131}I, which is ten times higher than the normal prevalence of leukemia. To minimize the likelihood of leukemia, Beierwaltes advocates a 1-year interval between therapies while the total cumulative administered activity should not exceed 29.6 GBq [31]. Overall, the relatively low incidence of radiation-induced malignancies supports the benefit/risk ratio in favor of radioiodine therapy.

References

1. Gritzmann N, Koischwitz D, Rettenbacher T (2000) Sonography of the thyroid and parathyroid glands. Radiol Clin North Am 38:1131–1145

2. Hegedus L (2001) Thyroid ultrasound. Endocrinol Metab Clin North Am 30:339–360

3. Solbiati L, Osti V, Cova L, Tonolini M (2001) Ultrasound of thyroid, parathyroid glands and neck lymph nodes. Eur Radiol 11:2411–2424

4. Baskin MD, Face HJ (1997) Thyroid ultrasonography: a review. Endocr Pract 3:153–157

5. Baldini M, Castagnone D, Rivolta D, et al (1997) Thyroid vascularisation by color Doppler ultrasonography in Graves disease. Changes related to different phases and to long-term outcome of the disease. Thyroid 7:823–828

6. Birchall IW, Chow CC, Metreweli C (1990) Ultrasound appearances of de Quervain's thyroiditis. Clin Radiol 41:57–59

7. Sostre S, Reyes MM (1991) Sonographic diagnosis and grading of Hashimoto's thyroiditis. J Endocrinol Invest 14:115–121

8. Papi G, LiVolsi VA (2004) Current concepts on Riedel thyroiditis. Am J Clin Pathol 121(suppl):50–63

9. Kobayashi T, Naka W, Harada T, Nishikawa T (1995) Association of the acral type of pustular psoriasis, Sjogren's syndrome, systemic lupus erythematosus, and Hashimoto's thyroiditis. J Dermatol 22125–22128

10. Tutuncu NB, Erbas T, Bayraktar M, Gedik O (2000) Multifocal idiopathic fibrosclerosis manifesting with Riedel's thyroiditis. Endocr Pract 6:447–449

11. Wiesner W, Engel H, von Schulthess GK, Krestin GP, Bicik I (1999) FDG PET-negative liver metastases of a malignant melanoma and FDG PET-positive Hürthle cell tumor of the thyroid. Eur Radiol 9:975–978

12. Gertner ME, Kebebew E (2004) Multiple endocrine neoplasia type 2.Curr Treat Options Oncol 5:315–325

13. Michelow PM, Leiman G (1995) Metastases to the thyroid gland: diagnosis by aspiration cytology. Diagn Cytopathol 13:209–213

14. do Rosario PW, Fagundes TA, Maia FF, Franco AC, Figueiredo MB, Purisch S (2004) Sonography in the diagnosis of cervical recurrence in patients with differentiated thyroid carcinoma. J Ultrasound Med 23:915–920

15. Rodriguez JM, Reus M, Moreno A, Martinez M, Soria T, Carrasco L, Parrilla P (1997) High-resolution ultrasound associated with aspiration biopsy in the follow-up of patients with differentiated thyroid cancer. Otolaryngol Head Neck Surg 117:694–697

16. Simeone JF, Daniels GH, Hall DA, McCarthy K, Kopans DB, Butch RJ, Mueller PR, Stark DD, Ferrucci JT Jr, Wang CA (1987) Sonography in the follow-up of 100 patients with thyroid carcinoma. AJR Am J Roentgenol 148:45–49

17. Mazzaferri EL, Jhiang SM (1994) Long-term impact of initial surgical and medical therapy on papillary and follicular thyroid cancer. Am J Med 97:418–428

18. DeGroot LJ, Kaplan EL, McCormick M, et al (1990) Natural history, treatment and course of papillary thyroid carcinoma. J Clin Endocrinol Metab 71:414–424

19. Wong JB, Kaplan MM, Meyer KB, et al (1990) Ablative radioiodine therapy for apparently localized thyroid carcinoma: a decision analytic perspective. Endocrinol Metab Clin North Am 19:741–760

20. Samaan NA, Schultz PN, Hickey RC, et al (1992) The results of various modalities of treatment of well differentiated thyroid carcinoma: a retrospective review of 1599 patients. J Clin Endocrinol Metab 75:714–720

21. Cooper DS, Specker B, Ho M, et al (1998) Thyrotropin suppression and disease progression in patients with differentiated thyroid cancer: results from the National Thyroid Cancer Treatment Cooperative Registry. Thyroid 8:737–744

22. Ross DS (1994) Hyperthyroidism, thyroid hormone therapy and bone. Thyroid 4:319–326

23. Sawin CT, Geller A, Wolf PA, et al (1994) Low serum thyrotropin concentrations as a risk factor for atrial fibrillation in older persons. N Engl J Med 331:1249–1252

24. Biondi B, Fazio S, Carella C, et al (1994) Control of adrenergic overactivity by beta blockade improves the quality of life in patients receiving long term suppressive therapy with levothyroxine. J Clin Endocrinol Metab 78:1028–1033

25. Biermann M, Pixberg MK, Schuck A, Heinecke A, Kopcke W, Schmid KW, Dralle H, Willich N, Schober O (2003) Multicenter study differentiated thyroid carcinoma (MSDS). Diminished acceptance of adjuvant external beam radiotherapy. Nuklearmedizin 42:244–250

26. Brierley JD, Tsang RW (1996) External radiation therapy in the treatment of thyroid malignancy. Endocrinol Metab Clin North Am 25:141–157

27. Van Tol KM, Jager PL, Piers DA, et al (2002) Better yield of 18fluorodeoxyglucose positron emission tomography in patients with metastatic differentiated thyroid carcinoma during thyrotropin stimulation. Thyroid 12:381–387

28. Chin BB, Patel P, Cohade C, et al (2004) Recombinant human thyrotropin stimulation of fluoro-d-glucose positron emission tomography uptake in well differentiated thyroid carcinoma. J Clin Endocrinol Metab 89:91–95

29. Grigsby PW, Baglan K, Siegel BA (1999) Surveillance of patients to detect recurrent thyroid carcinoma. Cancer 85:945–951

30. Maxon HR, Smith HS (1990) Radioiodine-131 in the diagnosis and treatment of metastatic well differentiated thyroid cancer. Endocrinol Metab Clin North Am 19:685–719

31. Beierwaltes WH (1978) The treatment of thyroid carcinoma with radioactive iodine. Semin Nucl Med 8:79–94

5 Evaluation of Thyroid Nodules

Michel Procopiou and Christoph A. Meier

5.1 Introduction

Thyroid nodules are very frequent findings and their prevalence steadily increases with age. However, clinically significant thyroid cancer is a rare malignancy and death from thyroid cancer is even less common with an estimated annual death rate of 0.25 per 100,000 in the US population. Moreover, the ever-increasing discovery of thyroid nodules by high-resolution radiological imaging procedures performed for other indications raises the problem of how incidentally discovered lesions should be investigated in a cost-effective and safe manner to identify the rare patient with a clinically significant malignancy.

In the present chapter the clinical criteria prompting the evaluation of thyroid nodules are reviewed, as is the currently recommended diagnostic approach that principally relies on fine-needle aspiration (FNA) biopsies. The clinical implications of the different cytological diagnoses are discussed, with special emphasis on the management of indeterminate, microfollicular lesions. Finally, the evidence for and against suppressive thyroid hormone therapy for benign thyroid nodules and multinodular goiters is presented, with particular consideration of high-risk patients with prior external radiation therapy to the neck region.

5.2 Frequency of Thyroid Nodularity

Thyroid nodules, either solitary or within a multinodular gland, are very frequent occurrences. In autopsy series, 30–60% of thyroids are found to harbor nodules, with nearly 40% of these nodules being larger than 2 cm (see [15] and references therein). With modern ultrasonographic techniques detecting thyroid nodules of a few millimeters, the frequency of nodularity was estimated at 16–67% in unselected subjects [98]. From such population studies it becomes apparent that thyroid nodules are extremely frequent in the normal population, and their prevalence increases with advancing age. Starting at the age of 20, the prevalence of nodules detected by palpation increases by 1% for each decade of age or by 10% per decade if detected by ultrasound [59]. About half of such patients present with a solitary nodule, while the other half harbors multiple nodules. When palpation is used as the mode of detection, nodules are found in 5–20% of the normal population, most of which exceed the size of 1 cm, which is usually the threshold for detection by physical examination. As for the nodules detected by ultrasonography, nearly 50% of patients with a clinically solitary nodule have in fact a multinodular gland on echographic examination [13]. The prevalence of thyroid nodules and multinodular goiters strongly depends on the iodine intake, and it is lower in iodine-replete areas, such as the USA. However, even in iodine-sufficient regions the occurrence of clinically detectable nodular thyroids or sporadic goiters is observed in up to 4–7% of the population [75,101].

5.3   Etiology of Thyroid Nodules and Risk for Malignancy

The histological nature of thyroid nodules reveals in the vast majority either a cystic or solid adenoma or a colloid nodule, both of which represent various stages of nodule formation and degeneration within a nodular thyroid gland (Table 5.1). Indeed, 30% of nodules represent a mixture of solid and cystic components, with pure thin-walled cysts being very rare. Graves' disease and chronic lymphocytic Hashimoto's thyroiditis can give rise to nodules, as may subacute de Quervain's thyroiditis or an infection. Less than 10% of palpable thyroid nodules are malignant and with the increasing use of FNA biopsy for ever smaller lesions, this figure is closer to 5%. The risk of a concomitant thyroid cancer within a longstanding multinodular gland has been well investigated and is similar to that in a solitary thyroid nodule, i.e., less than 5–10% [8,19,20,33,34,72,99]. Over 80% of the malignancies present in palpable nodules are papillary cancers, followed by follicular cancers and the much rarer anaplastic carcinomas. The non-epithelial cancers such as thyroid medullary carcinoma and thyroid lymphomas are even less frequent tumors, the latter being associated with Hashimoto's thyroiditis.

The low prevalence of thyroid cancer within palpable nodules contradicts the prevalence of cancers in autopsy and surgical series with careful histological analysis, describing foci of mostly papillary cancers in up to 17% and 13% of the glands, respectively [15,47,61,74,82,83,97]. If one estimates that 20% of the population have a multinodular thyroid and that 5% of these patients harbored a thyroid cancer, the estimated prevalence in the general population would be around 10 per 1,000 [45,94]. However, the prevalence of clinically relevant thyroid malignancies is only 0.025–0.050 cases per 1,000 persons, strongly suggesting that less than 1 of 200–400 histological microcarcinomas leads to clinically relevant disease. Hence, the histological definition of a thyroid cancer is not always predictive of clinically relevant malignant biological behavior of the lesion within the life span of the patient. This is particularly true for non-palpable thyroid lesions below 1 cm, which are incidentally detected by radiological or ultrasonographic procedures for other indications and which harbor cancers as frequently as larger nodules [72]. Clinicians should always keep in mind these fundamental epidemiological figures while trying to exclude cancer in a given nodule. It has been estimated that among the US population, 10–18 million persons have palpable nodules, a number rising to 75–125 million persons when ultrasound detection is used [58]. However, only 12,000 thyroid cancers are diagnosed in the USA, with 1,000 persons dying as a consequence of thyroid cancer per year. As stated by Mazzaferri, looking for aggressive thyroid cancer in thyroid nodules resembles "finding a needle in the haystack" [58].

Table 5.1 Etiology of thyroid nodules

Benign lesions (90–95%)	Malignant lesions (5–10%)
Adenomas (follicular, microfollicular, Hürthle cell neoplasms)	Primary thyroid cancers:
Colloid nodule	Epithelial cancers: papillary, follicular, anaplastic
Chronic lymphocytic thyroiditis (Hashimoto)	Other cancers: medullary thyroid cancer, primary thyroid lymphoma, other rare cancer types
Rare causes:	Metastatic cancer to the thyroid gland:
True epithelial cyst	Renal, breast, lung, colon, melanoma, and other cancer types
Infections (bacterial, tuberculosis)	
Acute thyroiditis (de Quervain's thyroiditis)	
Infiltrative (sarcoidosis, amyloidosis, lipomatosis)	

5.4 Pathogenesis of Thyroid Nodularity

5.4.1 Clinical Conditions Predisposing to the Formation of Nodules and Goiters

5.4.1.1 Iodine Deficiency

Iodine deficiency is the most frequent factor contributing to the development of multinodular goiters, affecting over 1.5 billion persons worldwide, i.e., nearly 30% of the world's population in 1990 [23]. In 1990, over 650 million people were estimated to be affected by goiter due to iodine deficiency, which is particularly severe and prevalent in central Africa and some areas of China. However, efforts by the WHO and private organizations were successful in reducing the number of persons with inadequate iodine intake by ascertaining a minimal supply of 150 µg iodine per day [31].

The pathogenesis of nodular goiter formation has been intensively studied and debated over the past decades. Classically it was thought that the presence of a persistent, although often only marginal, elevation of thyroid-stimulating hormone (thyrotropin, TSH) levels, for example in situations of iodine deficiency, was the prime stimulus leading to thyrocyte proliferation and the formation of a diffusely enlarged gland already during childhood and adolescence [25,30]. Subsequently, nodules appear as the patient ages, finally leading to a multinodular goiter. While the important role of iodine deficiency and the growth-promoting contribution of TSH are uncontested, a modified concept has emerged over the past decade, whereby the thyroid has an inherent propensity to form nodules with age, and that this phenomenon is amplified by the presence of additional factors, such as iodine deficiency and elevated TSH levels, further promoting thyrocyte proliferation and nodule formation [24].

5.4.1.2 External Radiation

External radiation to the neck during childhood is the best established environmental risk factor for the development of thyroid cancer [86]. In addition, the increased thyroid cancer incidence in children exposed to the fall-out from the Chernobyl accident has shown that radioiodine is equally carcinogenic, although this does not appear to be the case for the doses used in the diagnosis and treatment of thyroid disorders [69,77].

Patients, and particularly women, are most sensitive to external radiation before adolescence, where an increase in thyroid nodules and cancers is observed already at doses of 10 cGy, and which persists for at least four decades after the initial exposure [89,90]. Nearly 40% of such patients develop nodules with a maximal incidence 20–30 years after irradiation, and over one third of these lesions were found to be malignant after thyroidectomy [27,87,88].

5.5 Clinical Presentation of Thyroid Nodules

The size and nodularity of the thyroid gland increases over time and the presence of a nodular gland is often first detected either by the patients themselves or by the physician during a routine physical examination or a radiological examination of the neck. Most patients with nodular goiters are asymptomatic and the medical concerns essentially revolve around three questions: (1) the presence of thyroid dysfunction, (2) the presence of a malignancy, and (3) the likelihood of a progressive increase in size of the nodule ultimately leading to symptoms. Some patients can present with a rapidly enlarging, and sometimes painful, thyroid mass, which may reflect degeneration and hemorrhage into a previously undetected adenomatous nodule or cancer, or alternatively may indicate the presence of an aggressive malignancy, particularly anaplastic carcinoma or lymphoma.

5.6 Relevance of Clinical Risk Factors for Malignancy in Nodular Thyroid Disease

Belfiore et al. examined different risk factors for malignancy in a series of 5,637 patients from Sicily (Italy) with cold thyroid nodules [8]. The global rate of non-medullary thyroid cancer was 4.6% (259 cancers). The risk of malignancy was greater in males (8.2% versus 4.2%) but as nodules were much more frequent in women (female:male ratio = 8.3), more cancers were still found among women (female:male ratio = 4). Extreme ages also increased the risk of cancer for patients younger than 20 years (6.5% risk) and older than 60 (more than 6.6% risk). This finding was particularly striking for those older than 70 years (16.4% risk) in relation to an increased rate of anaplastic cancers. Sex and age interacted giving higher risks for older men (50% risk). The authors found no risk difference between single nodules and multinodular glands. These epidemiological risk factors are certainly not sensitive or specific enough to change clinical management when used in a given patient, with the exception of the combination of old age and male sex. Hamming and colleagues assigned patients on clinical grounds into three risk categories (high, moderate, and low risk for malignancy) [41]. The analysis was performed in 169 patients with histological confirmation of cytological FNA diagnosis with a total of 39 thyroid cancers (23%). Thirty-one patients were in the high-risk clinical group with a 71% rate of cancer. The remaining patients were in the moderate (38%) and low (44%) suspicion categories with a similar risk of cancer (14% and 11%, respectively). Clinical findings (fixation to adjacent structures, vocal cord paralysis, and enlarged lymph nodes) were the relevant criteria to the high-risk category but even when these ominous findings were present a final benign diagnosis was made in 20–30% of cases. In conclusion, patients investigated for nodular thyroid disease rarely present with malignant signs but, when they do, they must be taken into account in evaluating the need for surgery or repeated FNA. Single epidemiological risk factors have low utility in individual patients. A list of risk factors for malignancy is given in Table 5.2.

Table 5.2 Clinical risk factors for malignancy in patients with nodular thyroid disease. Adapted from references [8,41]

History	Patient characteristics	Physical examination
Thyroid cancer in family history [a] or MEN type 2 [a]	Age <20 years	Firm nodule
Rapid nodule growth	Age >60 years	Fixation to adjacent neck structures [a]
History of neck irradiation before adolescence [a]	Male sex	Vocal cord paralysis [a]
		Enlarged regional lymph nodes [a]
		Nodule diameter >4 cm [a]

[a] When present these factors are probably the best clinical predictors of malignancy

5.7 Which Nodules Should be Evaluated for Malignancy?

Most experts would agree that palpable solitary nodules above 1 cm should be investigated in euthyroid patients [34,98]. This limit is justified by the very low recurrence rate and the virtually absent mortality for differentiated thyroid cancers below 10 mm [60]. Since the presence of an autonomous nodule, Graves' disease, or Hashimoto's thyroiditis may result in erroneous cytological diagnoses, it is important to rule out hyper- or hypothyroidism by measuring a serum TSH level before proceeding further with the evaluation of a nodule. The prevalence of multinodular glands in elderly persons from marginally iodine-sufficient regions (such as certain parts of Europe) is still considerable, and the risk for a malignancy in these patients without additional risk factors is no higher than that observed for a solitary nodule [8,19,20,33,72,99]. Hence, a reasonable approach consists in the evaluation of the dominant nodule in a multinodular gland of a euthyroid patient, with the term dominant referring here to either the largest nodule or the one that has recently increased significantly in size. In elderly patients with multinodular goiters without a radiation history before adolescence and without recent changes in the size of the existing nodules or the appearance of new lesions, we usually only evaluate nodules above 1.5 cm, while following the evolution clinically. It would be erroneous to assume that the best quality of care is delivered by evaluating all thyroid nodules, including FNA, irrespective of their size and their clinical context (multinodular gland, age of the patient, radiation history), since the probability for the presence of a cytologically "suspicious" (i.e., microfollicular) lesion is 20% and since most of these patients will eventually undergo a thyroidectomy to exclude the presence of a follicular cancer that is present in 10–20% of all microfollicular lesions. Hence, once the decision is made to aspirate a nodule, the patient has an a priori probability of 10–20% for a thyroidectomy, which is unnecessary in 80–90% of the cases! From these considerations and the clinical irrelevance of most occult papillary microcarcinomas, it can be concluded that nodules below 1 cm (or <1.5 cm within a multinodular goiter) should not require further evaluation in most patients and that these lesions can be followed clinically unless the patient presents with specific risk factors for malignancy (such as local or distant metastases of unknown origin, family history of thyroid cancer, or irradiation before adolescence). This strategy applies to thyroid incidentalomas, nodules that are discovered on an imaging study ordered for a non-thyroid disease (usually an ultrasound) or as part of the evaluation of a clinically solitary apparent thyroid nodule [15]. A new way of finding thyroid incidentalomas has been recently reported in patients undergoing positron emission tomography (PET) using the radiotracer fluorodeoxyglucose (FDG). Normally the thyroid gland is not visualized on whole-body FDG-PET scan but incidental diffuse or focal increased uptakes have been reported in large series in 0.6% and 1.6% of cases, respectively. Diffuse uptake is indicative of a benign process (thyroiditis) but focal uptake is associated with a significantly increased thyroid cancer risk (30–50% in those selected for FNA) [91]. This latter uptake pattern may therefore warrant further investigation depending on the general and oncological condition of the patient.

While the above discussion is appropriate for patients with nodules below 4 cm, it is recommended to operate on non-functioning lesions above this size without necessarily performing a prior biopsy. This approach is justified by the high potential of such nodules to become locally symptomatic and the difficulty in confidently excluding a malignancy, present in more than 40% of lesions of this size, by aspiration cytology [102]. FNA in such nodules could give a higher rate of false-negative cytology potentially due to sampling issues.

Finally, patient preferences must be taken into account, for example when choices must be made between clinical follow-up, biopsy, and surgery. Clinicians must not forget in their cancer quest that death from cancer is a rare event and that microscopic cancers seldom lead to significant disease [105].

5.8 Diagnostic Approach to a Thyroid Nodule

Classically, thyroid scanning with radioiodine was used to distinguish between benign, hot nodules, with further evaluation being reserved for cold lesions. However, this approach is fraught with various problems: (1) 80–85% of the nodules are cold, hence requiring further work-up anyway, and, moreover, most patients with autonomous hot nodules can also be identified on the basis of a low TSH serum level; (2) thyroid scintigraphy may be falsely reassuring for cold nodules under 2 cm, where the overprojection of normal thyroid tissue may mimic the presence of a functioning nodule; and (3) the use of ^{99m}Tc pertechnetate is practical and economical, but it may result in 3–8% of cases in the false-positive capture of the tracer (see 5.8.3.1). For these reasons and with the perfection of the technique and interpretation of thyroid cytology, the preferred approach now consists of the biopsy of the nodule by FNA (Fig. 5.1). A thyroid scan is indicated in the small fraction of patients with a low or low-normal TSH as FNA can safely be

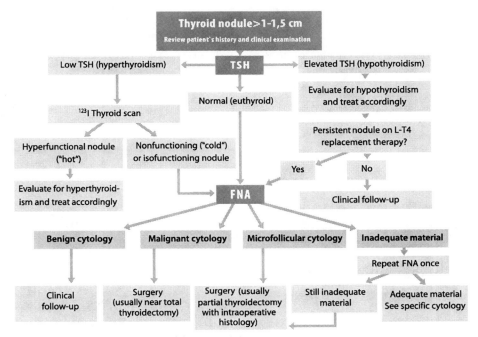

Fig. 5.1 Diagnostic algorithm for the evaluation of thyroid nodules

avoided if the nodule is clearly scintigraphically "hot" (see 5.8.3.1). Besides the clinical reasons discussed above, this algorithm is also more cost-effective, since a minority of the patients (less than 10%) will undergo both an FNA and a thyroid scan, as compared to 90% when the reverse order is followed. Experience of the physician performing the FNA and expertise of the cytopathologist are crucial in order to obtain proper sampling of the nodule and a correct cytological diagnosis.

5.8.1   Fine-needle Aspiration

After exclusion of hypo- or hyperthyroidism by measuring a TSH level, the FNA biopsy is the first and most important diagnostic procedure in the evaluation of a thyroid nodule. Aspiration cytology of the thyroid has an overall diagnostic accuracy of over 95%, with a sensitivity of typically over 95% and a specificity above 95% even in multinodular glands [19,33,35,50,52,53]. Since the technique and interpretation of FNA biopsies are described in detail in Chapter 6, only a brief summary of the clinically relevant conclusions is discussed here. The cytopathology laboratory should classify the sample into one of four categories, each of which is heterogeneous in etiology, but similar in the subsequent management

(Table 5.3). Such an approach based on FNA has been shown to reduce the number of unnecessary thyroidectomies while increasing the cancer yield in patients finally submitted to surgery [14,35]. Figure 5.2 gives an overview of cytological diagnosis after FNA and corresponding probabilities of malignant and benign histological diagnoses, which are further detailed below.

5.8.1.1   Unsatisfactory Sample

First, the sample may be unsatisfactory in its cellularity in 5–20% of the cases, although no universally accepted criteria exist defining the adequacy of a specimen. Criteria for adequate material vary from a minimum of five groups of cells to as many as ten groups on each of two slides [14]. The often quoted definition of Hamburger requires "at least six clusters of benign cells on each of two slides prepared from separate aspirates, for a diagnosis of benign" [40]. The rate of inadequate samples is largely dependent on the experience of the physician performing the aspiration and on the criteria used to judge adequacy, but even in the most experienced hands the rate of non-diagnostic biopsies is around 5%. Other factors that increase the rate of unsatisfactory samples are dilution of aspirated thyrocytes (either by blood in vascular-

Table 5.3 Classification of thyroid FNA biopsy results

Clinical relevance	Cytology	Management
Benign	Macrofollicular	Clinical follow-up
Malignant	Papillary cancer (or other cancers types, such as anaplastic carcinoma, medullary carcinoma, lymphoma)	Surgery (specific management for the anaplastic carcinoma and thyroid primary lymphoma)
Suspect	Microfollicular (= follicular neoplasm)	Surgery
Inadequate	Insufficient material	Repeat FNA

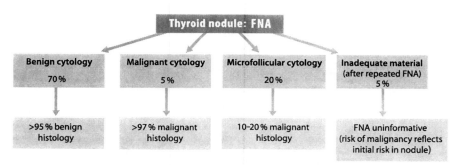

Fig. 5.2 Correlation between FNA cytology and histological diagnosis. Data from references [33,35]

ized nodules or by fluid in cystic lesions) or lesions technically difficult to biopsy [14]. While a possible explanation is the presence of a degenerated fibrotic or colloid nodule, it is important to emphasize that samples with insufficient material do not provide re-assurance and the procedure needs to be repeated. Indeed, in one surgical series around 10% of oper-ated nodules with previous non-diagnostic biopsies turned out to be cancers [62]. Performing more than one aspiration during the first FNA decreases the rate of unsatisfactory samples [7]. Repeat FNA is worth-while because it will provide adequate sampling in 50–70% of patients [8,33].

5.8.1.2 Benign Lesion

Around 70% of all aspirates will be interpreted as be-ing of a benign macrofollicular nature, reflecting the presence of an adenomatous or colloid nodule. Once the presence of a malignant lesion in a dominant nod-ule has been ruled out by FNA, such patients should be followed clinically. Since the false-negative rate for a malignancy is usually less than 5%, a rebiopsy is not warranted unless the nodule changes significantly in size (see 5.9.1).

5.8.1.3 Malignant Lesion

A reading of the biopsy sample as malignant occurs in about 5% of the aspirated nodules. A papillary thyroid cancer is present in the vast majority of these patients and thanks to its specific cytological features this diagnosis can be made with over 90–95% sen-sitivity and specificity. Hence, surgery is warranted in such patients without further tests or imaging. In rare cases, the cytology may suggest the presence of anaplastic cancer, medullary carcinoma, a metastasis, or a lymphoma. While the false-positive rate for the diagnosis of papillary cancer of FNA biopsies is typi-cally below 5%, the cytological features of aspirates from autonomous benign nodules may mimic those present in follicular cancers (microfollicular lesions, see below), emphasizing that the biopsy of nodules in hyperthyroid patients should be avoided. Finally, the lymphocytic infiltrates found in Hashimoto's thy-roiditis may erroneously indicate the presence of a thyroid lymphoma and hence the latter diagnosis re-quires careful evaluation by the pathologist using flow cytometry.

5.8.1.4 Microfollicular Lesion

The result of a microfollicular lesion (also called "fol-licular neoplasms," or simply "suspicious") is reported in 10–20% of aspirated thyroid nodules, leaving the clinician with the differential diagnosis between a follicular adenoma and a follicular cancer, the latter being present in less than 10–20% of microfollicular lesions [34,37,85]. This cancer rate can even be lower than 10% depending on the cytological criteria used to define microfollicular lesions. Since the cytological features of aspirates from autonomous benign nodules may mimic those present in follicular cancers (micro-follicular lesions), it is important to perform the cy-tological evaluation of a thyroid nodule only after the euthyroid state of the patient has been ascertained. Hence, in hyperthyroid patients with a low TSH a radioiodine scan should be performed and an FNA should only be done if the nodule is scintigraphically cold (see 5.8.3.1). It is generally recommended that patients with microfollicular lesions should undergo a partial thyroidectomy with intraoperative histology, which will allow the extension of the procedure to a near-total thyroidectomy if vascular or capsular inva-sion is found, i.e., the diagnosis of a follicular cancer is made. However, given the relatively low a priori likeli-hood for the presence of a malignancy in such lesions (typically 10–20%), this approach should be individu-alized, for example in elderly patients with increased surgical risk or a shortened life expectancy. In such patients the history of the growth of the nodule, its size and the presence of cervical lymph nodes allow a more refined, although subjective, assessment of the risk of malignancy, which should be balanced against the operative risk. It should also be kept in mind that the careful clinical follow-up of such surgically high-risk patients (for example by ultrasonographical meas-urements of the nodule size after 3, 6, and 12 months and then every 6–12 months) should allow the detec-tion of most, but certainly not all, clinically relevant malignant lesions, allowing then a reevaluation of the indication for surgery.

The management of patients with microfollicular lesions currently entailing an unnecessary thyroidec-tomy in 80–90% of the patients might potentially be improved by the advent of novel immunological and molecular markers.

While cytology alone is, by definition, incapable of distinguishing microfollicular adenomas from follic-ular cancers, with the latter being defined by capsular or vascular invasion, specific surface molecules and genetic rearrangements have recently been detected in follicular cancers. For example, the presence of the adhesion molecules galectin-3 and CD44v6 by immunocytochemistry was reported to distinguish adenomas and cancers with up to 95% specificity and 87% sensitivity [5,32,68]. The use of immunostaining for galectin-3 and CD44v6 was tested in a large multicenter study retrospectively on 1,009 thyroid tissues and cell blocks and prospectively on 226 fresh cytological samples [6]. In the prospective part of this study, galectin-3 immunostaining had excellent sensitivity (100%) and specificity (98%) allowing discrimination between benign and malignant lesions on preoperative FNA material. CD44v6 had a much lower diagnostic accuracy with 35% of benign lesions showing CD44v6 expression (false-positive results). Although most of the publications report detection of galectin-3 in nearly all cases of follicular or papillary carcinomas, some other studies have not reproduced these enthusiastic results. In one study, five of five follicular carcinomas were negative in galectin-3 immunochemistry [28]. Another group found that galectin-3 did not reliably distinguish benign from malignant follicular lesions [63]. Five of 19 follicular carcinomas had negative immunostaining for galectin-3 while 23 of 32 benign follicular adenomas where positive [63]. The results where much better for papillary carcinoma, but this thyroid cancer is usually readily identified with standard cytology.

The rearrangement and fusion of the PAX8 and PPARγ genes has the potential to become a specific, but apparently not very sensitive, genetic marker for malignancy in thyroidal cytological specimens [48]. Other molecular candidates (such as oncofetal fibronectin, telomerase, high mobility group 1 protein, and BRAF mutation) require further investigations [11,18].

In summary, while galectin-3 is a potentially promising marker for the differential diagnosis of microfollicular lesions, it currently awaits confirmatory studies for its routine use.

5.8.2 Cystic Lesions

Upon aspiration or ultrasound examination, a thyroid nodule may turn out to be a cystic nodule, rather than a solid one. Pure cysts lined by epithelial cells are very rare and the vast majority of thyroid cystic lesions contain a solid part. They result from degeneration of a solid lesion, most frequently from a benign adenoma or a papillary cancer (Table 5.4). Roughly 30% of thyroid nodules present a cystic component ranging from a small area to a predominant cystic part

with a minimal solid aspect in the cyst wall. The finding of a cystic component in a thyroid lesions does not give any information on the potential for malignancy of the nodule. The risk is neither increased nor reduced. Consequently, cystic nodules should be as a rule managed in the same way as purely solid nodules but a specific approach emphasizing some particularities is given in Fig. 5.3.

de los Santos and colleagues reported on a retrospective series of 221 thyroidectomies performed for nodular diseases [22]. Thirty-two percent ($n = 71$) were cystic lesions and 68% ($n = 150$) were purely solid. Malignancy rates were statistically not different between these two groups (14% versus 23%). There was no difference in the fluid color from benign and malignant lesions, and bloody fluid was seen in about 80% of cystic lesions. Among the cystic thyroid nodules, only 3 were true cysts and all of the cancers were papillary carcinomas. The fluid should be aspirated and evaluated cytologically. Any palpable residue after evacuation of the liquid component requires an FNA biopsy of this solid part. Recurring cystic lesions should be reaspirated with cytological evaluation. Surgery should be considered after multiple recurrences because of an increased risk of malignancy despite benign FNA or if repeated FNA do not reach sufficient material for proper cytological evaluation [1]. One concern with this approach is the number of inadequate samples, which is higher for cystic than purely solid nodules, particularly for large cysts (>3 cm). Recent studies have emphasized the role of ultrasound-guided FNA. In one study, fluid analysis after initial simple aspiration was non-diagnostic in 40 of 42 nodules, but the use of ultrasound-guided FNA yielded an adequate sample in 117 of 124 (94.4%) of cystic nodules (defined as more than 50% of the nodule filled with fluid) [12]. In this prospective series,

Table 5.4 Differential diagnosis of thyroid cystic lesions

Benign	Malignant
Adenoma (functioning or non-functioning)	Papillary cancer
Rare: true cyst, hydatid cyst	Rare: other types of thyroid cancer or metastases
Non-thyroidal (rare)	
Thyroglossal duct cyst (rarely carcinoma)	
Parathyroid cyst	
Cystic hygroma	
Brachial cleft cyst	

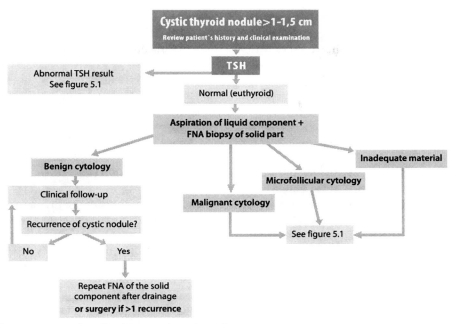

Fig. 5.3 Specific management algorithm for cystic thyroid nodules

the rate of malignancy was at least 4% (not all patients with inadequate or suspicious findings on FNA were operated on) and cystic nodules represented 25% of all nodules referred for FNA at this institution. However, this high FNA success rate was not confirmed in a retrospective series from Boston. Even with the use of systematic ultrasound guidance, initial FNA was non-diagnostic in more than 50% of cystic nodules (nodules with >50% of cystic component) [2].

5.8.3   Additional Tests

5.8.3.1   *Thyroid Scan*

With the advent of FNA biopsies, the importance of thyroid scans in the evaluation of nodular thyroids was greatly reduced. However, it has a role in patients with a low or low-normal TSH level, indicating developing thyroid autonomy and hence the possible presence of a toxic adenoma which is associated with microfollicular cytology. Therefore, such patients should undergo a thyroid scan to exclude the presence of a truly autonomous thyroid nodule, appearing "hot" on a ^{123}I scan, as these nodules are almost never malignant [14]. Since the use of ^{99m}Tc pertechnetate results in the false-positive capture of the tracer in 3–8% of thyroid cancers, ^{123}I is the preferred isotope for this examination. [123]I is devoid of this problem because it requires an intact organification step after trapping [14].

In patients with nodules <2 cm the overprojection of normally functioning thyroid tissue may hide the presence of a cold nodule. Alternatively, an autonomous nodule not yet resulting in a suppressed TSH level may display no enhancement of tracer uptake compared to the surrounding follicles (indeterminate scan). Only the finding of a clearly "hot" (hyperfunctional) nodule is reassuring and such a nodule does not need to be biopsied.

5.8.3.2   *Ultrasonography*

The role and use of ultrasonography in the initial evaluation of nodular thyroids is controversial and its routine use is not universally recommended [64,93]. Certain ultrasonographic features have been associated with malignancy (hypoechogenicity, microcalcifications, irregular margins, and intranodular vascularization) while other findings are suggestive of benignity (coarse calcifications, thin and well-defined halo, regular margin, and low or absent intranodular flow) [42,72]. However, the echographic criteria and their accuracy for determining the benign or malignant nature of a nodule are insufficient even in the opinion of authors who use it systematically [42]. In one study no single echographic sign was predictive for malignancy in patients with non-palpable nodules, although the combination of hypoechogenicity with another ultrasound "malignancy" sign could be effective in selecting high-risk nodules for FNA [72]. The utility and reproducibility of these echographic signs should be confirmed in other centers before widespread use. The ultrasound examination adds to the cost of the evaluation of a thyroid nodule without providing clinically relevant decisional support in most patients with a palpable nodule [76,93,95]. Additional drawbacks of ultrasound examination are the added costs and most significantly its high operator dependency.

Recent studies evaluating the use of ultrasound have reached unexpected conclusions. Papini et al. evaluated prospectively 494 patients with non-palpable nodules referred for ultrasound examination and ultrasound-guided FNA [72]. The authors found 31 cancers among the 402 patients with adequate samples (8%) and the incidence was similar in nodules measuring 8–10 mm compared with nodules of 11–15 mm. Eleven of these cancers showed extracapsular invasion (36%). While these results might be interpreted as justifying a more aggressive approach toward nodules below 10 mm, one has to keep in mind the very low incidence of clinically significant cancers. If the results of this study were extrapolated to the whole US population where as many as 50% of patients have thyroid nodules on ultrasound examination, more than *2 million* American citizens should be living with an "invasive" thyroid cancer, while we know that the true US annual incidence of thyroid cancer and death from thyroid cancer are much lower (around 12,000 and 1,000 per year, respectively). Possible explanations for these findings are: (1) a referral bias in the population examined and (2) that the detected cancers, although showing capsular invasion, might not have an aggressive clinical behavior [100]. In a study evaluating the usefulness of ultrasonography in the management of nodular thyroid disease, the authors found that it altered clinical management for 63% of patients (109 of 173), but they compared their echographic findings to the referring physicians' examination, 61% of them being primary care physicians [2]. Besides, some of the changes in management would probably not have been judged necessary in other centers.

In contrast, ultrasonography may be an important tool in determining the origin of an unclear neck mass, as well as in assisting in the diagnosis of a multinodular gland and the definition of the "dominant" nodule(s), which require cytological evaluation [65]. Similarly, the ultrasound-guided FNA biopsy of incidentally discovered, but non-palpable thyroid nodules above 1 cm is helpful in obtaining a representative specimen and may more generally be considered when a repeated FNA has to be performed because

of a first inadequate sample. However, we are unconvinced that the *systematic* use of thyroid ultrasound significantly improves patient care beyond clinical management by an expert physician in nodular disease [57]. Thyroid ultrasound might in fact not only add to costs, but also increase patient anxiety with the disclosure of incidental and insignificant findings, a phenomenon known as "labeling".

5.8.3.3   Calcitonin Level

Medullary carcinoma of the thyroid (MTC) is a rare tumor derived from the neuroendocrine thyroid C cells [66]. Twenty percent of cases occur as hereditary tumors (MEN type 2A, rarely type 2B or familial MTC) while the majority of cases are sporadic [92]. Fifty percent of sporadic cases present with metastatic cervical adenopathy at diagnosis and 10-year disease-specific survival is about 50% for patients older than 40 years [92]. More than 50% of cases are diagnosed only after a surgical procedure has been performed to rule out thyroid carcinoma [66]. Except for families with inherited tumor syndromes, medullary thyroid cancers are present in less than 0.5% of thyroid nodules, corresponding to about 5% of all thyroid cancers. In order to detect these sporadic cases earlier and to perform the appropriate surgical intervention, some groups have advocated screening patients with thyroid nodular disease with serum calcitonin. Calcitonin is secreted by the thyroid C cells and is a sensitive marker of MTC. In one series from France of 1,167 solitary nodules, 16 medullary cancers (1.4%) were present, 3 of which were detected by FNA [67]. Nearly 60% of these medullary cancers were <1 cm in size. Although only 25% of these medullary cancers were detected by cytology, calcitonin levels were elevated in nearly 90%. This has led to the claim that serum calcitonin should be routinely measured in patients with thyroid nodules. However, 20 of the 1,151 patients without a medullary cancer also had elevated serum calcitonin concentrations, resulting in a false-positive rate of 59% for this test. A recent prospective series from Italy of 10,864 patients found 44 cases of MTC with only 3 false-positive tests [26]. This is the lowest rate of false-positive tests (6.4%) so far published in a prospective study. In the series from Vierhapper, the rate of false-positive tests for basal calcitonin was 81% and still 57% after pentagastrin stimulation [104]. The reasons for these differences are unclear. They might be due to different cut-offs or selection of the populations screened. Interestingly, Vierhapper et al. note that the number of MTC diagnosed by screening during their study was higher than the predicted incidence by their institution's past experience [104]. Systematic screening could therefore diagnose indolent forms of MTC earlier (with an "apparent" benefit), while really aggressive MTC would still present at an advanced stage. Given the high probability for a false-positive result that would lead to a thyroidectomy despite a reassuring cytological result, as well as the unknown clinical relevance of sporadic medullary microcarcinomas, most experts would currently not recommend the routine measurement of basal serum calcitonin levels [92]. However, any cytological suspicion for an MTC should prompt an immunocytological staining for calcitonin on FNA, which has an excellent sensitivity and specificity.

In the event of a patient referred to the surgeon with an elevated calcitonin serum level, the value should be confirmed with a validated assay and reference range. In case of a borderline abnormal result, a stimulation test with pentagastrin should be used and the patient evaluated for an alternative cause of a false-positive result, such as renal failure. FNA should then be performed with appropriate immunohistochemical staining for calcitonin. However, it should be kept in mind that the calcitonin serum dosage may result from an occult medullary carcinoma different from the nodular lesion that prompted the initial evaluation.

5.8.3.4   Thyroglobulin Levels

It is important to note that the measurement of thyroglobulin levels is not helpful for the exclusion of a thyroid cancer, since there is substantial overlap between thyroglobulin levels in patients with any thyroid disorder (particularly multinodular disease) and thyroid cancer [21,56,96]. However, in a patient presenting with metastatic disease of unknown origin and a nodular thyroid, the measurement of a thyroglobulin level can be a helpful tool in the exclusion of a differentiated thyroid cancer as the underlying malignancy.

5.9   Treatment and Follow-up of Benign Thyroid Nodules

5.9.1   Natural History of Nodules and Role of Repeat FNA

In a series of 532 patients found to have benign thyroid nodules after FNA, 134 (25%) could be reevaluated 9–11 years later [49]. On clinical examination, around 35% of nodules did not change in size and 45% either decreased or disappeared while only 20% enlarged. FNA was repeated in 116 cases (87%) and showed suspicious findings in 4 patients, but only 1 follicular cancer was confirmed after surgery (plus two incidental papillary carcinomas discovered in nodules different from the ones biopsied). Similarly, 22% of patients in the control groups of trials of levothyroxine-suppressive therapy, had significant reduction in nodule size without therapy [36]. Alexander and colleagues evaluated 268 patients in a follow-up study with a mean interval of 20 months after the diagnosis of benign thyroid nodule based on FNA [3]. Thyroid ultrasound showed an increase in volume (volume change ≥15%) in 39% but only in 4% using a different criterion (>50% change in maximal diameter). However, no patient or physician is likely to notice a 15% or 30% change in the volume of a nodule and these small increases are of no clinical relevance. In this series, 61 patients underwent repeated FNA (74 FNA) with only one suspicious result confirmed at surgery as a papillary carcinoma. Grant et al. from the Mayo Clinic reported follow-up on 680 patients who underwent FNA in 1980, the first year this technique was used in their institution. Among the 94% of the patients for whom information was available 6 years later, only 0.7% of initially benign nodules were demonstrated to be malignant [39]. Similarly, Lucas et al. studied the value of routine repeated FNA in 116 females with benign nodular disease [55]. All patients had a second FNA after a 1-year interval without any change to a suspicious or malignant finding.

In conclusion, data from follow-up series show that 20–40% of nodules will show an increase in size during follow-up. After a first FNA with benign cytology, even nodules that grow have a very low risk of malignancy (<2%) because of the very high sensitivity of FNA. In spite of the low predictive value for malignancy of nodule growth after a cytological diagnosis of benignity, a new evaluation should be considered. Hence, when the clinical suspicion for a malignancy is high (see Table 5.2 and subsection 5.8.3), such as in patients with otherwise unexplained suspicious cervical lymph nodes, a history of prior radiation therapy to the neck during childhood or adolescence, or the presence of a rapidly enlarging nodule or gland, repeat FNA or surgery should be considered even if the first cytology is reassuring [52]. We do not recommend systematic repeat FNA because of its low yield (<2%) and its potential risk of increasing the rate of unnecessary thyroidectomies.

The follow-up of patients with a history of external neck irradiation in childhood is conceptually similar, but it requires the annual palpation and/or ultrasound examination of the thyroid gland for at least four decades, even if no nodules are initially present.

5.9.2   Role of Levothyroxine (L-T$_4$) Suppressive Therapy

Several studies examined the effect of suppressive T$_4$ therapy on the evolution of solitary nodules, some demonstrating a lack of efficacy and others showing a reduction in the volume of a small fraction of nodules. Some studies were non-randomized or uncontrolled trials and varied in methodological issues such as inclusion criteria (truly solitary nodules or multinodular goiters, cystic lesions), doses and length of therapy, documentation of TSH suppression during therapy, and assessment of the response to therapy. A recent meta-analysis found 14 randomized controlled trials addressing the issue of T$_4$ suppression for solitary thyroid nodules [79]. Nine studies met the selection criteria representing a total of 596 patients (mostly women, mean age 36–48 years old) [4,17,38,51,70,71,78,106,108]. The mean nodule volume or diameter reduction were not statistically significant between the L-T$_4$-treatment group and the control group as measured by ultrasound. In five pooled studies, 39 of 180 patients (22%) in the L-T$_4$ group and 18 of 178 patients (10%) in the control group had a nodule volume reduction defined as greater or equal to 50%, but the difference did not reach statistical significance. In six studies reporting the proportion of patients with nodule growth, increase of nodule volume was observed in 59 of 237 patients in the L-T$_4$ group (25%) and 89 of 234 patients in the control group (38%). This inhibition of nodule growth by TSH suppression in 34% (CI 14–49%) of the subjects was statistically significant. Another meta-analysis of six trials (five of six included in the Richter et al. paper [79]) also concluded [16] that L-T$_4$ suppressive therapy is not effective in decreasing the volume of solitary nodules.

According to these meta-analyses, L-T$_4$ suppressive therapy may be somewhat effective in inhibiting the growth of new or existing nodules and has at best a very modest effect in reducing the size of solitary thyroid nodules. However, no study has evaluated the clinical relevance of this treatment on outcomes that matter for the patients (patient satisfaction, impact on health-related quality of life, reduction in the number of unnecessary thyroidectomies, costs). Follow-up in these studies were in general very short (12–18 months) and side effects poorly documented. Indeed, a low TSH has been documented to be associated with an increased risk for osteoporosis [103],

atrial fibrillation [84], and cardiovascular death [73]. Moreover, any effect of the treatment disappears when the treatment is stopped [36,46].

Data are even scarcer for non-toxic multinodular goiter, with only three controlled studies being available [9,54,107]. In the most recent trial, Wesche et al. compared the efficacy of ^{131}I versus suppressive L-T$_4$ treatment in sporadic non-toxic nodular goiter (57 patients completed follow-up) [107]. Forty-three percent of the patients in the L-T$_4$ group responded to therapy with a modest 22% mean decrease in goiter size. A significant loss of bone mass density was observed in this group. Treatment with ^{131}I was more effective with a 46% goiter reduction in responders (97% of the group). However, large doses of ^{131}I are required (around 50 mCi) leading to long hospital stays in most countries, depending on their regulatory requirements. In conclusion, surgery is the therapeutic option of choice for patients with goiters if they need any treatment. The vast majority of patients with asymptomatic goiters can be followed without specific treatment [44].

For all these reasons (see Table 5.5), like other experts, we do not advocate L-T$_4$ suppression therapy for benign nodular thyroid disease [36,44] except for very particular situations.

Finally, the question of therapy with suppressive, rather than replacement doses of L-T$_4$ needs to be considered, which is particularly relevant since the long-term recurrence rate of nodular goiters is above

Table 5.5 Reasons why L-T$_4$ suppressive therapy is not a useful treatment in benign nodular thyroid disease

- Natural history of thyroid nodules shows clinically detectable growth in a minority of patients (<20%). Most nodules either shrink spontaneously or do not grow significantly in size

- Results from prospective studies are contradictory. Meta-analyses conclude to no or at best to a very modest effect of L-T$_4$ suppressive therapy on the size or volume of nodule or growth of new nodules

- No study addressed the issue of the clinical relevance of the treatment on outcomes that matter to the patients (symptoms, reduction in the number of unnecessary thyroidectomies versus osteoporosis and cardiovascular side effects)

- Studies included mostly middle-aged women (mean age 36–48 years old) and follow-up was short (usually less than 18 months)

- Any effect of suppressive therapy regresses when treatment is stopped

40% over 30 years after partial thyroidectomy [80]. In randomized trials the suppressive treatment with thyroxine was generally ineffective, except for a possible benefit in iodine-deficient areas [10,43,80,81]. However, one notable exception may be patients with a nodular thyroid and with a history of external irradiation to the neck, where suppressive therapy with T_4 reduced the postoperative recurrence rate 2.5-fold after correction for the extent of surgery and sex [29]. When such high-risk patients require surgery for benign nodules, a total, rather than partial, thyroidectomy is often the wiser procedure. Apart from this exception, thyroxine suppressive therapy failed to prevent postoperative recurrence of nodular thyroid disease and is not recommended as postoperative prophylaxis except for treatment of hypothyroidism [36].

References

1. Abbas G, Heller KS, Khoynezhad A, Dubner S, Sznyter LA (2001) The incidence of carcinoma in cytologically benign thyroid cysts. Surgery 130:1035–1038
2. Alexander EK, Heering JP, Benson CB, Frates MC, Doubilet PM, Cibas ES, Marqusee E (2002) Assessment of non-diagnostic ultrasound-guided fine-needle aspirations of thyroid nodules. J Clin Endocrinol Metab 87:4924–4927
3. Alexander EK, Hurwitz S, Heering JP, Benson CB, Frates MC, Doubilet PM, Cibas ES, Larsen PR, Marqusee E (2003) Natural history of benign solid and cystic thyroid nodules. Ann Intern Med 138:315–318
4. Badillo J, Shimaoka K, Lessmann EM, Marchetta FC, Sokal JE (1963) Treatment of nontoxic goiter with sodium liothyronine. A double-blind study. JAMA 184:29–36
5. Bartolazzi A (2000) Improving accuracy of cytology for nodular thyroid lesions. Lancet 355:1661–1662
6. Bartolazzi A, Gasbarri A, Papotti M, Bussolati G, Lucante T, Khan A, Inohara H, Marandino F, Orlandi F, Nardi F, Vecchione A, Tecce R, Larsson O (2001) Application of an immunodiagnostic method for improving preoperative diagnosis of nodular thyroid lesions. Lancet 357:1644–1650
7. Belfiore A, La Rosa GL (2001) Fine-needle aspiration biopsy of the thyroid. Endocrinol Metab Clin North Am 30:361–400
8. Belfiore A, La Rosa GL, La Porta GA, Giuffrida D, Milazzo G, Lupo L, Regalbuto C, Vigneri R (1992) Cancer risk in patients with cold thyroid nodules: relevance of iodine intake, sex, age, and multinodularity [see comments]. Am J Med 93:363–369
9. Berghout A, Wiersinga WM, Drexhage HA, Smits NJ, Touber JL (1990) Comparison of placebo with L-thyroxine alone or with carbimazole for treatment of sporadic non-toxic goitre. Lancet 336:193–197
10. Bistrup C, Nielsen JD, Gregersen G, Franch P (1994) Preventive effect of levothyroxine in patients operated for non-toxic goitre: a randomized trial of one hundred patients with nine years follow-up. Clin Endocrinol (Oxf) 40:323–327
11. Bojunga J, Zeuzem S (2004) Molecular detection of thyroid cancer: an update. Clin Endocrinol (Oxf) 61:523–530
12. Braga M, Cavalcanti TC, Collaco LM, Graf H (2001) Efficacy of ultrasound-guided fine-needle aspiration biopsy in the diagnosis of complex thyroid nodules. J Clin Endocrinol Metab 86:4089–4091
13. Brander A, Viikinkoski P, Nickels J, Kivisaari L (1991) Thyroid gland: US screening in a random adult population. Radiology 181:683–687
14. Burch HB (1995) Evaluation and management of the solid thyroid nodule. Endocrinol Metab Clin North Am 24:663–710
15. Burguera B, Gharib H (2000) Thyroid incidentalomas. Prevalence, diagnosis, significance, and management. Endocrinol Metab Clin North Am 29:187–203
16. Castro MR, Caraballo PJ, Morris JC (2002) Effectiveness of thyroid hormone suppressive therapy in benign solitary thyroid nodules: a meta-analysis. J Clin Endocrinol Metab 87:4154–4159
17. Cheung PS, Lee JM, Boey JH (1989) Thyroxine suppressive therapy of benign solitary thyroid nodules: a prospective randomized study. World J Surg 13:818–821
18. Ciampi R, Knauf JA, Kerler R, Gandhi M, Zhu Z, Nikiforova MN, Rabes HM, Fagin JA, Nikiforov YE (2005) Oncogenic AKAP9-BRAF fusion is a novel mechanism of MAPK pathway activation in thyroid cancer. J Clin Invest 115:94–101
19. Clark KC, Moffat FL, Ketcham AS, Legaspi A, Robinson DS (1991) Nonoperative techniques for tissue diagnosis in the management of thyroid nodules and goiters. Semin Surg Oncol 7:76–80
20. Cole WH (1991) Incidence of carcinoma of the thyroid in nodular goiter. Semin Surg Oncol 7:61–63
21. Date J, Feldt-Rasmussen U, Blichert-Toft M, Hegedus L, Graversen HP (1996) Long-term observation of serum thyroglobulin after resection of nontoxic goiter and relation to ultrasonographically demonstrated relapse. World J Surg 20:351–357
22. de los Santos ET, Keyhani-Rofagha S, Cunningham JJ, Mazzaferri EL (1990) Cystic thyroid nodules. The dilemma of malignant lesions. Arch Intern Med 150:1422–1427
23. Delange F (2000) Iodine deficiency. In: Braverman LE, Utiger RD (eds) Werner & Ingbar's the thyroid. Lippincott Williams & Wilkins, Philadelphia, pp 295–316
24. Derwahl M, Studer H (2000) Multinodular goitre: "much more to it than simply iodine deficiency". Baillieres Best Pract Res Clin Endocrinol Metab 14:577–600
25. Dumont JE, Ermans AM, Maenhaut C, Coppee F, Stanbury JB (1995) Large goitre as a maladaptation to iodine deficiency. Clin Endocrinol (Oxf) 43:1–10

26. Elisei R, Bottici V, Luchetti F, Di Coscio G, Romei C, Grasso L, Miccoli P, Iacconi P, Basolo F, Pinchera A, Pacini F (2004) Impact of routine measurement of serum calcitonin on the diagnosis and outcome of medullary thyroid cancer: experience in 10,864 patients with nodular thyroid disorders. J Clin Endocrinol Metab 89:163–168

27. Favus MJ, Schneider AB, Stachura ME, Arnold JE, Ryo UY, Pinsky SM, Colman M, Arnold MJ, Frohman LA (1976) Thyroid cancer occurring as a late consequence of head-and-neck irradiation. Evaluation of 1056 patients. N Engl J Med 294:1019–1025

28. Feilchenfeldt J, Totsch M, Sheu SY, Robert J, Spiliopoulos A, Frilling A, Schmid KW, Meier CA (2003) Expression of galectin-3 in normal and malignant thyroid tissue by quantitative PCR and immunohistochemistry. Mod Pathol 16:1117–1123

29. Fogelfeld L, Wiviott MB, Shore-Freedman E, Blend M, Bekerman C, Pinsky S, Schneider AB (1989) Recurrence of thyroid nodules after surgical removal in patients irradiated in childhood for benign conditions. N Engl J Med 320:835–840

30. Foley TPJ (1993) Goiter in adolescents. Endocrinol Metab Clin North Am 22:593–606

31. Gaitan E (1990) Intervention policy in endemic goitre areas. Thyroidology 2:113–119

32. Gasbarri A, Martegani MP, Del Prete F, Lucante T, Natali PG, Bartolazzi A (1999) Galectin-3 and CD44v6 isoforms in the preoperative evaluation of thyroid nodules. J Clin Oncol 17:3494–3502

33. Gharib H (1994) Fine-needle aspiration biopsy of thyroid nodules: advantages, limitations, and effect. Mayo Clin Proc 69:44–49

34. Gharib H (1997) Changing concepts in the diagnosis and management of thyroid nodules. Endocrinol Metab Clin North Am 26:777–800

35. Gharib H, Goellner JR (1993) Fine-needle aspiration biopsy of the thyroid: an appraisal. Ann Intern Med 118:282–289

36. Gharib H, Mazzaferri EL (1998) Thyroxine suppressive therapy in patients with nodular thyroid disease. Ann Intern Med 128:386–394

37. Gharib H, Goellner JR, Zinsmeister AR, Grant CS, van Heerden JA (1984) Fine-needle aspiration biopsy of the thyroid. The problem of suspicious cytologic findings. Ann Intern Med 101:25–28

38. Gharib H, James EM, Charboneau JW, Naessens JM, Offord KP, Gorman CA (1987) Suppressive therapy with levothyroxine for solitary thyroid nodules. A double-blind controlled clinical study. N Engl J Med 317:70–75

39. Grant CS, Hay ID, Gough IR, McCarthy PM, Goellner JR (1989) Long-term follow-up of patients with benign thyroid fine-needle aspiration cytologic diagnoses. Surgery 106:980–986

40. Hamburger JI (1994) Diagnosis of thyroid nodules by fine-needle biopsy: use and abuse. J Clin Endocrinol Metab 79:335–339

41. Hamming JF, Goslings BM, van Steenis GJ, van Ravenswaay Claasen H, Hermans J, van de Velde CJ (1990) The value of fine-needle aspiration biopsy in patients with nodular thyroid disease divided into groups of suspicion of malignant neoplasms on clinical grounds. Arch Intern Med 150:113–116

42. Hegedus L (2001) Thyroid ultrasound. Endocrinol Metab Clin North Am 30:339–360

43. Hegedus L, Nygaard B, Hansen JM (1999) Is routine thyroxine treatment to hinder postoperative recurrence of nontoxic goiter justified? J Clin Endocrinol Metab 84:756–760

44. Hegedus L, Bonnema SJ, Bennedbaek FN (2003) Management of simple nodular goiter: current status and future perspectives. Endocr Rev 24:102–132

45. Henneman G (2000) Multinodular goiter. The thyroid and its diseases. www.thyroidmanager.org

46. Koc M, Ersoz HO, Akpinar I, Gogas-Yavuz D, Deyneli O, Akalin S (2002) Effect of low- and high-dose levothyroxine on thyroid nodule volume: a crossover placebo-controlled trial. Clin Endocrinol (Oxf) 57:621–628

47. Koh KB, Chang KW (1992) Carcinoma in multinodular goitre. Br J Surg 79:266–267

48. Kroll TG, Sarraf P, Pecciarini L, Chen C, Mueller E, Spiegelman BM, Fletcher JA (2000) PAX8-PPARγ1 fusion in oncogenic human thyroid carcinoma. Science 289:1357–1360

49. Kuma K, Matsuzuka F, Yokozawa T, Miyauchi A, Sugawara M (1994) Fate of untreated benign thyroid nodules: results of long-term follow-up. World J Surg 18:495–498

50. La Rosa GL, Belfiore A, Giuffrida D, Sicurella C, Ippolito O, Russo G, Vigneri R (1991) Evaluation of the fine-needle aspiration biopsy in the preoperative selection of cold thyroid nodules. Cancer 67:2137–2141

51. La Rosa GL, Lupo L, Giuffrida D, Gullo D, Vigneri R, Belfiore A (1995) Levothyroxine and potassium iodide are both effective in treating benign solitary solid cold nodules of the thyroid. Ann Intern Med 122:1–8

52. Levy EG, Greenlee C, Mandel S, Kaplan M (2000) Should you always trust FNA interpretations? Thyroid 10:279–280

53. Liel Y (1999) The yield of adequate and conclusive fine-needle aspiration results in thyroid nodules is uniform across functional and goiter types. Thyroid 9:25–28

54. Lima N, Knobel M, Cavaliere H, Sztejnsznajd C, Tomimori E, Medeiros-Neto G (1997) Levothyroxine suppressive therapy is partially effective in treating patients with benign, solid thyroid nodules and multinodular goiters. Thyroid 7:691–697

55. Lucas A, Llatjos M, Salinas I, Reverter J, Pizarro E, Sanmarti A (1995) Fine-needle aspiration cytology of benign nodular thyroid disease. Value of re-aspiration. Eur J Endocrinol 132:677–680

56. Madeddu G, Casu AR, Marrosu A, Marras G, Langer M (1984) Serum thyroglobulin in patients with autonomous thyroid nodules. Clin Endocrinol (Oxf) 21:377–382

57. Mandel SJ (2004) A 64-year-old woman with a thyroid nodule. JAMA 292:2632–2642

58. Mazzaferri EL (1992) Thyroid cancer in thyroid nodules: finding a needle in the haystack. Am J Med 93:359–362

59. Mazzaferri EL (1993) Management of a solitary thyroid nodule. N Engl J Med 328:553–559

60. Mazzaferri EL, Jhiang SM (1994) Long-term impact of initial surgical and medical therapy on papillary and follicular thyroid cancer. Am J Med 97:418–428

61. McCall A, Jarosz H, Lawrence AM, Paloyan E (1986) The incidence of thyroid carcinoma in solitary cold nodules and in multinodular goiters. Surgery 100:1128–1132

62. McHenry CR, Walfish PG, Rosen IB (1993) Non-diagnostic fine-needle aspiration biopsy: a dilemma in management of nodular thyroid disease. Am Surg 59:415–419

63. Mehrotra P, Okpokam A, Bouhaidar R, Johnson SJ, Wilson JA, Davies BR, Lennard TW (2004) Galectin-3 does not reliably distinguish benign from malignant thyroid neoplasms. Histopathology 45:493–500

64. Meier CA (2000) Thyroid nodules: pathogenesis, diagnosis and treatment. Baillieres Best Pract Res Clin Endocrinol Metab 14:559–575

65. Mikosch P, Gallowitsch HJ, Kresnik E, Jester J, Wurtz FG, Kerschbaumer K, Unterweger O, Dinges HP, Lind P (2000) Value of ultrasound-guided fine-needle aspiration biopsy of thyroid nodules in an endemic goitre area. Eur J Nucl Med 27:62–69

66. Modigliani E, Franc B, Niccoli-Sire P (2000) Diagnosis and treatment of medullary thyroid cancer. Baillieres Best Pract Res Clin Endocrinol Metab 14:631–649

67. Niccoli P, Wion-Barbot N, Caron P, Henry JF, de Micco C, Saint Andre JP, Bigorgne JC, Modigliani E, Conte-Devolx B (1997) Interest of routine measurement of serum calcitonin: study in a large series of thyroidectomized patients. The French Medullary Study Group. J Clin Endocrinol Metab 82:338–341

68. Orlandi F, Saggiorato E, Pivano G, Puligheddu B, Termine A, Cappia S, De Giuli P, Angeli A (1998) Galectin-3 is a presurgical marker of human thyroid carcinoma. Cancer Res 58:3015–3020

69. Pacini F, Vorontsova T, Demidchik EP, Molinaro E, Agate L, Romei C, Shavrova E, Cherstvoy ED, Ivashkevitch Y, Kuchinskaya E, Schlumberger M, Ronga G, Filesi M, Pinchera A (1997) Post-Chernobyl thyroid carcinoma in Belarus children and adolescents: comparison with naturally occurring thyroid carcinoma in Italy and France. J Clin Endocrinol Metab 82:3563–3569

70. Papini E, Bacci V, Panunzi C, Pacella CM, Fabbrini R, Bizzarri G, Petrucci L, Giammarco V, La Medica P, Masala M (1993) A prospective randomized trial of levothyroxine suppressive therapy for solitary thyroid nodules. Clin Endocrinol (Oxf) 38:507–513

71. Papini E, Petrucci L, Guglielmi R, Panunzi C, Rinaldi R, Bacci V, Crescenzi A, Nardi F, Fabbrini R, Pacella CM (1998) Long-term changes in nodular goiter: a 5-year prospective randomized trial of levothyroxine suppressive therapy for benign cold thyroid nodules. J Clin Endocrinol Metab 83:780-783

72. Papini E, Guglielmi R, Bianchini A, Crescenzi A, Taccogna S, Nardi F, Panunzi C, Rinaldi R, Toscano V, Pacella CM (2002) Risk of malignancy in nonpalpable thyroid nodules: predictive value of ultrasound and color-Doppler features. J Clin Endocrinol Metab 87:1941–1946

73. Parle JV, Maisonneuve P, Sheppard MC, Boyle P, Franklyn JA (2001) Prediction of all-cause and cardiovascular mortality in elderly people from one low serum thyrotropin result: a 10-year cohort study. Lancet 358:861–865

74. Pelizzo MR, Piotto A, Rubello D, Casara D, Fassina A, Busnardo B (1990) High prevalence of occult papillary thyroid carcinoma in a surgical series for benign thyroid disease. Tumori 76:255–257

75. Pinchera A, Aghini-Lombardi F, Antonangeli L, Vitti P (1996) Multinodular goiter. Epidemiology and prevention. Ann Ital Chir 67:317–325

76. Radecki PD, Arger PH, Arenson RL, Jennings AS, Coleman BG, Mintz MC, Kressel HY (1984) Thyroid imaging: comparison of high-resolution real-time ultrasound and computed tomography. Radiology 153:145–147

77. Read CH Jr, Tansey MJ, Menda Y (2004) A 36-year retrospective analysis of the efficacy and safety of radioactive iodine in treating young Graves' patients. J Clin Endocrinol Metab 89:4229–4233

78. Reverter JL, Lucas A, Salinas I, Audi L, Foz M, Sanmarti A (1992) Suppressive therapy with levothyroxine for solitary thyroid nodules. Clin Endocrinol (Oxf) 36:25–28

79. Richter B, Neises G, Clar C (2002) Pharmacotherapy for thyroid nodules. A systematic review and meta-analysis. Endocrinol Metab Clin North Am 31:699–722

80. Rojdmark J, Jarhult J (1995) High long term recurrence rate after subtotal thyroidectomy for nodular goitre. Eur J Surg 161:725–727

81. Rzepka AH, Cissewski K, Olbricht T, Reinwein D (1994) Effectiveness of prophylactic therapy on goiter recurrence in an area with low iodine intake: a sonographic follow-up study. Clin Investig 72:967–970

82. Sampson RJ, Key CR, Buncher CR, Iijima S (1969) Thyroid carcinoma in Hiroshima and Nagasaki. I. Prevalence of thyroid carcinoma at autopsy. JAMA 209:65–70

83. Sampson RJ, Woolner LB, Bahn RC, Kurland LT (1974) Occult thyroid carcinoma in Olmsted County, Minnesota: prevalence at autopsy compared with that in Hiroshima and Nagasaki, Japan. Cancer 34:2072–2076

84. Sawin CT, Geller A, Wolf PA, Belanger AJ, Baker E, Bacharach P, Wilson PW, Benjamin EJ, D'Agostino RB (1994) Low serum thyrotropin concentrations as a risk factor for atrial fibrillation in older persons. N Engl J Med 331:1249–1252

85. Schlinkert RT, van Heerden JA, Goellner JR, Gharib H, Smith SL, Rosales RF, Weaver AL (1997) Factors that predict malignant thyroid lesions when fine-needle aspiration is suspicious for follicular neoplasm. Mayo Clin Proc 72:913–916

86. Schneider AB (1990) Radiation-induced thyroid tumors. Endocrinol Metab Clin North Am 19:495–508

87. Schneider AB, Favus MJ, Stachura ME, Arnold J, Arnold MJ, Frohman LA (1978) Incidence, prevalence and characteristics of radiation-induced thyroid tumors. Am J Med 64:243–252

88. Schneider AB, Shore-Freedman E, Ryo UY, Bekerman C, Favus M, Pinsky S (1985) Radiation-induced tumors of the head and neck following childhood irradiation. Prospective studies. Medicine (Baltimore) 64:1–15

89. Schneider AB, Recant W, Pinsky SM, Ryo UY, Bekerman C, Shore-Freedman E (1986) Radiation-induced thyroid carcinoma. Clinical course and results of therapy in 296 patients. Ann Intern Med 105:405–412

90. Schneider AB, Ron E, Lubin J, Stovall M, Gierlowski TC (1993) Dose-response relationships for radiation-induced thyroid cancer and thyroid nodules: evidence for the prolonged effects of radiation on the thyroid. J Clin Endocrinol Metab 77:362–369

91. Schoder H, Yeung HW (2004) Positron emission imaging of head and neck cancer, including thyroid carcinoma. Semin Nucl Med 34:180–197

92. Sherman SI (2003) Thyroid carcinoma. Lancet 361:501–511

93. Singer PA, Cooper DS, Daniels GH, Ladenson PW, Greenspan FS, Levy EG, Braverman LE, Clark OH, McDougall IR, Ain KV, Dorfman SG (1996) Treatment guidelines for patients with thyroid nodules and well-differentiated thyroid cancer. American Thyroid Association. Arch Intern Med 156:2165–2172

94. Sokal JE (1957) A long term follow-up of non-toxic nodular goitre. JAMA 99:60

95. Solbiati L, Volterrani L, Rizzatto G, Bazzocchi M, Busilacci P, Candiani F, Ferrari F, Giuseppetti G, Maresca G, Mirk P (1985) The thyroid gland with low uptake lesions: evaluation by ultrasound. Radiology 155:187–191

96. Spencer CA (2000) Thyroglobulin. In: Braverman LE, Utiger RD (eds) Werner & Ingbar's the thyroid. Lippincott Williams & Wilkins, Philadelphia, pp 402–413

97. Stoffer RP, Welch JP, Hellwig CA, Chesky WE, McCusker EN (1960) Nodular goitre. Arch Intern Med 106:10

98. Tan GH, Gharib H (1997) Thyroid incidentalomas: management approaches to nonpalpable nodules discovered incidentally on thyroid imaging. Ann Intern Med 126:226–231

99. Tollin SR, Mery GM, Jelveh N, Fallon EF, Mikhail M, Blumenfeld W, Perlmutter S (2000) The use of fine-needle aspiration biopsy under ultrasound guidance to assess the risk of malignancy in patients with a multinodular goiter. Thyroid 10:235–241

100. Topliss D (2004) Thyroid incidentaloma: the ignorant in pursuit of the impalpable. Clin Endocrinol (Oxf) 60:18–20

101. Tunbridge WM, Evered DC, Hall R, Appleton D, Brewis M, Clark F, Evans JG, Young E, Bird T, Smith PA (1977) The spectrum of thyroid disease in a community: the Whickham survey. Clin Endocrinol (Oxf) 7:481–493

102. Tuttle RM, Lemar H, Burch HB (1998) Clinical features associated with an increased risk of thyroid malignancy in patients with follicular neoplasia by fine-needle aspiration. Thyroid 8:377–383

103. Uzzan B, Campos J, Cucherat M, Nony P, Boissel JP, Perret GY (1996) Effects on bone mass of long term treatment with thyroid hormones: a meta-analysis. J Clin Endocrinol Metab 81:4278–4289

104. Vierhapper H, Raber W, Bieglmayer C, Kaserer K, Weinhausl A, Niederle B (1997) Routine measurement of plasma calcitonin in nodular thyroid diseases. J Clin Endocrinol Metab 82:1589–1593

105. Wang C, Crapo LM (1997) The epidemiology of thyroid disease and implications for screening. Endocrinol Metab Clin North Am 26:189–218

106. Wemeau JL, Caron P, Schvartz C, Schlienger JL, Orgiazzi J, Cousty C, Vlaeminck-Guillem V (2002) Effects of thyroid-stimulating hormone suppression with levothyroxine in reducing the volume of solitary thyroid nodules and improving extranodular nonpalpable changes: a randomized, double-blind, placebo-controlled trial by the French Thyroid Research Group. J Clin Endocrinol Metab 87:4928–4934

107. Wesche MF, Tiel VBMM, Lips P, Smits NJ, Wiersinga WM (2001) A randomized trial comparing levothyroxine with radioactive iodine in the treatment of sporadic nontoxic goiter. J Clin Endocrinol Metab 86:998–1005

108. Zelmanovitz F, Genro S, Gross JL (1998) Suppressive therapy with levothyroxine for solitary thyroid nodules: a double-blind controlled clinical study and cumulative meta-analyses. J Clin Endocrinol Metab 83:3881–3885

6 Fine-needle Aspiration Cytology of the Thyroid

Anne E. Busseniers and Susan A. Silver

CONTENTS

6.1 Introduction

Thyroid nodules are common in the general population and their incidence increases with age. An estimated 40% of the United States population harbors thyroid nodules, approximately half of which are solitary on physical examination [17,34]. An increasing number of these are found incidentally on imaging studies of the neck (e.g., magnetic resonance imaging, full-body scan, carotid Doppler) performed for unrelated reasons. Only about 12,000 new thyroid cancers are diagnosed each year in the United States with approximately 1,000 deaths from the disease. Many more people, though, have clinically silent thyroid cancers. The latter represent clinically insignificant papillary carcinomas found in up to 35% of thyroid glands evaluated at autopsy or at surgery [62,91], manifest as small subcentimeter-sized nodules [99]. It would therefore be clinically and fiscally irresponsible to remove all thyroid nodules surgically. Fine-needle aspiration (FNA) has become the ultimate test, in conjunction with clinical judgment, to triage those individuals who will most benefit from surgery.

The summary of our experience and practice with FNA of the thyroid is presented in this chapter. This practice includes obtaining a detailed, targeted history from the patient, reviewing relevant imaging studies if applicable, doing a targeted physical examination, performing the aspiration procedure, reviewing the adequacy of the sample prior to the patient leaving the office, rendering a diagnosis, and communicating it to the referring physician. The latter is generally accomplished within 24 hours of the procedure. The preliminary pathology results and their implications are often discussed with the patient at the end of the consultation, particularly when the diagnosis is benign. We serve as consultants both to our patients and to our clinicians and, therefore, the final cytopathology report often includes a recommendation based on the sum total of information gleaned from the patient's office visit [20]. We concur with Lawrence and Kaplan [80] that the person obtaining the history, performing the physical examination, reviewing pertinent records, and performing and interpreting the FNA is in a unique position to make such a recommendation.

6.2   FNA of the Thyroid

6.2.1   Accuracy

Arriving at an accurate FNA diagnosis involves a systematic chain of events, not all of which are in the control of the aspirator/cytopathologist. A demarcated, accessible target must be identified. The composition of the nodule must be amenable to penetration by a thin needle; for example, densely fibrotic and calcified lesions generally do not yield cells. The size of the nodule must be within a certain range to allow representative sampling; specifically, very small nodules may be missed by aspiration and very large nodules may harbor an unsampled malignancy. Proper technique must be used to obtain an adequate sample. Proper preparation of the sample is necessary to minimize artifacts. Accurate interpretation requires an experienced cytopathologist. The final diagnosis must be communicated clearly, using consistent terminology, to ensure proper treatment. A deficiency in any link in the chain may result in an inaccurate diagnosis, with sampling and interpretative errors accounting for the majority of such cases [41,122].

The early literature on FNA of the thyroid focused primarily on what the procedure could achieve, namely, providing a sensitive and cost-effective tool for the detection of malignancy [59]. With refined diagnostic and technical acumen, the current success of thyroid FNA has accomplished a twofold increase in

the detection of thyroid cancers during neck exploration, with a concomitant 50% reduction in the number of thyroid surgical procedures performed [51,59]. Recent publications have focused more on limitations of the FNA technique, namely, inadequate and inconclusive samples. For a number of reasons, an accuracy rate of 100% has not been achieved and is likely not achievable; as such, histologic evaluation of the surgically resected lesion remains the gold standard.

Reported sensitivity and specificity rates of FNA for the diagnosis of thyroid neoplasia differ widely [30]. The latter is primarily due to how these rates are calculated. For example, in some studies, carcinomas and benign neoplasms are evaluated as one category [74], indeterminate/suspicious cases are variably considered [5,11], and not all reports include only histologically confirmed cases [22]. Studies using histologically verified cases show mean sensitivity and specificity rates of 77.7% and 85.4%, respectively [1,5,68,76,103,112]. Table 6.1 summarizes the sensitivity, specificity, positive predictive value, negative predictive value, and accuracy rates published in the recent literature. Clearly, the wide ranges depicted here are contributed to by wide variability in experience and training of the aspirator and/or diagnostician. When one keeps sight of the fact that the purpose of thyroid FNA is to triage patients for surgery, the relatively low specificity rates cited in the literature are not as problematic as the reported sensitivity rates. The latter, as alluded to elsewhere in this chapter, is largely a function of interpretative and sampling errors.

Although the yield of obtaining a malignant diagnosis on repeat FNA in the follow-up of a presumably benign thyroid nodule may be low, rebiopsy reportedly reduces the rate of false-negative diagnoses from a mean of 5.2% to less than 1.3% [29,42]. The routine performance of repeat FNA in the follow-up of patients with benign nodular thyroid disease with or without any clinical changes is, however, of limited value [44]. Clinical factors rather than repeat FNA

Table 6.1 Statistical parameters of FNA of the thyroid [1, 5, 22, 68, 73, 76, 103, 112, 116, 121]

	Range
Sensitivity	38–100%
Specificity	67–98.2%
Positive predictive value	34–99%
Negative predictive value	66.3–100%
Accuracy	72–94.4%

may hold precedence in surgical management of patients with benign nodular thyroid disease [83,94].

As the study of thyroid disease at the molecular level evolves, its application to FNA samples will undoubtedly continue to refine the triaging of patients for surgery. Currently, these methods are not applicable to everyday practice.

6.2.2 Indications

There are numerous diagnostic procedures available to aid in rendering a diagnosis of a thyroid lesion. If these procedures are not used rationally, it will undoubtedly lead to an unjustifiable increase in cost with little practical gain [103]. The utilization of FNA varies considerably among experienced surgeons and on different continents. Chen et al. [32] recently compared the utilization of FNA in a center in the United Kingdom to one in the United States. FNA was more commonly employed in the US (84%) than in the UK (52%). In a retrospective analysis of all thyroid carcinomas using the Netherlands Pathology Database, it was determined that only 66% of patients were analyzed using FNA prior to surgery [55].

Rational indications for performing FNA of the thyroid in the United States include the initial diagnostic test of a solitary cold nodule, a dominant new or enlarging cold nodule in a gland showing multinodularity, thyroiditis, clinically inoperable carcinoma, and metastatic disease to the thyroid. In addition, it may provide psychologic reassurance of benign disease and relieve neck pain caused by sudden enlargement of a cyst.

6.2.3 Contraindications

There are no specific contraindications to the procedure. The needles are sufficiently thin (23 gauge or smaller) that the procedure can be performed safely on patients who are anticoagulated. In patients with mitral valve prolapse, prophylactic antibiotic therapy is not indicated.

6.3 The FNA Procedure for Palpable Lesions

The reader is referred to a detailed description of the procedure as it pertains to palpable thyroid nodules in a chapter by Busseniers [19]. With practice and increasing competency, and provided the target is not located in the posterior aspect of a lobe, one should be able to detect and aspirate nodules as small as 4–5 mm, without the added expense of ultrasound guidance.

6.3.1 Equipment

The following equipment is recommended: 10-cc syringe holder; 10-cc syringes; 23- and 25-gauge needles, short and long; alcohol pads; gauze; glass slides with frosted end; grease pencil; Xylocaine gel and/or ice pack; hair dryer; liquid medium (e.g., Cytolyte) for needle rinses; rapid stain (e.g., Diff-Quik stain, rapid H&E); microscope (Fig. 6.1).

6.3.2 Preparation and Examination of the Patient

A properly informed patient is less anxious and will more readily tolerate multiple passes without the use of a local anesthetic (see further on). For this reason, we allow ample time to explain each step of the procedure in detail and answer any questions the patient may have.

Skillful palpation is a critical step in ensuring that the material is aspirated from the appropriate area. It takes practice and patience and, in our opinion, is of paramount importance in obtaining an adequate and representative sample. We initially examine the patient in an upright seated position, with shoulders down and neck muscles relaxed. Often, the nodule will be visible when the patient swallows, especially if he or she is not overweight. The "lump" appears as an asymmetric shadow that moves up and down when the patient is talking and/or swallowing. Nodules as small as 5 mm may be visible when located in the isthmus or anterior aspect of either lobe. The

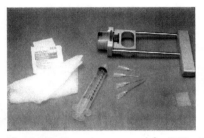

Fig. 6.1 Basic equipment used for FNA. Alcohol pads, gauze, syringe holder, 10-cc syringe, 25-gauge (5/8 and 1½ inch in length) needle, 23-gauge (1 and 1½ inch in length) needle, and glass slides

patient is then asked to lie back and a pillow is placed under his or her shoulders to hyperextend the neck. The chin, however, does not have to be lifted excessively since this may stretch the skin at the base of the neck to such an extent that the nodule is more difficult to feel. We keep the table at a mild upward incline to diminish vertigo. When the nodule is located in the lateral or posterior aspect of the lobe, we have found it useful to have an assistant push down on the contralateral lobe. This will often result in the nodule assuming a more superficial location, facilitating the insertion of the needle.

We do not advocate injection of a local anesthetic. It not only results in an additional needle stick, but, in our experience, the actual injection of the anesthetic is painful, produces a secondary lump overlying the one to be sampled, and makes insertion of the needle at the proper depth more difficult. Furthermore, if the anesthetic becomes admixed with the aspirated sample, it may distort the cells due to osmosis, rendering cytologic interpretation difficult. For a particularly anxious patient, a topical gel or a small ice pack may be applied over the site to be aspirated.

6.3.3   FNA with Aspiration Device (Aspiration Technique)

After definitively defining the nodule by palpation, the aspirator's middle and ring fingers of one hand are placed at the superior and inferior edge of the lump, and the patient is asked to swallow. The latter is useful in confirming the location of the nodule and also reduces the likelihood of the patient swallowing during the procedure, which could result in a tear in the thyroid capsule.

The aspiration site is cleaned with alcohol and dried prior to insertion of the needle. The needle is then inserted into the center of the lump, perpendicular to the skin and just medial to the sternocleidomastoid

muscle. The placement of the needle is easily guided using the thumb of the other hand (Fig. 6.2a). We do not recommend lifting the lump between index finger and thumb and inserting the needle laterally through the sternocleidomastoid muscle. Once inserted, the needle is moved rapidly back and forth in the same plane as its insertion, while applying minimal or no suction. This may be done in only one direction or in a tight circular fashion, with the beveled edge of the needle used as a small cutting device to dislodge cells and tissue fragments. Material will quickly appear in the needle hub. If the contents are noted to be bloody, suction should be released immediately and the needle withdrawn. Pressure is then applied at the puncture site. The entire procedure lasts approximately 10–15 seconds.

6.3.3.1   Amount of Suction

The thyroid gland is vascular and so are the majority of lesions occurring in it (notable exceptions are inflammatory conditions and cysts composed of colloid). Therefore, one must be attentive to applying suction gradually, and only when indicated, in order to prevent a sudden rupture of capillaries resulting in a sample diluted by blood. If one encounters resistance to the insertion of the needle and little material appears in the needle hub after a few seconds, one is most likely dealing with a thyroiditis, a papillary cancer, or some other type of sclerotic lesion. In this instance, gradual suction may be applied, which usually does not require more than 3–5 cc of pressure.

6.3.3.2   Directions of the Needle

It is best to maintain the needle in one direction while obtaining a sample. It is, however, our practice to use small circular movements as explained above. With

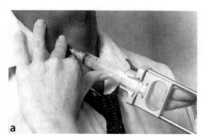

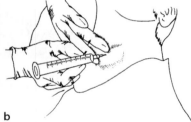

Fig. 6.2 Technique. **a** Aspiration technique. Second and third fingers of one hand immobilize the lump while the thumb guides the needle into the lesion, perpendicular to the skin. **b** Non-aspiration technique. The plunger is removed from the syringe, the lesion is immobilized with the third and fourth fingers of one hand, while the other hand holds the syringe as one would grip a pencil

a
b

increasing experience, nodules may be sampled multidirectionally, with redirection of the needle undertaken when the needle tip is just beneath the surface of the lesion.

6.3.3.3   Number of Passes

We usually perform one aspirate per palpable centimeter of the lesion, ensuring that each pass is performed in a different area. For a 3-cm nodule, for example, we obtain samples from the upper, middle, and lower aspects of the lesion. Larger nodules may require more samples to reduce the possibility of a false-negative result due to sampling error.

6.3.3.4   Sampling of a Multinodular Gland

Careful evaluation of the multinodular thyroid is indicated, as the presence of one pathologic process by no means excludes the possibility of a second concurrent pathologic entity. In one series of 1,330 cases involving the FNA of two or more palpable nodules, two different pathologic diagnoses were rendered in 1% of cases [124].

Multinodular thyroid disease carries a risk of malignancy in the range of 5–13.7%, comparable to that which exists for solitary thyroid nodules [49,117]. Many of these malignancies represent occult carcinomas, usually papillary carcinoma, which by convention are smaller than 10–15 mm. Of note, occult carcinomas account for up to 60% of all cases of papillary carcinoma [24].

6.3.4   Non-aspiration Technique

When using the non-aspiration technique, a syringe holder is not required. The plunger is removed from the syringe to which the needle is attached. The lump is immobilized with one hand, in the same fashion as described earlier. The hand used to perform the procedure holds the syringe at its base close to the needle hub, much like holding a pen or pencil (Fig. 6.2b). The remainder of the procedure is similar to the aspiration technique. Once material is visible in the needle hub, the needle is withdrawn and pressure is applied at the puncture site. The plunger is then placed back into the syringe and used to expel small drops of material onto the slides.

The greatest advantage of the non-aspiration technique is that it allows the aspirator better control with greater proximity to the nodule. It allows for increased precision when aspirating very small nodules (under 5 mm), and it is also less threatening to patients.

If one knows that the lesion is at least partially cystic, we recommend using the aspiration technique to take the first sample. Fluid from large cysts can easily be removed. The non-aspiration technique may then be performed on any remaining solid component of the nodule.

6.3.5   Complications

The following complications are possible: local infection, hematoma, localized pain, and vasovagal episodes. In our experience and that of others, these complications are exceedingly rare [10]. We encourage our patients to resume their normal activities following the procedure, and recommend the use of an ice pack or a non-steroidal anti-inflammatory drug to alleviate any local discomfort.

6.3.6   Preparation of the Aspirated Sample

Sample preparation varies considerably among laboratories, and is largely dependent on the experience and preferences of the pathologists who interpret the FNA material. An otherwise adequate sample may be wasted if the material is not smeared or handled properly. The importance of having properly prepared smears consisting of a thin, even layer of material cannot be overemphasized.

In our laboratory we prepare, on average, three to six smears per pass, and rinse the remainder of the material in Cytolyte for preparation of thin-layer (ThinPrep; Cytyc, Marlborough, MA) slides. If tissue fragments are visible floating in the fluid, a cell block is prepared. To prepare the smears, small drops of material are placed in the middle of one edge of the long axis of a slide. The edge of another slide is used to spread the material evenly across the slide (Fig. 6.3a). If the material is highly viscous or bloody, an additional slide may be placed on top of the drop of material to facilitate the gentle spreading of the material across the slide (Fig. 6.3b).

Depending largely on the preferences of the cytopathologist, the cytologic smears may then be air-dried and subsequently stained using Diff-Quik, or alternatively, alcohol-fixed and stained with Papanicolaou or hematoxylin and eosin stains. Some laboratories prepare both air-dried and alcohol-fixed smears. Fixation must be immediate if the slides are to be alcohol-

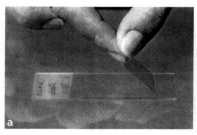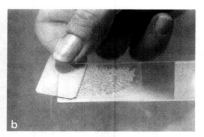

Fig. 6.3 Slide preparation. **a** A small drop of aspirated material is placed at the edge of the slide, while the edge of another slide or coverglass is used to drag the material along to spread it evenly. **b** If the material is highly viscous or bloody, an additional slide may be placed on top of the drop of material to facilitate gentle spreading of the material across the slide

fixed. This is necessary to prevent air-drying artifact which may result in an inconclusive diagnosis.

6.3.7 Types of Aspirated Material and Clues to Their Origin

Colloid: Colloid appears viscous, pale yellow, and shiny when smeared on slides. Care must be taken so that the material does not wash off the slide during slide preparation.

Cyst fluid: The fluid varies from straw-colored to pale or dark green/brown to a cloudy dark-brown.

Dry tap: This occurs when no material appears in the needle hub after a few seconds of aspiration. It generally indicates placement of the needle into soft tissue/skeletal muscle of the neck, and is associated with acute discomfort. A dry tap may also indicate fibrosis within the nodule.

Blood: Blood appears immediately upon insertion of the needle due to sampling a highly vascular lesion or puncturing a vessel. The aspiration should be stopped immediately and pressure applied to the puncture site. The procedure may be repeated with a smaller gauge needle and with the patient in an upright seated position.

6.3.8 The Final Report

A complete final report typically includes:
- Patient demographics
- Clinical history: signs and symptoms associated with thyroid disease and their duration, ultrasound and uptake scan findings, family history of thyroid disease, history of exposure to irradiation
- Physical examination: location and size of nodule(s), status of cervical lymph nodes
- Procedure: size of needles used, aspiration mode (aspiration versus non-aspiration technique),

number of passes performed, type of sample obtained (hemorrhagic, amount of cyst fluid if any), number of smears prepared, needle rinse preparation, and types of any ancillary tests performed
- Findings of on-site evaluation for specimen adequacy
- Microscopic description
- Final diagnosis
- Recommendations

6.4 Cytologic Diagnostic Categories

Four diagnostic categories are traditionally used to classify FNA specimens: benign, malignant, suspicious/indeterminate, and unsatisfactory (Table 6.2). Percentages of each of these categories may vary widely for a given laboratory depending upon a number of factors including the patient population, the experience and skill of the aspirator, and the experience and skill of the pathologist interpreting the sample.

6.5 Cytologic Diagnoses

6.5.1 Approach

The best approach is to evaluate each aspirate smear in a consistent fashion for four basic components: (1)

Table 6.2 Distribution of cytologic diagnostic categories [20, 40, 110, 116]

	Literature range	Busseniers
Benign	22–75%	82.5%
Malignant	10–32%	3.5%
Suspicious/indeterminate	15–42%	13%
Unsatisfactory	5–43.1%	1%

smear background, (2) cellularity, (3) architectural patterns, and (4) cellular detail.

Our approach is to first scan the background of the smears at low power for the presence of blood, colloid, thin cystic fluid, granular material, inflammatory cells, and a tumor cell diathesis. Once the background is assessed, the cellularity and composition of the cells present are evaluated. These cells may include follicular epithelial cells including those with Hürthle cell change, squamous metaplastic cells, lymphocytes, and histiocytes. Note is made of any atypical cells, and cells present that are not typically seen in primary lesions of the thyroid. The dimension of each cellular component is evaluated relative to the standard red blood cell; with respect to the follicular cell population, the degree of nuclear monotony is also noted. Malignant cytologic features are assessed as well. As part of the smear evaluation, architectural patterns assumed by the cells are noted. Finally, any specific cellular features such as the presence of intracytoplasmic nuclear pseudoinclusions and nuclear grooves are noted.

6.5.2 Terminology Used in Microscopic Descriptions

Acinar structures or rosettes: Follicular epithelial cells arranged in a circular two-dimensional fashion without definite central lumen formation. They probably represent tubules (see further on) in cross-section (Fig. 6.4).

Fire flares: Rounded empty spaces bordered by cytoplasm at the periphery of a sheet of follicular epithelial cells (Fig. 6.5).

Intranuclear pseudoinclusion: Invagination of the cytoplasm into the nucleus which creates the illusion of an empty hole in the nucleus (Fig. 6.6).

Microfollicles: Follicular epithelial cells arranged in a small circular cluster with lumina which may or may not contain colloid. When seen three-dimensionally, the circular arrangement is still prominent but, unlike spherules, the nuclei show marked overlap and the borders are irregular (Fig. 6.7).

Oxyphilic cells: Follicular epithelial cells with abundant, finely granular cytoplasm. The cytoplasm of these cells contain numerous mitochondria which account for the granularity seen by light microscopy (Fig. 6.8).

Psammoma bodies: Round calcified structures with well-demarcated concentric lamellations (Fig. 6.9).

Sheets: Monolayers of follicular epithelial cells with delicate cytoplasm, ill-defined cytoplasmic borders, and evenly spaced nuclei arranged in a so-called honeycomb fashion (Fig. 6.10).

Spherules: Three-dimensional representation of non-neoplastic thyroid follicles. They appear as round to ovoid cellular structures, with smooth contours and evenly spaced, round and regular nuclei. Colloid may be seen within them (Fig. 6.11).

Tubules: Follicular cells arranged in parallel arrays (Fig. 6.12).

6.5.3 The Unsatisfactory Aspirate

Unsatisfactory aspirates include samples containing:
- Blood only
- Hemodiluted samples with a paucity of thyroid epithelial cells
- Thyroid follicular epithelial cells entrapped in a blood clot
- Minimal thyroid material, such as scant colloid and rare follicular cells
- Cyst contents with a scanty follicular epithelial cell component

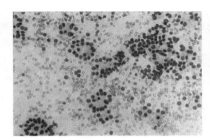

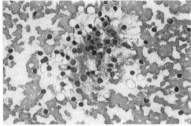

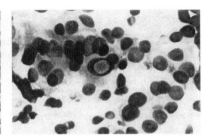

Fig. 6.4 Acinar structures or rosettes. Follicular epithelial cells are arranged in a small circular fashion without definite central lumen formation (Diff-Quik stain)

Fig. 6.5 Fire flares. Rounded empty spaces bordered by cytoplasm at the periphery of a sheet of follicular epithelial cells (Diff-Quik stain)

Fig. 6.6 Intranuclear pseudoinclusion. The inclusion occupies at least one third of the nuclear surface, has a dense rim of chromatin, and the same hue as the cytoplasm (Diff-Quik stain)

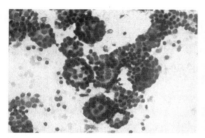

Fig. 6.7 Microfollicles. Follicular epithelial cell nuclei are relatively monotonous in size, and arranged in small spherical structures with nuclear overlap, scalloped edges, and little cytoplasm (Diff-Quik stain)

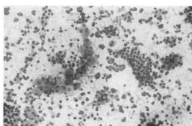

Fig. 6.8 Sheet of oxyphilic cells (*left of center*) as seen in adenomatoid nodule, admixed with follicular epithelial cells showing small, regular nuclei. Note the prominent granularity of the oxyphilic cell cytoplasm (Diff-Quik stain)

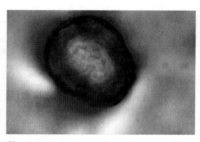

Fig. 6.9 Psammoma body shown at high magnification to illustrate the concentric calcific lamellations (Diff-Quik stain)

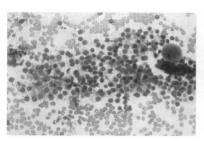

Fig. 6.10 Sheets of follicular epithelial cells. Note the delicate cytoplasm with paravacuolar granules, ill-defined cytoplasmic borders, and evenly spaced nuclei within these sheets. The nuclear size is predictable and approximates the size of a red blood cell (Diff-Quik stain)

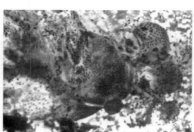

Fig. 6.11 Spherules of varying sizes as seen in adenomatoid nodule and cellular adenomatoid nodule. The follicular epithelial cells have delicate cytoplasm, and evenly spaced nuclei. The edge of the spherules is smooth; some internal colloid is also noted (Diff-Quik stain)

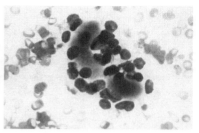

Fig. 6.12 Tubules as seen in a follicular neoplasm. The follicular epithelial cells are arranged in longitudinal, parallel arrays. Note the thick, inspissated colloid located centrally, and nuclear enlargement with nuclear rim irregularity (Diff-Quik stain)

- Only material of non-thyroid origin (e.g., skeletal muscle)

There exist no specific criteria for classifying a thyroid aspirate as satisfactory. Some authors have suggested using a minimal number of follicular epithelial cells present on the smears [8]. It is our position, however, that if so few cells are present, the sample is likely to be unsatisfactory. On the other hand, a diagnosis of papillary carcinoma, for example, can be rendered on just a few groups of cells, if all cytologic criteria are met.

Unsatisfactory samples should not be construed as benign. Likewise, microscopic descriptions in an FNA report should be interpreted with caution; a report stating "no malignant cells present" is worthless if the microscopy describes a paucicellular sample. If there is a clinical or radiologic indication to aspirate a nodule and the FNA is unsatisfactory, repeat FNA will yield adequate material in at least 50% of these cases

[105]. In one study, 44% of nodules resected following an FNA classified as unsatisfactory proved to be neoplastic, 50% of which were malignant [18]. Subsequent studies have reported malignancies in 37–51% following an initially non-diagnostic FNA [13,33].

It is generally accepted that on-site evaluation of the specimen for adequacy, prior to discharging the patient, decreases the unsatisfactory rate. However, it should be noted that obtaining an adequate sample for cytologic interpretation is size-dependent. Carpi et al. [26] reported an improved FNA adequacy rate from 64% to 87% with increase in mean nodule size from 0.7 to 1.1 cm. Suggestions for minimizing the number of unsatisfactory samples include selecting individuals to aspirate and interpret samples who are qualified and maintain expertise [116].

6.5.4   Benign Lesions

6.5.4.1   *Subacute Granulomatous Thyroiditis (de Quervain's Thyroiditis)*

Although the diagnosis is typically made clinically, some patients present with unilateral enlargement of the gland or a solitary palpable nodule that is usually hard in consistency and not necessarily painful to palpation.

The smears may be highly cellular with bare follicular epithelial nuclei and small groups and sheets of follicular epithelial cells exhibiting small, regular nuclei, some with degenerative change and others with reactive features. There are abundant histiocytes, aggregates of epithelioid histiocytes (granulomas), and multinucleated giant cells, some with engulfed colloid [56,67]. These multinucleated cells may be quite large and composed of 10–30 oval-shaped nuclei. Inflammatory cells including mature lymphocytes and occasional neutrophils may also be present. Colloid is usually abundant and fragmented, and, along with the inflammatory cells, creates a background of granularity and cell debris (Fig. 6.13a,b) [50].

6.5.4.2   *Hashimoto's Thyroiditis*

On palpation, the thyroid gland is generally moderately enlarged with a nodular surface and a meaty consistency. However, up to 25% of aspirated cases of chronic thyroiditis present as a clinically solitary nodule [48]. Although the gland is usually not tender on palpation, painful Hashimoto's thyroiditis has been reported [78].

The classic smear of Hashimoto's thyroiditis (Fig. 6.14a,b) has an admixture of follicular cells, oxyphilic cells, and lymphoid cells including small, mature lymphocytes, follicular center cells, and plasma cells [101]. Lymphocytes being fragile, may be crushed, appearing as a tangle of threads. Germinal centers may be seen as well as histiocytes and multinucleated giant cells. The latter usually contain less than 10–12 nuclei. The follicular cells and oxyphilic (Hürthle) cells are arranged in sheets, groups, and acinar structures. Microfollicles may also be seen. The amount of colloid in the smears is moderate to scant. The diagnosis of chronic lymphocytic (Hashimoto's) thyroiditis rests upon finding a combination of follicular epithelial cells with oxyphilic cell change, and lymphoid cells including plasma cells.

6.5.4.3   *Riedel's Thyroiditis*

The thyroid gland is hard and often small on palpation.

The smears are generally paucicellular and notable for fragments of fibrous tissue with bland spindle-shaped cells and myofibroblasts [63]. Follicular epithelial cells are scanty. Hürthle cells and lymphoid

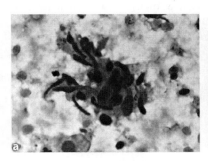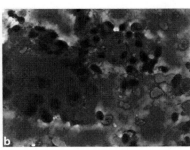

Fig. 6.13 Subacute granulomatous thyroiditis. **a** Group of loosely cohesive spindle-shaped cells in a background of inflammatory debris. **b** Multinucleated giant cells on the left. The background shows dense colloid (Diff-Quik stain)

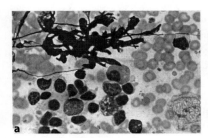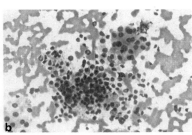

Fig. 6.14 Chronic lymphocytic (Hashimoto's) thyroiditis. **a** Pleomorphic population of lymphoid cells includes small, mature lymphocytes, a plasma cell, and follicular center cells. A lymphoid tangle is present at 12 o'clock. **b** Oxyphilic epithelial cells admixed with lymphoid cells (Diff-Quik stain)

follicular center cells are not conspicuous. The FNA is often deemed unsatisfactory [3].

6.5.4.4   *Adenomatoid Nodule*

The nodule is non-tender and soft to rubbery on palpation.

The smears show abundant colloid, either dense or watery. Colloid is best appreciated on air-dried direct smears, with the classic "cracking" artifact or in a mosaic/flowery pattern (Fig. 6.15). Colloid may be difficult to appreciate on slides prepared from liquid-based medium, where it appears as fragments of paper-thin, transparent, pale gray-blue material. When aspirated by an experienced individual, the smears may be highly cellular. Follicular epithelial cells are arranged in sheets, small groups resembling clusters of grapes, and in spherules of variable sizes, individually or in tissue fragments (Figs. 6.10, 6.11). Bare follicular cell nuclei may be present in the background (Fig. 6.15). The follicular cell nuclei are small, approximating the size of red blood cells, and have thin, transparent cytoplasm. An admixture of spindle-shaped cells, histiocytes, and follicular cells with oxyphilic (Hürthle) cell change are commonly seen in the background [21].

6.5.4.5   *Cellular Adenomatoid Nodule*

On palpation, the lesion may seem harder or more rubbery than the ordinary adenomatoid nodule because of a predominance of follicular epithelial cells relative to the amount of colloid.

The smears are often described as cellular, consisting of follicular epithelial cells arranged in spherules, sheets, groups, rosettes, and tubules. The cells may

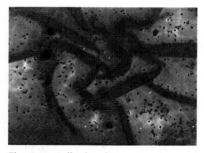

Fig. 6.15 Colloid with a mosaic pattern (cracking due to drying artifact) seen in adenomatoid nodule with abundant colloid (colloid cyst). Note the small, bare follicular cell nuclei in the background (Diff-Quik stain)

overlap or may show lack of cohesiveness. Tissue fragments may be evident. Microfollicles usually are absent. Cytoplasm is abundant, often delicate, frayed, and pale blue to gray. The follicular epithelial cell nuclei may show variability in size, up to two to three times the size of red blood cells. Cytoplasmic fire flares are a common finding [21].

6.5.5   Indeterminate Neoplasms

6.5.5.1   *Follicular Neoplasm*

An inherent limitation of thyroid FNA is its inability to distinguish follicular adenoma from follicular carcinoma. The reason for this limitation is that the diagnostic distinction between follicular adenoma and carcinoma is based on the presence or absence of thyroid capsular and/or vascular invasion by the neoplastic cells. This determination requires evaluation of the resected neoplastic tissue. The more important distinction to make as a cytopathologist is between a non-neoplastic adenomatoid nodule and a follicular neoplasm.

A lesion with an FNA diagnosis of follicular neoplasm has a high probability (80–95%) of representing a follicular neoplasm at surgery, but overall, only 20–24% of these represent follicular carcinoma [4,15,27,46,48,52,53,58,64,74,75,81,88,114]. A higher incidence of malignancy is found in men, in nodules larger than 3 cm, and in patients over age 40; these features may be useful in planning and triaging patients for surgery [12]. Similarly, nodules that are hard to palpation or that are solitary and hypoechoic may help define a subset of patients with an FNA diagnosis of follicular neoplasm who are at increased risk of malignancy [102]. Some studies, however, have not shown age and gender to correlate with malignancy in follicular neoplasms [6].

Smears prepared from FNAs of follicular adenoma and follicular carcinoma are strikingly similar, as a result of overlapping histologic appearances between these two entities. Indeed, the follicular cells comprising follicular adenoma and carcinoma are indistinguishable cytologically.

Smears prepared from the FNA of a follicular neoplasm generally fall into three categories: (1) extremely cellular with scant colloid; (2) hemorrhagic; and (3) cystic, due to degenerative change. In our experience, abundant colloid may rarely be present and is usually associated with a predominantly macrofollicular or mixed micro- and macrofollicular adenoma. The striking amount of colloid seen in such

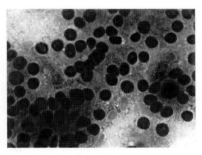

Fig. 6.16 Follicular neoplasm with a monotonous population of follicular epithelial cells showing enlarged, overlapping nuclei, rosettes, and a microfollicle with inspissated colloid at 3 o'clock (Diff-Quik stain)

neoplasms emphasizes the necessity of both adequate and representative sampling.

The classic appearance of a follicular neoplasm on FNA smears has minimal colloid in the background. If present at all, it is seen in small, dense, round or oval-shaped fragments (so-called casts), representing colloid expelled from microfollicles by the smearing technique. The smears are usually cellular and composed of a monotonous population of follicular epithelial cells with mild to moderate nuclear enlargement [21]. An exception is the rare atypical adenoma in which enlarged, hyperchromatic nuclei may be seen, similar to that described in other endocrine neoplasms. The cytoplasm of the follicular cells is nearly transparent, sometimes inconspicuous, and typically not abundant due to a relatively increased nuclear to cytoplasmic ratio. As such, the nuclei are the prominent feature in these smears and are arranged as acini (Fig. 6.4), tubules (Fig. 6.12), and microfollicles (Fig. 6.7) seen singly or within tissue fragments. Microfollicles may or may not contain central dense colloid (Fig. 6.16). A prominent capillary network may also be seen in the background or within these tissue fragments and, when seen in contiguity with microfollicles, should not be misinterpreted as a papillary architecture.

6.5.5.2 Hürthle Cell Neoplasm

As with follicular neoplasms, a distinction between Hürthle cell adenoma and Hürthle cell carcinoma cannot be reliably made by FNA as it requires evaluation for the presence or absence of capsular and/or vascular invasion on the resected neoplasm (in the absence of metastatic disease).

Approximately 10–15% of thyroid neoplasms diagnosed as Hürthle cell neoplasm by FNA are malignant [53,92]. It has been suggested by Chen et al. [31] that Hürthle cell carcinomas are more likely to be larger than Hürthle cell adenomas; the authors reported a 65% incidence of carcinoma among Hürthle cell neoplasms ≥4 cm.

Hürthle cell neoplasms are typically soft on palpation. Aspirates generally yield high cellularity with little colloid [118]. Since Hürthle cell neoplasms represent a variant of follicular neoplasm, the architectural arrangement of the neoplastic cells is similar in aspirates of both. Hürthle (oxyphilic) cells are arranged in microfollicles with or without inspissated colloid. Three-dimensional tissue fragments are common with a sense of cellular disorganization [104]. The Hürthle cells have a relatively monotonous appearance with minimal pleomorphism and fairly abundant cytoplasm with characteristic granularity [66]. The nuclei may be binucleated, are often eccentrically located, and typically have macronucleoli.

While Hürthle cells may be a prominent feature in FNAs of non-neoplastic Hürthle cell lesions, including adenomatoid nodules and Hashimoto's thyroiditis, features reported to be specific for Hürthle cell neoplasms include a predominance (>90%) of discohesive Hürthle cells with abundant granular cytoplasm, macronucleoli, intracytoplasmic lumina, and abundant capillaries (Fig. 6.17) [113,120]. Of note, the degree of cellularity or presence of microfollicles are not useful in the distinction between non-neoplastic and neoplastic Hürthle cell lesions [113]. Aspi-

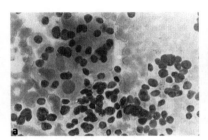
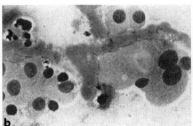
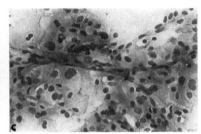

Fig. 6.17 Hürthle cell neoplasm. **a** Discohesive sheets of oxyphilic cells, some with intracytoplasmic vacuoles. **b** Binucleated oxyphilic cells with prominent nucleoli. **c** Prominent capillary network within tissue fragments composed of oxyphilic cells (Diff-Quik stain)

rates of Hürthle cell neoplasms usually do not contain ordinary follicular cells or lymphoid cells. However, if a Hürthle cell neoplasm undergoes cystic degenerative change, foamy and pigmented histiocytes may be present along with scant cellularity.

6.5.6   Malignant Neoplasms

6.5.6.1   *Papillary Carcinoma*

On palpation, the nodule is usually well defined and has a rubbery consistency. One may encounter some resistance upon insertion of the needle. In such cases, increased suction may be required in order to obtain material in the needle hub. If the tumor is calcified, a gritty sensation may be appreciated when moving the needle; it is even possible to hear the scraping of the needle within the lesion. The neoplasm may be soft to palpation if a significant cystic component is present.

Microscopically, the smears consist primarily of neoplastic cells. Aspirates of papillary carcinoma usually contain sparse colloid, and the colloid that is present is of a different nature than that seen in other thyroid lesions. The colloid in papillary carcinoma is typically described as dense, pasty, or bubblegum-like (Fig. 6.18). The architectural arrangement of the neoplastic cells varies from the classic papillary finger-like projections, which may or may not contain a fibrovascular core (Fig. 6.19), to sheets of cells with nuclei in close proximity but not overlapping (Fig. 6.20a), to single cells [70,95].

The cells of papillary carcinoma are generally uniformly enlarged with minimal pleomorphism. Marked cellular pleomorphism is rare and suggests anaplastic transformation. The cells have either finely granular cytoplasm resembling oxyphilic cells or dense cytoplasm with well-defined cytoplasmic borders (Fig. 6.20b) [70]. The cytoplasm often contains septate vacuoles, which have been likened to soap bubbles (Fig. 6.20b) [95]. Increased nuclear to cytoplasmic ratio, with nuclei enlarged up to four times the size of red blood cells, is characteristic (Fig. 6.19). However, it is the morphology of the nuclei that is the single most important diagnostic feature. The nuclei exhibit fine, powdery chromatin with a solitary, inconspicuous, eccentrically located nucleolus [106]. The chromatin may be seen dispersed to the periphery of the nucleus (Fig. 6.20). Intranuclear cytoplasmic pseudoinclusions are generally readily appreciated (Fig. 6.6). Note that intranuclear inclusions encompass at least one third of the nuclear surface and do not extend beyond the nuclear rim. It is important to apply these criteria in recognizing these inclusions since a number of artifacts may mimic them, namely, red blood cells superimposed on follicular epithelial nuclei, and degenerative vacuoles (most often seen in cystic lesions). With careful scrutiny, intranuclear pseudoinclusions are found in up to 90% of adequately sampled papillary carcinomas [70,82]. In most cases of papillary carcinoma, longitudinal grooves are visible in the nuclei, imparting a coffee bean or cerebriform appearance [87]. The latter

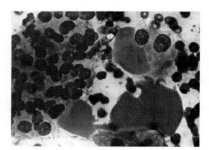

Fig. 6.18 Papillary carcinoma showing characteristic dense colloid described as bubble gum-like (Diff-Quik stain)

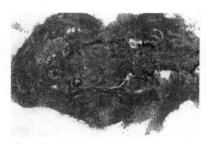

Fig. 6.19 Papillary carcinoma. At low magnification, a central fibrovascular core of a papilla is conspicuous, with papillary carcinoma cells arranged at its periphery (Diff-Quik stain)

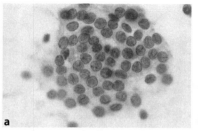

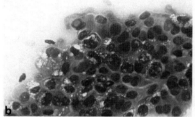

Fig. 6.20 Papillary carcinoma. **a** Note monotonously enlarged nuclei, increased nuclear to cytoplasmic ratio without nuclear overlap, dispersed chromatin with eccentric nucleolus, and nuclear grooves (hematoxylin and eosin stain). **b** The cells show nuclear enlargement, focal cytoplasmic vacuolization resembling soap bubbles, and dense cytoplasm with well-defined cytoplasmic borders. An intranuclear inclusion is present at 12 o'clock (Diff-Quik stain)

represent cytoplasmic invaginations through the full length of the nucleus (Fig. 6.18). Although nuclear grooves may be seen in a variety of benign thyroid lesions, when present in the majority of the nuclei this feature is highly suggestive of papillary carcinoma [111]. It should be noted that both nuclear grooves and chromatin dispersed to the periphery are best appreciated in fixed rather than air-dried smears.

Psammoma bodies, which represent concentric lamellated calcified bodies formed from the necrosed tips of papillae, are highly characteristic of any papillary neoplasm (Fig. 6.9); they are identified in 20–40% of papillary carcinomas [82,95]. Other features that may be seen in smears of papillary carcinoma include multinucleated giant cells, a lymphoid background, and cystic degenerative change.

Variants of Papillary Carcinoma

Follicular Variant of Papillary Carcinoma

Smears from the follicular variant of papillary carcinoma are cellular. The neoplastic cells are arranged in acinar structures and also as monolayered and/or branching sheets [47]. The cytologic diagnosis of this variant rests on the identification of the same characteristic nuclear features of usual papillary carcinoma, namely, monomorphism, powdery chromatin, intranuclear cytoplasmic pseudoinclusions, and longitudinal grooves. Psammoma bodies, multinucleated giant cells, and lymphocytes may be present [86].

The follicular variant of papillary carcinoma results in a "suspicious," equivocal diagnosis on FNA more frequently than does the usual papillary carcinoma [65]. The sensitivity of FNA for this variant (25%) is significantly lower than that for usual papillary carcinoma (74%) [84]. Fulciniti et al. [47], however, has reported the accuracy of FNA diagnosis of this variant to approach 90%.

Other Variants of Papillary Carcinoma

Other variants of papillary carcinoma include sclerosing, tall cell, columnar, Hürthle cell, Warthin-like, and the macrofollicular encapsulated variant. With the exception of the latter two entities, these variants are associated with a more aggressive behavior than usual papillary carcinoma [9,28,35,38,82,106]. Owing to the rarity of these lesions, their cytologic description falls outside the scope of this chapter.

6.5.6.2 Medullary Carcinoma

On palpation, the lesion usually presents as a hard, solitary, well-circumscribed mass with a predilection for the upper poles of the thyroid.

The aspirates yield cellular samples composed of neoplastic neuroendocrine cells and amyloid, seen in varied proportions. The neoplastic cells are loosely cohesive and are often seen as individual cells in smears (Fig. 6.21). The cells may form microfollicles and papillary projections and may therefore mimic other thyroid neoplasms [123]. A classic presentation is a combination of plasmacytoid and spindle cells with occasional bizarre tumor cells mimicking anaplastic giant cells [69]. The nuclei are often positioned eccentrically in the cytoplasm and have an evenly distributed chromatin pattern, as seen in other neuroendocrine neoplasms. Often, the nucleus is seen protruding beyond the cytoplasmic border. Intranuclear cytoplasmic pseudoinclusions are not uncommon. Mitotic activity is usually minimal. The cytoplasm is typically dense with well-defined borders, and may contain a fine dusting of red (neuroendocrine) granules, best appreciated on smears stained with Diff-Quik. When a cytologic diagnosis of medullary carcinoma is suggestive but not definitive, it may be helpful to stain an alcohol-fixed smear or cell block slide with calcitonin immunostain. A recommendation in the pathology report to obtain serum calcitonin and carcinoembryonic antigen (CEA) levels is also suggested to aid in confirming the diagnosis.

The amount of amyloid present is variable, and inversely correlates with the cellularity. It is reportedly present in 65–80% of aspirates [16,89,115]. Grossly, amyloid may be recognizable to the aspirator as a white, chalky substance. In smears, it has been compared to waxy candle drippings. As amyloid may closely resemble colloid, special histochemical stains (e.g., Congo red) are often required to confirm its presence. Coarse calcifications may also be seen, although psammoma bodies are seen in less than 10% of cases.

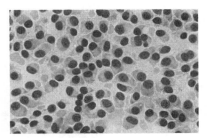

Fig. 6.21 Medullary carcinoma. The poorly cohesive malignant cells show plasmacytoid features with eccentric nuclei (Diff-Quik stain)

A number of variants of medullary carcinoma have been described including spindle cell, papillary, mixed follicular/medullary carcinoma, small cell, and giant cell variants [36,69,93].

6.5.6.3   Insular Carcinoma

Insular carcinoma is considered intermediate in behavior between the well-differentiated and less aggressive malignancies (papillary carcinoma and follicular carcinoma), and the more aggressive anaplastic carcinoma [23].

On palpation, the nodule is rubbery and averages larger than 2 cm.

The smears are highly cellular, populated by monomorphic follicular cells present singly and also arranged in acini, tubules, and follicles. Loose aggregates and groups with no distinguishing architecture are also observed. The cells have relatively bland, delicate, and ill-defined cytoplasm, oval to round nuclei, inconspicuous nucleoli, and a high nuclear to cytoplasmic ratio [97,100].

6.5.6.4   Giant and Spindle Cell (Anaplastic) Carcinoma

This diagnosis is often suspected clinically. Patients typically present with a rapidly enlarging mass, possibly resulting from malignant transformation of a preexisting thyroid neoplasm [25]. To palpation the mass is hard, and often quite large with an irregular nodular surface.

The smears of anaplastic carcinoma are usually very cellular, regardless of the experience of the aspirator. The neoplastic cells are large with extreme pleomorphism and readily apparent malignant features including irregular chromatin, macronucleoli, and mitoses. The cells may have a spindled and giant cell morphology (Fig. 6.22) [57]. The background frequently shows necrotic cellular debris (malignant diathesis) with inflammatory cells [54].

The differential diagnosis includes a high-grade sarcoma such as malignant fibrous histiocytoma [108], a variant of medullary carcinoma, and metastatic carcinoma.

6.5.6.5   Malignant Lymphoma

Secondary involvement of the thyroid, although rare, is more common than primary lymphoma involving the thyroid. Patients typically present with a rapidly

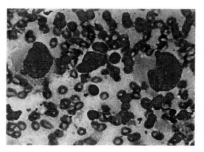

Fig. 6.22 Anaplastic carcinoma. Bizarre malignant giant cells have scant cytoplasm, nuclear pleomorphism, and nuclear rim irregularities (Diff-Quik stain)

enlarging thyroid gland and a preexisting history of a diffuse goiter. There is a strong association with Hashimoto's thyroiditis [60,90].

The cytologic appearance is similar to that of lymphomas at other sites. The most common type of lymphoma to arise in the thyroid gland is non-Hodgkin's lymphoma, B cell type [109]. The smears are relatively cellular with individual large lymphoid cells in the background. The lymphoid cells have scant cytoplasm that is blue-gray on Diff-Quik stain. Some subtypes, such as the immunoblastic type, show macronucleoli. Crushed chromatin (lymphoid tangles) is commonly seen as are groups of atypical lymphoid cells with individual cell necrosis. The smears contain very little to no colloid, and may show evidence of Hashimoto's thyroiditis in the background [37]. When a diagnosis of lymphoma is suspected in our laboratory, material is set aside for flow cytometric analysis.

6.5.6.6   Metastases to the Thyroid

Metastases to the thyroid are very uncommon. In one study, the incidence at autopsy and at thyroidectomy for metastatic malignancy was 0.5% and 1.2%, respectively [79]. Metastases are most likely to occur in the clinical setting of a patient with a known primary [119]. Clinically, renal cell carcinoma is the most common type of metastatic disease to the thyroid; at autopsy, colorectal, lung, breast, and renal cell carcinoma along with melanoma and malignant lymphoma prevail [43,96].

6.6   FNA of the Thyroid in Children and Adolescents

Thyroid nodules in children and adolescents are uncommon. FNA has been found to be as reliable in children as in adults for the definitive diagnosis of thyroid nodules [2]. Khurana et al. [72] reported a 24.6% prevalence of malignancy in their series of thyroid FNAs in 57 children and adolescents with surgical follow-up. Papillary carcinoma ($n = 11$) and follicular carcinoma ($n = 3$) accounted for the malignancies in this series.

6.7 FNA of the Thyroid in Pregnancy

The loss of iodine during pregnancy induces thyroid growth and hyperplasia which is usually diffuse [107]. A preexisting nodule may increase in size and present as an enlarging suspicious lump in a pregnant woman. The cytologic findings on FNA show similar features as those described for cellular adenomatoid nodules. The smears usually show increased cellularity in the background of thin, watery colloid. The follicular epithelial cells are arranged in groups, sheets, and spherules. Some hyperplastic papillary fragments may also be seen. The cells in these tissue fragments, however, lack the cytologic cellular criteria for papillary carcinoma.

6.8 Cytologic Diagnostic Challenges in FNA of the Thyroid

Cytologic diagnostic challenges pertaining to thyroid FNA arise from several situations including: (1) similar morphologic appearances between certain types of cells; (2) inexperience of the diagnostician; and (3) absence or paucity of diagnostic cells due to the inherent nature of the lesion.

It is our philosophy that it is the role of the cytopathologist to keep the number of indeterminate/suspicious cases to a minimum by consistently applying strict diagnostic criteria on diagnostic samples only. It is incumbent upon the surgeon to understand the diagnostic limitations of the FNA procedure, which are summarized below.

6.8.1 Cystic Lesion of Thyroid with Scant or Absent Follicular Cells

Cystic change occurs in a number of circumstances with the most common being: (1) degeneration of a long-standing goiter; (2) hemorrhage into a preexisting nodule; (3) colloid accumulation; and (4) degeneration of neoplasms, most notably papillary carcinoma

and follicular and Hürthle cell neoplasms. Parathyroid cysts, thyroglossal duct cysts, and branchial cleft cysts may also be aspirated in the vicinity of the thyroid. An estimated 9% of cysts are malignant when surgically excised [39,61]. A pre-FNA ultrasound, if available, may be useful to the aspirator in conveying the presence and extent of a cystic component. The FNA procedure may be therapeutic if the cyst fluid can be evacuated in its entirety. This, however, occurs infrequently. More commonly, a solid component remains after the fluid is aspirated, in which case sampling of this solid component is crucial for diagnosis.

Grossly, the color of the cyst fluid varies from pale yellow, to green, to dark brown. The color is not a reliable indicator of malignancy. However, if the fluid is watery, clear, and colorless, a parathyroid cyst should be considered and the fluid submitted for parathyroid hormone essay. In our practice of nearly 5,000 thyroid aspirates, we have encountered only two parathyroid cysts.

Microscopically, cyst contents may contain cholesterol crystals, foamy and pigmented histiocytes (the latter in the setting of hemorrhage), multinucleated giant cells, and follicular cells with shrunken, degenerative nuclei. Squamous metaplastic cell change, considered a reparative process, is not uncommon in cystic lesions (Fig. 6.23). These cells may appear quite atypical and lead to a false-positive diagnosis. Degenerative follicular epithelial cells may display cytoplasmic and nuclear vacuolization, also seen as a degenerative phenomenon in cystic papillary carcinoma. Careful attention to the nuclear cytologic features will enable one to make the distinction between benign follicular cells and cells of papillary carcinoma. The cyst contents of a neoplasm may also be paucicellular. If epithelial cells are present, they may show degenerative changes obscuring nuclear detail, which may lead to a false-negative result [7]. It is therefore imperative that a diagnosis not be rendered unless well-preserved epithelial cells are present in sufficient numbers.

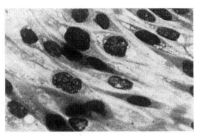

Fig. 6.23 Squamous metaplastic cell change in a benign cystic adenomatoid nodule. The cells are elongated with dense cytoplasm and discrete cytoplasmic borders (Diff-Quik stain)

6.8.2   Cellular Follicular Lesion

Thyroid lesions with a follicular architecture cover a broad range of diagnoses including hyperplastic epithelial changes, follicular neoplasms, and follicular variant of papillary carcinoma. Up to 30% of lesions diagnosed with a follicular pattern by FNA are carcinoma on final histologic review [14]. In our experience, 75% of lesions diagnosed in this gray-zone category of cellular follicular lesion harbor a neoplasm with near equal distribution between adenomas and carcinomas (unpublished data). Among the latter, both follicular carcinoma and follicular variant of papillary carcinoma are represented.

6.8.3   Prominent Hürthle Cell Proliferation

Hürthle cell change of non-neoplastic origin is relatively common in goiters and Hashimoto's thyroiditis [45]. As the differential diagnosis of a prominent Hürthle population includes a Hürthle cell neoplasm, obtaining a representative sample is crucial. Multiple passes from a neoplasm will yield similar cytologic findings of a monotonous cell population. In goiters and thyroiditis, multiple passes will likely show the varied cytologic components of these lesions.

Hashimoto's thyroiditis may be a source of both false-positive and false-negative results. In some cases, the oxyphilic (Hürthle) cell change is severe and the inflammatory component minor or not sampled [3]. This may lead to an erroneous diagnosis of follicular neoplasm of Hürthle cell type, emphasizing once again the importance of obtaining a representative sample. Additionally, inflammation may induce cellular epithelial changes including nuclear enlargement, nucleoli, and mild to moderate cellular pleomorphism (Fig. 6.24). In the setting of an inflamma-

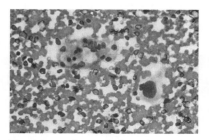

Fig. 6.24 Hashimoto's thyroiditis with cellular atypia. A small sheet of oxyphilic cells is surrounded by lymphoid cells and plasma cells. Note the markedly atypical cells with nuclear enlargement, abundant cytoplasm, and bland chromatin at 3 o'clock (Diff-Quik stain)

tory background, the cytopathologist must exercise extreme care not to overdiagnose such cases based on these findings.

Hashimoto's thyroiditis may occur concomitantly with various thyroid neoplasms including follicular adenoma, papillary carcinoma, and malignant lymphoma [56,77,85]. As such, careful and representative sampling of the lesion is necessary to reduce the possibility of a false-negative diagnosis.

6.8.4   Cytologically Atypical Cells

Atypia is difficult to define. It usually refers to the presence of some but not all of the cytologic criteria for malignancy, namely, nuclear enlargement, cellular pleomorphism, and hyperchromatism. Follicular epithelial cell atypia may be seen following radioactive iodine therapy as well as after radiation for cervical neoplasms of other than thyroid origin. Follicular cell atypia may also be seen in the atypical adenoma, Hashimoto's thyroiditis, subacute granulomatous thyroiditis (particularly in the acute stages), and in benign thyroid cysts. As previously discussed, inflammation may induce follicular epithelial cell atypia resulting in a false-positive diagnosis [98].

Focal epithelial atypia in the background of cystic degeneration or inflammation should be interpreted with caution. It should be noted that primary thyroid neoplasms typically yield a relatively monotonous cell population with minimal cellular pleomorphism. An exception are the bizarre and pleomorphic cells seen in high-grade malignant neoplasms, although such cases generally do not pose a diagnostic challenge [71].

6.8.5   Hürthle Cell Neoplasm Versus Papillary Carcinoma

Diffuse Hürthle (oxyphilic) cell change with formation of a Hürthle cell nodule may be a feature of Hashimoto's thyroiditis. Papillary carcinoma, the most common type of thyroid malignancy, is seen in immune-compromised glands, the most common cause of hypothyroidism. Oxyphilic cell change results in enlargement of follicular epithelial cells and cytoplasmic features that may resemble those seen in papillary carcinoma; the nuclear features, however, are different. Follicular lesions also occur in the background of Hashimoto's thyroiditis. When the inflammatory component is the dominant feature, it may obscure neoplasia [77].

6.8.6 Atypical Lymphoid Proliferation

The differential diagnosis includes Hashimoto's thyroiditis and malignant lymphoma. The florid lymphoid phase of Hashimoto's thyroiditis may mimic lymphoma. However, in the former, there is an admixture of small, mature lymphocytes, plasma cells, immature cells, and oxyphilic cell change. Lymphomatous transformation of an already immune-compromised gland shows increased monotony of the lymphoid component. When the FNA procedure is done with on-site evaluation for specimen adequacy, a diagnosis of lymphoma can be suspected and additional passes performed for flow cytometric analysis.

References

1. Al-Hureibi KA, Al-Hureibi AA, Abdulmughni YA, et al (2003) The diagnostic value of fine needle aspiration cytology in thyroid swellings in a university hospital, Yemen. Saudi Med J 24:499–503

2. Arda IS, Yildirim S, Demirhan B, et al (2001) Fine needle aspiration biopsy of thyroid nodules. Arch Dis Child 85:313–317

3. Atkinson BF (1993) Fine needle aspiration of the thyroid. Monogr Pathol 35:166–199

4. Atkinson BF, Ernst CS, LiVolsi VA (1986) Cytologic diagnoses of follicular tumors of the thyroid. Diagn Cytopathol 2:1–3

5. Aversa S, Pivano G, Vergano R, et al (1999) The accuracy of the fine-needle aspiration biopsy in 1250 thyroid nodules. Acta Otorhinolaryngol Ital 19:260–264

6. Bahar G, Braslavsky D, Shpitzer T, et al (2003) The cytological and clinical value of thyroid "follicular lesions." Am J Otolaryngol 24:217–220

7. Bakhos R, Selvaggi SM, De Jong S, et al (2000) Fine-needle aspiration of the thyroid: rate and causes of cytohistopathologic discordance. Diagn Cytopathol 23:233–237

8. Bakshi NA, Mansoor I, Jones BA (2003) Analysis of inconclusive fine-needle aspiration of thyroid follicular lesions. Endocr Pathol 14:167–175

9. Baloch ZW, LiVolsi VA (2000) Warthin-like papillary carcinoma of the thyroid. Arch Pathol Lab Med 124:1192–1195

10. Baloch ZW, LiVolsi VA (2004) Fine-needle aspiration of thyroid nodules: past, present and future. Endocr Pract 10:234–241

11. Baloch ZW, Sack MJ, Yu GH, et al (1998) Fine-needle aspiration of thyroid: and institutional experience. Thyroid 8:565–569

12. Baloch ZW, Fleisher S, LiVolsi VA, et al (2002) Diagnosis of "follicular neoplasm": a gray zone in thyroid fine-needle aspiration cytology. Diagn Cytopathol 26:41–44

13. Baloch Z, LiVolsi VA, Jain R, et al (2003) Role of repeat fine-needle aspiration biopsy (FNAB) in the management of thyroid nodules. Diagn Cytopathol 29:203–206

14. Blansfield JA, Sack MJ, Kukora JS (2002) Recent experience with preoperative fine-needle aspiration biopsy of thyroid nodules in a community hospital. Arch Surg. 137:818–821

15. Block, Dailey GE, Robb JA (1983) Thyroid nodules indeterminate by needle biopsy. Am J Surg 146:72–78

16. Bose S, Kapila K, Verma K (1992) Medullary carcinoma of the thyroid: a cytological, immunocytochemical, and ultrastructural study. Diagn Cytopathol 8:28–32

17. Brander A, Viikinkoski P, Nickels J, et al (1991) Thyroid gland: US screening in a random adult population. Radiology 181:683–687

18. Busseniers AE (1993) The "unsatisfactory" thyroid aspirate: facts and fiction. Acta Cytol 37:808

19. Busseniers AE (1996) Superficial fine needle aspiration. Introduction and technique. In: Erozan H, Bonfiglio TA (eds) Fine needle aspiration of subcutaneous organs and masses. Lippincott-Raven, Philadelphia, pp 1–6

20. Busseniers AE (2005) FNA of the thyroid: experience of one dedicated cytopathologist. Program and Abstract Book of the 87th Annual Meeting of the The Endocrine Society, San Diego, CA, 2005, p 319

21. Busseniers AE, Oertel YC (1993) "Cellular adenomatoid nodules" of the thyroid: review of 219 fine-needle aspirates. Diagn Cytopathol 9:581–588

22. Cap J, Ryska A, Rehorkova, et al (2000) Sensitivity and specificity of the fine needle aspiration biopsy of the thyroid: clinical point of view. Clin Endocrinol 51:509–515

23. Carcangiu ML, Zampi G, Rosai J (1984) Poorly differentiated (insular) thyroid carcinoma: a reinterpretation of Langhans'Wuchernde struma. Am J Surg Pathol 8:655–668

24. Carcangiu ML, Zampi G, Pupi A, et al (1985a) Papillary carcinoma of the thyroid: a clinicopathologic study of 241 cases treated at the University of Florence, Italy. Cancer 55:805–828

25. Carcangiu ML, Steeper T, Zampi G, et al (1985b) Anaplastic thyroid carcinoma: a study of 70 cases. Am J Clin Pathol 83:135–158

26. Carpi A, Nicolini A, Casara D, et al (2003) Nonpalpable thyroid carcinoma: clinical controversies on preoperative selection. Am J Clin Oncol 26:232–235

27. Caruso D, Mazzaferri EL (1991) Fine needle aspiration biopsy in the management of thyroid nodules. Endocrinologist 1:194–202

28. Caruso G, Tabarri B, Lucchi I, et al (1990) Fine needle aspiration cytology in a case of diffuse sclerosing carcinoma of the thyroid. Acta Cytol 34:352–354

29. Chehade JM, Silverberg AB, Kim J, et al (2001) Role of repeated fine-needle aspiration of thyroid nodules with benign cytologic features. Endocr Pract 7:237–243

30. Chen H, Nicol TL, Rosenthal DL, Udelsman R (1997) The role of fine-needle aspiration in the evaluation of thyroid nodules. In: Norton JA (ed) Problems in general surgery: surgery of the thyroid gland. Lippincott-Raven, New York, pp 1–13

31. Chen H, Nicol TL, Zeiger MA, et al (1998) Hurthle cell neoplasms of the thyroid: are there factors predictive of malignancy? Ann Surg 227:542–546

32. Chen H, Dudley NE, Westra WH, et al (2003) Utilization of fine-needle aspiration in patients undergoing thyroidectomy at two academic centers across the Atlantic. World J Surg 27:208–211

33. Chow LS, Gharib H, Goellner JR, et al (2001) Nondiagnostic thyroid fine-needle aspiration cytology: management dilemmas. Thyroid 11:1147–1151

34. Christensen SB, Eriscsson UB, Janzon L, et al (1984) The prevalence of thyroid disorders in a middle-aged female population, with special reference to the solitary thyroid nodule. Acta Chir Scand 150:13–19

35. Damiani S, Dina R, Eusebi V (1994) Cytologic grading of aggressive and nonaggressive variants of papillary thyroid carcinoma. Am J Clin Pathol 101:651–655

36. Das A, Gupta SK, Banerjee AK, et al (1992) Atypical cytologic features of medullary carcinoma of the thyroid: a review of 12 cases. Acta Cytol 36:137–141

37. Das DK, Gupta SK, Franci IM, et al (1993) Fine-needle aspiration cytology diagnosis of non-Hodgkin lymphoma of thyroid: a report of four cases. Diagn Cytopathol 9:639–645

38. Das DK, Mallik MK, Sharma P, et al (2004) Papillary thyroid carcinoma and its variants in fine needle aspiration smears. A cytomorphologic study with special reference to tall cell variant. Acta Cytol 48:325–336

39. de los Santos ET, Keyhani-Rofagha S, Cunningham JJ, et al (1990) Cystic thyroid nodules: the dilemma of malignant lesions. Arch Intern Med 150:1422–1427

40. DeMay RM (1996) In the art and science of cytopathology. ASCP Press, Chicago, p 711

41. De Vos tot Nederveen Cappel RJ, Bouvy ND, Bonjer HJ, et al (2001) Fine needle aspiration cytology of thyroid nodules: how accurate is it and what are the causes of discrepancy cases? Cytopathology 12:399–405

42. Dwarakanathan AA, Staren ED, D'Amore MJ, et al (1993) Importance of repeat fine-needle biopsy in the management of thyroid nodules. Am J Surg 166:350–352

43. Elliott RHE Jr, Frantz VK (1960) Metastatic carcinoma masquerading as primary thyroid cancer: a report of author's 14 cases. Am Surg 151:551–561

44. Erdogan MF, Kamel N, Aras D, et al (1998) Value of re-aspirations in benign nodular thyroid disease. Thyroid 8:1087–1090

45. Flint A, Lloyd RV (1990) Hurthle-cell neoplasms of the thyroid gland. Pathol Annu 25:37–52

46. Frable MA, Frable WJ (1980) Fine needle aspiration biopsy of the thyroid: histopathologic and clinical correlations. Prog Surg Pathol 1:105–118

47. Fulciniti F, Benincasa G, Vetrani A, et al (2001) Follicular variant of papillary carcinoma: cytologic findings on FNAB samples: experience with 16 cases. Diagn Cytopathol 25:86–93

48. Gagneten CB, Roccatagliata G, Lowenstein A, et al (1987) The role of fine needle aspiration biopsy cytology in the evaluation of the clinically solitary thyroid nodule. Acta Cytol 31:713–716

49. Gandolfi PP, Frisina A, Raffa M, et al (2004) The incidence of thyroid carcinoma in multinodular goiter: retrospective analysis. Acta Biomed Ateneo Parmense 75:114–117

50. Garcia Solano J, Gimenez Bascunana A, Sola Perez J, et al (1997) Fine-needle aspiration of subacute granulomatous thyroiditis (de Quervain's thyroiditis): a clinico-cytologic review of 36 cases. Diagn Cytopathol 16:214–220

51. Gharib H (1994) Fine needle aspiration biopsy of thyroid nodules: advantages, limitations, and effect. Mayo Clin Proc 69:44–49

52. Gharib H, Goellner JR (1993) Fine-needle aspiration biopsy of the thyroid: an appraisal. Ann Intern Med 118:282–289

53. Gharib H, Goellner JR, Zinsmeister AR, et al (1984) Fine-needle aspiration biopsy of the thyroid: the problem of suspicious cytologic findings. Ann Intern Med 101:25–28

54. Gharib H, Goellner JR, Johnson DA (1993) Fine-needle aspiration cytology of the thyroid: a 12-year experience with 11,000 biopsies. Clin Lab Med 13:699–709

55. Giard RW, Hermans J (2000) Use and accuracy of fine-needle aspiration cytology in histologically proven thyroid carcinoma: an audit using a national pathology database. Cancer 90:330–334

56. Guarda LA, Baskin HJ (1987) Inflammatory and lymphoid lesions of the thyroid gland: cytomorphology by fine-needle aspiration. Am J Clin Pathol 87:14–22

57. Guarda LA, Peterson CE, Hall W, et al (1991) Anaplastic thyroid carcinoma. Cytomorphology and clinical implications of fine-needle aspiration. Diagn Cytopathol 7:63–67

58. Hamburger JI, Hamburger SW (1986) Fine needle biopsy of thyroid nodules: avoiding the pitfalls. NY State J Med 86:241–249

59. Hamburger B, Gharib H, Melton LF III, et al (1982) Fine needle aspiration biopsy of thyroid nodules: impact on thyroid practice and cost of care. Am J Med 73:381–384

60. Hamburger JL, Miller JM, Kini SR, et al (1983) Lymphoma of the thyroid. Ann Intern Med 99:685–693

61. Hammer M, Wortsman J, Folse R (1982) Cancer in cystic lesions of the thyroid. Arch Surg 117:1020–1023

62. Harach HR, Franssila KO, Wasenius V-M, et al (1985) Occult papillary carcinoma of the thyroid: a "normal" finding in Finland. A systematic autopsy study. Cancer 56:531–538

63. Harigopal M, Sahoo S, Recant WM, et al (2004) Fine-needle aspiration of Riedel's disease: report of a case and review of the literature. Diagn Cytopathol 30:193–197

64. Hsu C, Boey J (1987) Diagnostic pitfalls in the fine needle aspiration of thyroid nodules: a study of 555 cases in Chinese patients. Acta Cytol 31:699–704

65. Jain M, Khan A, Patwardhan N, et al (2001) Follicular variant of papillary thyroid carcinoma: a comparative study of histopathologic features and cytology results in 141 patients. Endocr Pract 7:139–142

66. Jayaram G (1983) Problems in the interpretation of Hurthle cell populations in fine needle aspirates from the thyroid. Acta Cytol 27:84–85

67. Jayaram G, Marwaha RK, Gupta RK, et al (1987) Cytomorphologic aspects of thyroiditis: a study of 51 cases with functional, immunologic and ultrasonographic data. Acta Cytol 31:687–693

68. Jayaram G, Razak A, Ghan SK, et al (1999) Fine needle aspiration cytology of the thyroid: a review of experience in 1854 cases. Malays J Pathol 21:17–27

69. Kaur A, Jayaram G (1990) Thyroid tumors: cytomorphology of medullary, clinically anaplastic, and miscellaneous thyroid neoplasms. Diagn Cytopathol 6:383–389

70. Kaur A, Jayaram G (1991) Thyroid tumors: cytomorphology of papillary carcinoma. Diagn Cytopathol 7:462–472

71. Kelman AS, Rathan A, Leibowitz J, et al (2001) Thyroid cytology and the risk of malignancy in thyroid nodules: importance of nuclear atypia in indeterminate specimens. Thyroid 11:271–277

72. Khurana KK, Labrador E, Izquierdo R, et al (1999) The role of fine-needle aspiration biopsy in the management of thyroid nodules in children, adolescents, and young adults: a multi-institutional study. Thyroid 9:383–386

73. Kim SJ, Kim EK, Park CS, et al (2003) Ultrasound-guided fine-needle aspiration biopsy in nonpalpable thyroid nodules: is it useful in infracentimetric nodules? Yonsei Med J 44:635–640

74. Kini SR, Miller JM, Hamburger JI, et al (1985) Cytopathology of follicular lesions of the thyroid gland. Diagn Cytopathol 1:123–132

75. Klemi PJ, Joensuu H, Nylamo E (1991) Fine needle aspiration biopsy in the diagnosis of thyroid nodules. Acta Cytol 35:434–438

76. Ko HM, Jhu IK, Yang SH, et al (2003) Clinicopathologic analysis of fine needle aspiration cytology of the thyroid. A review of 1,613 cases and correlation with histopathologic diagnoses. Acta Cytol 47:727–732

77. Kollur SM, El Sayed S, El Hag IA (2003) Follicular thyroid lesions coexisting with Hashimoto's thyroiditis: incidence and possible sources of diagnostic errors. Diagn Cytopathol 28:35–38

78. Kon YC, DeGroot LJ (2003) Painful Hashimoto's thyroiditis as an indication for thyroidectomy: clinical characteristics and outcome in seven patients. J Clin Endocrinol Metab 88:2667–2672

79. Lam KY, Lo CY (1998) Metastatic tumors of the thyroid gland. Arch Pathol Lab Med 122:37–41

80. Lawrence W Jr, Kaplan BJ (2002) Diagnosis and management of patients with thyroid nodules. J Surg Oncol 80:157–170

81. Layfield LJ, Reichman A, Bottles K, et al (1992) Clinical determinants for the management of thyroid nodules by fine-needle aspiration cytology. Arch Otolaryngol Head Neck Surg 118:717–721

82. Leung C-S, Hartwick RWJ, Bedard YC (1993) Correlation of cytologic and histologic features in variants of papillary carcinoma of the thyroid. Acta Cytol 37:645–650

83. Liel Y, Ariad S, Barchana M (2001) Long-term follow-up of patients with initially benign thyroid fine needle aspirations. Thyroid 11:775–778

84. Lin HS, Komisar A, Opher E, et al (2000) Follicular variant of papillary carcinoma: the diagnostic limitation of preoperative fine-needle aspiration and intraoperative frozen section evaluation. Laryngoscope 110:1431–1436

85. Liu LH, Bakhos R, Wojcik EM (2001) Concomitant papillary thyroid carcinoma and Hashimoto's thyroiditis. Semin Diagn Pathol 18:99–103

86. LiVolsi VA (1992) Papillary neoplasms of the thyroid: pathologic and prognostic features. Anat Pathol 97:426–434

87. LiVolsi VA, Gupta PK (1992) Thyroid fine-needle aspiration: intranuclear inclusions, nuclear grooves and psammoma bodies-paraganglioma-like adenoma of the thyroid. Diagn Cytopathol 8:82–84

88. Lo Gerfo P, Starker P, Weber C, et al (1985) Incidence of cancer in surgically treated thyroid nodules based on method of selection. Surgery 98:1197–1201

89. Lowhagen T, Sprenger E (1974) Cytologic presentation of thyroid tumors in aspiration biopsy smear: a review of 60 cases. Acta Cytol 18:192–197

90. Matsuzuka F, Miyauchi A, Katayama S, et al (1993) Clinical aspects of primary thyroid lymphoma: diagnosis and treatment based on our experience of 119 cases. Thyroid 3:93–99

91. Mazzaferri EL, de los Santos ET, Rofagha-Keyhani S, et al (1988) Solitary thyroid nodule: diagnosis and management. Med Clin North Am 72:1177–1211

92. McHenry CR, Thomas SR, Slusarczyk SJ, et al (1999) Follicular or Hurthle cell neoplasm of the thyroid: can clinical factors be used to predict carcinoma. Surgery 126:798–802

93. Mendelsohn G, Bigner SH, Eggleston JC, et al (1980) Anaplastic variants of medullary thyroid carcinoma: a light-microscopic and immunohistochemical study. Am J Surg Path 4:333–341

94. Merchant SH, Izquierdo R, Khurna KK (2000) Is repeated fine-needle aspiration cytology useful in the management of patients with benign nodular thyroid disease? Thyroid 10:489–492

95. Miller TR, Bottles K, Holly EA, et al (1986) A step-wise logistic regression analysis of papillary carcinoma of the thyroid. Acta Cytol 30:285–293

96. Mirallie E, Rigaud J, Mathonnet M, et al (2005) Management and prognosis of metastases to the thyroid gland. J Am Coll Surg 200:203–207

97. Nguyen GK, Akin MR (2001) Cytopathology of insular carcinoma of the thyroid. Diagn Cytopathol 25:325–330

98. Ofner C, Hittmair A, Kroll I, et al (1994) Fine needle aspiration cytodiagnosis of subacute (de Quervain's) thyroiditis in an endemic goiter area. Cytopathology 5:33–40

99. Pelizzo MR, Piotto A, Rubello D, et al (1990) High prevalence of occult papillary thyroid carcinoma in a surgical series for benign thyroid disease. Tumori 76:255–257

100. Pietribiasi F, Sapino A, Papotti M, et al (1990) Cytologic features of poorly differentiated 'insular' carcinoma of the thyroid, as revealed by fine-needle aspiration biopsy. Am J Clin Pathol 94:687–692

101. Poropatich C, Marcus D, Oertel YC (1994) Hashimoto's thyroiditis: fine-needle aspiration of 50 asymptomatic cases. Diagn Cytopathol 11:141–145

102. Raber W, Kaserer K, Niederle B, et al (2000) Risk factors for malignancy of thyroid nodules initially identified as follicular neoplasia by fine-needle aspiration: results of a prospective study of one hundred twenty patients. Thyroid 10:109–112

103. Ravetto C, Colombo L, Dottorini ME (2000). Usefulness of fine-needle aspiration in the diagnosis of thyroid carcinoma: a retrospective study in 37,895 patients. Cancer 90:357–363

104. Ravinsky E, Safneck JR (1988) Differentiation of Hashimoto's thyroiditis from thyroid neoplasms in fine needle aspirates. Acta Cytol 32:854–861

105. Renshaw AA (2001) Accuracy of fine-needle aspiration using receiver operator characteristic curves. Am J Clin Pathol 117:493–494

106. Rosai J (1993) Papillary carcinoma. Monogr Pathol 35:138–163

107. Rosen IB, Walfish PG, Nikore V (1985) Pregnancy and surgical thyroid disease. Surgery 98:1135–1140

108. Samaan NA, Ordonez NG (1990) Uncommon types of thyroid cancer. Endocrinol Metab Clin North Am 19:637–648

109. Sangalli G, Serio G, Zampatti C, et al (2001) Fine needle aspiration cytology of primary lymphoma of the thyroid: a report of 17 cases. Cytopathology 12:257–264

110. Sclabas GM, Staerkel GA, Shapiro SE (2003) Fine-needle aspiration of the thyroid and correlation with histopathology in a contemporary series of 240 patients. Am J Surg 186:702–709

111. Scopa CD, Melachrinous M, Saradopoulou C, et al (1993) The significance of the grooved nucleus in thyroid lesions. Mod Pathol 6:691–694

112. Settakorn J, Chaiwun B, Thamprasert K, et al (2001) Fine needle aspiration of the thyroid gland. J Med Assoc Thai 84:1401–1406

113. Silver SA, Bussenuers AE (1995) Cytologic criteria for differentiating neoplastic from nonneoplastic Hurthle cell lesions by fine needle aspiration. Mod Pathol 8:44A

114. Silverman JF, West RL, Larkin EW, et al (1986) The role of fine needle aspiration biopsy in the rapid diagnosis and management of thyroid neoplasm. Cancer 57:1164–1170

115. Suen KS, Quenville NF (1983) Fine needle aspiration biopsy of the thyroid gland: a study of 304 cases. J Clin Pathol 36:1036–1045

116. Tabaqchali MA, Hanson JM, Johnson SJ, et al (2000) Thyroid aspiration cytology in Newcastle: a six year cytology/histology correlation study. Ann R Coll Surg Engl 82:149–155

117. Tollin SR, Mery GM, Jelveh N, et al (2000) The use of fine-needle aspiration biopsy under ultrasound guidance to assess the risk of malignancy in patients with multinodular goiter. Thyroid 10:235–241

118. Vodanoviv S, Crepinko I, Smoje J (1993) Morphologic diagnosis of Hurthle cell tumors of the thyroid gland. Acta Cytol 37:317–322

119. Watts NB (1987) Carcinoma metastatic to the thyroid: prevalence and diagnosis by fine-needle aspiration cytology. Am J Med Sci 293:13–17

120. Yang YJ, Khurana KK (2001) Diagnostic utility of intracytoplasmic lumen and transgressing vessels in evaluation of Hurthle cell lesions by fine-needle aspiration. Arch Pathol Lab Med 125:1031–1035

121. Yang GC, Liebeskind D, Messina AV (2001) Ultrasound-guided fine-needle aspiration of the thyroid assessed by Ultrafast Papanicolaou stain: data from 1135 biopsies with a two to six-year follow-up. Thyroid 11:581–589

122. Ylagan LR, Farkas T, Dehner LP (2004) Fine needle aspiration of the thyroid: a cytohistologic correlation and study of discrepant cases. Thyroid 14:35–41

123. Zeppa P, Vetrani A, Marino M, et al (1990) Fine needle aspiration cytology of medullary thyroid carcinoma: a review of 18 cases. Cytopathology 1:35–44

124. Zeppa P, Benincasa G, Lucariello A, et al (2001) Association of different pathologic processes of the thyroid gland in fine needle aspiration samples. Acta Cytol 45:347–352

7 Technique of Thyroidectomy

Daniel Oertli

CONTENTS

7.1 Introduction

Thyroidectomy is the most frequent intervention in endocrine surgery. When performed in specialized centers, the operation is safe with low morbidity and a virtually 0% mortality [1]. Complications of thyroid surgery are directly correlated to the extent of resection and inversely proportional to the experience of the operating surgeon [1–4]. Thus, the cornerstones of safe and effective thyroid surgery are an adequate training, the understanding of the anatomy and pathology, as well as a meticulous dissection technique. The dissection must be based on a sound knowledge of three-dimensional topographic anatomy, typical landmarks, and possible anatomic variations. The meticulous dissection technique is achieved by a proper exposure of all fine anatomic structures in a bloodless dry surgical field. The use of magnifying glasses (magnification 2.5–3.5×), bipolar coagulation, and fine titan clips or ligatures is highly recommended. Neuromonitoring has proved useful for identifying the recurrent laryngeal nerve (RLN), in particular if the anatomic situation is complicated by prior surgery [5]. However, neuromonitoring does not reliably predict postoperative outcome [6,7]. A recent study based on 288 patients undergoing thyroid surgery with intraoperative identification and intraoperative neuromonitoring showed that the incidence of recurrent nerve lesions in benign, malignant, and recurrent thyroid disease was not lowered by the use of intraoperative neuromonitoring [8]. Although an intact nerve function can be verified by this method, we do not recommend the routine use of RLN neuromonitoring.

The endocrine surgeon's success depends completely on his or her devotion to a stepwise meticulous and fine dissection technique. Several dissection devices have recently been propagated for thyroid surgery. The harmonic scalpel using ultrasonic frictional heating to seal vessels is widely used in laparoscopic and open abdominal surgery. It is documented to be safe and fast for cutting and coagulating tissue. Its use for dissection during thyroidectomy has been evaluated in several studies and has been compared to the conventional clamp-and-tie technique. Two randomized studies [9,10] and two case-controlled studies [11,12] have shown that the harmonic scalpel significantly shortens the operative time compared to the conventional technique. This reduction of up to 20% in operative time has proved to be cost-effective [13].

Thyroidectomy using the electrothermal sealing technique has also been introduced and tested [14,15]. However, this technique did not significantly reduce operative time, blood loss, or the complication rate compared to conventional knot-tying but it increased operative costs in one study [15]. All mentioned studies compared new ultrasonic or diathermy dissection devices with the conventional clamp-and-tie technique. However, no comparison with the utilization of hemoclips to secure smaller vessels was done. Personally, I make liberal use of hemoclips for thyroid and parathyroid surgery and I am convinced that this speeds up the operation similarly to the use of the quite costly new devices.

7.2   Extent of Surgery and Definitions

Until 2000 there was no uniformly applied definition in the literature regarding the extent of thyroidectomy that should be performed for benign and malignant pathologies. To fill this gap, Kebebew and Clark formulated such a classification (Table 7.1) [16]. Lumpectomy or nodulectomy refer to removal of a thyroid nodule alone with minimal surrounding thyroid tissue. Partial thyroidectomy involves removal of a nodule with a larger margin of normal thyroid tissue. The definition of subtotal thyroidectomy belongs to the bilateral removal of more than 50% of each lobe including the isthmus. Lobectomy or hemithyroidectomy refers to the complete removal of one lobe with the isthmus. Near total thyroidectomy is defined as the total extracapsular removal of one lobe including the isthmus with less than 10% of the contralateral lobe left behind. During total thyroidectomy both lobes and the isthmus are completely removed leaving behind only viable parathyroid glands.

7.3   Preoperative Measures

All patients should be rendered euthyroid before surgery. Preoperative preparation of patients with thyrotoxicosis is particularly critical to avoid operative or postoperative thyroid storm. The planned procedure should be discussed with the patient and informed consent must be obtained. Routine preoperative laryngoscopy is not necessary if the patient does not report voice changes [17]. However, if patients have previously undergone any type of neck surgery or if the voice appears to be altered, laryngoscopy is indicated. The tentative skin incision is marked preoperatively using a permanent marker pen on the awake patient with reclined neck. This is done in a symmetric fashion along the Langer's skin lines or in a skin crease in

between the medial borders of the sternocleidomastoid muscles. The appropriate position of the neck incision is approximately two finger breadths above the sternal notch or in the middle between the sternal notch and the thyroid cartilage. If the incision is too low, the tendency to keloid formation and resulting unsatisfactory cosmesis is increased.

7.4   Positioning and Draping

The patient is positioned with the neck extended. Rolled towels are placed under the shoulders which allow sufficient neck extension. A sponge doughnut is placed under the occiput for adequate head support. In order to prevent venous congestion in the neck, the head of the table is elevated to a 30° position during surgery. Disinfection is performed using an alcoholic agent without iodine which might interfere with postoperative radionuclear scanning and ablative therapy. The surgical field is draped from below the sternal notch up to the chin and on the posterior margin of the sternocleidomastoid muscles.

7.5   Surgical Steps

Every surgeon should adopt a stepwise, standardized strategy for thyroidectomy. One possible way (the author's recommendation) for a successful thyroidectomy is presented below. Modifications may be necessary in the case of perithyroidal inflammation, large goiters, or unexpected intraoperative findings.

7.5.1   Skin Incision and Creation of Skin Flaps

A curvilinear collar-type incision is placed transversally along the Langer's line of the skin, i.e., the

Table 7.1 Definition of extent of resection

Thyroidectomy procedure	Removal of:	Indications
Partial (nodulectomy, lumpectomy)	Nodule + margin of normal tissue	Benign lesion
Subtotal	More than one half of the thyroid gland and isthmus	Benign lesion
Lobectomy (= hemithyroidectomy)	One entire lobe and isthmus	Standard initial treatment for all indeterminate nodules
Near-total	Lobectomy on one side, isthmectomy and subtotal resection of contralateral lobe	Papillary carcinoma in a low-risk patient, not requiring radioiodine ablation
Total	Both lobes and isthmus	Any other type of thyroid carcinoma

standard Kocher's incision. The use of a natural skin crease if present seems attractive. In order to optimize cosmesis, the skin incision should be as long as necessary but as short as possible. Personally, the author believes that a 4- to 5-cm incision allows safe thyroidectomy in most cases and results in excellent cosmesis. However, patients with larger tumors or goiters or those with short necks will require a larger incision for optimal exposure. The incision is carried out through the skin and the subcutaneous layer through the platysma muscle to the lateral extent of the skin incision. The two skin flaps are created by dissecting them away from the strap muscles upward to the thyroid cartilage and downward to the sternal border. Elevation of the two flaps is almost bloodless if the layer beneath the platysma is followed and dissected. The cranial flap is transfixed using stay sutures that are secured on two hooks placed on a horizontal rod which is placed above the patient's head (Fig. 7.1). The caudal flap is pulled downward using a Roux retractor enabling optimal exposure to the strap muscles.

7.5.2 Strap Muscles

The approach to the thyroid capsule is done by splitting the strap muscles in the midline. Small crossing vessels are treated with bipolar coagulation. For a bilateral approach, the left thyroid lobe is first dissected. This is usually the more cumbersome preparation when the operating surgeon is positioned on the right side of the patient. By predominantly blunt dissection, the anterior aspect of the respective thyroid gland is exposed. Caution should be applied while retracting the strap muscles to avoid disrupting the medial thyroid veins. These veins are isolated and either ligated or clipped and divided. Proper exposure to the lateral aspects of the thyroid gland is achieved using right-angled (de Quervain) retractors. Division of the strap muscles may be necessary in the case of a very large goiter, when a central neck dissection is indicated, or in reoperative cases. The two muscles (sternohyoid and sternothyroid) are separated using diathermia. Their borders are secured with 2-0 threads that serve as stay sutures.

7.5.3 Upper Pole

Using Kocher's forceps, lateral retraction of the upper pole of the thyroid lobe is applied in order to open up the avascular space [18] between the lobe and the cricothyroid muscle, thus exposing the external branch of the superior laryngeal nerve [19,20]. This nerve can sometimes be identified as it descends with the vessels and anterior to the cricoid muscle but is often not visible (Fig. 7.2). A recent study showed that the identification and dissection of the superior laryngeal nerve do not lower the risk of damage compared with the simple transection of the superior vein and ar-

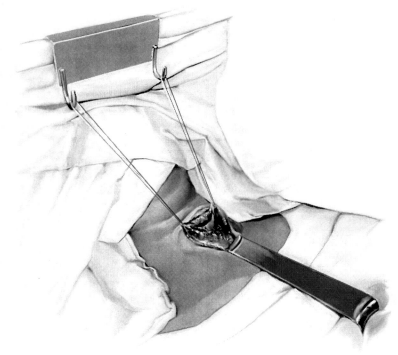

Fig. 7.1 Intraoperative situation after creation of the superior skin-platysma flap which is secured with threads. The inferior flap is retracted using a Roux retractor

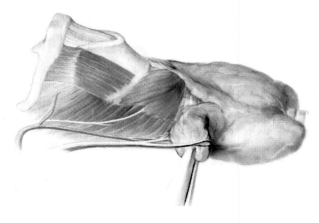

Fig. 7.2 Lateral and caudal retraction of the upper pole of the thyroid in order to open up the avascular space between the lobe and the cricothyroid muscle, thus exposing the external branch of the superior laryngeal nerve

tery close to the thyroid [21]. The superior vessels are usually ligated with transfixing sutures. Large goiters with prominent superior poles often require more than one transection step.

7.5.4   Isthmus and Pyramidal Lobe

By blunt dissection, the isthmus is freed from the underlying trachea and divided between transfixing ligatures. If subtotal or total thyroidectomy is performed, the division of the isthmus is often not necessary. The pyramidal lobe, which originates more often from the left thyroid lobe, is traced upward and removed as completely as possible.

7.5.5   Hilum of the Gland

Only the complete division of the superior vessels enables the surgeon to medially rotate and anteriorly mobilize the gland which results in optimal exposure of the hilar structures. Capsular dissection, as described by Thompson et al. [22], refers to the development of a plane between the thyroid capsule and the tertiary branches of the inferior thyroid artery. The branches are ligated or clipped individually directly on the surface of the thyroid gland. This method, which is widely practiced today, minimizes surgical damage to both the parathyroid glands and the RLN [23]. Meticulous dissection steps will then enable identification of the RLN where it crosses the inferior thyroid artery, as well as the two parathyroid glands. It is wise to preserve as much of the inferior thyroid artery and its branches as possible, since it supplies the blood to the two parathyroid glands. Truncal ligation of the inferior thyroid artery should be omitted. However, it is sometimes helpful to hold the trunk of the artery

using a vessel loop in order to facilitate further exposure of the RLN. The nerve may easily be found at its constant landmark, the so-called Zuckerkandl tuberculum [24,25], where it crosses beneath the thyroid gland and enters below Berry's ligament of the thyroid cartilage (Fig. 7.3). The RLN can always be identified laterodorsally to the ligament of Berry; it never penetrates the ligament [26]. The left RLN leaves the vagus nerve as the vagus crosses over the arch of the aorta. It hooks around the aorta and ascends again, similarly to the right RLN, laterally to the trachea to its terminal branches within the laryngeal muscles. This explains why the left RLN runs closer to the tracheoesophageal groove than the right RLN [27]. The RLN may pass posteriorly or superficially to the inferior thyroid artery or its branches intertwine with many variations. Although several methods of localizing the RLN have been described, surgeons should be aware of the variations and must have a thorough knowledge of the normal anatomy to achieve a high standard of care. This will ensure the integrity and safety of the RLN during thyroid surgery. The identification of the RLN may be assisted by palpation; it may be felt like a cord that can be rolled against the trachea [28]. The nerve appears as a white cord commonly accompanied by a small artery. To clearly identify the RLN, dissection of its crossing point with the inferior thyroid artery is critical. Gentle dissection, best performed with a fine curved jaw hemostat, is necessary at this point. Although there are many different anatomic relationships between the nerve and the artery, the crossing point is one constant anatomic landmark where the RLN can usually be identified. One exception to this rule is the non-recurrent inferior laryngeal nerve (Fig. 7.4). This anomaly is found virtually only on the right side and is associated with an anomalous right subclavian artery with a reported frequency of 0.2–0.8% [29–31].

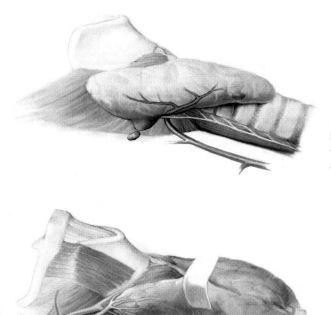

Fig. 7.3 Topographic relationship between the inferior thyroid artery and the tubercle of Zuckerkandl to the recurrent laryngeal nerve and the superior parathyroid gland

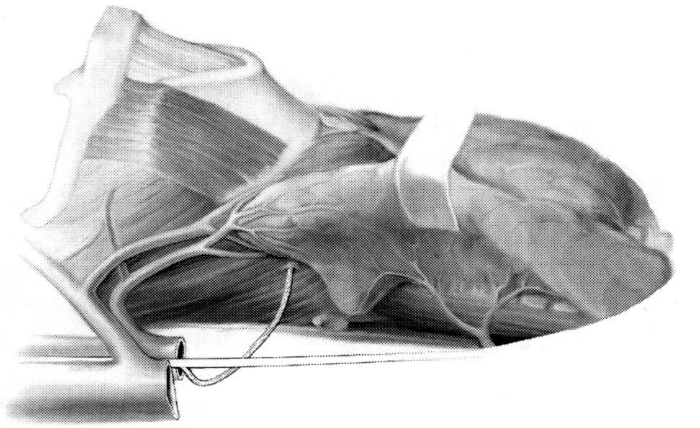

Fig. 7.4 Intraoperative finding of a non-recurrent inferior laryngeal nerve

7.5.6 Handling of the Parathyroid Glands

Regardless of whether a unilateral lobectomy or total thyroidectomy is performed, all identified parathyroid tissue should be preserved on its native blood supply. If a gland is devascularized during dissection, it should be transplanted. Although there have been sporadic reports of parathyroid autotransplantation, it has only been in the last 30 years that the technique has become used and only recently has it become accepted as part of routine clinical practice during total thyroidectomy [32]. The best way to preserve the parathyroid glands in situ is the extracapsular dissection of the thyroid gland. With the utilization of the extracapsular dissection, the parathyroid glands are swept off the thyroid capsule and are left in situ with their vascular pedicles. The superior parathyroid gland is usually found after mobilization of the superior pole of the thyroid. The lateral aspect of the thyroid gland superior to the inferior thyroid artery usually reveals a fat pad where the parathyroid can be found. This fat pad including the parathyroid gland should be mobilized off the lateral aspect of the thyroid starting at its superior medial edge and sweeping the pad inferiorly and laterally. It is important not to disrupt the fat pad

and not to dissect the gland further than just beyond the edge of the thyroid to preserve its blood supply. The inferior parathyroid gland is usually found at the inferior pole of the thyroid or within the tongue of the thymus. Once identified, it is taken off the inferior pole in a similar fashion to the superior gland. Disruption of the thyroid-thymic ligament should be avoided as it provides most of the blood supply to the inferior parathyroid gland.

All normal but devascularized parathyroid tissue should be transplanted into the sternocleidomastoid muscle or other convenient muscle at the time of thyroidectomy. Sometimes, the gland is partly devascularized and should then be trimmed back to the area of good arterial flow and viability. The remaining portion is removed, minced, and autotransplanted. Histologic confirmation of parathyroid tissue is crucial in the setting of thyroid cancer. Nodal metastases from thyroid cancer can mimic parathyroid tissue and should not be transplanted. There are principally two ways to do a parathyroid autotransplantation. First, the gland tissue is removed and minced into tiny cubes that are smaller than 1 mm^3. By separating the muscle fibers of the sternocleidomastoid muscle, a pocket containing about a 1-ml space is created using blunt dissection. The minced tissue is then transplanted into the pocket which is closed and marked by hemostatic clips or a non-absorbable thread. It is essential to leave a completely dry pocket behind since hematoma formation within the pocket would be prone to phagocytosis including the parathyroid tissue. The second possibility to achieve the parathyroid transplantation is the creation of a parathyroid suspension using saline which is then aspirated with a 2-ml syringe and injected into the sternocleidomastoid muscle with an 18-gauge needle.

7.5.7   Lower Thyroid Pole

The transection of the vessels running to the lower pole is usually done after proper exposition of the RLN. Veins from the anterior superior mediastinum are exposed and divided very close to the thyroid gland. In up to 12% of cases an accessory ima artery may spread into the lower pole. This vessel may originate either from the brachiocephalic trunk, the right carotid artery, directly from the aortic arch, the internal thoracic artery, or from a mediastinal artery. This vessel may cause intraoperative bleeding especially when a large retrosternal goiter is bluntly mobilized.

7.5.8   Removal of the Lobe

During the final steps of the thyroidectomy, the lobe is dissected away from the trachea under constant exposure and preservation of the RLN. The dense attachments at the level of the posterior suspensory ligament (Berry) usually require sharp dissection. Attention must then be paid to the relatively constant superior branch of the inferior thyroid artery (criminal branch) that often crosses underneath the RLN and spreads medially from beneath the nerve into the

thyroid gland. This small artery should be isolated and clipped before cutting (Fig. 7.5). The use of any cautery or other thermal dissection device should be avoided at this step due to the potential for thermal injury of the RLN that is in close proximity to the inferior thyroid artery. Inadvertent bleeding from this artery and uncontrolled attempts of hemostasis at this point of dissection may harm the RLN. Sudden bleeding is best handled, with the aid of suction, by identifying the vessel stump, and clamping or clipping, being constantly aware of the presence of the RLN. If oozing occurs at this point, the placement of a hemostyptic gelatine sponge is advised.

7.5.9   Wound Closure

A postoperative drain can never replace accurate hemostasis and is of little or no use if severe postoperative bleeding occurs. Two randomized trials did not show any advantage of drainage after thyroidectomy [33,34]. The strap muscles are sutured continuously with a 3-0 absorbable thread, the platysma with a 4-0 thread, and the skin is closed by an intradermal running suture using 5-0 absorbable thread. A smooth collar may be used for the first 24 hours postoperatively and the patient should be advised to keep a head up position of about 30° in order to minimize venous congestion and swelling of the soft tissues around the wound.

7.6   Reoperative Thyroid Surgery

Avoidance of RLN injury is best achieved by identification of the nerve early during reoperation. The best approach is the identification of the RLN in a previously undissected area and to follow the nerve into the dissected scarred region ("from the known

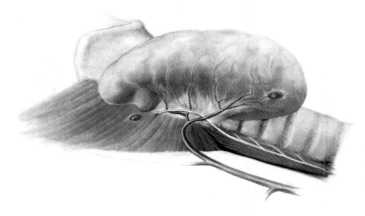

Fig. 7.5 Last steps of dissection for thyroid lobectomy: a small superior branch of the inferior thyroid artery usually crosses underneath the RLN and spreads medially from beneath the nerve into the thyroid parenchyma

toward the unknown"). Although the use of intra-operative neuromonitoring for confirmation of the RLN has some theoretical applications for a difficult dissection, visual identification of the RLN is still essential. Principally three distinct approaches exist for reoperative thyroid and parathyroid surgery.

First, the lateral or "back door" approach enters the thyroid bed between the anterior border of sternocleidomastoid and the strap muscles (Fig. 7.6). Lateral mobilizing of the sternocleidomastoid muscle exposes the sternohyoid and underlying sternothyroid muscles, whose fibers spread out inferiorly and laterally over the carotid artery and jugular vein. Gentle retraction of the carotid artery exposes the paratracheal soft tissue. This area, which is located inferolaterally to the inferior pole of the thyroid, is, if present, usually unchanged from previous interventions. Here, the RLN can usually be identified without difficulty.

Second, the low anterior approach enters the thyroid bed similarly to the primary operation. The strap muscles are separated in the midline down to the sternal notch and are reflected laterally. The dissection is then carried out in the paratracheal regions inferior to the area of previous dissection where the right or left RLN is identified.

Third, the anterior superior approach exposes the region between the superior pole of the thyroid, if present, and the larynx. The RLN can be identified as it enters the larynx with dissection in this avascular space between the superior thyroid pole and the larynx. This can even be realized without taking down the superior pole vessels. The RLN can be traced inferiorly and identified in the hilum of the thyroid which is often extensively scarred.

7.7　Minimally Invasive Thyroidectomy

Whereas minimally invasive parathyroidectomy has become popular among endocrine surgeons, experience with minimally invasive thyroidectomy remains limited. The feasibility and safety of fully endoscopic thyroidectomy or video-endoscopically assisted thyroidectomy have been proved in a few studies that reported a minor risk of complications and a low conversion rate of 3–11% [35–38]. The key to the success of these approaches is a rigorous selection of the patients. Inclusion criteria are solitary nodules smaller than or equal to 3 cm, thyroid volume less than 20 ml, absence of thyroiditis, absence of previous neck irradiation, and absence of previous neck surgery. Thus, minimally invasive thyroidectomies are valid alternatives to conventional surgery for patients with small solitary nodules [39]. However, only 10.6% of patients requiring thyroid surgery eventually qualify for this approach [40].

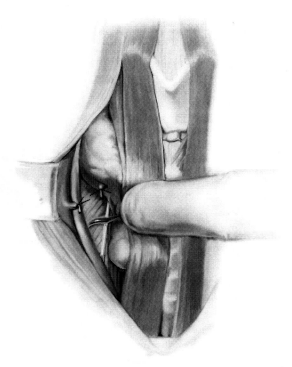

Fig. 7.6 With the "back door" approach, the surgeon enters the thyroid bed between the anterior border of the sternocleidomastoid muscle and the lateral border of the strap muscles

References

1.　Bliss RD, Gauger PG, Delbridge LW (2000) Surgeon's approach to the thyroid gland: surgical anatomy and the importance of technique. World J Surg 24:891–897

2.　Runkel N, Riede E, Mann B, Buhr HJ (1998) Surgical training and vocal-cord paralysis in benign thyroid disease. Langenbecks Arch Surg 383:240–242

3.　Lamade W, Renz K, Willeke F, Klar E, Herfarth C (1999) Effect of training on the incidence of nerve damage in thyroid surgery. Br J Surg 86:388–391

4.　Udelsman R (2004) Experience counts. Ann Surg 240:26–27

5.　Ito Y, Iwase H, Tanaka H, Yuasa H, Kureyama Y, Yamashita H, et al (2001) Metachronous primary hyperparathyroidism due to a parathyroid adenoma and a subsequent carcinoma: report of a case. Surg Today 31:895–898

6. Hermann M, Hellebart C, Freissmuth M (2004) Neuro-monitoring in thyroid surgery: prospective evaluation of intraoperative electrophysiological responses for the prediction of recurrent laryngeal nerve injury. Ann Surg 240:9–17

7. Zambudio AR, Rodriguez J, Riquelme J, Soria T, Canteras M, Parrilla P (2004) Prospective study of postoperative complications after total thyroidectomy for multinodular goiters by surgeons with experience in endocrine surgery. Ann Surg 240:18–25

8. Beldi G, Kinsbergen T, Schlumpf R (2004) Evaluation of intraoperative recurrent nerve monitoring in thyroid surgery. World J Surg 28:589–591

9. Voutilainen PE, Haglund CH (2000) Ultrasonically activated shears in thyroidectomies: a randomized trial. Ann Surg 231:322–328

10. Defechereux T, Rinken F, Maweja S, Hamoir E, Meurisse M (2003) Evaluation of the ultrasonic dissector in thyroid surgery. A prospective randomised study. Acta Chir Belg 103:274–277

11. Voutilainen PE, Haapiainen RK, Haglund CH (1998) Ultrasonically activated shears in thyroid surgery. Am J Surg 175:491–493

12. Siperstein AE, Berber E, Morkoyun E (2002) The use of the harmonic scalpel vs conventional knot tying for vessel ligation in thyroid surgery. Arch Surg 137:137–142

13. Ortega J, Sala C, Flor B, Lledo S (2004) Efficacy and cost-effectiveness of the U1traCision harmonic scalpel in thyroid surgery: an analysis of 200 cases in a randomized trial. J Laparoendosc Adv Surg Tech A 14:9–12

14. Dror A, Salim M, Yoseph R (2003) Sutureless thyroidectomy using electrothermal system: a new technique. J Laryngol Otol 117:198–201

15. Kiriakopoulos A, Dimitrios T, Dimitrios L (2004) Use of a diathermy system in thyroid surgery. Arch Surg 139:997–1000

16. Kebebew E, Clark OH (2000) Differentiated thyroid cancer: "complete" rational approach. World J Surg 24:942–951

17. Jarhult J, Lindestad PA, Nordenstrom J, Perbeck L (1991) Routine examination of the vocal cords before and after thyroid and parathyroid surgery. Br J Surg 78:1116–1117

18. Aina EN, Hisham AN (2001) External laryngeal nerve in thyroid surgery: recognition and surgical implications. Aust N Z J Surg 71:212–214

19. Monfared A, Gorti G, Kim D (2002) Microsurgical anatomy of the laryngeal nerves as related to thyroid surgery. Laryngoscope 112:386–392

20. Friedman M, LoSavio P, Ibrahim H (2002) Superior laryngeal nerve identification and preservation in thyroidectomy. Arch Otolaryngol Head Neck Surg 128:296–303

21. Bellantone R, Boscherini M, Lombardi CP, Bossola M, Rubino F, De Crea C, et al (2001) Is the identification of the external branch of the superior laryngeal nerve mandatory in thyroid operation? Results of a prospective randomized study. Surgery 130:1055–1059

22. Thompson NW, Olsen WR, Hoffman GL (1973) The continuing development of the technique of thyroidectomy. Surgery 73:913–927

23. Delbridge L, Reeve TS, Khadra M, Poole AG (1992) Total thyroidectomy: the technique of capsular dissection. Aust N Z J Surg 62:96–99

24. Mirilas P, Skandalakis JE (2003) Zuckerkandl's tubercle: Hannibal ad Portas. J Am Coll Surg 196:796–801

25. Pelizzo MR, Toniato A, Gemo G (1998) Zuckerkandl's tuberculum: an arrow pointing to the recurrent laryngeal nerve (constant anatomical landmark). J Am Coll Surg 187:333–336

26. Sasou S, Nakamura S, Kurihara H (1998) Suspensory ligament of Berry: its relationship to recurrent laryngeal nerve and anatomic examination of 24 autopsies. Head Neck 20:695–698

27. Liebermann-Meffert DM, Walbrun B, Hiebert CA, Siewert JR (1999) Recurrent and superior laryngeal nerves: a new look with implications for the esophageal surgeon. Ann Thorac Surg 67:217–223

28. Wheeler MH (1999) Thyroid surgery and the recurrent laryngeal nerve. Br J Surg 86:291–292

29. Proye CA, Carnaille BM, Goropoulos A (1991) Nonrecurrent and recurrent inferior laryngeal nerve: a surgical pitfall in cervical exploration. Am J Surg 162:495–496

30. Chow SM, Law SC, Au SK, Mang O, Yau S, Yuen KT, et al (2003) Changes in clinical presentation, management and outcome in 1348 patients with differentiated thyroid carcinoma: experience in a single institute in Hong Kong, 1960–2000. Clin Oncol (R Coll Radiol) 15:329–336

31. Defechereux T, Albert V, Alexandre J, Bonnet P, Hamoir E, Meurisse M (2000) The inferior non-recurrent laryngeal nerve: a major surgical risk during thyroidectomy. Acta Chir Belg 100:62–67

32. Wells SA Jr, Gunnells JC, Shelburne JD, Schneider AB, Sherwood LM (1975) Transplantation of the parathyroid glands in man: clinical indications and results. Surgery 78:34–44

33. Schoretsanitis G, Melissas J, Sanidas E, Christodoulakis M, Vlachonikolis JG, Tsiftsis DD (1998) Does draining the neck affect morbidity following thyroid surgery? Am Surg 64:778–780

34. Wihlborg O, Bergljung L, Martensson H (1988) To drain or not to drain in thyroid surgery. A controlled clinical study. Arch Surg 123:40–41

35. Yeh TS, Jan YY, Hsu BR, Chen KW, Chen NIE (2000) Video-assisted endoscopic thyroidectomy. Am J Surg 180:82–85

36. Gagner M, Inabnet WB III (2001) Endoscopic thyroidectomy for solitary thyroid nodules. Thyroid 11:161–163

37. Miccoli P, Bellantone R, Mourad M, Walz M, Raffaelli M, Berti P (2002) Minimally invasive video-assisted thyroidectomy: multi-institutional experience. World J Surg 26:972–975

38. Mourad M, Saab N, Malaise J, Ngongang C, Fournier B, Daumerie C, et al (2001) Minimally invasive video-assisted approach for partial and total thyroidectomy: initial experience. Surg Endosc 15:1108–1111

39. Bellantone R, Lombardi CP, Bossola M, Boscherini M, De Crea C, Alesina PF, et al (2002) Video-assisted vs conventional thyroid lobectomy: a randomized trial. Arch Surg 137:301–304

40. Miccoli P, Berti P, Materazzi G, Minuto M, Barellini L (2004) Minimally invasive video-assisted thyroidectomy: five years of experience. J Am Coll Surg 199:243–248

8 Surgery for the Solitary Thyroid Nodule

Prabhat K. Bhama and Gerard M. Doherty

8.1   Introduction

The solitary thyroid nodule must be carefully evaluated because of the risk of malignancy, however, selective management is paramount due to the high frequency of benign lesions. While 4–7% of the adult population in the USA have a palpable thyroid nodule [1], the vast majority of these patients have benign disease, and do not require surgical resection.

This chapter focuses on the use of lobectomy for nodules suspicious but not diagnostic for carcinoma, as well as algorithms for treatment of diagnosed thyroid carcinoma. The extent of surgery for malignant thyroid disease is also discussed, along with strategies for risk stratification for treatment of differentiated thyroid cancer. Follicular cell-derived thyroid cancers, including papillary thyroid cancer, follicular thyroid cancer, and Hürthle cell cancer are highlighted.

8.2   Lobectomy for Suspicious Lesions

Evaluation of a palpable solitary nodule in the thyroid gland should begin with a comprehensive history and physical examination. It is typically impossible to distinguish a benign nodule from a malignant nodule by palpation, however, there are some clinical findings that are indicative of malignant disease. A history of a hard and relatively fast growing nodule is associated with a higher risk for malignancy when compared with a soft and slowly growing nodule. Furthermore, the presence of a solitary nodule is more indicative of malignancy, whereas a multinodular thyroid is more consistent with benign disease. Thyroid function studies may also be useful, since a suppressed thyroid-stimulating hormone (TSH) level is suggestive of benign pathology, as it is uncommon for malignant lesions to cause thyrotoxicosis or thyroiditis [2].

Further evaluation of the solitary nodule is best done by ultrasound and fine-needle aspiration (FNA). The ultrasound examination of the thyroid gland allows accurate evaluation of the thyroid nodule itself as well as the surrounding thyroid tissue (Fig. 8.1). Characterization of the nodule includes the size, shape, solid versus cystic nature, the presence of calcifications in the nodule, and the nature of the borders (smooth, irregular, etc.). The use of ultrasound-guided FNA can improve the diagnostic accuracy (Fig. 8.2), but interpretation of the aspirate for definitive diagnosis may still not be possible. In cases of follicular neoplasia, FNA is limited in its ability to distinguish malignant from benign disease, since the diagnosis of follicular carcinoma is histological. Specifically, identification of capsular or vascular invasion is necessary for diagnosis of malignant disease. This scenario is similar when dealing with Hürthle cell neoplasms.

Although cytological findings of FNA are sufficient for diagnosis in approximately 85% of specimens, 15% of aspirates fail to yield satisfactory results [3,4]. In such cases, pathology reports may be suspicious for malignant disease, and approximately 20% of such suspicious lesions will actually be malignant Hürthle

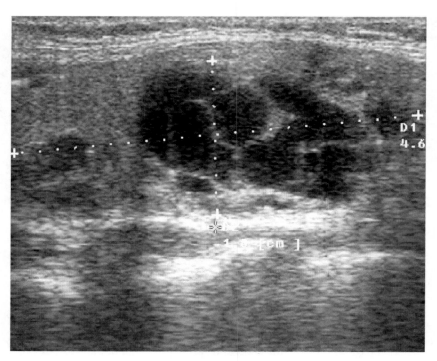

Fig. 8.1 Longitudinal view of the left thyroid lobe, with a complex cystic and solid lesion in the mid to lower portion of the lobe. There is a second smaller cystic lesion in the upper pole of the gland. The cystic nature of these lesions is emphasized by the posterior acoustic enhancement visible as the whiter areas posterior (*lower on the figure*) to the thyroid lobe

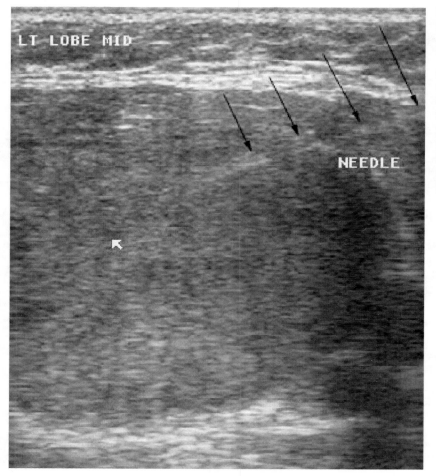

Fig. 8.2 Ultrasound-guided fine-needle aspiration (FNA) of a palpable left thyroid lobe lesion. The ultrasound technique is used to direct the needle (*arrows*) to the lesion that is to be sampled. Although ultrasound is not strictly necessary for the sampling of palpable lesions, it is helpful for directing the needle to a specific area within the target lesion. For non-palpable lesions, ultrasound in necessary for FNA cytology

or follicular neoplasms. While some have suggested the employment of ^{123}I scintigraphy in cases of suspicious nodules, this test is not sufficient for uncovering malignant disease. The presence of "hot" nodules on ^{123}I scintigraphy is suggestive of benign disease, since malignant neoplasms typically manifest as "cold" nodules. However, patients with "hot" nodules on ^{123}I scan have occasionally been found to have thyroid cancer upon further investigation [5].

Thus, there are currently no investigative procedures available to definitively distinguish benign from malignant disease in patients with suspicious lesions of indeterminate cytology. A recent study indicated that experienced pathologists may be accurate when predicting benign disease using FNA, however, the authors determined that the predictive value of the test was not enough to preclude surgical resection [6]. As such, suspicious lesions are considered to be positive for cancer, and should be treated with surgical resection to avoid the adverse consequences associated with untreated thyroid cancer. The principal surgical approach to solitary, undetermined nodule is ipsilateral lobectomy. The reason for primary removal of the entire ipsilateral thyroid lobe is to avoid serious complications, since if further surgery is needed a reoperation is difficult and may be harmful in scarred tissue.

8.3 Treatment for Differentiated Thyroid Cancers

8.3.1 Principles

Differentiated carcinoma of the thyroid includes both papillary and follicular variants. The primary treatment for these cancers is resection. Although surgical intervention is clearly indicated, controversy remains regarding the extent of thyroid tissue that should be removed during the initial operation. Whereas total thyroidectomy may help ensure removal of all neoplastic tissue, it leaves the patient with no thyroid tissue, necessitating lifelong thyroid hormone supplementation and exposing the patient to the risk of bilateral dissection of the adjacent normal neck structures. Alternatively, more conservative procedures may leave inconspicuous residual cancer within the patient. Unfortunately, there are no prospective randomized clinical trials evaluating the extent of thyroidectomy, adjuvant radioactive iodide therapy, and TSH suppressive therapy. Because of the relatively good prognosis and low incidence of papillary thyroid cancer (PTC), such a study would

require a large multicenter trial with long follow-up time. It is unlikely that such trials will ever be performed.

Three primary surgical strategies exist for the treatment of differentiated thyroid cancer: total thyroidectomy, near-total thyroidectomy, and lobectomy with isthmusectomy. Total thyroidectomy involves removal of the entire thyroid gland and its capsule, whereas near-total thyroidectomy preserves the posterior capsule of the thyroid contralateral to the neoplasm. These two procedures are generally considered together as completely ablative approaches to thyroid carcinoma. Unilateral lobectomy and isthmusectomy is removal of the lobe ipsilateral to the lesion, and removal of the thyroid isthmus. This approach allows preservation of normal thyroid tissue, thereby obviating the need for lifelong thyroid hormone supplementation. In addition, unilateral lobectomy with isthmusectomy essentially eliminates the risk for hypoparathyroidism and bilateral vocal cord paralysis. Subtotal thyroidectomy is a procedure in which preservation of several grams of thyroid tissue is involved. Due to higher complication rates encountered when subsequent surgery is indicated, subtotal thyroidectomy is not a recommended treatment option for patients with differentiated thyroid cancer [7].

Regardless of the surgical approach chosen, the function of the vocal cords should be assessed prior to surgery by noting any history of voice changes. Examination of the larynx by indirect laryngoscopy as a visual survey for vocal cord mobility is indicated whenever there is a history or examination finding of vocal changes. In the case of unilateral vocal cord paralysis, extreme caution should be taken to preserve the contralateral recurrent laryngeal nerve to avoid acute airway compromise. The surgical team should also be prepared to create an alternative airway (i.e., tracheostomy) if the need arises during surgery or postoperatively.

8.3.2 Treatment: Papillary Thyroid Cancer

8.3.2.1 Total Thyroidectomy

Total thyroidectomy is a safe and effective primary treatment for patients with PTC. In patients with high-risk lesions or extrathyroidal tumor extension, it is generally accepted that total thyroidectomy is the appropriate treatment. However, in patients with low-risk lesions, the extent of surgical resection is controversial. Two key justifications exist for the use of near-total or total thyroidectomy in patients with

PTC. First, removal of the entire thyroid gland may include the excision of cancer that was occult on the preoperative assessment, and second, the postoperative follow-up surveillance for recurrent disease is more sensitive if the entire thyroid is removed. After a total or near-total thyroidectomy, postoperative radioactive iodine can be used to identify and ablate any residual thyroid cancer, and serum thyroglobulin is a more accurate marker of recurrent or persistent PTC following total thyroidectomy when compared with more conservative resections of thyroid tissue.

Advocates of more conservative procedures contend that there is a higher risk of complications following total thyroidectomy. Nonetheless, complication rates less than 2% after total thyroidectomy have been reported by numerous surgeons with experience in total thyroidectomy (Table 8.1). Factors determining the risk for complication from total thyroidectomy include: the extent of thyroid disease, the experience of the surgeon, and the anatomic variation of the parathyroid glands, recurrent laryngeal nerves, and external laryngeal nerves [8–10]. Major complications of total thyroidectomy include vocal cord paralysis secondary to recurrent laryngeal nerve injury, and hypocalcemia due to injury or resection of the parathyroid glands. Regardless, many surgeons achieve comparable complication rates for total thyroidectomy, near-total thyroidectomy, and more conservative procedures [11,12]. Amongst the <2% of patients who had complications after total thyroidectomy, tumors were more likely to be more invasive and involve the recurrent laryngeal nerve, thereby necessitating resection of the nerve. While these data indicate that complications following total thyroidectomy are rare, they are reported from surgeons with extensive operative experience doing total thyroidectomy. In the hands of less experienced surgeons, complication rates may be higher. Therefore, for patients with PTC necessitating total or completion thyroidectomy, surgical treatment is best implemented by the experienced surgeon.

Papillary thyroid cancer often exists with intraglandular multifocal disease that may not be identified upon initial evaluation. In a study of 105 patients, Katoh et al. found that intraglandular cancer foci (other than the tumor regarded as the primary focus) were present in over 78% of patients. Moreover, these multicentric lesions were found in the contralateral lobe in 61%. The authors concluded that intraglandular metastasis is an important characteristic of PTC [13]. This has also been demonstrated in a high proportion of microcarcinomas of the thyroid, which harbor bilateral foci of disease [14].

A more recent study indicated that approximately 44% of 182 patients studied harbored histologically confirmed PTC at completion thyroidectomy. This bilaterality was independent of risk classification. Bilateral tumors at completion thyroidectomy were present in patients of both high- and low-risk classifications. This study suggests total thyroidectomy in order to eradicate all neoplastic tissue in patients with PTC. In addition, the authors recommended completion thyroidectomy for patients with a history of PTC that were initially treated with more conservative surgical therapy [15].

Hay et al., from the Mayo clinic, studied local recurrence, nodal and distant metastases in patients with low-risk PTC based on the AMES prognostic classification system. They found that patients who underwent lobectomy for PTC had a higher recurrence rate (14%) and nodal metastases (19%) than those patients treated with procedures involving both lobes. However, they found no significant difference in survival rate and distant metastases [16]. Other studies have demonstrated that between 5% and 10% of recurrences of thyroid cancer occur in the contralateral lobe [17], indicating that total thyroidectomy

Table 8.1 Complications reported after total thyroidectomy

Authors, year	Number of patients	Transient nerve paresis; number (%)	Permanent nerve paresis; number (%)	Transient hypoparathyroidism; number (%)	Permanent hypoparathyroidism; number (%)
Thompson, 1978 [44]	165	NR	0	NR	<2%
Clark, 1988 [45]	160	4 (2.5%)	3 (2%)	NR	1 (0.6%)
Ley, 1992 [12]	124	1 (0.8%)	1 (0.8%)	13 (10%)	2 (1.6%)
Tartaglia, 2003 [46]	1,636	31 (1.9%)	15 (0.9%)	NR	14 (0.9%)
Rosato, 2004 [26]	9,599	195 (2%)	94 (1%)	797 (8.3%)	163 (1.7%)

during the initial operation may have been beneficial in these patients. Moreover, complications due to central neck recurrence are the cause of death in 50% of patients who die from recurrent thyroid carcinoma [18]. In addition, a review of 1,599 patients with differentiated thyroid carcinoma concluded that patients with well-differentiated thyroid cancers who die from their disease most likely die secondary to local recurrence [19]. Such complications may best be avoided by implementation of total thyroidectomy and lymphadenectomy as the primary surgical treatment for differentiated thyroid cancers.

Finally, there is approximately a 1% risk of progression from a differentiated thyroid cancer to anaplastic thyroid cancer. Whereas the prognosis of PTC is very good, anaplastic thyroid cancer results in near uniform lethality. Therefore, elimination of all PTC via total thyroidectomy may prevent progression to anaplastic thyroid cancer from residual tissue left behind during thyroid lobectomy and isthmusectomy.

Total thyroidectomy and central neck lymph node dissection is indicated for virtually all patients with PTC when postoperative radioactive iodine is considered (see below for discussion of lymph node management). In patients with excellent prognosis (tumor size less than 1 cm, confined to the thyroid without evidence of any metastatic disease, in an otherwise healthy female less than 45 years of age), more conservative approaches may be used. However, lower recurrence and mortality rates are associated even with patients who have low-risk PTC and undergo total thyroidectomy [16,20]. Moreover, patients undergoing total thyroidectomy can also benefit from more accurate assessment of disease recurrence or residual disease using serum thyroglobulin levels. In addition, postoperative radioactive iodine scanning and ablation are more effective in patients after total thyroidectomy. In cases where injury to the recurrent laryngeal nerve or parathyroid glands cannot be avoided, near-total thyroidectomy can be employed to leave behind a small amount of thyroid tissue, followed by ablation of residual tissue with radioactive iodine.

8.3.2.2 Unilateral Lobectomy and Isthmusectomy

The use of unilateral lobectomy and isthmusectomy for the treatment of differentiated thyroid cancers is supported by two arguments. First, unilateral procedures can avoid the risk of some potential complications of bilateral procedures. Second, some studies have failed to demonstrate a survival benefit of total

thyroidectomy compared to lobectomy and isthmusectomy.

Because of the proximity of the recurrent laryngeal nerve with respect to the fascia surrounding the thyroid (the visceral portion of the pretracheal layer of deep cervical fascia), it seems plausible to assume that bilateral procedures place the recurrent laryngeal nerve at greater risk for injury than unilateral procedures. On the one hand, unilateral injury to the recurrent laryngeal nerve leaves the ipsilateral vocal cord paralyzed in the paramedian position, resulting in hoarseness of the voice. In addition, the voice may often appear breathy, secondary to incomplete adduction of the vocal cords. This complication can be treated with medialization of the paralyzed cord via type I thyroplasty. However, morbidity is substantially increased, along with healthcare costs. On the other hand, bilateral recurrent laryngeal nerve injury can result in acute airway obstruction. This may present as postoperative stridor and dyspnea, and may require endotracheal reintubation with establishment of an alternative airway via tracheostomy. The incidence of recurrent laryngeal nerve injury during total thyroidectomy is approximately 1–1.5% and likely much less in the hands of the experienced surgeon.

Total thyroidectomy also places the patient at risk for lifelong hypocalcemia if all parathyroid tissue is unintentionally resected with the thyroid gland, while unilateral procedures do not. In fact, the most common underreported morbidity that does occur following thyroidectomy is likely transient hypocalcemia [21] that can be monitored effectively without difficulty by frequent postoperative examinations of the patient. However, a recent study of over 450 patients who underwent total thyroidectomy demonstrated that permanent hypocalcemia occurred in only 0.7% of all patients. The authors noted that high serum phosphorus level on postoperative day 7 was the only independent factor predicting permanent hypoparathyroidism, and thus, permanent hypocalcemia [22].

One retrospective study of 109 patients with nonmedullary thyroid cancer with 5- to 30-year follow-up demonstrated that significantly more complications occur with total thyroidectomy when compared with partial thyroidectomy. Furthermore, no differences in cancer mortality or recurrence rates amongst patients treated with total thyroidectomy versus partial thyroidectomy were found. The authors therefore recommended the use of partial thyroidectomy for non-medullary thyroid cancers [23]. A more recent study demonstrated that there is no survival benefit with total thyroidectomy when compared with partial thyroidectomy in patients with PTC in both low- and high-risk prognostic groups [24].

A recent study of incidental multifocal papillary thyroid microcarcinomas (less than or equal to 1 cm) found that subtotal thyroidectomy followed by adjuvant radioiodine therapy is a therapeutic option for patients with incidental multifocal microcarcinomas. However, the authors did note that future studies should be pursued for further evaluation of this technique [25].

Despite the significant, life-changing complications reported in the literature secondary to total thyroidectomy, major complications occur in less than 2% of all thyroid procedures, and complications are significantly more likely in secondary procedures that may be necessary if there is a recurrence.

8.3.2.3 Recommendations for Extent of Surgery

In our opinion, it is important that patients with PTC be treated by a surgeon with extensive experience in performing total thyroidectomy. Despite the reported complications following total thyroidectomy, complication rates are minimal in the hands of experienced surgeons [26] Furthermore, the high incidence of bilateral foci in patients with PTC indicates that these patients are best treated initially with total thyroidectomy, rather than undergoing a follow-up completion thyroidectomy for recurrent or residual disease that was not appreciated at the primary evaluation. Moreover, total thyroidectomy allows for more accurate follow-up using thyroglobulin as a marker of residual or recurrent disease. Postoperative radioactive iodine scanning and ablation is also more effective in patients after total thyroidectomy compared with more conservative procedures. Finally, studies show that a lower recurrence rate and mortality are associated with total or near-total thyroidectomy in patients with even low-risk PTC.

Thus, in virtually all patients, excluding those with the very best prognosis (tumor size less than 1 cm, confinement to the thyroid without metastases, in an otherwise healthy woman under 45 years of age), total thyroidectomy is the treatment of choice for papillary thyroid carcinoma.

8.3.2.4 Lymph Node Dissection

As with any surgical procedure, lymph node dissection carries some risk of iatrogenic injury. Specifically, nodal metastases in patients with PTC often requires dissection in the proximity of the parathyroid glands, putting the glands at risk for injury secondary to surgical manipulation. Therefore, careful stratification of patients into groups requiring lymph node dissection and those not requiring lymph node dissection is important for minimizing morbidity.

Approximately 80% of patients with PTC also have microscopic regional lymph node metastases [16]. The optimal diagnostic and therapeutic approaches for this have not been entirely clear. Microscopic occult metastases may often be ablated by adjuvant radioactive iodine therapy, but they may also be a site of persistent disease that would have easily been removed at the initial operation. While patients with PTC and matted lymph nodes or tumor extending through the lymph node capsule have a worse prognosis, the prognostic significance of lymph node metastases is controversial. [20,27,28].

Gross nodal disease occurs in 20–30% of adult cases of PTC, and is certainly justification for lymph node dissection (Fig. 8.3) [29]. Moreover, lymph node metastases are also associated with a higher recurrence rate when patients are matched for age and gender. Therefore, nodal metastases confirmed by preoperative ultrasound or intraoperative exploration should be treated with node dissection [7]. Specifically, removal of ipsilateral central neck nodes and perithyroid lymph nodes (Delphian node and lymph nodes medial to the carotid sheath) or lateral compartment nodes (levels 2–5) is important for nodes that have identifiable involvement with disease. Compartment-based resections of lateral neck nodes are preferable to "berry-picking" if they are clinically involved. For lateral compartment disease, the best approach is to perform functional modified radical neck dissection, during which all fibrofatty tissue with lymph nodes is removed. This procedure spares motor and sensory nerves, the sternocleidomastoid muscle, and the internal jugular vein as well, unless they are involve by tumor.

Removal of central neck lymph nodes is associated with an improvement in the regional recurrence rate, and an improved survival rate in retrospective studies [30–32]. This also has the advantage of demonstrating which patients have involved nodes, to make the selection of radioiodine therapy clear, even for those who may have otherwise apparently good prognostic tumors (small size and lack of extrathyroidal extension). The current American Thyroid Association Guidelines for the management of differentiated thyroid cancer now call that a staging/prophylactic level 6 lymph node dissection for all patients undergoing thyroidectomy for thyroid carcinoma should be considered [33].

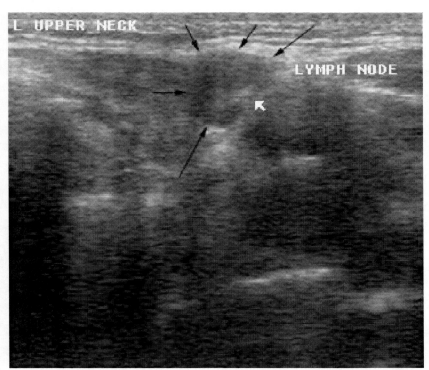

Fig. 8.3 Left cervical lymph node metastases detected on preoperative ultrasound examination of the neck (*arrows*). The node has the characteristics of replacement by metastatic disease, and was involved by FNA cytology. The node is globular and irregular in shape, compared to the typical smooth, fusiform node contour

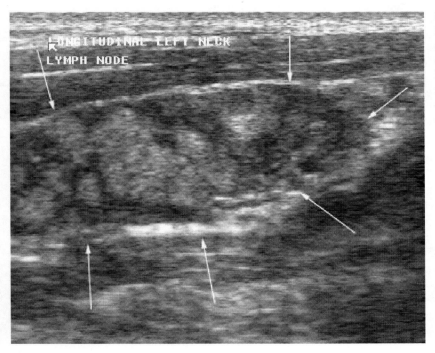

Fig. 8.4 Metastatic cancer causing lymphadenopathy in the left neck of a teenaged woman with thyroid carcinoma. Detected upon follow-up examination, this enlarged, irregular node (*arrows*) led to a compartmental node dissection for metastases

Prophylactic lateral neck node dissection is not recommended because in patients it is not associated with improved overall survival, and involves violation of additional planes by a substantially more extensive operation. However, follow-up of thyroid cancer patients by physical examination and ultrasound can identify patients with lateral neck nodal disease that can then be appropriately treated by therapeutic compartmental node dissection (Fig. 8.4).

8.3.3   Treatment: Follicular Thyroid Cancer

Despite differences in histological features, treatment for follicular thyroid carcinoma (FTC) is similar to that of PTC. Surgical resection remains the primary method of therapy for FTC of the thyroid. Moreover, the use of total thyroidectomy versus hemithyroidectomy is controversial. When dealing with disease confined to the thyroid (T_{1-2} N_0 M_0), total thyroidectomy or hemithyroidectomy with extirpation of central lymph nodes are both adequate.

For larger tumors (T_3–T_4), more extensive therapy is warranted. Total thyroidectomy along with postoperative radioactive iodine therapy is indicated in such cases. Proponents of unilateral procedures maintain that bilateral procedures carry an increased risk of morbidity, secondary to recurrent laryngeal nerve and parathyroid gland injury. Once again, morbidity is minimal in the hands of the experienced surgeon. Since follicular tumors spread primarily via hematogenous routes, cervical lymph node metastases are not as common in FTC when compared with PTC (35% versus 67%, respectively). However, therapeutic modified neck dissection is appropriate for patients with clinically apparent disease. Postoperative radioactive iodine scans and radioiodine ablation are also essential to help detect any residual disease and eliminate it.

8.3.4   Treatment: Oncocytic (Hürthle Cell) Thyroid Cancer

A variant of FTC, oncocytic carcinoma, is also known as oxyphilic or Hürthle cell carcinoma. While treatment strategies are similar to those of FTC, it is important to distinguish the two entities. Radioactive iodine uptake in oncocytic carcinoma of the thyroid is much less than that of FTC, therefore, postoperative diagnosis and ablation of residual disease with radioactive iodine is more difficult in patients with oncocytic thyroid cancer. Because of similarities in the natural history and prognosis with FTC, treatment of oncocytic cell carcinoma is similar to that of FTC [34].

8.4   Risk Stratification for Cancer Treatment

Certain environmental and genetic factors play an important role in predisposing particular individuals to developing thyroid cancer. Chances of developing differentiated thyroid cancers are increased by exposure to radiation. Such exposures occurred more often in the 1940s and 1950s than they do now. For instance, external radiation therapy was used to treat conditions such as tinea capitis, hypertrophic thymus, tonsillitis, acne, and otitis externa. Multiple studies have confirmed the increased risk of thyroid cancers and benign thyroid nodules in children exposed to low doses of radiation therapy [35–38]. It is important to note that exposure to external radiation beam therapy increases the risk of developing PTC, but it is not associated with the occurrence of FTC.

It has also been found that patients with familial adenomatous polyposis (FAP) have a predisposition toward developing benign and malignant thyroid neoplasms, specifically, differentiated tumors [39,40]. FTCs in particular have been associated with FAP, Gardner's syndrome, and Cowden's syndrome, but are most often sporadic.

Furthermore, studies have shown that diets both high and low in iodine can also increase the risk of developing thyroid cancer. When iodine uptake is sufficient, it is likely that a diagnosed differentiated thyroid carcinoma will be of the papillary type. FTCs are more common in areas that suffer from iodine deficiency and endemic goiter. Regions of the world suffering from iodine deficiency can exacerbate goiters by consumption of large quantities of cruciferous vegetables, which block iodine uptake [41].

Whereas certain environmental and innate factors can influence one's chance of developing thyroid cancer, the characteristics of a specific tumor or individual can dictate the prognosis of the patient. The age at initial diagnosis, patient age, gender, and family history are all important factors in determining one's prognosis. Specifically, increased recurrence rates are observed amongst patients under age 20 and over age 60. Moreover, mortality rates increase steadily after age 40 [42]. Nuclear atypia, tumor necrosis, vascular invasion, and other characteristics of histological grade are also influential prognostic factors in patients with thyroid cancer [43].

8.5   Summary

Thyroid nodules are quite common, and the basis of their evaluation is the FNA cytology. However, some tumors cannot be completely characterized by FNA, and so require at minimum a diagnostic ipsilateral thyroid lobectomy for definitive histology. In such cases, complete lobectomy is the minimum procedure, to avoid the potential need for further operation on that side of the trachea.

Differentiated thyroid carcinoma is best treated by total thyroidectomy, which is safe in experienced hands. The best prognosis cancers can be managed by lobectomy alone with careful surveillance of the remaining lobe. Lateral neck dissection is reserved for clinically evident cancer involvement of that compartment, though central neck (level 6) node dissection should be a part of every initial thyroid cancer operation.

References

1. Singer PA, et al (1996) Treatment guidelines for patients with thyroid nodules and well-differentiated thyroid cancer. American Thyroid Association. Arch Int Med 156:2165–2172
2. Kumar H, et al (1999) Gender, clinical findings, and serum thyrotropin measurements in the prediction of thyroid neoplasia in 1005 patients presenting with thyroid enlargement and investigated by fine-needle aspiration cytology. Thyroid 9:1105–1109
3. Gharib H, Goellner JR, Johnson DA (1993) Fine-needle aspiration cytology of the thyroid. A 12-year experience with 11,000 biopsies. Clin Lab Med 13:699–709
4. Cersosimo E, et al (1993) "Suspicious" thyroid cytologic findings: outcome in patients without immediate surgical treatment. Mayo Clin Proc 68:343–348
5. Nagai GR, et al (1987) Scintigraphic hot nodules and thyroid carcinoma. Clin Nucl Med 12:123–127
6. Smith J, et al (2005) Can cytology accurately predict benign follicular nodules? Am J Surg 189:592–5; discussion 595
7. Soh EY, Clark OH (1996) Surgical considerations and approach to thyroid cancer. Endocrinol Metab Clin North Am 25:115–139
8. Udelsman R, Shaha AR (2005) Is total thyroidectomy the best possible surgical management for well-differentiated thyroid cancer? Lancet Oncol 6:529–531
9. Udelsman R (2004) Experience counts [comment]. Ann Surg 240:26–27
10. Sosa JA, et al (1998) The importance of surgeon experience for clinical and economic outcomes from thyroidectomy. Ann Surg 228:320–330
11. Reeve T, Thompson NW (2000) Complications of thyroid surgery: how to avoid them, how to manage them, and observations on their possible effect on the whole patient. World J Surg 24:971–975
12. Ley PB, et al (1993) Safety and efficacy of total thyroidectomy for differentiated thyroid carcinoma: a 20-year review. Am Surg 59:110–114
13. Katoh R, et al (1992) Multiple thyroid involvement (intraglandular metastasis) in papillary thyroid carcinoma. A clinicopathologic study of 105 consecutive patients. Cancer 70:1585–1590
14. Pellegriti G, et al (2004) Clinical behavior and outcome of papillary thyroid cancers smaller than 1.5 cm in diameter: study of 299 cases [see comment]. J Clin Endocrinol Metab 89:3713–3720
15. Pacini F, et al (2001) Contralateral papillary thyroid cancer is frequent at completion thyroidectomy with no difference in low- and high-risk patients [see comment]. Thyroid 11:877–881
16. Hay ID, et al (1998) Unilateral total lobectomy: is it sufficient surgical treatment for patients with AMES low-risk papillary thyroid carcinoma? Surgery 124:958–964; discussion 964–966
17. Tollefson HR, Shah JP, Huvos AJ (1972) Papillary carcinoma of the thyroid. Recurrence in the thyroid gland after initial treatment. Am J Surg 124:468–472
18. Silverberg SG, Hutter RV, Foote FW Jr (1970) Fatal carcinoma of the thyroid: histology, metastases, and causes of death. Cancer 25:792–802
19. Samaan NA, et al (1992) The results of various modalities of treatment of well differentiated thyroid carcinomas: a retrospective review of 1599 patients. J Clin Endocrinol Metab 75:714–720
20. DeGroot LJ, et al (1990) Natural history, treatment, and course of papillary thyroid carcinoma. J Clin Endocrinol Metab 71:414–424
21. Flynn MB, et al (1994) Local complications after surgical resection for thyroid carcinoma. Am J Surg 168:404–407
22. Pisanu A, et al (2005) Hypocalcemia following total thyroidectomy: early factors predicting long-term outcome. Giornale di Chirurgia 26:131–134
23. Schroder DM, Chambous A, France CJ (1986) Operative strategy for thyroid cancer, is total thyroidectomy worth the price? Cancer 58:2320
24. Haigh PI, Urbach DR, Rotstein LE (2005) Extent of thyroidectomy is not a major determinant of survival in low- or high-risk papillary thyroid cancer. Ann Surg Oncol 12:81–89
25. Dietlein M, et al (2005) Incidental multifocal papillary microcarcinomas of the thyroid: is subtotal thyroidectomy combined with radioiodine ablation enough? Nucl Med Commun 26:3–8
26. Rosato L, et al (2004) Complications of thyroid surgery: analysis of a multicentric study on 14,934 patients operated on in Italy over 5 years. World J Surg 28:271–276
27. Akslen LA (1993) Prognostic importance of histologic grading in papillary thyroid carcinoma. Cancer 72:2680–2685
28. Akslen LA, et al (1991) Survival and causes of death in thyroid cancer: a population-based study of 2479 cases from Norway. Cancer Res 51:1234–1241

29. Mirallie E, et al (1999) Localization of cervical node metastasis of papillary thyroid carcinoma. World J Surg 23:970–973; discussion 973–974

30. Gemsenjager E, et al (2003) Lymph node surgery in papillary thyroid carcinoma. J Am Coll Surg 197:182–190

31. Tisell LE (1998) Role of lymphadenectomy in the treatment of differentiated thyroid carcinomas. Br J Surg 85:1025–1026

32. Tisell LE, et al (1996) Improved survival of patients with papillary thyroid cancer after surgical microdissection. World J Surg 20:854–859

33. Cooper D, et al (2006) Treatment guidelines for patients with thyroid nodules and well-differentiated thyroid cancer. American Thyroid Association. Thyroid 16:109–42

34. Cooper DS, Schneyer CR (1990) Follicular and Hürthle cell carcinoma of the thyroid. Endocrinol Metab Clin North Am 19:577–591

35. Ron E, et al (1995) Thyroid cancer after exposure to external radiation: a pooled analysis of seven studies. Radiat Res 141:259–277

36. Ron E, Modan B (1980) Benign and malignant thyroid neoplasms after childhood irradiation for tinea capitis. J Natl Cancer Inst 65:7–11

37. Shore RE (1992) Issues and epidemiological evidence regarding radiation-induced thyroid cancer. Radiat Res 131:98–111

38. Shore RE, et al (1993) Thyroid cancer among persons given X-ray treatment in infancy for an enlarged thymus gland. Am J Epidemiol 137:1068–1080

39. Cetta F, et al (2001) Thyroid carcinoma usually occurs in patients with familial adenomatous polyposis in the absence of biallelic inactivation of the adenomatous polyposis coli gene. J Clin Endocrinol Metab 86:427–432

40. Cetta F, et al (2000) Germline mutations of the APC gene in patients with familial adenomatous polyposis-associated thyroid carcinoma: results from a European cooperative study. J Clin Endocrinol Metab 85:286–292

41. Bacher-Stier C, et al (1997) Incidence and clinical characteristics of thyroid carcinoma after iodine prophylaxis in an endemic goiter country. Thyroid 7:733–741

42. Mazzaferri EL, Jhiang SM (1994) Long-term impact of initial surgical and medical therapy on papillary and follicular thyroid cancer [see comment] [erratum appears in Am J Med 1995 98:215]. Am J Med 97:418–428

43. Akslen LA, LiVolsi VA (2000) Prognostic significance of histologic grading compared with subclassification of papillary thyroid carcinoma [see comment]. Cancer 88:1902–1908

44. Thompson NW, Nishiyama RH, Harness JK (1978) Thyroid carcinoma: current controversies. Curr Probl Surg 15:1–67

45. Clark OH, et al (1988) Thyroid cancer: the case for total thyroidectomy. Eur J Cancer Clin Oncol 24:305–313

46. Tartaglia F, et al (2003) Complications in total thyroidectomy: our experience and a number of considerations. Chir Ital 55:499–510

9 Modified Radical Neck Dissection

Robert Udelsman

9.1 Introduction

Neck dissections play an essential role in the management of head and neck cancer. Their role in the management of thyroid cancer is somewhat controversial and limited by the absence of prospective clinical trials. The dilemma is further complicated by the indolent history of most well-differentiated thyroid cancers and the common occurrence of both clinically significant and occult cervical lymph node metastases particularly in young patients with papillary carcinoma of the thyroid. A strong indication for modified radical neck dissection in the setting of well-differentiated thyroid cancer is the finding of cervical lymphadenopathy by either palpation or an imaging study. Confirmation of metastatic disease can be obtained by a preoperative fine-needle aspiration (FNA) which can be performed under ultrasound guidance.

Cervical lymphadenopathy is not uncommon in the setting of well-differentiated thyroid cancer. A recent series reported the frequent occurrence of metastases in both the central (64.1%) and lateral (44.5%) neck [1]. In the past many surgeons advocated local "berry picking" resections designed to remove grossly enlarged nodes [2,3]. These "berry picking" procedures are associated with a higher local recurrence rate necessitating remedial surgery that is associated with a higher complication rate [4]. The complication rate associated with functional neck dissections is no higher than that associated with "berry picking" procedures [4]. It is noteworthy that limited modified neck dissections in which the superior extent of surgery is limited to the spinal accessory nerve are also associated with residual and recurrent disease due to skip metastases [5]. A carefully performed modified radical neck dissection is well-tolerated and results in excellent cosmetic, functional, and oncologic outcomes [6,7].

The technique of radical neck dissection was described by George Crile in 1906 [8]. This extirpative procedure was often used in the setting of metastatic head and neck cancers, often of squamous cell origin, with metastases to the cervical lymph nodes. The operation encompassed removal of the cervical nodes and sacrifice of the internal jugular vein, spinal accessory and greater auricular nerves, as well as the sternocleidomastoid, digastric, and stylohyoid muscles. This radical neck dissection was modified to encompass an oncologically equivalent cervical lymphadenectomy while preserving functional structures including the sternocleidomastoid muscle, internal jugular vein, spinal accessory and greater auricular nerves, as well as the digastric and stylohyoid muscles. Accordingly, a modified radical neck dissection is also referred to as a functional or Bocca neck dissection [9].

Patients with thyroid cancer are usually treated with a total or near-total thyroidectomy followed by radioactive iodine therapy and life-long thyroid hormone suppression. A subset of patients either present with metastatic nodal disease or develop metachronous nodal disease later in their course. The most frequent sites of metastases are the central cervical nodes (level VI) bounded by the hyoid bone superiorly, the innominate vein inferiorly, and bilaterally by the carotid sheath [10]. Small lymph nodes are frequently encountered in this central region during initial thyroidectomy and should be resected when they are suspicious for metastatic disease as evidenced by enlargement, firmness, or irregularity by palpation.

A modified radical neck dissection refers to resection of the lymph nodes in levels II through V and often including the central nodes in level VI. This chapter describes the operation in detail. It can be performed as an isolated procedure or in combination with a total thyroidectomy. It can also be performed bilaterally. It is often performed for well-differentiated thyroid cancers, most commonly papillary carcinoma of the thyroid. Occasionally patients with follicular or Hürthle cell carcinoma also require modified neck dissections. Patients with medullary carcinoma of the thyroid present a unique set of challenges and, due to the absence of effective adjuvant therapy, surgery plays an even more dominant role in their management. Furthermore, medullary cancer of the thyroid has an early predilection for both central and lateral nodal dissemination. The detailed management plan for medullary carcinoma of the thyroid is beyond the scope of this chapter. The description of the operative procedure for a modified radical neck dissection performed in isolation is described, as the technique of thyroidectomy is illustrated in Chapter 7.

9.2   Operative Technique

The patient is placed on the operating table with the head extended and the neck and anterior chest are prepared for surgery (Fig. 9.1). An inflatable thyroid pillow is placed behind the patient's back. A linear incision is made that extends from the mid-neck as a continuation of a Kocher incision extending superiorly to approximately 1 inch below the left earlobe. If a bilateral neck dissection is required this incision is extended bilaterally and an apron flap is raised superiorly. Because the spinal accessory nerve is superficial it is important for the surgeon to note the surface landmarks depicting the course of the accessory nerve. If one were to connect a line between the angle of the mandible and the mastoid process and transect this line at a right angle in its mid-portion, the inferior course of that line would be a close approximation of the course of the spinal accessory nerve. It is well worth drawing this on the patient's skin at the time of surgery. The marginal mandibular nerve is protected superiorly but is rarely seen in this exposure. Once the incision is made skin hooks are utilized to develop the anterior flap which is raised with an electrocautery.

In Fig. 9.2 the anterior and posterior flaps are completed and the underlying anatomy is demonstrated. The anterior flap is created in the subplatysmal layer and developed as the skin is pulled toward the medial neck. Once the anterior flap has been developed, the posterior flap is developed. The sternocleidomastoid muscle, external jugular vein, and greater auricular nerve are shown. The greater auricular nerve anatomy is extremely important serving as a landmark as the nerve emerges from the lateral aspect of the sterno-

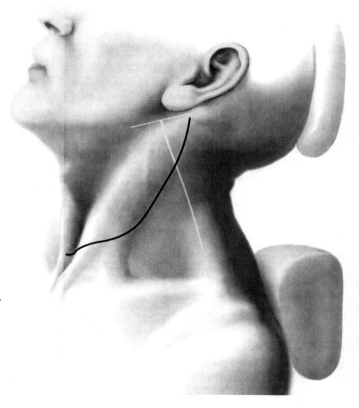

Fig. 9.1 An inflatable pillow is placed behind the patient's back and the head is extended and supported by a head ring. The course of the spinal accessory nerve is marked on the patient's skin. The most commonly employed incision for thyroid cancer is a continuation of a Kocher incision along the posterior border of the sternocleidomastoid muscle superiorly to approximately 1 inch below the ipsilateral ear lobe

cleidomastoid muscle at Erb's point. The nerve then traverses upward over the muscle going toward the earlobe. Preservation of this nerve is readily accomplished thereby preserving sensation to the earlobe. As the posterior flap is developed, great care and attention must be focused on protecting the spinal accessory nerve which is superior to the greater auricular nerve. The trapezius muscle is identified posterolaterally and the accessory nerve will course from behind the sternocleidomastoid muscle eventually innervating the trapezius muscle. A nerve stimulator is quite useful in locating the accessory nerve. Once the flaps have been completed, a self-retaining retractor is used to hold the skin and platysma in place. Frequently the skin is sewn to the retractor for added exposure. At this point, the external jugular vein is identified superiorly and ligated to form the apex of the tissues that will be unwrapped from the sternocleidomastoid muscle.

The fascial sheath covering the sternocleidomastoid muscle is shown being unwrapped in Fig. 9.3. The flap, once developed, is mobilized from superior to inferior (Fig. 9.4). Once this has been performed (Fig. 9.4) a Penrose drain is placed around the sternocleidomastoid muscle (note there are two heads, a sternal head and a clavicular head) and the muscle is pulled medially. If the patient is particularly muscular, it is useful to place separate drains around each head facilitating enhanced exposure. The omohyoid muscle is identified and deep to it the carotid sheath is located. A thin Penrose drain is placed around the omohyoid and in the majority of cases this muscle is preserved. The three structures of the sheath, the common carotid artery, vagus nerve, and internal jugular vein, are carefully protected. Frequently vessel loops are placed around these structures to assist with mobilization. One must be very careful not to injure the sympathetic trunk that lies deep to the common carotid artery as injury to this structure will result in Horner's syndrome. Occasionally, it is necessary to sacrifice the internal jugular vein due to tumor invasion; however, this is unusual in the setting of well-differentiated thyroid cancer. Maintaining the integrity of the anterior jugular veins is important as they become an effective collateral drainage system when the internal jugular vein is sacrificed.

At this point the cervical fat pad extending below the clavicle is mobilized from inferior to superior. The

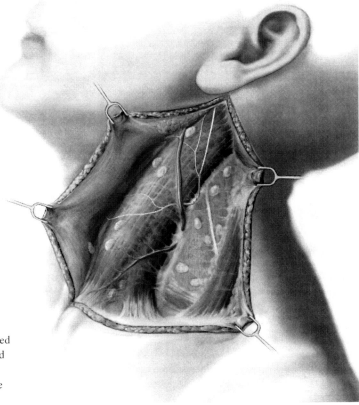

Fig. 9.2 The subplatysmal flaps have been developed anteriorly and posteriorly. The greater auricular and spinal accessory nerves have been identified and preserved. The sternocleidomastoid muscle and the external jugular vein are visualized

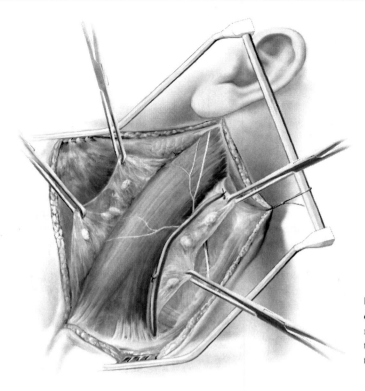

Fig. 9.3 The external jugular vein is ligated superiorly and the fascial sheath covering the sternocleidomastoid muscle is unwrapped. Lymph nodes along the great vessels of the neck are commonly encountered at this point

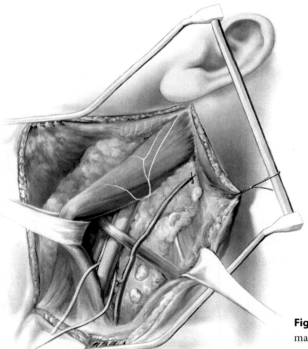

Fig. 9.4 A Penrose drain is placed around the sternocleidomastoid and the muscle is pulled anteriorly. The omohyoid muscle is preserved and the carotid sheath is identified

carotid sheath structures and particularly the thoracic duct are protected. An unrecognized injury to the thoracic duct can cause a troublesome postoperative lymphatic leak which often leads to a lymphocele and infection. It is prudent to tie the lymphatic tissues inferiorly to minimize lymphatic leaks.

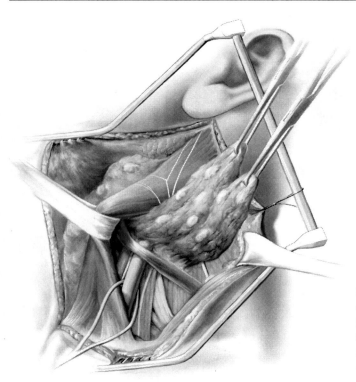

Fig. 9.5 The cervical fat pad containing lymphatics and nodes is mobilized from below the clavicle and pulled superiorly. The thoracic duct, phrenic nerve, and brachial plexus are protected. As the specimen is mobilized it is passed under the omohyoid muscle and traction is applied to the specimen superiorly

The next step is to identify the phrenic nerve which lies lateral to the vagus nerve (Fig. 9.5). This is an important landmark to identify as it innervates the diaphragm. It also represents the deep margin of the specimen lying superficial to the anterior scalene muscle. All superficial fat and lymph node-bearing tissues are resected anterior to the phrenic nerve as this block of tissue is swept from inferior to superior. The specimen is then passed beneath the omohyoid muscle as the dissection continues as shown and the specimen is pulled superiorly. The omohyoid muscle and phrenic nerve are shown, the brachial plexus is identified laterally, and superiorly the accessory nerve is seen. Branches of the transverse cervical nerves are usually sacrificed. However, it is not difficult to preserve one or more of these branches and thereby maintain sensation to the skin of the ipsilateral shoulder. The soft tissues underneath the accessory nerve are mobilized and included with the specimen.

Figure 9.6 shows the specimen has now been mobilized off the sternocleidomastoid muscle and has been passed from the lateral aspect of the muscle underneath the muscle belly anteriorly. At this point, a thyroid retractor is placed underneath the mandible and the mandible is pulled superiorly. The parotid and submandibular glands are preserved and the digastric muscle is identified. Inferior to the digastric muscle is the hypoglossal nerve which must be identified.

A useful trick to help locate the hypoglossal nerve is to follow the branch of the ansa cervicalis nerve as it courses superiorly along the anterior surface of the carotid artery until it joins the hypoglossal nerve at a right angle. Stimulation of the hypoglossal nerve will result in a movement of the tongue. In addition, the proximal accessory nerve must be identified at the medial aspect of the sternocleidomastoid muscle as soft tissues along the accessory nerve are included with the specimen. The nerve can be felt like a violin string if one distracts the sternocleidomastoid muscle posteriorly. It is extremely important to protect this nerve. All tissues inferior to the digastric muscle and hypoglossal nerve are resected in continuity with the specimen as the final tissues are removed from the great vessels and vagus nerve.

At the completion of the operation, shown in Fig. 9.7, a Penrose drain has been placed around the sternocleidomastoid muscle and the omohyoid muscle; the common carotid artery, vagus nerve, internal jugular vein, phrenic nerve, brachial plexus, accessory nerve, and greater auricular nerve are all preserved. Closure is obtained by reapproximating the platysma muscle with interrupted sutures and a subcuticular closure of the skin. A drain is always placed due to the extensive lymphadenectomy.

The operation is well-tolerated and the vast majority of patients are extubated in the operating room.

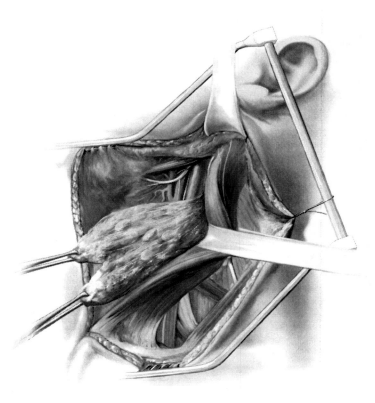

Fig. 9.6 The specimen is passed from its lateral position underneath the sternocleidomastoid muscle and is pulled from an inferior-medial direction. A thyroid retractor is used to pull the mandible superiorly and the digastric muscle is identified. The hypoglossal and proximal spinal accessory nerves are identified and preserved. The cervical fat tissues with their contained lymphatics are resected in continuity as the specimen is pulled off the great vessels

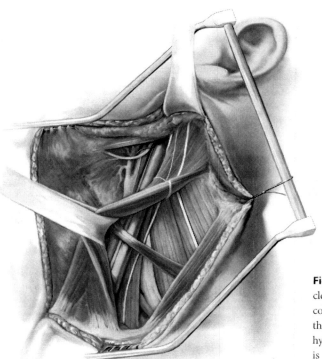

Fig. 9.7 The specimen has been removed. The sterno-cleidomastoid and omohyoid muscles are intact. The common carotid artery, internal jugular vein, as well as the vagus, phrenic, spinal accessory, greater auricular, and hypoglossal nerves are all preserved. The brachial plexus is intact

References

1. Wada N, et al (2003) Lymph node metastases from 259 papillary thyroid microcarcinomas. Ann Surg 237:399–407
2. Raina S, et al (1983) Current attitudes in the management of thyroid cancer. Am Surg 49:110–112
3. Nicolosi A, et al (1993) The role of node-picking lymphadenectomy in the treatment of differentiated carcinoma of the thyroid. Minerva Chir 48:459–463
4. Munacchio MJ, et al (2003) Greater local recurrence occurs with "berry picking" than neck dissection in thyroid cancer. Am Surg 69:191–197
5. Pingpank JF, et al (2002) Tumor above the spinal accessory nerve in papillary thyroid cancer that involves lateral neck nodes. Arch Otolaryngol Head Neck Surg 128:1275–1278
6. Gemsenjäger E, et al (2003) Lymph node surgery in papillary carcinoma. J Am Coll Surg 197:182–190
7. Kupferman ME, et al (2004) Safety of modified radical neck dissection for differentiated thyroid carcinoma. Laryngoscope 114:403–406
8. Crile G (1906) Excision of cancer of the head and neck. JAMA 47:1786–1789
9. Bocca E, et al (1980) Functional neck dissection: a description of operative technique. Arch Otolaryngol 106:524–527
10. Greene FL, et al (eds) (2002) AJCC cancer staging manual, 6th edn. Springer, New York, pp 77–87

10 Thyroid Pathology

Zubair W. Baloch and Virginia A. LiVolsi

10.1   Normal Thyroid

The normal thyroid is a bilobed gland, connected by an isthmus. It is encased by a thin capsule that does not strip easily and contains sizable venous channels. The weight of normal thyroid in the United States ranges from 10 to 20 g. The follicle is the functional unit of the thyroid and averages about 20 μm in diameter [1,2,3,4]. A thyroid lobule consists of 20–40 follicles bound together by a thin sheath of connective tissue and supplied by a lobular artery [3,5]. The thyroid follicles are formed by a single layer of low cuboidal epithelium. The nucleus of the follicular cell is round to ovoid in shape; it is usually centrally placed with an inconspicuous nucleolus. The follicle is enveloped by a basal lamina and is surrounded by numerous capillaries and lymphatics [5,6]. The follicular lumen contains colloid, partly composed of thyroglobulin, which is evenly applied to the luminal cell borders. Calcium oxalate crystals are common in the colloid of adults.

Electron microscopy demonstrates that the normal flat to low cuboidal follicular cells interdigitate and overlap one another, and that they are intimately related to the capillaries that surround the follicle; microvilli on the apical surface are numerous near the cellular margins [6,7].

C cells are intrafollicular and are seen next to the follicular cells and within the basal lamina that surrounds each follicle of the normal gland. C cells are most numerous in the central portions of the middle and upper thirds of the thyroid lobes [3]. They are believed to originate from the C cells that arise from the neural crest and migrate with the ultimobranchial body into the thyroid. C cells are typically more numerous in thyroids of infants as compared to adult glands [8,9]. They are polygonal to spindle shaped, have "light" or low density, cytoplasm, and contain numerous membrane-bound cytoplasmic granules containing calcitonin. A small number of C cells (or cells similar to them) contain somatostatin and can increase in number in some patients [10–13].

C cell aggregates can be sizeable (hyperplastic) in some adults without any known endocrinologic abnormality [14]. C cell hyperplasia is defined as consisting of more than 40 C cells/cm² and the presence of at least three low-power microscopic fields containing more than 50 C cells [15]. The small solid cell nests of ovoid to spindled epidermoid cells in thyroid are also considered to be of ultimobranchial origin [15]. Typically, the nests have about the same distribution in the thyroid lobes as the C cells [16,17]. The term "mixed follicles" [18] applies to follicles which are lined by follicular cells and epidermoid cells (and sometimes C cells) and contain both colloid and mucoid material. The ultimobranchial structures probably also give rise to a small proportion of normal thyroid follicles [18].

Oxyphil cells (oncocytes, Askanazy cells, Hürthle cells) are altered/metaplastic follicular cells; they are enlarged, have granular eosinophilic cytoplasm, and have large, hyperchromatic, or bizarre nuclei [19]. The cytoplasm is filled with enlarged mitochondria. They are common in longstanding Graves' disease, autoimmune thyroiditis, thyroids affected by radiation, follicular-derived neoplasms, and some adenomatous nodules [19–21].

Small aggregates of lymphoid cells in the thyroid stroma can be seen in normal thyroid gland [22]. Also present in the interstitial tissue are antigen-presenting dendritic cells; these are sparse in the normal gland but are increased in autoimmune thyroid disease [23,24].

10.2   Developmental Variations

The thyroglossal tract extends in the midline from the foramen cecum at the base of the tongue to the isthmus of the normal gland [25]. The tract consists of connective tissue, the thyroglossal duct, lymphoid tissue, and thyroid follicles; it is attached to and may extend through the center of the hyoid bone and is intimately related to the surrounding skeletal muscle. Thyroid tissue may persist at the base of the tongue and in some patients may be the only thyroid present [25,26]. The thyroglossal duct is typically lined by ciliated pseudostratified epithelium. If the duct is traumatized or infected, the epithelium may undergo alteration to transitional or squamous type, or maybe totally be replaced by fibrous tissue. Foreign body reaction and chronic inflammation may be conspicuous. If fluid accumulates in part of the thyroglossal duct, a thyroglossal cyst may develop [3,27,28].

Any type of diffuse thyroid disease can involve lingual thyroid and the thyroid tissue along the thyroglossal tract [28–30]. In rare instances portions of thyroglossal duct are included within the thyroid

gland proper and, rarely, can serve as the origin of an intrathyroidal cyst [25]. Parathyroid glands, thymic tissue, small collections of cartilage, and glands lined by ciliated cells may be seen in normal thyroids, presumably related to defective development of the branchial pouches [31–33].

Because of the intimate relationship that exists in the embryo between the immature thyroid tissue and the adjacent developing skeletal muscle, strips of striated muscle are occasionally included within the thyroid [34–36].

Thyroid tissue can be found in close proximity or within the perithyroidal skeletal muscle. Such collections of thyroid tissue are particularly prominent when the gland is hyperplastic or is affected by chronic lymphocytic thyroiditis; these should not be confused with carcinoma [34,37].

Groups of thyroid follicles in lateral cervical lymph nodes always represent metastatic carcinoma (papillary carcinoma) [34,37,38]. A few experienced pathologists state normal thyroid follicles rarely occur in cervical lymph nodes [39]. Hence normal thyroid tissue lying only within the capsule of a midline node may represent an embryologic remnant and not metastatic cancer [39,40].

10.3   Goiter

Goiter is a diffuse or nodular enlargement of the gland usually resulting from a benign process or a process of unknown origin [41–43]. When there is a deficiency of circulating thyroid hormone because of inborn errors of metabolism, iodine deficiency, or goitrogenic agents, and if the hypothalamic-pituitary axis is intact, production of thyroid-stimulating hormone (TSH; thyrotropin) is increased; consequently, cellular activity and increased glandular activity and glandular mass result in an attempt to achieve the euthyroid state [43–45].

Worldwide, the most common cause for a deficient output of thyroid hormone is an inadequate amount of iodine in the diet, leading to iodine-deficiency goiter (endemic goiter) [46,47]. Other causes of hyperplasia include inborn errors of thyroid metabolism (dyshormonogenetic goiter) [48,49], dietary goitrogens, and goitrogenic drugs and chemicals [50–53].

The pathologic changes of simple non-toxic goiter include one or more of the following: (1) hyperplasia, (2) colloid accumulation, and (3) nodularity [41,54,55]. Hyperplasia represents the response of the thyroid follicular cells to TSH, other growth factors, or to circulating stimulatory antibodies [34,55,56]. The hyperplasia may compensate for thyroid hormonal deficiency, but in some cases, even severe hyperplasia does not lead to sufficient hormonal output to avoid development of hypothyroidism.

If the deficiency of thyroid hormone occurs at birth or early in life, cretinism or juvenile myxedema may result, even though the gland is enlarged and hyperplastic; this is especially likely when an inborn error of thyroidal metabolism is present [57,58]. A hyperplastic gland is diffusely enlarged, and not nodular [34,41,56].

Thyroid follicles are collapsed and contain only scanty colloid. The follicular cells are enlarged and columnar in shape with nuclear enlargement, hyperchromasia, and even pleomorphism. When the hyperplastic stage is extreme and prolonged, there may be confusion with carcinoma because of the degree of cellularity and the presence of enlarged cells. Because of follicular collapse and epithelial hyperplasia and hypertrophy, papillary formation can occur [59]. This pattern occurs most often in untreated dyshormonogenetic goiter [48]. The recognition of the benign nature of this process is possible because of its diffuse nature [59], unlike carcinoma, in which the tumors grow as localized groups of abnormal cells with a background of non-neoplastic parenchyma.

Thyroid follicles may not remain in a state of continuous hyperplasia but instead undergo a process called involution, with the hyperplastic follicles reaccumulating colloid. The epithelium becomes low cuboidal or flattened and resembles that of the normal gland. The gland is diffusely enlarged, soft, and has a glistening cut surface because of the excess of stored colloid. In addition to large follicles filled with colloid, there are foci in the gland where hyperplasia is still evident (Fig. 10.1). This phase of non-toxic goiter is often termed colloid goiter [60,61].

Patients with long-standing thyroid disorders associated with deficiency of circulating thyroid hormone typically develop nodular goiters that result from overdistention of some involuted follicles, and persistence of the zones of epithelial hyperplasia. The new follicles form nodules and may be heterogeneous in their appearance, in their capacity for growth and function, and in their responsiveness to TSH. The vascular network is altered through the elongation and distortion of vessels leading to hemorrhage, necrosis, inflammation, and fibrosis. These localized degenerative and reparative changes produce some nodules that are poorly circumscribed, and others that are well demarcated and resemble true adenomas (adenomatous goiter) [62,63]. Because the nodules distort vascular supply to some areas of the gland, some zones will contain larger than normal amounts of TSH and/or iodide and others will have relative

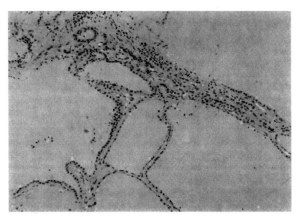

Fig. 10.1 Thyroid follicles lined by low cuboidal epithelium and expanded by thin colloid consistent with colloid goiter

TSH and/or iodide deficiency. Growth of goiters therefore may be related to focally excess stimulation by TSH, stimulation by growth factors, focally abnormal iodide concentration, growth-promoting thyroid antibodies, and poorly understood intrathyroidal factors [47].

Nodular goiter is essentially a process involving the entire gland, but the nodularity may be asymmetric, and individual nodules within the same gland may vary greatly in size. If one nodule is much larger or more prominent than the others (dominant nodule), distinguishing it from a true neoplasm (such as adenoma) may not be possible [37,63]. Several studies have shown that about 70% of dominant nodules in nodular goiter are indeed clonal proliferations [64,65]. The formation of cysts, hemorrhage, fibrosis, and calcification further complicates the assessment of the gland [34,37].

The heterogeneity of the generations of replicating follicular cells, in response to outside stimuli, functional capacity, and rate of growth, forms groups of cells that are hyperfunctional or autonomous, or both. These form "hot" nodules that may cause hyperthyroidism (Plummer's disease) [66].

10.3.1 Graves' Disease

This disorder is also termed diffuse toxic goiter; it is characterized by diffuse enlargement of the thyroid up to several times normal size. The capsule is smooth and the gland is hyperemic. The cut surfaces are fleshy and lack normal translucence because of loss of colloid. If the patient is untreated, the microscopic appearance shows cellular hypertrophy and hyperplasia [34,67]. The follicular cells are tall columnar and are arranged into papillary formations that extend into

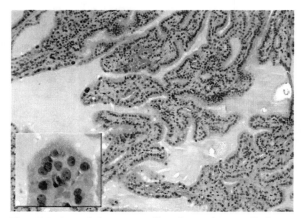

Fig. 10.2 Graves' disease, papillary hyperplasia. Cells lining the papillae show eosinophilic cytoplasm and round nuclei with even chromatin pattern (*inset*)

the lumina of the follicles (Fig. 10.2). Blood vessels are congested. At the ultrastructural level, microvilli are increased in number and elongated, the Golgi apparatus and endoplasmic reticulum are enlarged, and mitochondria are numerous [56,67]. Lymphoid infiltrates are seen between the follicles, ranging from minimal to extensive. T cells predominate among the epithelial cells (cytotoxic suppressor cells) and in the interstitial tissue (helper inducer cells) where there are no lymphoid follicles [68]. B cells are numerous in the lymphoid follicles. Class II major histocompatibility complex antigens are expressed on the epithelial cells, and these epithelial cells induce the proliferation of T cells, helping to perpetuate the process [68–71].

Lymphoid hyperplasia may occur elsewhere in the body: thymus, lymph nodes, and spleen [72,73].

Because nearly all patients now receive antithyroid medication before surgery, the glands can display varying degrees of involution. In some cases they appear almost normal except for numerous large follicles filled with colloid. A few papillae may remain. The hyperemia is notably decreased, especially if there has been preoperative administration of iodide [63]. If the patient has only been treated for symptoms, i.e., with beta-blockers, the histology of the gland resembles that of the untreated state [74,75].

If hyperplasia continues for many months or several years, oxyphilic/oncocytic metaplasia of the cells begins to occur, the amount of stroma increases in an irregular fashion, and nodularity develops, just as in euthyroid goiter. If the process subsides spontaneously or because of the maintenance on antithyroid medication, the involution may be remarkably complete or irregular (with some foci of hyperplasia evident) [74,75].

In some patients the lymphocytic infiltration is very prominent and resembles the gland affected by chronic lymphocytic thyroiditis [34].

10.3.2   Dyshormonogenetic Goiter

When an inborn error of thyroid metabolism exists, and a sufficient amount of circulating thyroid hormone is not available, the normal physiologic response of the pituitary to increase TSH causes a larger, more active thyroid that may or may not be able to produce enough hormones to reach a euthyroid state. The prolonged and marked TSH stimulation leads to an enlarged and nodular thyroid; microscopically there is enlargement of follicular cells, virtual absence of colloid, and increased stroma [49,76].

Large follicular cells with bizarre, hyperchromatic nuclei may be numerous. The enlarged gland, the bizarre cells, and the cellular nodules have at times been mistaken for carcinoma [48] (Fig. 10.3). Cancer can occur in a dyshormonogenetic goiter, but it is very rare [48,77].

10.3.3   Iatrogenic and Related Hyperplasias

Chronic ingestion of excess iodide, for whatever reason, occasionally leads to diffuse hyperplasia. Small nodules with papillary formations may be numerous. Infiltration of lymphocytes may occur [78].

About 3% of patients given lithium salts for a prolonged period develop goiter or hypothyroidism, or both. Patients so treated have been reported to have diffuse hyperplasia with considerable cellular and nuclear pleomorphism [79].

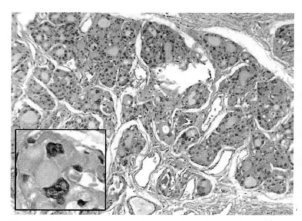

Fig. 10.3 Dyshormonogenetic goiter. Variably sized aggregates of follicular cells and enlarged pleomorphic nuclei (*inset*)

Bromide ingestion may lead to hypothyroidism because of loss of iodide from the gland. This leads to hyperplastic C cells, foci of papillary proliferation, and loss of colloid [80].

10.4 The Thyroiditides

Although occasionally presenting as nodules or asymmetric enlargement of the gland, thyroiditis commonly involves the thyroid diffusely.

10.4.1 Acute Thyroiditis

Acute thyroiditis is rare and is almost always due to infection, although acute thyroiditis may be encountered in the thyroid shortly following radiation exposure [81,82]. The disease is most commonly encountered in malnourished children, elderly debilitated adults, immunocompromised individuals, or in otherwise healthy patients following trauma to the neck [81,83]. Most patients present with painful enlargement of the gland. Microscopically acute inflammation with microabscess formation is present. Microorganisms may be seen. A variety of organisms cause thyroiditis including bacteria, fungi, and viruses [84].

10.4.2 Granulomatous Thyroiditis

Granulomatous subacute thyroiditis, also referred to as non-suppurative thyroiditis or de Quervain's disease, is a rare entity that usually presents in women and has been associated with HLA Bw35 [85]. The changes seen in the gland are most likely due to the response of the thyroid to systemic viral infection [86–88]; some authors suggest that it represents actual viral infection of the gland. Most patients with subacute thyroiditis recover without any permanent damage to the thyroid. However, some studies have reported end stage hypothyroidism in 5–9% of patients [89]. Microscopically, early in the disease, there is loss of the follicular epithelium and colloid depletion. The inflammatory response, composed initially of polymorphonuclear leukocytes and even microabscesses, progresses until lymphocytes, plasma cells, and histiocytes become the major inflammatory cells. A rim of histiocytes and giant cells replaces the follicular epithelium. A central fibrotic reaction occurs [90]. Recovery is associated with regeneration of follicles from the viable edges of the involved areas [91].

10.4.3 Palpation Thyroiditis

Palpation thyroiditis (multifocal granulomatous folliculitis) is found in 85–95% of surgically resected thyroids, and probably represents the thyroid's response to minor trauma. The histologic features of this lesion include multiple isolated follicles or small groups of follicles that show partial or circumferential loss of epithelium and replacement of the lost epithelium by inflammatory cells, predominantly macrophages [92,93].

10.4.4 Autoimmune Thyroiditis

Common synonyms for autoimmune thyroiditis include Hashimoto's thyroiditis, lymphocytic thyroiditis, and struma lymphomatosa [94]. The disorder, most common in women, encompasses a spectrum of clinical and pathologic changes, ranging from an absence of symptoms of thyroid dysfunction to hypothyroidism and rarely, hyperthyroidism, from a large goiter to an atrophic gland, and from scattered clusters of infiltrating lymphocytes to extensive chronic inflammation and scarring with almost complete loss of follicular epithelium [94,95].

Various circulating antithyroid antibodies and other immune phenomena occur, including in situ immune complex deposition and basement membrane changes in the gland and expression of major histocompatibility complex antigens on the thyroid cells [96,97]. The thyroiditis may be found in the same families in which idiopathic hypothyroidism and Graves' disease are common. It may follow typical Graves' disease [98].

The hyperthyroid variant of autoimmune thyroiditis is closely related to Graves' disease and may be almost identical in its gross and microscopic appearance to the latter condition, suggesting that this variant may indeed be Graves' disease [99].

The presence of lymphoid cells in the substance of the thyroid parenchyma probably reflects an abnormal immunologic state. However, the interrelationships among classic chronic thyroiditis, its variants, and "non-specific" thyroiditis are problematic [34]. The morphologic and immunopathologic overlap between non-specific lymphocytic thyroiditis and Hashimoto's disease suggest that they represent a spectrum of autoimmune injury [34,94,100].

In Hashimoto's thyroiditis the gland is firm and symmetrically enlarged weighing from 25 to 250 g [94]. The thyroid has a tan yellow appearance attributed to the abundant lymphoid tissue. The thyroid

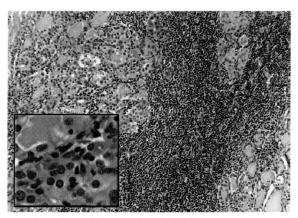

Fig. 10.4 Chronic lymphocytic thyroiditis (Hashimoto's thyroiditis). Oncocytic follicular cells (*inset* showing high power) arranged in nodular pattern with a concomitant lymphocytic infiltrate

follicles are small and atrophic. Colloid appears dense or may be absent. Follicular cells are metaplastic and include oncocytic (Hürthle cell), clear cell, and squamous types. In the stroma and in atrophic follicles, a lymphoplasmacytic infiltration with well-developed germinal centers is found (Fig. 10.4). Variable degrees of interlobular fibrosis are seen [34,94]. The lymphocytic infiltrate is composed of both T and B cells in an almost 1:1 ratio; this differs from the peripheral blood, which shows T cell predominance [101–103]. T lymphocytes within the thyroid are predominantly suppressor type [104,105], whereas the peripheral blood of these patients contains mostly helper T cells. The B cells are usually of the IgG kappa subclass [103].

Patients with Hashimoto's thyroiditis are at increased risk of neoplasia with the most common malignancy being malignant lymphoma, B cell type [106,107]. In addition, patients with Hashimoto's disease may be prone to the development of plasmacytomas within the gland [107]. A peculiar variant of mucoepidermoid carcinoma known as sclerosing mucoepidermoid carcinoma with eosinophilia has been recognized in patients with Hashimoto's disease [108].

10.4.5 Chronic Lymphocytic Thyroiditis Classification

Mizukami et al. established a new classification of chronic lymphocytic thyroiditis [94]. This classification is useful because it allows one to see that the mere presence of lymphocytes in the thyroid does not

indicate autoimmune disease. They basically divided their patients into four groups:

1. *Chronic thyroiditis, oxyphilic.* This group contains patients with classic Hashimoto's disease histology.
2. *Chronic thyroiditis, mixed.* This group shows less of an infiltrate than group 1 with minimal fibrosis. Patients demonstrate either eu-, hyper-, or hypothyroidism.
3. *Chronic thyroiditis, hyperplastic.* This group shows glandular hyperplasia associated with only a small lymphocytic reaction. Most patients are hyperthyroid.
4. *Chronic thyroiditis, focal.* This group shows only a focal lymphocytic reaction and most patients are euthyroid.

10.4.6 Fibrosing Variant of Hashimoto's Thyroiditis

The fibrous or fibrosing variant of Hashimoto's thyroiditis comprises approximately 10–13% of all cases of Hashimoto's disease. Pathologically, the thyroid architecture is destroyed with severe follicular atrophy, dense keloid-like fibrosis, and prominent squamous or epidermoid metaplasia of the follicular epithelium [109,110]. Surgery in this setting can be extremely difficult.

10.4.7 Painless/Silent Thyroiditis

Painless thyroiditis is an autoimmune disease that causes painless enlargement of the thyroid gland along with brief hyperthyroidism followed by hypothyroidism. It can occur in the postpartum period and is termed postpartum thyroiditis [111–113]. Most cases show follicular disruption and lymphocytic infiltration, but stromal fibrous and oxyphilic changes are rare [111].

10.4.8 Focal Non-specific Thyroiditis

Lymphocytic infiltration of the thyroid is found more frequently at autopsy and in surgical specimens since the addition of iodide to the water supplies of the United States about 60 years ago [114,115]. It has been suggested that iodide (iodine) may combine with a protein, act as an antigen, and evoke an immune response localized to the thyroid gland [116]. Postmortem studies indicate an incidence of focal lymphocytic thyroiditis of about 15–20% in women and rarely in men [114]. These cases show focal aggregates of lymphocytes, occasional germinal center formation, but oncocytes are rarely present. Follicular atrophy is also rare [100].

10.4.9 Riedel's Thyroiditis

Riedel's thyroiditis (Riedel's disease, invasive fibrous thyroiditis, Riedel's struma) has been incorrectly included among the thyroiditides [117]. This is really not a disorder of the thyroid but one that involves the thyroid as well as other structures in the neck or even systemic structures; sclerosing mediastinitis, retroperitoneal fibrosis, pseudotumor of the orbit, and sclerosis of the biliary tract (sclerosing cholangitis) [118–121]. Riedel's disease is an extremely rare entity with an incidence of 0.05% of surgical thyroid diseases and showing a female predominance [122]. Most patients are euthyroid, although hypothyroidism and hyperthyroidism have been reported [117,122].

Descriptions of the thyroid range from stony hard to woody fixed ("ligneous" thyroiditis). Histologically, the involved portions of the gland are destroyed and replaced by keloid-like fibrous tissue associated with lymphocytes and plasma cells [122,123]. The fibrous tissue extends into muscle, nerves, and fat, and entraps blood vessels. In about 25% of cases, the parathyroid glands are also encased [123,124]. There is an associated vasculitis (predominantly a phlebitis) with frequent thrombosis [125].

Quantitative studies of the immunoglobulin-containing cells in fibrous Hashimoto's thyroiditis show that cells containing kappa light chains outnumber lambda-containing cells (64% versus 36%) whereas in Riedel's disease lambda-containing cells comprise >70% of the immunocyte population. In Hashimoto's thyroiditis, IgA cells make up about 15% of the lymphocytes, whereas IgA-containing plasma cells comprise about 45% of the immunocyte population in Riedel's disease. The immunologic evaluation supports the separation of the distinctive Riedel's lesion from other thyroiditides [126].

10.4.10 Combined Riedel's Disease and Hashimoto's Thyroiditis

In rare instances the thyroid gland can show features of both Riedel's disease and Hashimoto's thyroiditis. The histologic picture resembles Riedel's disease, whereas the serology shows thyroglobulin and microsomal antibodies seen in Hashimoto's thyroiditis [127].

10.5 Amiodarone Injury with Thyrotoxicosis

Administration of amiodarone may cause thyrotoxicosis, primarily due to the large quantity of iodine in the drug [78,128]. Tissue changes are usually focal. Groups of follicles contain degenerated follicular cells (with granular or vacuolated cytoplasm); some follicles have lost follicular cells, and there is partial or complete loss of colloid. Zones of fibrosis are evident. The intervening thyroid tissue is normal [129].

10.6 Miscellaneous Disorders

10.6.1 Radiation Effects

Ionizing radiation delivered in small doses to the thyroid glands of infants, children, and adolescents causes a marked increase in the later incidence of benign and malignant neoplasms [130]. Larger doses produce more numerous nodules; many of these nodules are particularly cellular, and some are atypical in their structure and cytologic features, suggesting premalignant characteristics [131]. The cancers that develop after small doses of radiation are mostly papillary carcinomas, are often multicentric or bilateral, and are frequently small [130]. In addition to the nodules and neoplasms that occur, other changes are believed to be more common as well, including focal epithelial hyperplasia (possibly incipient nodules), chronic lymphocytic thyroiditis, oxyphilic metaplasia of follicular cells, and slight fibrosis [132,133].

Large doses of ionizing radiation (e.g., therapeutic radiation for head and neck cancer, or radioiodine therapy) can initially cause vascular injury and follicular cell necrosis. Hemorrhages, edema, and small numbers of the usual inflammatory cells appear. The damaged is healed by scarring and the follicular epithelium can show a mixture of atrophic, hyperplastic, and metaplastic changes [134,135].

10.6.2 Amyloidosis

The thyroid may be involved by primary or secondary amyloidosis. The amyloid deposition may be sufficiently uneven to produce a mass. Such an accumulation must be differentiated from that occurring in some cases of medullary carcinoma [136,137].

10.6.3 Black Thyroid

Prolonged therapy with tetracycline antibiotics, especially minocycline, may cause the accumulation of sufficient pigment in the follicular cells to produce a dark brown to black gland. Much of the pigment is lipofuscin, but part may be a metabolite of the drug. Rarely, there may be interference with thyroid function [138,139].

10.7 Neoplasms

Thyroid neoplasms demonstrate a variety of morphologic patterns that complicate their pathologic interpretation [140]. All neoplasms that arise from thyroid epithelial cells may have some functional capacities. They may respond to TSH and may even produce excessive amounts of thyroid hormones or, if medullary carcinoma, release abnormal quantities of calcitonin or other hormones [34]. Localization of thyroglobulin or calcitonin by immunohistochemistry aids in the classification of unusual thyroidal tumors and in providing definite identification of metastatic thyroid carcinomas [37].

10.7.1 Benign Neoplasms

10.7.1.1 Adenomas and Adenomatous Nodules

A follicular adenoma or solitary adenomatous or adenomatoid nodule is defined as a benign encapsulated mass of follicles, usually showing a uniform pattern throughout the confined nodule [35,37]. Follicular adenomas with papillary hyperplasia (some of which are functional) should not be classified as papillary adenomas [141], but as papillary hyperplastic nodules [142]. Adenomas are solitary; indeed, if there are multiple nodules in a lobe or a thyroid gland, it is probably more appropriate to diagnose multinodular goiter with adenomatous change (adenomatous hyperplasia). The features that distinguish histologically between adenoma and adenomatous nodules included encapsulation, uniformity of pattern within the adenoma, and compression of the surrounding gland by the adenoma and its capsule (Fig. 10.5) [143].

Descriptive terms that have been used to delineate the patterns seen in follicular adenomas include macrofollicular, simple, microfollicular, fetal, embryonal,

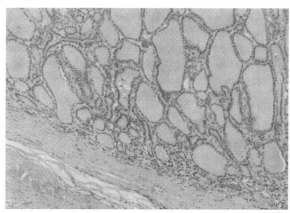

Fig. 10.5 Follicular adenoma. Thinly encapsulated follicular patterned lesion and lack of capsular or vascular invasion

and trabecular [35]. However, since these patterns have no clinical importance, it is not necessary to subdivide thyroid adenomas. Relatively common changes found in adenomas include hemorrhage, edema, and fibrosis, especially in the central portions of the tumor [35]. Calcification may be seen. Lesions that have undergone fine-needle aspiration biopsy may show necrosis, increased mitotic activity, and cellular atypia in the area of the needle tract [144].

Whether or not some solitary follicular nodules have the biologic potential to become carcinoma is unknown; the findings of aneuploid cell populations in 27% of such lesions suggest that some of these may represent carcinoma in situ [145,146]. The solitary follicular lesion that is removed by lobectomy and when adequately studied shows no evidence of invasion, will neither recur nor metastasize [35]. (Enucleation of follicular adenomas or nodulectomy should be condemned as a surgical procedure and considered suboptimal care. The pathologic evaluation of these lesions requires analysis of the tumor capsule–thyroid interface [143].)

Hyalinizing Trabecular Adenoma/Neoplasm of the Thyroid

The hyalinizing trabecular adenoma is a distinct patterned follicular-derived lesion of the thyroid; i.e., it expresses thyroglobulin, thyroid transcription factor (TTF1) and not calcitonin [147]. Microscopically, these adenomas grow in nests that are surrounded by dense hyaline stroma. The nested histology of the tumor cells is reminiscent of that seen in paragangliomas (thus termed by some authors as paraganglioma-like adenoma of thyroid—PLAT) [148]. The nuclear features of the follicular cells are similar to those seen

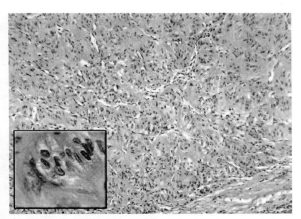

Fig. 10.6 Hyalinizing trabecular neoplasm. Tumor mainly of elongated cells (*inset*) and hyalinized stroma

in papillary carcinoma (Fig. 10.6) [149]. By immunohistochemistry, the cells of hyalinizing trabecular adenoma stain positive for thyroglobulin and cytokeratin 19 and negative for calcitonin, although the presence of other neuroendocrine markers has been described [150].

Some authors have proposed that these adenomas actually represent a variant of papillary carcinoma. This is due to similar nuclear cytology, immunoprofile, and RET oncogene rearrangements in both tumors [151]. However, a benign behavior has so far been described in all cases of hyalinizing trabecular adenoma. Therefore, we believe until metastatic behavior is described in a case of hyalinizing trabecular adenoma with classic histology, these tumors can be designated as hyalinizing trabecular neoplasm as proposed by the World Health Organization [149].

Atypical Follicular Adenoma

The term atypical follicular adenoma includes those follicular tumors that show pathologically disturbing features (spontaneous necrosis, infarction, numerous mitoses, or unusual cellularity), but do not show invasive characteristics on careful examination. The overwhelming majority of the atypical adenomas behave in a benign fashion clinically [152–154].

10.7.2   Malignant Neoplasms

The most common malignant neoplasms of the thyroid origin are the well-differentiated carcinomas of follicular epithelial origin: up to 80% of these are papillary carcinomas [35]. Most non-neoplastic diseases of the thyroid do not seem to be precursors of malignant diseases, with the exception that autoimmune thyroiditis may predispose to malignant lymphoma [37]. Anaplastic carcinomas have often arisen in goitrous thyroids, and careful examination of the resected tissues has frequently demonstrated benign tumors or well-differentiated carcinomas in close association with the anaplastic neoplasm. Such findings have led to suggestions that the benign tumor or low-grade carcinoma can "transform" into the anaplastic carcinoma [155].

10.7.2.1 Papillary Carcinoma

This is the most common malignant tumor of the gland in countries having iodine-sufficient or iodine-excess diets, and comprises about 80% of thyroid malignancies in the United States [156–158]. Papillary thyroid carcinoma (PTC) clinically behaves in an indolent fashion and carries an excellent prognosis (>90% survival at 20 years) [158]. It invades lymphatics leading to multifocal lesions and to regional lymph node metastases [156,158]. Venous invasion rarely occurs and metastases outside the neck are unusual (5–7% of cases) [159].

Papillary thyroid carcinoma can occur at any age and rarely has been diagnosed as a congenital tumor [160]. Most tumors are diagnosed in patients in the third and fifth decades. Women are affected more than men in ratios of 2:1 to 4:1 [161].

Etiologic Factors

Etiologic factors for PTC are not well established; various cellular and genetic mechanisms/targets have been studied in the development of PTC.

Iodide

The addition of iodine to the diet in endemic goiter areas in Europe has been associated with a decreased incidence of follicular cancer and an increase in PTC [162,163].

External Radiation

External radiation probably plays a role in the development of PTC [164,165]. The average time from radiation exposure to tumor development has classically been reported as 20 years; however, development time can be variable [130,165]. The Chernobyl nuclear accident has induced a great increase in the incidence of PTC in Belarus, Russia, and Ukraine [130]. The increased incidence is seen predominantly in young children. Most reported tumors following this nuclear disaster have been PTC, some of which show aggressive features including extracapsular extension and vascular invasion; however, mortality is extremely low [130,166].

Autoimmune Disease

Many studies indicate that up to one third of PTCs arise in the setting of chronic thyroiditis. Follow-up studies of patients with documented thyroiditis indicate that the tumor that arises much more frequently in these glands is malignant lymphoma, not PTC (see below) [167]. Since papillary cancer and thyroiditis are both common conditions, the possibility of coincidental coexistence is more likely than an etiologic relationship [167,168]. However, loss of heterozygosity for various tumor suppressor genes has been demonstrated in the cytologically atypical areas/nodules in chronic lymphocytic thyroiditis [169]. Thus, a link may exists between chronic lymphocytic thyroiditis and PTC.

Hormonal and Reproductive Factors

Papillary thyroid carcinoma is more common in women than men. Some studies have suggested the role of various hormonal factors in the development of PTC; these include increased parity, late age at the onset of first pregnancy, fertility problems, and oral contraceptives [170]. However, studies of steroid hormone receptors have been disappointing since about 50% of normal thyroid, and benign and malignant nodules can contain estrogen and/or progesterone receptors and smaller numbers of androgen receptors. No correlation with age or gender has been identified [171].

Genetic Syndromes

Papillary carcinomas have been described in patients with familial adenomatous polyposis coli (FAP), Cowden's syndrome, non-polyposis colon cancer syndrome (HNPCC), Peutz Jeghers' syndrome, and ataxia telangiectasia [172–174].

Familial adenomatous polyposis coli is caused by germline mutations of adenomatous polyposis coli (APC) gene. PTC (>95% of cases) occurs in 12% of patients with FAP; all these patients do show germline mutations of the APC gene, however, somatic mutations or loss of heterozygosity for the APC gene are not found in thyroid tumors. Interestingly, a majority of these tumors do show activation of ret/ptc1 in thyroid tumors suggesting a possible association between APC and ret/ptc in the development of this particular subset of familial papillary carcinoma [172–177].

Cowden's syndrome is characterized by formation of hamartomas in several organs and a high risk of developing breast and thyroid cancer. The genetic locus for Cowden's syndrome has been mapped to chromosome 10q23.3 and is also known as PTEN, which is a protein tyrosine phosphatase and exerts its tumor suppressor effects by antagonizing protein tyrosine kinase activity. Interestingly, PTEN mutation or gene deletion is noted in 26% of benign tumors but only in 6.1% of malignant tumors of the thyroid [178,179].

Thyroid/Parathyroid Adenomas

Occasionally, papillary cancers arise in benign nodules or adenomas. It is believed that this is likely to be a random event of location and does not indicate a casual relationship [143]. Several authors have described the association of PTC and parathyroid adenoma and/or hyperplasia [180,181]. Both types of lesions are associated with a history of low-dose external radiation to the neck.

Pathology

The gross appearance of PTC is quite variable. The lesions may appear anywhere within the gland. By definition, clinical papillary carcinomas are >1.0 to 1.5 cm in size often averaging 2–3 cm, although lesions may be quite large. The lesions are firm and usually white in color with an invasive appearance. Tumoral calcification is a common feature. Because of extensive sclerosis, the tumor may grossly resemble a scar. In addition, cyst formation may be observed [34,35,156].

Microscopically, PTC displays papillae containing a central core of fibrovascular tissue lined by one or occasionally several layers of cells with crowded/overlapping oval nuclei. The nuclei of papillary cancer have been described as clear, ground glass, empty, or Orphan Annie eyed. These nuclei are larger and more oval than normal follicular nuclei and contain hypodense chromatin. Intranuclear inclusions of

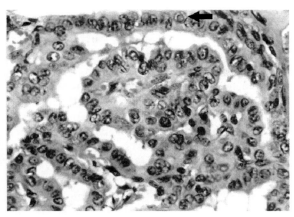

Fig. 10.7 Papillary carcinoma, classic type. Tumor cells arranged in papillary groups and showing chromatin clearing, intranuclear grooves, and inclusions (*arrow*)

cytoplasm are often found. Another characteristic of the papillary cancer nucleus is the nuclear groove (Fig. 10.7) [37,156,157]. Nuclear grooves may be seen in other thyroid lesions including Hashimoto's disease, adenomatous hyperplasia, and diffuse hyperplasia as well as in follicular adenomas (particularly hyalinizing trabecular neoplasm) [182]. Hence, the mere presence of nuclear grooves is not diagnostic for papillary carcinoma.

Psammoma bodies are lamellated round to oval structures that represent the "ghosts" of dead papillae and are formed by focal areas of infarction of the tips of papillae attracting calcium that is deposited upon the dying cells. These are seen within the cores of papillae or in the tumor stroma [35,156]; only rarely are psammoma bodies found in benign conditions in the thyroid [183,184]. Psammoma bodies are found in about 40–50% of cases, but their presence in thyroid tissue indicates that a papillary carcinoma is most likely present somewhere in the gland [35,37]. The finding of psammoma bodies in a cervical lymph node is strong evidence of a papillary cancer in the thyroid [185].

Scattered lymphocytes are common at the invasive edges of the tumor [186,187]. Cyst formation may occur and in fact may be so striking that the diagnosis of PTC is difficult to make particularly if the lesion has metastasized to neck lymph nodes making the distinction clinically from a branchial cleft cyst difficult [34,188,189].

Papillary thyroid carcinoma early in its development invades the glandular lymphatics [34], which accounts for the high incidence of regional node metastases [156]. The tumors can also present multifocally within the same gland [156]. It has been shown by molecular biology techniques that papillary carcinomas are clonal proliferations [190]. In view of these studies it is believed that multifocality of papillary carcinoma must be due to intrathyroidal lymphatic spread rather than multifocal primary tumors [64,190]. Recent RET/PTC and LOH studies have shown that multifocal papillary microcarcinomas can be separate primaries instead of intraglandular spread from one tumor source [191,192].

Venous invasion can be identified in up to 7% of papillary cancers [193]. Whether this finding alone is predictive of a more aggressive behavior is unclear [194,195].

Regional lymph node metastases are extremely common (50% or more) at initial presentation of usual papillary cancer (Fig. 10.8) [158]. Some patients will present with cervical node enlargement and will have no obvious thyroid tumor [196]. Not infrequently the nodal metastasis will involve one node that may be cystic. The histology of the nodal metastases in papillary cancer may appear papillary, mixed, or follicular. This feature does not adversely affect long-term prognosis [156,157]. Hence, attempts at staging of papillary carcinoma may have minimal clinical significance.

Tumor grading is of no use in this tumor since over 95% of these lesions are grade 1 [194]. In some tumors, either in the primary site or in recurrences, areas of poorly differentiated cancer characterized by solid growth of tumor, mitotic activity, and cytologic atypia can be found. Such lesions have a much more guarded prognosis [197]. Anaplastic change in a papillary cancer can occur, although it is uncommon [155].

Distant metastases of papillary carcinoma to lungs, bones, and brain occur in 5–7% of cases [198]. Despite the presence of multiple metastases, however, survival

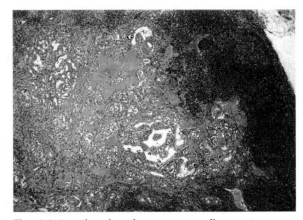

Fig. 10.8 Lymph node with metastatic papillary carcinoma

may still be prolonged, especially if the metastases can be treated with radioiodine [199]. In ordinary papillary carcinoma, death is uncommon [199].

Immunohistochemistry

Immunostaining shows that most papillary cancers express thyroglobulin, TTF1, and not calcitonin [37]. Several reports have been published regarding the use of various immunohistochemical markers that can differentiate papillary carcinoma from other follicular-derived lesions of the thyroid. From an extensive list of these markers the ones that have shown some promise include cytokeratin 19, HBME1, and galectin 3 [200–205]. However, none of these have proven to be specific since all can be expressed in some benign lesions of the thyroid. Therefore, some authors have proposed that diagnosis of PTC by immunohistochemistry should be carried out by using the markers mentioned above in an immunopanel [202,206].

The other markers that have been explored in the diagnosis of PTC include: S100 protein, blood group antigens, estrogen receptors, CD10, CD15, and CD57. The proliferation of markers indicates that no one of them is useful for the daily practice of pathology [207–210].

Flow Cytometry

Although the great majority of papillary thyroid cancers are diploid, the literature suggests up to 20% may show aneuploid or at least non-diploid subpopulations. It has been shown that aneuploid tumors are often associated with a more aggressive clinical course; however, multivariate analysis has not shown that ploidy is an independent prognostic factor [146,157,211].

Molecular Pathology

In the decade since 1995 the literature on thyroid has been focused mainly on the role of various biologic events and genetic determinants in the pathogenesis of various thyroid tumors. Rearrangements of RET gene, known as RET/PTC have been identified in papillary carcinoma of the thyroid [212,213]. The RET protooncogene is normally expressed in cells of neural crest origin and plays a role in kidney and gastrointestinal neuronal development. It is located on chromosome 10q11.2 and cell membrane receptor tyrosine kinase [212,214]. In normal thyroid wild-type

RET is only expressed in C cells and not follicular cells. RET/PTC seen in papillary carcinomas occurs due to fusion of the tyrosine kinase domain of RET to the 5′ portion of the various genes. To date more than ten novel types of rearrangements have been described in papillary carcinoma. RET/PTC1 and 3 are the most common forms that occur in sporadic papillary carcinoma. RET/PTC1 is formed by fusion of RET to H4 and RET/PTC3 occurs due to fusion of RET to ELE1 gene [214–216].

RET/PTC expression in thyroid follicular cells of transgenic mice leads to development of thyroid tumors with histologic features of papillary thyroid carcinoma [217]. Similarly, transfection of follicular cells in tissue culture by RET/PTC causes the cells to demonstrate nuclear features of papillary carcinoma [218]. The prevalence of RET/PTC in papillary carcinoma varies significantly among various geographic regions; in the United States it ranges from 11% to 43% [216]. In sporadic tumors RET/PTC1 is the most common form of rearrangement (60–70%) followed by RET/PTC3 (20–30%) [216,219]. The other rare forms of RET/PTC rearrangements have been mainly found in radiation-induced papillary carcinomas. Several studies have shown a strong association between radiation-induced papillary carcinoma and expression of RET/PTC; in papillary carcinoma in children affected by the Chernobyl nuclear accident, RET/PTC3 was found to be the commonest form of rearrangement followed by RET/PTC1 [220,221].

Recently it has been shown that RET/PTC expression can also occur in some benign lesions. These include hyalinizing trabecular neoplasm [151], Hashimoto's thyroiditis [222,223], and hyperplastic nodules and follicular adenoma [224].

Several authors have suggested an association between Hashimoto's thyroiditis and PTC; however, others have suggested that this association is most likely incidental since both are common. Recently two independent studies have shown high prevalence of RET/PTC in histologically benign thyroid tissue affected by Hashimoto's thyroiditis; these studies concluded that thyroiditic glands harbor multiple foci of papillary carcinoma that are not identified by histologic examination only [222,223]. However, a more recent study failed to reproduce these results [168].

RET/PTC has been identified in benign thyroid nodules, especially the ones that are seen in patients with a history of external radiation [224]. However, this still remains controversial and needs to be further elucidated by examination of a large cohort of cases.

Activation of the ras oncogene-signaling pathway is considered to be an important mechanism by which human cancer develops. Ras has been shown to regulate several pathways that contribute to cellular transformation including the Raf/MEK/ERK pathways. Numerous studies confirm that the Raf/MEK/ERK pathway is a significant contributor to the malignant phenotype associated with deregulated Ras signaling [225,226].

Recently, an activating mutation in the serine/threonine kinase BRAF was described of human PTCs. BRAF-activating mutations in thyroid cancer are almost exclusively the BRAF V600E mutation, and have been found in 29–69% of papillary thyroid cancers, 13% of poorly differentiated cancers, and 10% of anaplastic cancers [226–229]. These data identify that BRAF is an oncogene in human cancer. The high frequency of BRAF mutations in thyroid cancer suggests that inhibition of BRAF activity may represent an important new strategy in the treatment of patients with thyroid cancer.

Prognostic Factors

Poor prognostic factors in papillary carcinoma include older age at diagnosis, male sex, large tumor size, and extrathyroidal growth [158,199]. Pathologic variables associated with a more guarded prognosis include less differentiated or solid areas, vascular invasion, and aneuploid cell population [194]. Some authors have found varying prognostic factors in males and females. In men, age and presence of gross lymph node metastases were important, while in females age, presence of gross lymph node metastases, tumor size, and the number of structures adhered to the gland were important [199,230].

Some studies have shown that RET/PTC expression in papillary carcinoma can be associated with aggressive biologic behavior; conversely, others have reported that its expression is more commonly seen in slow growing and clinically indolent tumors [231,232]. It is also suggested that different rearrangements of RET/PTC are associated with different biologic behavior. Nikiforov et al. found a significant difference in local recurrence and distant metastases between tumor with RET/PTC1 and RET/PTC3 expression [216]. Cetta et al. reported similar findings [233]. Besides RET/PTC, several other biologic markers have been suggested as prognostic predictors in papillary carcinoma; these include p53, Ki67, cell cycle proteins, proliferating cell nuclear antigen (PCNA), bcl2, cathepsin D, and topoisomerase II [234–238].

Subtypes of Papillary Carcinoma

Papillary Microcarcinoma (Occult Papillary Carcinoma)

According to the WHO, papillary microcarcinoma is defined as tumor measuring 1 cm or less; however, some experts have also defined tumors measuring up to 1.5 cm as microcarcinomas (Fig. 10.9) [239,240]. These lesions are quite common as incidental findings at autopsy or in thyroidectomy for benign disease or in completion thyroidectomies in patients with a history of carcinoma involving the opposite thyroid lobe [241]. The incidence of these lesions has varied significantly with the study, but papillary microcarcinoma has been reported in up to 36% of carefully sectioned thyroid specimens [241]. Lymph node metastases from papillary microcarcinoma can occur; metastases from lesions less than 0.5 cm have been reported [240,241]. Distant metastases, although very rare, are also documented [242]. Histologically, the tumors may be totally follicular or show papillary areas as well. Sclerosis may be prominent; the lesions infiltrate the surrounding thyroid [34]. A familial form of papillary microcarcinoma has been recognized; these tumors are characterized by multifocality with increase tendency toward vascular and lymphatic invasion, distant metastasis, and even death [243,244]. It is important to recognize that the incidentally found microcarcinoma confined within the thyroid is probably of no clinical importance and should not be overtreated.

Follicular Variant of Papillary Cancer

The follicular variant of papillary carcinoma is a distinctive papillary carcinoma variant that shows follic-

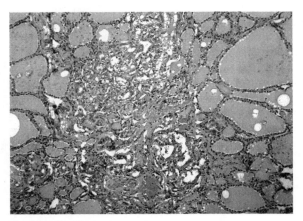

Fig. 10.9 Papillary microcarcinoma

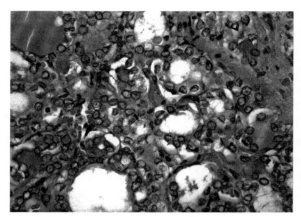

Fig. 10.10 Follicular variant of papillary carcinoma. Variably sized follicles lined by cells showing nuclear features of papillary carcinoma

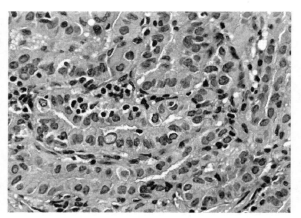

Fig. 10.11 Tall cell variant of papillary carcinoma. Enlarged tumor cells with oncocytic cytoplasm and nuclear features of papillary carcinoma

ular growth pattern and diagnostic nuclear features of papillary carcinoma (Fig. 10.10) [245,246]. The incidence of this variant is difficult to determine since in the past some of these lesions have been classified as follicular carcinomas or adenomas [247]. Grossly and histologically, the tumor may appear encapsulated [248]. The prognosis of the follicular variant is apparently similar to usual papillary cancer although there may be a greater risk for this variant to metastasize outside the neck and for vascular invasion; regional nodal metastases are less common than in classic papillary cancer [249,250].

Two distinct types of follicular variant are the diffuse and the encapsulated follicular variants. In the diffuse follicular variant, the gland is diffusely replaced by tumor [251]. Lymph node and distant metastases are common in these patients. The prognosis appears to be poor in these patients, although only a handful of cases have been described [252,253].

The encapsulated follicular variant refers to the follicular variant that is characterized by the presence of a capsule around the lesion. These lesions are associated with an excellent prognosis [251]. In some cases the diagnosis of this particular variant of papillary carcinoma can be difficult due to the presence of multifocal rather than diffuse distribution of nuclear features of papillary thyroid carcinoma. Because of this peculiar morphologic presentation, these tumors can be misdiagnosed as adenomatoid nodule or follicular adenoma [143,251]. Some authors have suggested that these tumors be classified as "tumors of undetermined malignant potential" due to their excellent prognosis [254]; however, others have shown that some cases belonging in this category can lead to distant metastasis [249].

Tall Cell Variant

The tall cell variant is an aggressive variant of papillary carcinoma that tends to occur in elderly patients. These tumors are usually large (>6 cm), extend extrathyroidally, and show mitotic activity and vascular invasion more often than usual papillary cancer. The tall cell variant of PTC consists of tumor cells twice as tall as they are wide and shows eosinophilic cytoplasm; because of this these tumors are referred to as the "pink cell" variant of papillary carcinoma (Fig. 10.11) [255,256]. Dedifferentiation to squamous cell carcinoma has been described in the tall cell variant of PTC [257]. The prognosis for this variant is less favorable than for usual papillary cancer, although it is believed that the poor outcome is secondary to the fact that these tumors are often associated with poor prognostic variables such as older age, extrathyroidal spread, necrosis, high mitotic rate, and distant metastases [258–260].

Columnar Cell Variant

The columnar cell variant is a rare form of papillary carcinoma [261]. (Some authors believe it is so unusual a tumor that it deserves its own category and should not be placed in the papillary group. The tumor needs to be distinguished from other papillary carcinomas since this lesion is associated with an extremely poor outcome with most deaths occurring within 5 years of diagnosis. Extrathyroidal extension is common as are distant metastases [261–263]. Encapsulated variants, which may have a better prognosis, have been described [264].

Warthin-like Variant

By light microscopy these tumors resemble "Warthin's tumor" of the salivary gland. These tumors usually arise in a background of lymphocytic thyroiditis and show papillary architecture. Limited follow-up has shown that these tumors in their pure form follow a clinical course similar to conventional papillary carcinoma [265,266].

Diffuse Sclerosis Variant

The diffuse sclerosis variant of papillary carcinoma is rare; it most often affects children and young adults, and may present as bilateral goiter. The tumor permeates the gland outlining the intraglandular lymphatics. The lesions tend to recur in the neck and have a somewhat more serious prognosis than usual childhood papillary cancer. These lesions appear to represent 10% of the papillary carcinomas seen in children exposed to the radioactive iodine released following the Chernobyl accident. While the tumors often show extracapsular extension, distant and nodal metastases, and a decreased disease-free survival when compared to the usual type of papillary carcinoma, mortality is low [267–270].

Solid Variant of Papillary Carcinoma

The solid variant of PTC is most commonly seen in children and has been reported in greater than 30% of patients with papillary carcinoma following the Chernobyl nuclear accident [271,272]. It is important to recognize these lesions as papillary carcinomas and not to classify them as more aggressive tumors such as insular carcinoma (discussed below). The prognosis is controversial with some studies showing outcomes similar to typical papillary carcinoma and other studies showing more aggressive behavior [271,273].

Other Variants of Papillary Carcinoma

Rare variants of papillary cancer in which prognostic data are not well established include the spindle cell variant [274], the clear cell type [275], the oxyphilic (Hürthle cell) variant [275,276], papillary carcinoma with lipomatous stroma [277,278], papillary carcinoma with fasciitis-like stroma [279], and the cribriform variant [280–281]. The last of these is often seen in patients with familial adenomatous polyposis although it may occur as a sporadic tumor. It is overwhelmingly common in women [175,282].

10.7.2.2 Follicular Carcinoma

Follicular carcinoma comprises about 5% of thyroid cancers; however, in iodide-deficient areas, this tumor is more prevalent making up 25–40% of thyroid cancers [283,284]. The true incidence of follicular carcinoma is difficult to determine since the follicular variant of papillary carcinoma may still be placed into this category [247]. Risk factors include iodine deficiency, older age, female gender, and radiation exposure (although the relationship of radiation to follicular carcinoma is far less strong than with papillary cancer) [162,285]. Clinically, follicular carcinoma usually presents as a solitary mass in the thyroid [283].

Follicular carcinoma has a marked propensity for vascular invasion and avoids lymphatics; hence, true embolic lymph node metastases are exceedingly rare. Follicular carcinoma disseminates hematogenously and metastasizes to bone, lungs, brain, and liver [283,286,287].

Patients who have follicular carcinoma that is widely invasive fare poorly [284,288]; however, those individual with encapsulated follicular tumors confined to the thyroid enjoy a prolonged survival (greater than 80% at 10 years) [289–292]. Studies using multivariate analysis have identified age >45, extrathyroidal extension, distant metastases, and tumor size >4 cm as independent prognostic factors in follicular carcinoma [286,291,293]. An extremely significant complication that may occur in patients with follicular cancer is transformation into anaplastic cancer; this may occur de novo in an untreated follicular lesion, or in metastatic foci [294].

The *widely invasive follicular carcinoma* is a tumor that is clinically and surgically recognized as a cancer; the role of the pathologist in its diagnosis is to confirm that it is of thyroid origin and is a follicular neoplasm. Up to 80% of the patients with widely invasive cancers can develop metastases, and a 50% fatality rate for widely invasive tumors compared with only 3% for those with minimal invasion has been reported.

The pathologist can only diagnose the minimally invasive follicular carcinoma by examining well-fixed histologic sections. These lesions are not diagnosable by fine-needle aspiration cytology since the diagnosis requires the demonstration of invasion at the edges of the lesion; therefore, sampling of the center, as in obtaining a cytologic sample, cannot be diagnostic [283–287,295–297].

The *minimally invasive follicular carcinoma* is an encapsulated tumor that grossly resembles a follicular adenoma and only on microscopic examination shows evidence of capsular and/or vascular invasion (Figs. 10.12, 10.13). On microscopic examination, follicular carcinomas most often have a microfollicular pattern and resemble a cellular follicular adenoma. Trabecular or solid patterns are fairly common and often accompany the microfollicular pattern [143,291].

What are the minimum criteria for making this diagnosis? Invasion of the capsule, invasion through the capsule, and invasion into veins in or beyond the capsule represent the diagnostic criteria for carcinoma in a follicular thyroid neoplasm [143,247,291]. The criterion for vascular invasion applies solely and strictly to veins in or beyond the capsule, whereas, the definition of capsular invasion is controversial [143,254]. Some authors require penetration of the capsule to diagnose a follicular tumor as carcinoma, while others need tumor invasion through the capsule into the surrounding normal thyroid [254,292]. Is capsular invasion insufficient for the diagnosis of follicular cancer? Distant metastases have been reported in follicular carcinoma diagnosed only on the basis of capsular and not vascular invasion, however, in some cases, metastases were already present at initial diagnosis [290,298]. The presence of vascular invasion is also indicative of malignancy in a follicular tumor. Invasion of vessels within or beyond the lesional capsule is necessary for a definitive diagnosis of vascular invasion [35]. The lesions with vascular invasion should be separated from the minimally invasive follicular carcinomas that show capsular invasion only, because angioinvasive lesions have a greater probability of recurrence and metastasis [251].

In our practice, we use the terms minimally invasive and angioinvasive carcinoma. The former is applied to those cases that show only capsular or transcapsular invasion, while the latter is used for tumors in which vascular invasion is found with or without capsular invasion. As mentioned above, we propose this distinction based on the belief that angioinvasive tumors have a greater propensity toward distant metastasis.

Similar problems exist in evaluating such lesions by frozen section [299,300]. Some authors recommend that intraoperative assessment of such lesions involves the examination of frozen sections from three or four separate areas of the nodule [301]. This wastes resources and rarely gives useful diagnostic information. The surgeon should have removed the lobe involved by the nodule and if it is a follicular carcinoma that is only minimally invasive, the appropriate therapy has probably already been accomplished. Since a only small number of these lesions will show evidence of invasion at the time of permanent section, i.e., the majority of them are benign, and since overdiagnosis is more dangerous for the patient than is the delay in making a definitive diagnosis [299], we discourage frozen section evaluation of these nodules.

None of the ancillary techniques assist in defining benign from malignant follicular tumors. Ultrastructural, morphometric, and flow cytometric analyses have not helped in distinguishing these lesions [145,302]. About 60% of follicular carcinomas will show aneuploid cell populations [145]. Backdahl analyzed 65 follicular thyroid tumors (26 benign and 39 carcinomas). He noted that of the 20 patients with cancer who survived, 19 had diploid tumors, whereas

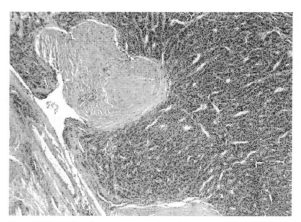

Fig. 10.12 Follicular carcinoma. Thickly encapsulated follicular and solid patterned lesion invading into the capsule in a mushroom-shaped growth

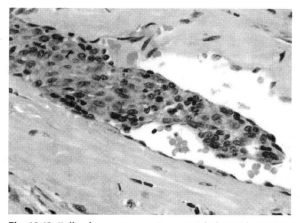

Fig. 10.13 Follicular carcinoma. Tumor embolus within a capsular vessel

17 of 19 patients who died of carcinoma had tumors with aneuploid DNA patterns [303].

All follicular carcinomas express thyroglobulin and show a similar cytokeratin profile to normal thyroid parenchyma. Some authors have shown that HBME1 is exclusively expressed in 90–100% of follicular carcinomas and not adenomas. However, others have reported HBME1 expression in adenomatoid nodules and follicular adenomas [204,210,304,305].

Molecular Biology of Follicular Carcinoma

A specific translocation t(2;3) leads to the expression of PAX8 peroxisome proliferator activated receptor gamma (PPAR gamma) chimeric protein; initial studies by Kroll et al. demonstrated that this translocation is specific to follicular carcinoma [306]. However, follow-up studies employing immunohistochemistry and molecular biology have shown that PPAR gamma expression can occur in some cases of follicular adenoma, follicular variant of papillary thyroid carcinoma, and even benign thyroid parenchyma [307,308]. *Ras* mutations are more frequent in follicular carcinoma as compared to follicular adenoma; some authors have found an association between *ras* mutations and clinically aggressive follicular carcinomas [309–311]. Loss of heterozygosity on chromosomes 10q and 3p can be seen in follicular carcinoma suggesting a role of tumor suppressor genes in its pathogenesis [312,313].

Well-differentiated Follicular "Tumors of Undetermined Malignant Potential"

This designation has been recently proposed in thyroid pathology for follicular patterned encapsulated tumors that have been controversial and difficult to diagnose due to: (1) questionable or minimal nuclear features of papillary thyroid carcinoma or (2) questionable or one focus of capsular invasion that is confined to tumor capsule and does not traverse the entire thickness of capsule and lacks any nuclear features of papillary thyroid carcinoma [254].

This terminology may be extremely helpful to pathologists in the diagnoses of certain follicular patterned lesions; however, these terms are proposed on the basis of data that lack complete clinical follow-up. Therefore, clinicians may find it problematic to establish treatment strategies [143].

Oncocytic (Hürthle Cell) Tumors

Hürthle cells are derived from follicular epithelium and are characterized morphologically by large size, distinct cell borders, voluminous granular cytoplasm, large nucleus, and prominent nucleolus. Ultrastructural studies have shown that the cytoplasmic granularity is produced by huge mitochondria filling the cell [314,315]. Hürthle cells can be found in a number of conditions in the thyroid [nodular goiter, non-specific chronic thyroiditis, longstanding hyperthyroidism, and chronic lymphocytic thyroiditis (Hashimoto's disease)] [19].

Perhaps no thyroid neoplasm has elicited more confusion or debate than Hürthle cell (oncocytic) neoplasms. Clinicians and pathologists alike have considered that such tumors do not "follow the rules" for histopathologic diagnosis of malignancy. Some authors cite 80% or more of these lesions as benign, whereas others consider all such lesions malignant [316,317]. Over the decade since 1995, studies from numerous institutions throughout the world have shown that oncocytic or Hürthle cell tumors can be divided into benign and malignant categories by careful adherence to strict pathologic criteria [318,319].

Since most Hürthle cell neoplasms are follicular in pattern, the criterion for distinguishing benign from malignant is the same as for follicular neoplasms, i.e., the identification of capsular and/or vascular invasion [318,319]. However, the pathologic criterion for malignancy is met more frequently for tumors composed of Hürthle cells than for their non-Hürthle counterparts. Thus, whereas 2–3% of solitary encapsulated follicular tumors of the thyroid show invasive characteristics, 30–40% of such lesions showing Hürthle cell cytology will show such features [315,318,320]. In addition, whereas true follicular carcinomas of the thyroid rarely, if ever, metastasize embolically to lymph nodes, about 30% of Hürthle cell carcinomas do [34,321].

Most Hürthle cell neoplasms of the thyroid are solitary mass lesions that show complete or partial encapsulation. They are distinguished from the surrounding thyroid by their distinctive brown to mahogany color [34,35,318]. Rarely, a Hürthle cell neoplasm may undergo spontaneous infarction. Extensive infarction may also be seen following fine-needle aspiration biopsy.

The claim that all Hürthle cell neoplasms should be considered malignant or potentially malignant, especially if 2 cm or greater in size, is no longer considered valid. Many studies from the United States and Europe indicate that benign Hürthle cell neoplasms exist. Size, nuclear atypia, multinucleation, cellular pleomorphism, mitoses, or histologic pattern of the lesion are not predictive of behavior [315,318,319].

By immunohistochemistry, Hürthle cell lesions are positive for thyroglobulin. Carcinoembryonic antigen (CEA) expression has been described in some, but not all series. Hürthle cell lesions are positive for S100 protein [318,322].

DNA ploidy studies have shown aneuploid DNA patterns in biologically and histologically benign Hürthle tumors of the thyroid. These findings do not indicate malignant behavior, however, about 20–50% of Hürthle cell tumors that are histologically malignant and aneuploid are more aggressive biologically and clinically than diploid Hürthle cell cancers [323].

Molecular Biology of Hürthle Cell Tumors

Hürthle cell tumors are biologically different from other follicular-derived tumors. H-*ras* mutations are more frequent in Hürthle cell carcinoma than follicular carcinoma [324,325], and a high percentage of allelic alterations occur as compared to other follicular-derived tumors. A study by Maximo et al. showed that Hürthle cell tumors display a relatively higher percentage of common deletions of mitochondrial DNA as compared to other follicular-derived tumors. In addition, Hürthle cell tumors also showed germline polymorphisms of ATPase 6 gene, which is required for the maintenance of mitochondrial DNA [326].

Clear Cell Tumors

Clear cell change of the cytoplasm can occur in many follicular-derived lesions of the thyroid, thyroiditis, nodules, and neoplasms [278,327,328]. Of greatest importance is the differentiation of clear cell change in follicular thyroid lesions from clear cell renal cell carcinomas metastatic to the thyroid [329]. Immunostains for thyroglobulin are usually helpful in sorting out this diagnostic problem.

Poorly Differentiated Carcinoma/ Insular Carcinoma

This heterogeneous group of malignant thyroid tumors includes carcinomas that are recognizable as originating from follicular epithelium (often with evidence of coexistent papillary or follicular carcinoma),

but that have moderate to high rates of mitotic activity, are composed of solid masses or trabeculae of relatively uniform epithelial cells, have tiny follicles present in varying numbers, may contain regions of acute necrosis, and are more aggressive than the usual well-differentiated carcinomas [197]. Included among these lesions are insular carcinoma, columnar cell, tall cell, and trabecular types of papillary cancer, and "poorly differentiated" carcinoma of Sakamoto [330].

Insular carcinoma or poorly differentiated thyroid carcinoma is a follicular-derived carcinoma with a prognosis between well-differentiated thyroid carcinomas (papillary or follicular) and anaplastic thyroid carcinoma. The term "insular" is used to describe the lesion's histologic growth pattern, which is somewhat "carcinoid-like." The incidence of this tumor appears to vary with differing geographic locations with incidence as high as 5% described in Italy, while the incidence in the United States is much lower [331].

The lesions are often large, gray-white in color, infiltrative, and show extensive necrosis. Microscopically the tumor is composed of small nests of cells that have a neuroendocrine growth pattern. Necrosis, vascular invasion, and mitoses are prominent features. By immunohistochemistry the tumor cells express thyroglobulin and not calcitonin. Insular carcinoma is associated with a worse prognosis than well-differentiated thyroid carcinomas, but is significantly better than anaplastic thyroid carcinoma [331–333]. The extent of the poorly differentiated component in a well-differentiated thyroid tumor can affect the prognosis; tumors with >10% of the poorly differentiated component are associated with frequent regional recurrences, distant metastases, and poor prognosis [334].

10.7.2.3 Anaplastic Thyroid Tumors

Anaplastic carcinomas are a group of high-grade thyroid carcinomas that are usually undifferentiated histologically and advertly have a lethal outcome [155,335]. Synonyms for anaplastic carcinoma include: undifferentiated, dedifferentiated, and sarcomatoid carcinoma. These tumors have represented approximately 10% of thyroid malignancies in older publications [155,336]. The tumor is more commonly seen in elderly females who present with a rapidly enlarging mass that often results in dyspnea. Risk factors are largely unknown but may include history of radiation and iodine deficiency [155]. A precursor well-differentiated thyroid carcinoma (papillary, follicular, or Hürthle cell) may be observed [337].

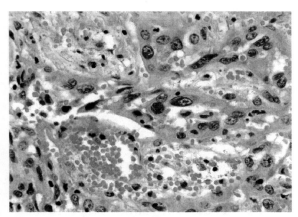

Fig. 10.14 Anaplastic carcinoma. Pleomorphic spindle-shape and epitheloid tumor cells

Grossly, the tumors are large with extensive intra-thyroidal and extrathyroidal invasion. Surgical resection is often not performed because of the lesion's extent and diagnosis is commonly made on biopsy. Necrosis, vascular invasion, and mitoses are quite prominent [337]. Histologically, a variety of patterns have been described. The tumors are usually made up of a variety of cell types (Fig. 10.14). Most tumors are composed of giant cells and spindle cells although "squamoid" differentiation is seen in about one third of cases [338]. Osteoclast-like giant cells are a common feature [339]. A "paucicellular" variant of anaplastic carcinoma has been described; it is characterized by dense fibrosis, calcification, and a poor patient outcome [340]. Spindle cell squamous anaplastic carcinoma may be the result of transformation of tall cell papillary carcinoma [257]. Carcinosarcoma of the thyroid has been described [341,342].

Electron microscopic and immunohistologic studies have indicated that almost all anaplastic thyroid tumors are indeed epithelial in nature [338,343]. By immunohistochemistry, anaplastic thyroid carcinomas should be positive for cytokeratin. Thyroglobulin immunostaining is often negative and thyroid transcription factor can be rarely positive in anaplastic carcinoma [343].

10.7.2.4 Thyroid Sarcoma

Sarcomas of the thyroid are rare; fibrosarcomas, leiomyosarcomas, and angiosarcomas have been described [344,345]. Angiosarcoma of thyroid has been most commonly described from the mountainous regions of the world (Alpine regions of Europe, the Andes in South America, and the Himalayas in Asia)

[344,346]. Clinically, the affected patients resemble those with anaplastic carcinoma. By gross and histologic examination these tumors resemble angiosarcomas of soft tissue. These tumors generally lack the usual histologic features and exceptional aggressiveness of anaplastic carcinomas, but they are neither typical follicular nor papillary carcinomas.

10.7.2.5 Squamous Cell Carcinoma, Mucoepidermoid Carcinoma, and Intrathyroidal Thymoma-like Neoplasms

Squamous cell carcinoma in thyroid occurs usually in association with papillary or anaplastic carcinoma [257]. Rarely, squamous cell carcinoma appears as an entity independent of any other form of thyroid cancer and behaves in an aggressive fashion with poor prognosis [347]. The major differential diagnosis is metastatic squamous carcinoma, especially from the head and neck, lungs, or esophagus.

Mucoepidermoid carcinoma is a distinctive variant of thyroid carcinoma. It is composed of solid masses of squamoid cells and mucin-producing cells, sometimes forming glands [348]. Some authors consider that this lesion is a variant of papillary carcinoma; all cases show thyroglobulin expression [108,349]. The prognosis of thyroid mucoepidermoid carcinoma is quite good. Lesions may metastasize to regional nodes and rarely distantly. Death from disease is rare [108].

Sclerosing mucoepidermoid carcinoma with eosinophilia is usually seen in a background of lymphocytic thyroiditis and is characterized by tumor cells arranged in small sheets, anastomosing trabeculae, and narrow strands associated with dense fibrosis and numerous eosinophils. While these lesions may metastasize to lymph nodes and show extracapsular spread, vascular invasion, and perineural invasion, death due to disease is uncommon. The tumor cells stain negative for thyroglobulin and calcitonin and positive for cytokeratin [108,350,351].

There is no consensus regarding the origin of these tumors. Some studies have suggested that on the basis of immunoprofile both these tumors have different origins; mucoepidermoid carcinoma shows follicular derivation, and sclerosing mucoepidermoid carcinoma is derived from ultimobranchial body nests/solid cell nests [108].

Rare thyroid tumors composed of spindled epithelial cells arranged in nests, sometimes associated with mucous microcysts, and resembling thymomas (*spindled and epithelial tumor with thymus-like dif-*

ferentiation; SETTLE) have been reported [352,353]. Neoplasms resembling thymic carcinomas have also been described (*carcinoma with thymus-like differentiation; CASTLE*) in thyroid. These lesions may originate from branchial pouch remnants within and adjacent to the thyroid [352,354–356].

10.7.2.6 Medullary Carcinoma

Medullary thyroid carcinoma comprises less than 10% of all thyroid malignancies [357–361]. This tumor is of great diagnostic importance because of its aggressiveness, its close association with multiple endocrine neoplasia syndromes (MEN2A and 2B), and a relationship to a C cell hyperplasia, a probable precursor lesion [362]. While the majority of medullary carcinomas are sporadic, about 10–20% are familial [362]. Since these familial cases have been identified, a gene associated with medullary carcinoma has been identified on chromosome 10 and involves mutations in the RET oncogene [363–365].

Medullary carcinoma can affect patients of any age; most affected individuals are adults with an average age of about 50 years. However, in familial cases, children can be affected; also in these instances the age of diagnosis tends to be younger (mean age about 20 years) [361,366]. Although sporadic medullary carcinomas are seen more commonly in women, familial cases have a slight female to equal sex ratio, since an autosomal dominant mode of inheritance is present [367,368].

Clinically sporadic medullary carcinoma will present with a thyroid nodule that is painless but firm. In up to 50% of cases, obvious nodal metastases will be present at the time of diagnosis. Distant metastases, such as to lung, bone, or liver, may also be noted initially in about 15–25% of cases. When the tumor produces excess hormone other than calcitonin, the presenting symptoms may be related to that hormone hypersecretion [adrenocorticotropic hormone (ACTH), prostaglandin] [369,370].

In the familial lesions there are associated endocrine and/or neuroendocrine lesions. Sipple's syndrome [multiple endocrine neoplasia (MEN) type 2A] [371] consists of medullary thyroid cancer and C cell hyperplasia, adrenal pheochromocytoma and adrenal medullary hyperplasia, and parathyroid hyperplasia [372]. Studies have shown that the gene responsible for familial medullary carcinoma is RET [373,374]; mutations in RET (different from the RET translocation in papillary carcinoma) are found in the tumors and the germline of patients with familial medullary

carcinomas and the MEN type 2 syndromes [373–375]. Mutations in specific codons have been correlated with clinical behavior and symptomatology in some families [374]. MEN type 2B consists of medullary thyroid carcinoma and C cell hyperplasia, pheochromocytoma and adrenal medullary hyperplasia, mucosal neuromas, gastrointestinal ganglioneuromas, and musculoskeletal abnormalities [376–379]. These patients may have familial disease (over 50% do), and some cases arise apparently as spontaneous mutations. These patients have biologically aggressive medullary carcinoma and may succumb to metastases at an early age. MEN2B shows similarity to von Recklinghausen's disease since in neurofibromatosis similar lesions are found in the gastrointestinal tract, and pheochromocytomas are common [378,379]. Nerve growth factor has been identified in some medullary carcinomas of these patients; it has been postulated that this product of the tumor may be responsible for the neural lesions seen in the MEN type 2B patients [380]. However, the neural lesions often precede by many years the development of medullary cancer. In MEN type 2B, the tumors and germline mutations in RET are found on codon 918—an intracellular focus of the RET oncogene [381,382].

Medullary carcinoma is usually located in the area of highest C cell concentration, i.e., the lateral upper two thirds of the gland. In familial cases, multiple small nodules may be detected grossly and, rarely, lesions may be found in the isthmus. The tumors range in size from barely visible to several centimeters. Many medullary carcinomas are grossly circumscribed but some will show infiltrative borders. The typical medullary carcinoma may be microscopically circumscribed or more likely will be infiltrating into the surrounding thyroid. The pattern of growth is of tumor cells arranged in nests separated by varying amounts of stroma. The tumor nests are composed of round, oval, or spindle-shaped cells; often there is isolated cellular pleomorphism or even multinucleated cells (Fig. 10.15) [383,384]. The tumor stroma characteristically contains amyloid although this is not necessary for the diagnosis as about 25% of medullary carcinomas do not contain amyloid (Fig. 10.15) [361,385,386]. The amyloid is most likely derived from procalcitonin and indeed immunohistochemical stains for calcitonin often stain the amyloid [37,386]. Calcifications in areas of amyloid deposition are characteristically present. The tumors commonly invade lymphatics and veins [384].

Several variants of medullary carcinoma on the basis of growth pattern have been described. These include: papillary variant, follicular variant, encap-

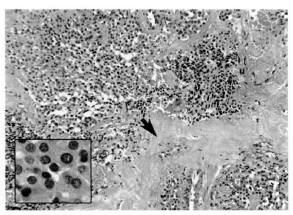

Fig. 10.15 Medullary carcinoma. Tumor cells arranged in nests and round nuclei with finely granular chromatin (*inset*) in a background of stroma and amyloid (*arrow*)

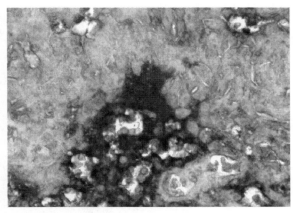

Fig. 10.16 Medullary carcinoma showing positive immunostaining with calcitonin antibody. The tumor is staining dark, and light staining is seen in the background amyloid

sulated variant, small cell variant, giant cell variant, oncocytic variant, and clear cell variant [389–391].

By immunohistochemistry, the majority of medullary carcinomas express low molecular weight cytokeratin, calcitonin (Fig. 10.16), calcitonin gene-related peptide, and thyroid transcription factor (TTF1). In addition, many tumors express CEA, which may also be elevated in the serum [392–394]. A variety of other peptides may be found in tumor cells including somatostatin, vasoactive intestinal peptide, and synaptophysin [395,396]. Some studies have also identified polysialic acid (neural cell adhesion molecule) in medullary carcinomas but not in other thyroid tumors [397].

Occasional lesions (and often these are small cell type) do not contain immunoreactive calcitonin. In order to accept a calcitonin-free tumor of the thyroid

as a medullary carcinoma, it should arise in a familial setting or occur in a thyroid with unequivocal C cell hyperplasia [398]. Immunoreactivity for calcitonin gene-related peptide would add proof to the histogenetic nature of such a lesion.

Prognostic Factors

From the clinical standpoint, stage is the most important variable for prognosis [399–401]. A tumor confined to the thyroid without nodal or distant metastases is associated with prolonged survival. Several workers have found that younger patients (under age 40), especially women, fare somewhat better than the whole group of medullary cancer patients [399,402]. Patients who are discovered by screening because they are members of affected families often have very small tumors and can be cured by thyroidectomy. Patients with Sipple's syndrome tend to have less aggressive tumors than the sporadic group whereas the patients with MEN type 2B have aggressive lesions [401,403,404]. Pathologic features that have been related to prognosis include tumor pattern, amyloid content, pleomorphism, necrosis, mitotic activity, and DNA aneuploidy [405].

Mixed Follicular and Medullary Carcinoma

These controversial tumors show thyroglobulin and calcitonin immunoreactivity and ultrastructural evidence of differentiation along two cell lines. Some of the series of these tumors may have been confusing, with trapping of follicles at the invading edge of the medullary carcinoma and diffusion of thyroglobulin into the medullary carcinoma; this may result in diagnosis of mixed tumors showing immunostaining for both hormones. Caution should be taken when making the diagnosis of mixed medullary and follicular-derived carcinomas [406–409].

Micromedullary Carcinoma

A few medullary carcinomas are discovered incidental to thyroid operations for other conditions, at autopsy, or because of an elevated serum calcitonin. The so-called *micromedullary carcinomas* (equivalent to micropapillary carcinoma and defined as tumors of 1 cm or less) have an excellent prognosis if confined to the gland [410,411]. Some of the micromedullary cancers arise in the background of chronic thyroiditis and may be associated with C cell hyperplasia even in the absence of familial disease [412]. Some of these patients have hypothyroidism and elevated TSH levels. Hence this type of C cell hyperplasia and micromedullary carcinoma may represent a secondary "reactive" phenomenon leading to early neoplastic change [410,412–414]. The non-tumoral parenchyma should be examined for evidence of C cell hyperplasia in a thyroid removed for a medullary carcinoma. Occasionally, the gland contains moderate to severe autoimmune thyroiditis, adenomatoid nodules, or another follicular-derived thyroid cancer [414–416].

10.7.3   Lymphoma

Secondary involvement of the thyroid by lymphoma has been reported in 20% of patients dying from generalized lymphoma. Primary lymphoma of the thyroid is uncommon but not rare. Most patients may have a history of diffuse goiter (probably the result of autoimmune thyroiditis) that has suddenly increased in size.

Most thyroid lymphomas are diffuse in type. Virtually all examples are B cell types; many may be extranodal lymphomas that arise in mucosa-associated lymphoid tissue (MALT) especially in the gastrointestinal tract. Some patients have typical plasmacytomas and these have a good prognosis. Hodgkin's disease is extremely rare. Malignant lymphoma should be differentiated from advanced autoimmune thyroiditis; this distinction requires assessment of lymphocyte clonality by special studies (e.g., flow cytometry, gene rearrangement) [106,107,417–419].

10.7.4   Thyroid Tumors in Unusual Locations

Although clinically significant *lingual thyroid* is an unusual disorder, and microscopic remnants of thyroid tissue have been described in 9.8% of tongues examined at autopsy. Rare cases of thyroid carcinoma arising in lingual thyroid are recorded [420].

Neoplasms arising in association with the *thyroglossal duct* might be expected to be squamous carcinomas, but these are extremely rare; indeed, most tumors occurring in this setting have been thyroid carcinomas and most are described as papillary. Medullary carcinoma has not been described; since the parafollicular cells are not found in the median thyroid, this is not unexpected. The clinical presentation of thyroglossal duct carcinoma is identical to that of benign thyroglossal duct cysts, i.e., a swelling in the anterior neck [27,421,422].

When the diagnosis of thyroglossal cyst-associated thyroid cancer is made, the question of its origin arises. Does this tumor represent a metastasis from a primary lesion in the gland, or is the primary site in the region of the gland, or is the primary site in the region of the cyst? In rare cases in which the thyroid was examined pathologically, areas of papillary carcinoma were found in the gland [30,423]. Most authors studying this problem conclude that the thyroglossal carcinoma is a primary tumor arising in remnants of thyroid associated with the duct; in those few cases where intrathyroidal tumor has been found, this was considered a separate primary [30,421] although molecular analyses have not yet been reported to settle this question.

Malignant tumors arising in thyroid tissue located within the trachea or larynx are very rare, but have been reported [424].

Carcinomas, usually papillary subtype, and lesions that resemble carcinoid tumors can arise in struma ovarii [425–427].

10.7.5   Metastatic Neoplasms

Tumors metastasize to the thyroid via direct extension from tumors in adjacent structures, by retrograde lymphatic spread, or hematogenously. Carcinomas of the larynx, pharynx, trachea, and esophagus can invade the thyroid directly. In these cases the distinction from a thyroid primary is usually not difficult. Retrograde extension via lymphatic routes into the thyroid is unusual. In theory, at least, any tumor involving cervical lymph nodes could extend into the thyroid by this mechanism. Hematogenous metastases to the thyroid vary according to tumor type [329]. Carcinomas of the kidney, lung, and colon and melanoma are most commonly found [329]. Such lesions are often solitary, circumscribed masses; they may appear quite compatible with a primary tumor. Resemblance to colonic adenocarcinoma, breast cancer, or pigmented melanoma reassures that this is a metastasis. However, clear cell carcinoma of the kidney, as noted above, may present a problem [329,428–430].

10.8   Frozen Section Diagnosis and the Thyroid

Before the advent of fine- and large-needle biopsy, the method most often used in diagnosis of thyroid nodules was intraoperative frozen section. The nodule or preferably the thyroid lobe was excised and a representative portion (preferably encompassing nodule capsule–thyroid interface) was prepared for frozen section and interpretation by a pathologist. In those cases in which the diagnosis of papillary, medullary, or anaplastic cancer was given, appropriate surgery was immediately undertaken.

Even with frozen section, however, despite recommendations of sampling two or even four different areas, the diagnosis of follicular carcinomas was notoriously difficult. In many cases, the diagnosis rendered is "follicular lesion diagnosis deferred to permanent sections" [299,300,431].

Several studies have evaluated frozen section and fine-needle aspirate (FNA) diagnostic results for thyroid nodules [432–434]. Although frozen section diagnosis may be specific (90–97%), it is not sensitive (60%). In addition, deferred diagnoses at frozen section do nothing to alter the operative procedure or guide the surgeon [299]. Frozen section results influenced the surgical approach in only a small percentage of cases. Also, in the era of cost containment, it does not seem justified to perform frozen sections for the intraoperative diagnosis of thyroid nodules; the initial approach to a thyroid nodule should be an aspiration biopsy (FNA) [299,435,436]. If the diagnosis rendered on FNA is definitely malignant, the surgeon should proceed with the appropriate surgery for that malignant diagnosis. If the FNA diagnosis is suspicious for malignancy, and that the suspected lesion is papillary carcinoma or a variant thereof, intraoperative frozen section may be useful since the diagnosis relies on the nuclear morphology and not the finding of invasion. If the FNA diagnosis is "neoplasm" and therefore non-committal as to the type, frozen section will not provide a definitive diagnosis and therefore should not be requested [37,248,251,437].

References

1. Dozois RR, Beahrs OH (1977) Surgical anatomy and technique of thyroid and parathyroid surgery. Surg Clin North Am 57:647–661
2. Akimova RN, Zotikov LA (1969) [An electron microscope study of thyroid gland cells under normal conditions and during the carcinogenic process in golden hamsters]. Vopr Onkol 15:68–75
3. Mansberger AR, Jr., Wei JP (1993) Surgical embryology and anatomy of the thyroid and parathyroid glands. Surg Clin North Am 73:727–746
4. Miller FR (2003) Surgical anatomy of the thyroid and parathyroid glands. Otolaryngol Clin North Am 36:1–7, vii
5. Zampi G, Bianchi S, Amorosi A, Vezzosi V (1994) [Thyroid cancer: anatomy and pathologic histology]. Chir Ital 46:4–7
6. Kondalenko VF, Kalinin AP, Odinokova VA (1970) [Ultrastructure of the normal and pathologic human thyroid gland]. Arkh Patol 32:25–34
7. Nesland JM, Sobrinho-Simoes M, Johannessen JV (1987) Scanning electron microscopy of the human thyroid gland and its disorders. Scanning Microsc 1:1797–1810
8. Sugiyama S (1971) The embryology of the human thyroid gland including ultimobranchial body and others related. Ergeb Anat Entwicklungsgesch 44:3–111
9. Kovalenko AE (1999) [Contemporary concepts of embryology and surgical anatomy of the thyroid gland]. Klin Khir 1999:38–42
10. Gibson W, Peng T, Croker B (1980) C-cell nodules in adult human thyroid: a common autopsy finding. Am J Clin Pathol 73:347–351
11. Wolfe H, DeLellis R, Voelkel E, Tashjian A (1975) Distribution of calcitonin containing cells in the normal neonatal human thyroid gland: a correlation of morphology with peptide content. J Clin Endocrinol Metab 41:1076–1081
12. Baschieri L, Castagna M, Fierabracci A, Antonelli A, Del Guerra P, Squartini F (1989) Distribution of calcitonin- and somatostatin-containing cells in thyroid lymphoma and in Hashimoto's thyroiditis. Appl Pathol 7:99–104
13. Dhillon AP, Rode J, Leathem A, Papadaki L (1982) Somatostatin: a paracrine contribution to hypothyroidism in Hashimoto's thyroiditis. J Clin Pathol 35:764–770
14. O'Toole K, Fenoglio-Preiser C, Pushparaj N (1985) Endocrine changes associated with the human aging process. III. Effect of age on the number of calcitonin immunoreactive cells in the thyroid gland. Hum Pathol 16:991–1000
15. Guyetant S, Rousselet MC, Durigon M, et al (1997) Sex-related C cell hyperplasia in the normal human thyroid: a quantitative autopsy study. J Clin Endocrinol Metab 82:42–47
16. Harach H (1986) Solid cell nests of the human thyroid in early stages of postnatal life. Acta Anat (Basel) 127:262–264
17. Harach H (1988) Solid cell nests of the thyroid. J Pathol 155:191–200
18. Harach HR (1987) Mixed follicles of the human thyroid gland. Acta Anat (Basel) 129:27–30
19. Baloch ZW, LiVolsi VA (1999) Oncocytic lesions of the neuroendocrine system. Semin Diagn Pathol 16:190–199
20. Weiss ML, Deckart H, Pilz R, Deckart E, Kleinau E (1984) [Oncocytes in thyroid gland aspirates. Differential diagnostic problem: tumor/thyroiditis]. Radiobiol Radiother (Berl) 25:765–768
21. Mikhailov IG, Vasil'ev NB, Smirnova EA (1980) [Comparative quantitative electron-microscopic study of the nucleoli of human thyroid oncocytes and follicular cells]. Arkh Patol 42:32–36
22. Mitchell JD, Kirkham N, Machin D (1984) Focal lymphocytic thyroiditis in Southampton. J Pathol 144:269–273

23. Kabel PJ, Voorbij HA, van der Gaag RD, Wiersinga WM, de Haan M, Drexhage HA (1987) Dendritic C-cells in autoimmune thyroid disease. Acta Endocrinol Suppl (Copenh) 281:42–48

24. Nakamura Y, Watanabe M, Matsuzuka F, Maruoka H, Miyauchi A, Iwatani Y (2004) Intrathyroidal CD4+ T lymphocytes express high levels of Fas and CD4+ CD8+ macrophages/dendritic C-cells express Fas ligand in autoimmune thyroid disease. Thyroid 14:819–824

25. Katz AD, Hachigian M (1988) Thyroglossal duct cysts. A thirty year experience with emphasis on occurrence in older patients. Am J Surg 155:741–744

26. Sturgis EM, Miller RH (1988) Thyroglossal duct cysts. J La State Med Soc 145:459–461

27. Topf P, Fried MP, Strome M (1988) Vagaries of thyroglossal duct cysts. Laryngoscope 98:740–742

28. Allard R (1982) The thyroglossal cyst. Head Neck Surg 5:134–140

29. Baughman R (1972) Lingual thyroid and lingual thyroglossal tract remnants. Oral Surg Oral Med Oral Pathol 34:781–798

30. Heshmati HM, Fatourechi V, van Heerden JA, Hay ID, Goellner JR (1997) Thyroglossal duct carcinoma: report of 12 cases. Mayo Clin Proc 72:315–319

31. Apel RL, Asa SL, Chalvardjian A, LiVolsi VA (1994) Intrathyroidal lymphoepithelial cysts of probable branchial origin [see comments]. Hum Pathol 25:1238–1242

32. Carpenter GR, Emery JL (1976) Inclusions in the human thyroid. J Anat 122:77–89

33. Harach HR, Vujanic GM, Jasani B (1993) Ultimobranchial body nests in human fetal thyroid: an autopsy, histological, and immunohistochemical study in relation to solid cell nests and mucoepidermoid carcinoma of the thyroid. J Pathol 169:465–469

34. LiVolsi VA (1990) Surgical pathology of the thyroid. Saunders, Philadelphia

35. Rosai J, Carcangui ML, DeLellis RA (1992) Tumors of the thyroid gland, vol 3rd series, fascicle 5. Armed Forces Institute of Pathology, Washington, DC

36. Hathaway BM (1965) Innocuous accessory thyroid nodules. Arch Surg 90:222–227

37. Baloch Z, LiVolsi VA (2002) Pathology of the thyroid gland. Churchill Livingston, Philadelphia

38. Gerard-Marchant R (1964) Thyroid follicle inclusions in cervical lymph nodes. Arch Pathol Lab Med 77:637–643

39. Roth L (1065) Inclusions of nonneoplastic thyroid tissue within cervical lymph nodes. Cancer 18:105–111

40. Meyer J, Steinberg L (1969) Microscopically benign thyroid follicles in cervical lymph nodes. Cancer 24:301–311

41. Bataskis J, Nishiyama R, Schmidt R (1963) "Sporadic goiter syndrome": a clinicopathologic analysis. Am J Clin Pathol 30:241–251

42. Johnson J (1949) Adenomatous goiters with and without hyperthyroidism. Arch Surg 59:1088–1099

43. Struder H, Ramelli F (1982) Simple goiter and its variants: euthyroid and hyperthyroid. Endocr Rev 3:40–61

44. Weaver D, Batsakis J, Nishiyama R (1969) Relationship of iodine to "lymphocytic goiter." Arch Surg 98:183–185

45. Brown R, Jackson I, Pohl S, Reichlin S (1978) Do thyroid stimulating immunoglobulins cause nontoxic and toxic multinodular goiter? Lancet 1:904–906

46. Gaitan E, Nelson NC, Poole GV (1991) Endemic goiter and endemic thyroid disorders. World J Surg 15:205–215

47. Braverman LE (2001) The physiology and pathophysiology of iodine and the thyroid. Thyroid 11:405

48. Ghossein RA, Rosai J, Heffess C (1997) Dyshormonogenetic goiter: a clinicopathologic study of 56 cases. Endocr Pathol 8:283–292

49. Rosenthal D, Carvalho-Guimaraes DP, Knobel M, Medeiros-Neto GA (1990) Dyshormonogenetic goiter: presence of an inhibitor of normal human thyroid peroxidase. J Endocrinol Invest 13:901–904

50. Bala TS, Janardanasarma MK, Raghunath M (1996) Dietary goitrogen-induced changes in the transport of 2-deoxy-d-glucose and amino acids across the rat blood-brain barrier. Int J Dev Neurosci 14:575–583

51. Fenwick GR, Griffiths NM (1981) The identification of the goitrogen (-)5-vinyloxazolidine-2-thione (goitrin) as a bitter principle of cooked Brussels sprouts (*Brassica oleracea* L. var. gemmifera). Z Lebensm Unters Forsch 172:90–92

52. Gabrilove JL, Dorrance WR, Soffer LJ (1952) Effect of corticotropin, cortisone and desoxycorticosterone on thyroid weight of the goitrogen-treated rat. Am J Physiol 169:565–567

53. Amdisen A, Jensen SE, Olsen T, Schou M (1968) [Development of goiter during lithium treatment]. Ugeskr Laeger 130:1515–1518

54. Maloof F, Wang CA, Vickery AL, Jr (1975) Nontoxic goiter-diffuse or nodular. Med Clin North Am 59:1221–1232

55. Struder H, Peter H, Gerber H (1987) Morphologic and functional changes in developing goiters. In: Hall R, Kobberling J (eds) Thyroid disorders associated with iodine deficiency and excess. Raven, New York

56. Murray D (1998) The thyroid gland. Blackwell Science, Malden, MA

57. Barsano C, DeGroot L (1979) Dyshormonogenetic goiter. Baillieres Clin Endocrinol Metab 8:145–165

58. Medeiros-Neto G, Bunduki V, Tomimori E, et al (1997) Prenatal diagnosis and treatment of dyshormonogenetic fetal goiter due to defective thyroglobulin synthesis. J Clin Endocrinol Metab 82:4239–4242

59. Ramelli F, Studer H, Bruggisser D (1982) Pathogenesis of thyroid nodules in multinodular goiter. Am J Pathol 109:215–223

60. Fialho NJ, de Oliveira CA (1971) [Colloid goiter (observations on 100 operated and treated cases)]. Rev Bras Med 28:314–326

61. Greer MA, Studer H, Kendall JW (1967) Studies on the pathogenesis of colloid goiter. Endocrinology 81:623–632

62. Nair K (1951) Adenoma of thyroid: simple adenomatous goiter. Antiseptic 48:716–724

63. Hirosawa H, Noguchi M, Sakata N, Tanaka S, Miyazaki I (1983) [Adenoma or adenomatous goiter with the clinical symptoms of hyperthyroidism]. Horumon To Rinsho 31(suppl):95–98

64. Apel RL, Ezzat S, Bapat BV, Pan N, LiVolsi VA, Asa SL (1995) Clonality of thyroid nodules in sporadic goiter. Diagn Mol Pathol 4:113–121

65. Hicks DG, LiVolsi VA, Neidich JA, Puck JM, Kant JA (1990) Clonal analysis of solitary follicular nodules in the thyroid. Am J Pathol 137:553–562

66. Miller JM (1975) Plummer's disease. Med Clin North Am 59:1203–1216

67. LiVolsi VA (1994) The pathology of autoimmune thyroid disease: a review. Thyroid 4:333–339

68. Margolick JB, Hsu SM, Volkman DJ, Burman KD, Fauci AS (1984) Immunohistochemical characterization of intrathyroid lymphocytes in Graves' disease. Interstitial and intraepithelial populations. Am J Med 76:815–821

69. Misaki T, Konishi J, Nakashima T, et al (1985) Immuno-histological phenotyping of thyroid infiltrating lymphocytes in Graves' disease and Hashimoto's thyroiditis. Clin Exp Immunol 60:104–110

70. Totterman TH (1978) Distribution of T-, B-, and thyro-globulin-binding lymphocytes infiltrating the gland in Graves' disease, Hashimoto's thyroiditis, and de Quervain's thyroiditis. Clin Immunol Immunopathol 10:270–277

71. Misaki T, Konishi J, Arai K, et al (1987) HLA-DR antigen expression on intrathyroidal lymphocytes and thyrocytes in Hashimoto's thyroiditis and Graves' disease: an immu-nohistological study. Endocrinol Jpn 34:257–262

72. Weetman AP, Gunn C, Hall R, McGregor AM (1985) Thyroid autoantigen-induced lymphocyte proliferation in Graves' disease and Hashimoto's thyroiditis. J Clin Lab Immunol 17:1–6

73. Brinkane A, Ounadi-Corbille W, Bellamy J, Leroy-Ter-quem E (2004) [Hyperplasia of the thymus in Graves' disease. A case report]. Rev Pneumol Clin 60:239–241

74. Kawai K, Tamai H, Mori T, et al (1993) Thyroid histol-ogy of hyperthyroid Graves' disease with undetectable thyrotropin receptor antibodies. J Clin Endocrinol Metab 77:716–719

75. Hirota Y, Tamai H, Hayashi Y, et al (1986) Thyroid func-tion and histology in forty-five patients with hyperthyroid Graves' disease in clinical remission more than ten years after thionamide drug treatment. J Clin Endocrinol Metab 62:165–169

76. Cassano C (1971) [Dyshormonogenetic goiter caused by altered synthesis of thyroglobulin]. Recenti Prog Med 50:9–23

77. Vickery AL, Jr (1981) The diagnosis of malignancy in dyshormonogenetic goitre. Clin Endocrinol Metab 10:317–335

78. Roti E, Uberti ED (2001) Iodine excess and hyperthyroid-ism. Thyroid 11:493–500

79. Strauss A, Trujillo M (1986) Lithium-induced goiter and voice changes. J Clin Psychopharmacol 6:120–121

80. Mizukami Y, Funaki N, Hashimoto T, Kawato M, Michi-gishi T, Matsubara F (1988) Histologic features of thyroid gland in a patient with bromide-induced hypothyroidism. Am J Clin Pathol 89:802–805

81. Imai C, Kakihara T, Watanabe A, et al (2002) Acute sup-purative thyroiditis as a rare complication of aggressive chemotherapy in children with acute myelogenous leuke-mia. Pediatr Hematol Oncol 19:247–253

82. Lambert MJ 3rd, Johns ME, Mentzer R (1980) Acute sup-purative thyroiditis. Am Surg 46:461–463

83. Golshan MM, McHenry CR, de Vente J, Kalajyian RC, Hsu RM, Tomashefski JF (1997) Acute suppurative thy-roiditis and necrosis of the thyroid gland: a rare endocrine manifestation of acquired immunodeficiency syndrome. Surgery 121:593–596

84. Leesen E, Janssen L, Smet M, Breysem L (2001) Acute suppurative thyroiditis. JBR-BTR 84:68

85. Hnilica P, Nyulassy S (1985) Plasma cells in aspirates of goitre and overt permanent hypothyroidism following subacute thyroiditis. Preliminary report. Endocrinol Exp 19:221–226

86. Weetman AP, Smallridge RC, Nutman TB, Burman KD (1987) Persistent thyroid autoimmunity after subacute thyroiditis. J Clin Lab Immunol 23:1–6

87. Greene J. Subacute thyroiditis (1971) Am J Med 51:97–108

88. Bastenie P, Bonnyns M, Neve P (1972) Subacute and chronic granulomatous thyroiditis. In: Bastenie PA, Er-mans AM (eds) Thyroiditis and thyroid function, clinical, morphological and physicological studies. Pergamon, Ox-ford, pp 69–97

89. Cordray JP, Nys P, Merceron RE, Augusti A (2001) [Fre-quency of hypothyroidism after de Quervain thyroiditis and contribution of ultrasonographic thyroid volume measurement]. Ann Med Interne (Paris) 152:84–88

90. Harach HR, Williams ED (1990) The pathology of gran-ulomatous diseases of the thyroid gland. Sarcoidosis 7:19–27

91. Meachim G, Young M (1963) De Quervain's subacute granulomatous thyroiditis: histological identification and incidence. J Clin Pathol 16:189–199

92. Carney JA, Moore SB, Northcutt RC, Woolner LB, Still-well GK (1975) Palpation thyroiditis (multifocal granulo-matous folliculitis). Am J Clin Pathol 64:639–647

93. Harach HR (1993) Palpation thyroiditis resembling C cell hyperplasia. Usefulness of immunohistochemistry in their differential diagnosis. Pathol Res Pract 189:488–490

94. Mizukami Y, Michigishi T, Kawato M, et al (1982) Chronic thyroiditis: thyroid function and histologic correlations in 601 cases. Hum Pathol 23:980

95. Hayashi Y, Tamai H, Fukata S, et al (1985) A long term clinical, immunological, and histological follow-up study of patients with goitrous chronic lymphocytic thyroiditis. J Clin Endocrinol Metab 61:1172–1178

96. Roitt IM, De Carvalho LC (1982) The immunological basis of autoimmune disease. Ciba Found Symp 1982:22–34

97. Podleski WK (1971) Quantitative distribution of IgG, IgM and IgA immunoglobulins in lymphocytic thyroiditis of the Hashimoto type. Arch Immunol Ther Exp 19:431–438

98. Tomer Y, Ban Y, Concepcion E, et al (2003) Common and unique susceptibility loci in Graves and Hashimoto diseases: results of whole-genome screening in a data set of 102 multiplex families. Am J Hum Genet 73:736–747

99. Fatourechi V, McConahey WM, Woolner LB (1971) Hyperthyroidism associated with histologic Hashimoto's thyroiditis. Mayo Clin Proc 46:682–689

100. Mizukami Y, Michigishi T, Hashimoto T, et al (1988) Silent thyroiditis: a histologic and immunohistochemical study. Hum Pathol 19:423–431

101. Aozasa M, Amino N, Iwatani Y, et al (1989) Intrathyroidal HLA-DR-positive lymphocytes in Hashimoto's disease: increases in CD8 and Leu7 cells. Clin Immunol Immunopathol 52:516–522

102. Iwatani Y, Amino N, Mori H, et al (1983) T lymphocyte subsets in autoimmune thyroid diseases and subacute thyroiditis detected with monoclonal antibodies. J Clin Endocrinol Metab 56:251–254

103. Iwatani Y, Hidaka Y, Matsuzuka F, Kuma K, Amino N (1993) Intrathyroidal lymphocyte subsets, including unusual CD4+ CD8+ cells and CD3loTCR alpha beta lo/-CD4-CD8 cells, in autoimmune thyroid disease. Clin Exp Immunol 93:430–436

104. Weetman AP, Volkman DJ, Burman KD, et al (1986) The production and characterization of thyroid-derived T-cell lines in Graves' disease and Hashimoto's thyroiditis. Clin Immunol Immunopathol 39:139–150

105. McIntosh RS, Watson PF, Weetman AP (1997) Analysis of the T cell receptor V alpha repertoire in Hashimoto's thyroiditis: evidence for the restricted accumulation of CD8+ T cells in the absence of CD4+ T cell restriction. J Clin Endocrinol Metab 82:1140–1146

106. Kossev P, Livolsi V (1999) Lymphoid lesions of the thyroid: review in light of the revised European-American lymphoma classification and upcoming World Health Organization classification. Thyroid 9:1273–1280

107. Lam KY, Lo CY, Kwong DL, Lee J, Srivastava G (1999) Malignant lymphoma of the thyroid. A 30-year clinicopathologic experience and an evaluation of the presence of Epstein-Barr virus. Am J Clin Pathol 112:263–270

108. Baloch ZW, Solomon AC, LiVolsi VA (2000) Primary mucoepidermoid carcinoma and sclerosing mucoepidermoid carcinoma with eosinophilia of the thyroid gland: a report of nine cases. Mod Pathol 13:802–807

109. Katz SM, Vickery AL Jr (1974) The fibrous variant of Hashimoto's thyroiditis. Hum Pathol 5:161–170

110. Papi G, Corrado S, Carapezzi C, De Gaetani C, Carani C (2003) Riedel's thyroiditis and fibrous variant of Hashimoto's thyroiditis: a clinicopathological and immunohistochemical study. J Endocrinol Invest 26:444–449

111. LiVolsi VA (1993) Postpartum thyroiditis. The pathology slowly unravels. Am J Clin Pathol 100:193–195

112. Weetman AP, Fung HY, Richards CJ, McGregor AM (1990) IgG subclass distribution and relative functional affinity of thyroid microsomal antibodies in postpartum thyroiditis. Eur J Clin Invest 20:133–136

113. Papi G, Corrado S, Carapezzi C, Corsello SM (2003) Postpartum thyroiditis presenting as a cold nodule and evolving to Graves' disease. Int J Clin Pract 57:556–558

114. Williams ED, Doniach I (1962) The post-mortem incidence of focal thyroiditis. J Pathol Bacteriol 83:255–264

115. Weaver DR, Deodhar SD, Hazard JB (1966) A characterization of focal lymphocytic thyroiditis. Cleve Clin Q 33:59–72

116. Vollenweider R, Stolkin I, Hedinger C (1982) [Focal lymphocytic thyroiditis and iodized salt prophylaxis. Comparative studies on goiter specimens at the Institute of Pathology of Zurich University]. Schweiz Med Wochenschr 112:482–488

117. Katsikas D, Shorthouse A, Taylor S (1976) Riedel's thyroiditis. Br J Surg 63:929–931

118. Arnott E, Greaves D (1965) Orbital involvement in Riedel's thyroiditis. Br J Ophthalmol 491:1–5

119. Bartholomew L, Cain J, Woolner L, Utz D, Ferris D (1963) Sclerosing cholangitis. Its possible association with Riedel's struma and fibrous retroperitonitis. N Engl J Med 269:8–12

120. Davies D, Furness P (1984) Riedel's thyroiditis with multiple organ fibrosis. Thorax 39:959–960

121. Rao C, Ferguson G, Kyle V (1973) Retroperitoneal fibrosis associated with Riedel's struma. Can Med Assoc J 108:1019–1021

122. Schwaegerle S, Bauer T, Esselstyn C (1988) Riedel's thyroiditis. Am J Clin Pathol 90:715–722

123. Papi G, Corrado S, Cesinaro AM, Novelli L, Smerieri A, Carapezzi C (2002) Riedel's thyroiditis: clinical, pathological and imaging features. Int J Clin Pract 56:65–67

124. Casoli P, Tumiati B (1999) Hypoparathyroidism secondary to Riedel's thyroiditis. A case report and a review of the literature. Ann Ital Med Int 14:54–57

125. Meij S, Hausman R (1978) Occlusive phlebitis, a diagnostic feature in Riedel's thyroiditis. Virchows Arch [A]. 377:339–349

126. Harach HR, Williams ED (1983) Fibrous thyroiditis: an immunopathological study. Histopathology 7:739–751

127. Baloch ZW, Feldman MD, LiVolsi VA (2000) Combined Riedel's disease and fibrosing Hashimoto's thyroiditis: a report of three cases with two showing coexisting papillary carcinoma. Endocr Pathol 11:157–163

128. Bogazzi F, Bartalena L, Gasperi M, Braverman LE, Martino E (2001) The various effects of amiodarone on thyroid function. Thyroid 11:511–519

129. Smyrk T, Goellner J, Brennan M, Carney J (1987) Pathology of the thyroid in amiodarone associated thyrotoxicosis. Am J Surg Pathol 11:197–204

130. Cetta F, Montalto G, Petracci M, Fusco A (1997) Thyroid cancer and the Chernobyl accident. Are long-term and long-distance side effects of fall-out radiation greater than estimated? J Clin Endocrinol Metab 82:2015–2017

131. Carr RF, LiVolsi VA (1989) Morphologic changes in the thyroid after irradiation for Hodgkin's and non-Hodgkin's lymphoma. Cancer 64:825–829

132. Aizawa T, Watanabe T, Suzuki N, et al (1998) Radiation-induced painless thyrotoxic thyroiditis followed by hypothyroidism: a case report and literature review. Thyroid 8:273–275

133. Avetisian IL, Gulchiy NV, Demidiuk AP, Stashuk AV (1996) Thyroid pathology in residents of the Kiev region, Ukraine, during pre- and post-Chernobyl periods. J Environ Pathol Toxicol Oncol 15:233–237

134. Nishiyama K, Kozuka T, Higashihara T, Miyauchi K, Okagawa K (1996) Acute radiation thyroiditis. Int J Radiat Oncol Biol Phys 36:1221–1224

135. Lindsay S, Dailey M, Jones M (1954) Histologic effects of various types of ionizing radiation on normal and hyperplastic human thyroid glands. J Clin Endocrinol Metab 14:1179–1219

136. Goldsmith JD, Lai ML, Daniele GM, Tomaszewski JE, LiVolsi VA (2000) Amyloid goiter: report of two cases and review of the literature. Endocr Pract 6:318–323

137. Hamed G, Heffess CS, Shmookler BM, Wenig BM (1995) Amyloid goiter. A clinicopathologic study of 14 cases and review of the literature. Am J Clin Pathol 104:306–312

138. Pastolero GC, Asa SL (1994) Drug-related pigmentation of the thyroid associated with papillary carcinoma. Arch Pathol Lab Med 118:79–83

139. Gordon G, Sparano B, Kramer A, Kelly R, Latropoulos M (1984) Thyroid gland pigmentation and minocycline therapy. Am J Pathol 117:98–109

140. LiVolsi VA, Feind CR (1976) Parathyroid adenoma and nonmedullary thyroid carcinoma. Cancer 38:1391–1393

141. Mai KT, Landry DC, Thomas J, et al (2001) Follicular adenoma with papillary architecture: a lesion mimicking papillary thyroid carcinoma. Histopathology 39:25–32

142. LiVolsi VA (1996) Well differentiated thyroid carcinoma. Clin Oncol (R Coll Radiol) 8:281–288

143. LiVolsi VA, Baloch ZW (2004) Follicular neoplasms of the thyroid: view, biases, and experiences. Adv Anat Pathol 11:279–287

144. LiVolsi VA, Merino MJ (1994) Worrisome histologic alterations following fine-needle aspiration of the thyroid (WHAFFT). Pathol Annu 29:99–120

145. Oyama T, Vickery AL Jr, Preffer FI, Colvin RB (1994) A comparative study of flow cytometry and histopathologic findings in thyroid follicular carcinomas and adenomas. Hum Pathol 25:271–275

146. Harlow SP, Duda RB, Bauer KD (1992) Diagnostic utility of DNA content flow cytometry in follicular neoplasms of the thyroid. J Surg Oncol 50:1–6

147. Carney JA, Ryan J, Goellner JR (1987) Hyalinizing trabecular adenoma of the thyroid gland. Am J Surg Pathol 11:583–591

148. Chetty R, Beydoun R, LiVolsi VA (1994) Paraganglioma-like (hyalinizing trabecular) adenoma of the thyroid revisited. Pathology 26:429–431

149. LiVolsi VA (2000) Hyalinizing trabecular tumor of the thyroid: adenoma, carcinoma, or neoplasm of uncertain malignant potential? Am J Surg Pathol 24:1683–1684

150. Fonseca E, Nesland J, Sobrinho-Simoes M (1997) Expression of stratified epithelial type cytokeratins in hyalinizing trabecular adenoma supports their relationship with papillary carcinoma of the thyroid. Histopathology 31:330–335

151. Papotti M, Volante M, Giuliano A, et al (2000) RET/PTC activation in hyalinizing trabecular tumors of the thyroid. Am J Surg Pathol 24:1615–1621

152. Hazard JB, Kenyon R (1954) Atypical adenoma of the thyroid. Arch Pathol 58:554–563

153. Fukunaga M, Shinozaki N, Endo Y, Ushigome S (1992) Atypical adenoma of the thyroid. A clinicopathologic and flow cytometric DNA study in comparison with other follicular neoplasms. Acta Pathol Jpn 42:632–638

154. Lang W, Georgii A, Atay Z (1977) [Differential diagnosis between atypical adenoma and follicular carcinoma of the thyroid gland (author's translation)]. Verh Dtsch Ges Pathol 61:275–279

155. Carcangiu ML, Steeper T, Zampi G, Rosai J (1985) Anaplastic thyroid carcinoma. A study of 70 cases. Am J Clin Pathol 83:135–158

156. Carcangui ML ZG, Pupi A, Castagnoli A, Rosai J (1985) Papillary carcinoma of the thyroid: a clinico-pathologic study of 241 cases treated at the University of Florence, Italy. Cancer 55:805–828

157. LiVolsi VA (1992) Papillary neoplasms of the thyroid. Pathologic and prognostic features. Am J Clin Pathol 97:426–434

158. Mazzaferi EYR (1981) Papillary thyroid carcinoma: a 10-year follow-up report of the impact of therapy in 576 patients. Am J Med 70:511–518

159. Furlan JC, Bedard YC, Rosen IB (2004) Clinicopathologic significance of histologic vascular invasion in papillary and follicular thyroid carcinomas. J Am Coll Surg 198:341–348

160. Mills SE, Allen MS Jr (1986) Congenital occult papillary carcinoma of the thyroid gland. Hum Pathol 17:1179–1181

161. Schottenfeld D, Gershman ST (1977) Epidemiology of thyroid cancer, part II. Clin Bull 7:98–104

162. Williams ED, Doniach I, Bjarnason O, Michie W (1977) Thyroid cancer in an iodide rich area: a histopathological study. Cancer 39:215–222

163. Harach HR, Escalante DA, Day ES (2002) Thyroid cancer and thyroiditis in Salta, Argentina: a 40-yr study in relation to iodine prophylaxis. Endocr Pathol 13:175–181

164. Petrova GV, Tereshchenko VP, Avetis'ian IL (1996) [The dynamics of thyroid diseases in the inhabitants of Kiev and Kiev Province after the accident at the Chernobyl Atomic Electric Power Station]. Lik Sprava 1996:67–70

165. Ron E, Kleinerman RA, Boice JD, LiVolsi VA, Flannery JT, Fraumeni JF (1987) A population-based case-control study of thyroid cancer. J Natl Cancer Inst 79:1–12

166. Pacini F, Vorontsova T, Molinaro E, et al (1999) Thyroid consequences of the Chernobyl nuclear accident. Acta Paediatr Suppl 88:23–27

167. Tamimi DM (2002) The association between chronic lymphocytic thyroiditis and thyroid tumors. Int J Surg Pathol 10:141–146

168. Nikiforova MN, Caudill CM, Biddinger P, Nikiforov YE (2002) Prevalence of RET/PTC rearrangements in Hashimoto's thyroiditis and papillary thyroid carcinomas. Int J Surg Pathol 10:15–22

169. Hunt JL, Baloch Z, Barnes EL, et al (2002) Loss of heterozygosity mutations of tumor suppressor genes in cytologically atypical areas of chronic lymphocytic thyroiditis. Endocr Pathol 13:23–30

170. La Vecchia C, Ron E, Franceschi S, et al (1999) A pooled analysis of case-control studies of thyroid cancer. III. Oral contraceptives, menopausal replacement therapy and other female hormones. Cancer Causes Control 10:157–166

171. Diaz NM, Mazoujian G, Wick MR (1991) Estrogen-receptor protein in thyroid neoplasms. An immunohistochemical analysis of papillary carcinoma, follicular carcinoma, and follicular adenoma. Arch Pathol Lab Med 115:1203–1207

172. Cetta F, Montalto G, Gori M, Curia MC, Cama A, Olschwang S (2000) Germline mutations of the APC gene in patients with familial adenomatous polyposis-associated thyroid carcinoma: results from a European cooperative study. J Clin Endocrinol Metab 85:286–292

173. Harach HR, Soubeyran I, Brown A, Bonneau D, Longy M (1999) Thyroid pathologic findings in patients with Cowden disease. Ann Diagn Pathol 3:331–340

174. Haggitt RC, Reid BJ (1986) Hereditary gastrointestinal polyposis syndromes. Am J Surg Pathol 10:871–887

175. Cetta F, Toti P, Petracci M, et al (1997) Thyroid carcinoma associated with familial adenomatous polyposis. Histopathology 31:231–236

176. Cetta F, Olschwang S, Petracci M, et al (1998) Genetic alterations in thyroid carcinoma associated with familial adenomatous polyposis: clinical implications and suggestions for early detection. World J Surg 22:1231–1236

177. Cetta F, Chiappetta G, Melillo RM, et al (1998) The ret/ptc1 oncogene is activated in familial adenomatous polyposis-associated thyroid papillary carcinomas. J Clin Endocrinol Metab 83:1003–1006

178. Dahia PL, Marsh DJ, Zheng Z, et al (1997) Somatic deletions and mutations in the Cowden disease gene, PTEN, in sporadic thyroid tumors. Cancer Res 57:4710–4713

179. Wirtzfeld DA, Petrelli NJ, Rodriguez-Bigas MA (2001) Hamartomatous polyposis syndromes: molecular genetics, neoplastic risk, and surveillance recommendations. Ann Surg Oncol 8:319–327

180. Meshikhes AW, Butt MS, Al-Saihati BA (2004) Combined parathyroid adenoma and an occult papillary carcinoma. Saudi Med J 25:1707–1710

181. Dralle H, Altenahr E (1979) Pituitary adenoma, primary parathyroid hyperplasia and papillary (non-medullary) thyroid carcinoma. A case of multiple endocrine neoplasia (MEN). Virchows Arch A Pathol Anat Histol 381:179–187

182. Francis IM, Das DK, Sheikh ZA, Sharma PN, Gupta SK (1995) Role of nuclear grooves in the diagnosis of papillary thyroid carcinoma. A quantitative assessment on fine needle aspiration smears. Acta Cytol 39:409–415

183. Riazmontazer N, Bedayat G (1991) Psammoma bodies in fine needle aspirates from thyroids containing nontoxic hyperplastic nodular goiters. Acta Cytol 35:563–566

184. Hunt JL, Barnes EL (2003) Non-tumor-associated psammoma bodies in the thyroid. Am J Clin Pathol 119:90–94

185. Hosoya T, Sakamoto A, Kasai N, Sakurai K (1983) [Nodal psammoma body in thyroid cancer as an indicator of cancer metastasis to the lymph node]. Gan No Rinsho 29:1336–1339

186. Mancini A, Rabitti C, Conte G, Gullotta G, De Marinis L (1993) [Lymphocytic infiltration in thyroid neoplasms. Preliminary prognostic assessments]. Minerva Chir 48:1283–1288

187. Gomez Saez JM, Gomez Arnaiz N, Sahun de la Vega M, Soler Ramon J (1997) [Prevalence and significance of lymphocyte infiltration in papillary carcinoma of the thyroid gland]. Ann Med Interna 14:403–405

188. Ruiz-Velasco R, Waisman J, Van Herle AJ (1978) Cystic papillary carcinoma of the thyroid gland. Diagnosis by needle aspiration with transmission electron microscopy. Acta Cytol 22:38–42

189. de los Santos ET, Keyhani-Rofagha S, Cunningham JJ, Mazzaferri EL (1990) Cystic thyroid nodules. The dilemma of malignant lesions. Arch Intern Med 150:1422–1427

190. Namba H, Matsuo K, Fagin JA (1990) Clonal composition of benign and malignant human thyroid tumors. J Clin Invest 86:120–125

191. Fusco A, Chiappetta G, Hui P, et al (2002) Assessment of RET/PTC oncogene activation and clonality in thyroid nodules with incomplete morphological evidence of papillary carcinoma: a search for the early precursors of papillary cancer. Am J Pathol 160:2157–2167

192. Hunt JL, LiVolsi VA, Baloch ZW, et al (2003) Microscopic papillary thyroid carcinoma compared with clinical carcinomas by loss of heterozygosity mutational profile. Am J Surg Pathol 27:159–166

193. Petkov R, Gavrailov M, Mikhailov I, Todorov G, Kutev N (1995) [Differentiated thyroid cancer: a study of the pathomorphological variants in 216 patients]. Khirurgiia 48:11–12

194. Akslen LA, LiVolsi VA (2000) Prognostic significance of histologic grading compared with subclassification of papillary thyroid carcinoma [see comments]. Cancer 88:1902–1908

195. Paessler M, Kreisel FH, LiVolsi VA, Akslen LA, Baloch ZW (2002) Can we rely on pathologic parameters to define conservative treatment of papillary thyroid carcinoma? Int J Surg Pathol 10:267–272

196. Santini L, Pezzullo L, D'Arco E, De Rosa N, Guerriero O, Salza C (1989) Lymph node metastases from an occult sclerosing carcinoma of the thyroid. A case report. Ital J Surg Sci 19:277–279

197. Akslen LA, LiVolsi VA (2000) Poorly differentiated thyroid carcinoma: it is important. Am J Surg Pathol 24:310–313

198. Tachikawa T, Kumazawa H, Kyomoto R, Yukawa H, Yamashita T, Nishikawa M (2001) [Clinical study on prognostic factors in thyroid carcinoma]. Nippon Jibiinkoka Gakkai Kaiho 104:157–164

199. Mazzaferri EL (1987) Papillary thyroid carcinoma: factors influencing prognosis and current therapy. Semin Oncol 14:315–332

200. Prasad ML, Pellegata NS, Huang Y, Nagaraja HN, Chapelle Ade L, Kloos RT (2005) Galectin-3, fibronectin-1, CITED-1, HBME1 and cytokeratin-19 immunohistochemistry is useful for the differential diagnosis of thyroid tumors. Mod Pathol 18:48–57

201. Casey MB, Lohse CM, Lloyd RV (2003) Distinction between papillary thyroid hyperplasia and papillary thyroid carcinoma by immunohistochemical staining for cytokeratin 19, galectin-3, and HBME-1. Endocr Pathol 14:55–60

202. Cheung CC, Ezzat S, Freeman JL, Rosen IB, Asa SL (2001) Immunohistochemical diagnosis of papillary thyroid carcinoma. Mod Pathol 14:338–342

203. Eimoto T, Naito H, Hamada S, Masuda M, Harada T, Kikuchi M (1987) Papillary carcinoma of the thyroid. A histochemical, immunohistochemical and ultrastructural study with special reference to the follicular variant. Acta Pathol Jpn 37:1563–1579

204. van Hoeven KH, Kovatich AJ, Miettinen M (1998) Immunocytochemical evaluation of HBME-1, CA 19-9, and CD-15 (Leu-M1) in fine-needle aspirates of thyroid nodules. Diagn Cytopathol 18:93–97

205. Baloch ZW, Abraham S, Roberts S, LiVolsi VA (1999) Differential expression of cytokeratins in follicular variant of papillary carcinoma: an immunohistochemical study and its diagnostic utility. Hum Pathol 30:1166–1171

206. Baloch ZW, LiVolsi VA (2002) The quest for a magic tumor marker: continuing saga in the diagnosis of the follicular lesions of thyroid. Am J Clin Pathol 118:165–166

207. Batistatou A, Zolota V, Scopa CD (2002) S-100 protein+ dendritiC-cells and CD34+ dendritic interstitial cells in thyroid lesions. Endocr Pathol 13:111–115

208. Hiasa Y, Nishioka H, Kitahori Y, et al (1991) Immunohistochemical detection of estrogen receptors in paraffin sections of human thyroid tissues. Oncology 48:421–424

209. Khan A, Baker SP, Patwardhan NA, Pullman JM (1998) CD57 (Leu-7) expression is helpful in diagnosis of the follicular variant of papillary thyroid carcinoma. Virchows Arch 432:427–432

210. Miettinen M, Karkkainen P (1996) Differential reactivity of HBME-1 and CD15 antibodies in benign and malignant thyroid tumours. Preferential reactivity with malignant tumours. Virchows Arch 429:213–219

211. Zedenius J, Auer G, Backdahl M, et al (1992) Follicular tumors of the thyroid gland: diagnosis, clinical aspects and nuclear DNA analysis. World J Surg 16:589–594

212. Grieco M, Santoro M, Berlingieri MT, et al (1990) PTC is a novel rearranged form of the ret proto-oncogene and is frequently detected in vivo in human thyroid papillary carcinomas. Cell 60:557–563

213. Santoro M, Rosati R, Grieco M, et al (1990) The ret proto-oncogene is consistently expressed in human pheochromocytomas and thyroid medullary carcinomas. Oncogene 5:1595–1598

214. Santoro M, Dathan NA, Berlingieri MT, et al (1994) Molecular characterization of RET/PTC3: a novel rearranged version of the RET proto-oncogene in a human thyroid papillary carcinoma. Oncogene 9:509–516

215. Inaba M, Umemura S, Satoh H, et al (2003) Expression of RET in follicular cell-derived tumors of the thyroid gland: prevalence and implication of morphological type. Pathol Int 53:146–153

216. Nikiforov YE (2002) RET/PTC rearrangement in thyroid tumors. Endocr Pathol 13:3–16

217. Jhiang SM, Cho JY, Furminger TL, et al (1998) Thyroid carcinomas in RET/PTC transgenic mice. Recent Results Cancer Res 154:265–270

218. Fischer AH, Bond JA, Taysavang P, Eugene B, Wynford-Thomas D (1998) Papillary thyroid carcinoma oncogene (RET/PTC) alters the nuclear envelope and chromatin structure. Am J Pathol 153:1443–1450

219. Fusco A, Santoro M, Grieco M, et al (1995) RET/PTC activation in human thyroid carcinomas. J Endocrinol Invest 18:127–129

220. Nikiforov YE, Rowland JM, Bove KE, Monforte-Munoz H, Fagin JA (1997) Distinct pattern of ret oncogene rearrangements in morphological variants of radiation-induced and sporadic thyroid papillary carcinomas in children. Cancer Res 57:1690–1694

221. Bounacer A, Wicker R, Schlumberger M, Sarasin A, Suarez HG (1997) Oncogenic rearrangements of the ret proto-oncogene in thyroid tumors induced after exposure to ionizing radiation. Biochimie 79:619–623

222. Wirtschafter A, Schmidt R, Rosen D, et al (1997) Expression of the RET/PTC fusion gene as a marker for papillary carcinoma in Hashimoto's thyroiditis [see comments]. Laryngoscope 107:95–100

223. Sheils O, Smyth P, Finn S, Sweeney EC, O'Leary JJ (2002) RET/PTC rearrangements in Hashimoto's thyroiditis. Int J Surg Pathol 10:167–168; discussion 168–169

224. Elisei R, Romei C, Vorontsova T, et al (2001) RET/PTC rearrangements in thyroid nodules: studies in irradiated and not irradiated, malignant and benign thyroid lesions in children and adults. J Clin Endocrinol Metab 86:3211–3216

225. Cohen Y, Xing M, Mambo E, et al (2003) BRAF mutation in papillary thyroid carcinoma. J Natl Cancer Inst 95:625–627

226. Nikiforova MN, Kimura ET, Gandhi M, et al (2003) BRAF mutations in thyroid tumors are restricted to papillary carcinomas and anaplastic or poorly differentiated carcinomas arising from papillary carcinomas. J Clin Endocrinol Metab 88:5399–5404

227. Soares P, Trovisco V, Rocha AS, et al (2004) BRAF mutations typical of papillary thyroid carcinoma are more frequently detected in undifferentiated than in insular and insular-like poorly differentiated carcinomas. Virchows Arch 444:572–576

228. Puxeddu E, Moretti S, Elisei R, et al (2004) BRAF(V599E) mutation is the leading genetic event in adult sporadic papillary thyroid carcinomas. J Clin Endocrinol Metab 89:2414–2420

229. Begum S, Rosenbaum E, Henrique R, Cohen Y, Sidransky D, Westra WH (2004) BRAF mutations in anaplastic thyroid carcinoma: implications for tumor origin, diagnosis and treatment. Mod Pathol 17:1359–1363

230. Mazzaferri EL (1999) An overview of the management of papillary and follicular thyroid carcinoma. Thyroid 9:421–427

231. Kjellman P, Learoyd DL, Messina M, et al (2001) Expression of the RET proto-oncogene in papillary thyroid carcinoma and its correlation with clinical outcome. Br J Surg 88:557–563

232. Basolo F, Molinaro E, Agate L, et al (2001) RET protein expression has no prognostic impact on the long-term outcome of papillary thyroid carcinoma. Eur J Endocrinol 145:599–604

233. Cetta F, Gori M, Raffaelli N, Baldi C, Montalto G (1999) Comment on clinical and prognostic relevance of Ret-PTC activation in patients with papillary thyroid carcinoma. J Clin Endocrinol Metab 84:2257–2258

234. Kim JY, Cho H, Rhee BD, Kim HY (2002) Expression of CD44 and cyclin D1 in fine needle aspiration cytology of papillary thyroid carcinoma. Acta Cytol 46:679–683

235. Takeuchi Y, Daa T, Kashima K, Yokoyama S, Nakayama I, Noguchi S (1999) Mutations of p53 in thyroid carcinoma with an insular component. Thyroid 9:377–381

236. Basolo F, Caligo MA, Pinchera A, et al (2000) Cyclin D1 overexpression in thyroid carcinomas: relation with clinico-pathological parameters, retinoblastoma gene product, and Ki67 labeling index. Thyroid 10:741–746

237. Lee A, LiVolsi VA, Baloch ZW (2000) Expression of DNA topoisomerase IIalpha in thyroid neoplasia. Mod Pathol 13:396–400

238. Tallini G, Garcia-Rostan G, Herrero A, et al (1999) Downregulation of p27KIP1 and Ki67/Mib1 labeling index support the classification of thyroid carcinoma into prognostically relevant categories. Am J Surg Pathol 23:678–685

239. DeLellis RA, Lloyd RD, Heitz PU, Eng C (eds) (2004) WHO: pathology and genetics. Tumours of endocrine organs. In: Kleihues P, Sobin LE (eds) WHO classification of tumours. IARC Press, Lyon, France

240. Rodriguez JM, Moreno A, Parrilla P, et al (1997) Papillary thyroid microcarcinoma: clinical study and prognosis. Eur J Surg 163:255–259

241. Hay ID, Grant CS, van Heerden JA, Goellner JR, Ebersold JR, Bergstralh EJ (1992) Papillary thyroid microcarcinoma: a study of 535 cases observed in a 50-year period. Surgery 112:1139–1146; discussion 1146–1147

242. Braga M, Graf H, Ogata A, Batista J, Hakim NC (2002) Aggressive behavior of papillary microcarcinoma in a patient with Graves' disease initially presenting as cystic neck mass. J Endocrinol Invest 25:250–253

243. Fernandez-Real JM, Ricart W (1999) Familial papillary thyroid microcarcinoma. Lancet 353:1973–1974

244. Lupoli G, Vitale G, Caraglia M, et al (1999) Familial papillary thyroid microcarcinoma: a new clinical entity. Lancet 353:637–639

245. Lindsay S (1960) Carcinoma of the thyroid gland: a clinical and pathologic study of 239 patients at the University of California Hospital. Springfield, IL

246. Chen KTC, Rosai J (1977) Follicular variant of thyroid papillary carcinoma: a clinicopathologic study of six cases. Am J Surg Pathol 1:123–130

247. LiVolsi VA, Asa SL (1994) The demise of follicular carcinoma of the thyroid gland. Thyroid 4:233–236

248. Baloch ZW, Gupta PK, Yu GH, Sack MJ, LiVolsi VA (1999) Follicular variant of papillary carcinoma. Cytologic and histologic correlation. Am J Clin Pathol 111:216–222

249. Baloch Z, LiVolsi VA, Henricks WH, Sebak BA (2002) Encapsulated follicular variant of papillary thyroid carcinoma. Am J Clin Pathol 118:603–605; discussion 605–606

250. Tielens ET, Sherman SI, Hruban RH, Ladenson PW (1994) Follicular variant of papillary thyroid carcinoma. A clinicopathologic study. Cancer 73:424–431

251. Baloch ZW, Livolsi VA (2002) Follicular-patterned lesions of the thyroid: the bane of the pathologist. Am J Clin Pathol 117:143–150

252. Mizukami Y, Nonomura A, Michigishi T, Ohmura K, Noguchi M, Ishizaki T (1995) Diffuse follicular variant of papillary carcinoma of the thyroid. Histopathology 27:575–577

253. Ivanova R, Soares P, Castro P, Sobrinho-Simoes M (2002) Diffuse (or multinodular) follicular variant of papillary thyroid carcinoma: a clinicopathologic and immunohistochemical analysis of ten cases of an aggressive form of differentiated thyroid carcinoma. Virchows Arch 440:418–424

254. Williams ED, Abrosimov A, Bogdanova TI, Roasi J, Sidorov Y, Thomas GA (2000) Two proposals regarding the terminology of thyroid tumors. Guest Editorial. Int J Surg Pathol 8:181–183

255. Johnson THLR, Thompson NW, Beierwalters WH, Sisson JC (1988) Prognostic implications of the tall cell variant of papillary carcinoma. Am J Surg Pathol 12:22–27

256. Sobrinho-Simoes M, Sambade C, Nesland JM, Johannessen JV (1989) Tall cell papillary carcinoma. Am J Surg Pathol 13:79–80

257. Bronner MP, LiVolsi VA (1991) Spindle cell squamous carcinoma of the thyroid: an unusual anaplastic tumor associated with tall cell papillary cancer. Mod Pathol 4:637–643

258. Prendiville S, Burman KD, Ringel MD, et al (2000) Tall cell variant: an aggressive form of papillary thyroid carcinoma. Otolaryngol Head Neck Surg 122:352–357

259. Jobran R, Baloch ZW, Aviles V, Rosato EF, Schwartz S, LiVolsi VA (2000) Tall cell papillary carcinoma of the thyroid: metastatic to the pancreas [In Process Citation]. Thyroid 10:185–187

260. Terry J, St John S, Karkowski F, et al (1994) Tall cell papillary thyroid cancer: incidence and prognosis. Am J Surg 168:459–461

261. Sobrinho-Simoes M, Nesland JM, Johannessen JV (1988) Columnar-cell carcinoma. Another variant of poorly differentiated carcinoma of the thyroid. Am J Clin Pathol 89:264–267

262. Chan JK (1990) Papillary carcinoma of thyroid: classical and variants. Histol Histopathol 5:241–257

263. Wenig BM, Thompson LDR, Adair CF, Shmookler B, Heffess CF (1998) Thyroid papillary carcinoma of columnar cell type. A clinicopathologic study of 16 cases. Cancer 82:740–753

264. Evans HL (1996) Encapsulated columnar-cell carcinoma of the thyroid. A report of four cases suggesting a favorable outcome. Am J Surg Pathol 20:1205–1211

265. Apel RL, Asa SL, LiVolsi VA (1995) Papillary Hürthle cell carcinoma with lymphocytic stroma. "Warthin-like tumor" of the thyroid. Am J Surg Pathol 19:810–814

266. Baloch ZW, LiVolsi VA (2000) Warthin-like papillary carcinoma of the thyroid. Arch Pathol Lab Med 124:1192–1195

267. Chan JKC, Tsui MS, Tse CH (1987) Diffuse sclerosing variant of papillary thyroid carcinoma. A histological and immunohistochemical study of three cases. Histopathology 11:191–201

268. Peix JL, Mabrut JY, Van Box Som P, Berger N (1998) [Thyroid cancer in children and adolescents. Clinical aspects, diagnostic problems and special therapeutics]. Ann Endocrinol (Paris) 59:113–120

269. Santoro M, Thomas GA, Vecchio G, et al (2000) Gene rearrangement and Chernobyl related thyroid cancers. Br J Cancer 82:315–322

270. Soares J, Limbert E, Sobrinho-Simoes M (1989) Diffuse sclerosing variant of papillary thyroid carcinoma. A clinicopathologic study of 10 cases. Pathol Res Pract 185:200–206

271. Nikiforov YE, Erickson LA, Nikiforova MN, Caudill CM, Lloyd RV (2001) Solid variant of papillary thyroid carcinoma: incidence, clinical-pathologic characteristics, molecular analysis, and biologic behavior. Am J Surg Pathol 25:1478–1484

272. Thomas GA, Bunnell H, Cook HA, et al (1999) High prevalence of RET/PTC rearrangements in Ukrainian and Belarussian post-Chernobyl thyroid papillary carcinomas: a strong correlation between RET/PTC3 and the solid-follicular variant. J Clin Endocrinol Metab 84:4232–4238

273. Sywak M, Pasieka JL, Ogilvie T (2004) A review of thyroid cancer with intermediate differentiation. J Surg Oncol 86:44–54

274. Vergilio J, Baloch ZW, LiVolsi VA (2002) Spindle cell metaplasia of the thyroid arising in association with papillary carcinoma and follicular adenoma. Am J Clin Pathol 117:199–204

275. Dickersin G, Vickery AL Jr, Smith S (1980) Papillary carcinoma of the thyroid, oxyphil cell type, "clear cell" variant: a light and electron microscopic study. Am J Surg Pathol 4:501–509

276. Berho M, Suster S (1997) The oncocytic variant of papillary carcinoma of the thyroid: a clinicopathologic study of 15 cases. Hum Pathol 28:47–53

277. Bisi H, Longatto Filho A, de Camargo RY, Fernandes VS (1993) Thyroid papillary carcinoma lipomatous type: report of two cases. Pathologica 85:761–764

278. Schroder S, Bocker W (1985) Lipomatous lesions of the thyroid gland: a review. Appl Pathol 3:140–149

279. Chan JK, Carcangiu ML, Rosai J (1991) Papillary carcinoma of thyroid with exuberant nodular fasciitis-like stroma. Report of three cases. Am J Clin Pathol 95:309–314

280. Cameselle-Teijeiro J, Chan JK (1999) Cribriform-morular variant of papillary carcinoma: a distinctive variant representing the sporadic counterpart of familial adenomatous polyposis-associated thyroid carcinoma? Mod Pathol 12:400–411

281. Hirokawa M, Kuma S, Miyauchi A, et al (2004) Morules in cribriform-morular variant of papillary thyroid carcinoma: immunohistochemical characteristics and distinction from squamous metaplasia. APMIS 112:275–282

282. Xu B, Yoshimoto K, Miyauchi A, et al (2003) Cribriform-morular variant of papillary thyroid carcinoma: a pathological and molecular genetic study with evidence of frequent somatic mutations in exon 3 of the beta-catenin gene. J Pathol 199:58–67

283. Franssila KO, Ackerman LV, Brown CL, Hedinger CE (1985) Follicular carcinoma. Semin Diagn Pathol 2:101–122

284. Tollefson HR, Shah JP, Huvos AG (1973) Follicular carcinoma of the thyroid. Am J Surg 126:523–528

285. Wade JS (1975) The aetiology and diagnosis of malignant tumours of the thyroid gland. Br J Surg 62:760–764

286. Jorda M, Gonzalez-Campora R, Mora J, Herrero-Zapatero A, Otal C, Galera H (1993) Prognostic factors in follicular carcinoma of the thyroid. Arch Pathol Lab Med 117:631–635

287. Segal K, Arad A, Lubin E, Shpitzer T, Hadar T, Feinmesser R (1994) Follicular carcinoma of the thyroid. Head Neck 16:533–538

288. Crile G, Pontius K, Hawk W (1985) Factors influencing the survival of patients with follicular carcinoma of the thyroid gland. Surg Gynecol Obstet 160:409–412

289. Schmidt RJ, Wang CA (1986) Encapsulated follicular carcinoma of the thyroid: diagnosis, treatment, and results. Surgery 100:1068–1077

290. Evans HL (1984) Follicular neoplasms of the thyroid. A study of 44 cases followed for a minimum of 10 years with emphasis on differential diagnosis. Cancer 54:535–540

291. Thompson LD, Wieneke JA, Paal E, Frommelt RA, Adair CF, Heffess CS (2001) A clinicopathologic study of minimally invasive follicular carcinoma of the thyroid gland with a review of the English literature. Cancer 91:505–524

292. Carcangiu ML (1997) Minimally invasive follicular carcinoma. Endocr Pathol 8:231–234

293. Shaha AR, Loree TR, Shah JP (1995) Prognostic factors and risk group analysis in follicular carcinoma of the thyroid. Surgery 118:1131–1136; discussion 1136–1138

294. Moore JH Jr, Bacharach B, Choi HY (1985) Anaplastic transformation of metastatic follicular carcinoma of the thyroid. J Surg Oncol 29:216–221

295. D'Avanzo A, Treseler P, Ituarte PH, et al (2004) Follicular thyroid carcinoma: histology and prognosis. Cancer 100:1123–1129

296. Jakubiak-Wielganowicz M, Kubiak R, Sygut J, Pomorski L, Kordek R (2003) Usefulness of galectin-3 immunohistochemistry in differential diagnosis between thyroid follicular carcinoma and follicular adenoma. Pol J Pathol 54:111–115

297. Collini P, Sampietro G, Rosai J, Pilotti S (2003) Minimally invasive (encapsulated) follicular carcinoma of the thyroid gland is the low-risk counterpart of widely invasive follicular carcinoma but not of insular carcinoma. Virchows Arch 442:71–76

298. Kahn NF, Perzin KH (1983) Follicular carcinoma of the thyroid: an evaluation of the histologic criteria used for diagnosis. Pathol Ann 18:221–253

299. Udelsman R, Westra WH, Donovan PI, Sohn TA, Cameron JL (2001) Randomized prospective evaluation of frozen-section analysis for follicular neoplasms of the thyroid. Ann Surg 233:716–722

300. Leteurtre E, Leroy X, Pattou F, et al (2001) Why do frozen sections have limited value in encapsulated or minimally invasive follicular carcinoma of the thyroid? Am J Clin Pathol 115:370–374

301. Paphavasit A, Thompson GB, Hay ID, et al (1997) Follicular and Hürthle cell thyroid neoplasms. Is frozen-section evaluation worthwhile? Arch Surg 132:674–678; discussion 678–680

302. Johannessen JV, Sobrinho-Simoes M (1982) Follicular carcinoma of the human thyroid gland. An ultrastructural study with emphasis on scanning electron microscopy. Diagn Histopathol 5:113–127

303. Backdahl M (1985) Nuclear DNA content and prognosis in papillary, follicular, and medullary carcinomas of the thyroid. Doctoral thesis, Karolinska Medical Institute, Stockholm, Sweden

304. Papotti M, Rodriguez J, Pompa RD, Bartolazzi A, Rosai J (2004) Galectin-3 and HBME-1 expression in well-differentiated thyroid tumors with follicular architecture of uncertain malignant potential. Mod Pathol 18:541–546

305. Rosai J (2003) Immunohistochemical markers of thyroid tumors: significance and diagnostic applications. Tumori 89:517–519

306. Kroll TG, Sarraf P, Pecciarini L, et al (2000) PAX8–PPAR[gamma] 1 fusion in oncogene human thyroid carcinoma. Science 289:1357–1360

307. Marques AR, Espadinha C, Catarino AL, et al (2002) Expression of PAX8–PPAR gamma 1 rearrangements in both follicular thyroid carcinomas and adenomas. J Clin Endocrinol Metab 87:3947–3952

308. Gustafson KS, LiVolsi VA, Furth EE, Pasha TL, Putt ME, Baloch ZW (2003) Peroxisome proliferator-activated receptor gamma expression in follicular-patterned thyroid lesions. Caveats for the use of immunohistochemical studies. Am J Clin Pathol 120:175–181

309. Esapa CT, Johnson SJ, Kendall-Taylor P, Lennard TW, Harris PE (1999) Prevalence of Ras mutations in thyroid neoplasia. Clin Endocrinol 50:529–535

310. Basolo F, Pisaturo F, Pollina LE, et al (2000) N-ras mutation in poorly differentiated thyroid carcinomas: correlation with bone metastases and inverse correlation to thyroglobulin expression. Thyroid 10:19–23

311. Capella G, Matias-Guiu X, Ampudia X, de Leiva A, Perucho M, Prat J (1996) Ras oncogene mutations in thyroid tumors: polymerase chain reaction-restriction-fragment-length polymorphism analysis from paraffin-embedded tissues. Diagn Mol Pathol 5:45–52

312. Grebe SK, McIver B, Hay ID, et al (1997) Frequent loss of heterozygosity on chromosomes 3p and 17p without VHL or p53 mutations suggests involvement of unidentified tumor suppressor genes in follicular thyroid carcinoma. J Clin Endocrinol Metab 82:3684–3691

313. Matsuo K, Tang SH, Fagin JA (1991) Allelotype of human thyroid tumors: loss of chromosome 11q13 sequences in follicular neoplasms. Mol Endocrinol 5:1873–1879

314. Nesland JM, Sobrinho-Simoes MA, Holm R, Sambade MC, Johannessen JV (1985) Hürthle-cell lesions of the thyroid: a combined study using transmission electron microscopy, scanning electron microscopy, and immunocytochemistry. Ultrastruct Pathol 8:269–290

315. Gonzalez-Campora R, Herrero-Zapatero A, Lerma E, Sanchez F, Galera H (1986) Hürthle cell and mitochondrion-rich cell tumors. A clinicopathologic study. Cancer 57:1154–1163

316. Thompson N, Dun E, Batsakis J, Nishiyama R (1974) Hürthle cell lesions of the thyroid gland. Surg Gynecol Obstet 139:555–560

317. Gundry S, Burney R, Thompson N, Lloyd R (1983) Total thyroidectomy for Hürthle cell neoplasm of the thyroid gland. Arch Surg 118:529–553

318. Bronner M, LiVolsi V (1988) Oxyphilic (Askanazy/Hürthle cell) tumors of the thyroid: microscopic features predict biologic behavior. Surg Pathol 1:137–150

319. Carcangiu ML, Bianchi S, Savino D, Voynick IM, Rosai J (1991) Follicular Hürthle cell tumors of the thyroid gland. Cancer 68:1944–1953

320. Chen H, Nicol TL, Zeiger MA, et al (1998) Hürthle cell neoplasms of the thyroid: are there factors predictive of malignancy? Ann Surg 227:542–546

321. Janser JC, Pusel J, Rodier JF, Navarrete E, Rodier D (1989) [Hürthle cell tumor of the thyroid gland. Analysis of a series of 33 cases]. J Chir (Paris) 126:619–624

322. Kanthan R, Radhi JM (1998) Immunohistochemical analysis of thyroid adenomas with Hürthle cells. Pathology 30:4–6

323. Bronner MP, Clevenger CV, Edmonds PR, Lowell DM, McFarland MM, LiVolsi VA (1988) Flow cytometric analysis of DNA content in Hürthle cell adenomas and carcinomas of the thyroid. Am J Clin Pathol 89:764–769

324. Schark C, Fulton N, Yashiro T, et al (1992) The value of measurement of ras oncogenes and nuclear DNA analysis in the diagnosis of Hürthle cell tumors of the thyroid. World J Surg 16:745–751; discussion 752

325. Bouras M, Bertholon J, Dutrieux-Berger N, Parvaz P, Paulin C, Revol A (1998) Variability of Ha-ras (codon 12) proto-oncogene mutations in diverse thyroid cancers. Eur J Endocrinol 139:209–216

326. Maximo V, Soares P, Lima J, Cameselle-Teijeiro J, Sobrinho-Simoes M (2002) Mitochondrial DNA somatic mutations (point mutations and large deletions) and mitochondrial DNA variants in human thyroid pathology: a study with emphasis on Hürthle cell tumors. Am J Pathol 160:1857–1865

327. Variakojis D, Getz ML, Paloyan E, Straus FH (1975) Papillary clear cell carcinoma of the thyroid gland. Hum Pathol 6:384–390

328. Carcangiu ML, Sibley RK, Rosai J (1985) Clear cell change in primary thyroid tumors. A study of 38 cases. Am J Surg Pathol 9:705–722

329. Lam KY, Lo CY (1998) Metastatic tumors of the thyroid gland: a study of 79 cases in Chinese patients. Arch Pathol Lab Med 122:37–41

330. Sakamoto A, Kasai N, Sugano H (1983) Poorly differentiated carcinoma of the thyroid. Cancer 52:1849–1855

331. Carcangiu ML, Zampi G, Rosai J (1984) Poorly differentiated ("insular") thyroid carcinoma. A reinterpretation of Langhans' "wuchernde Struma." Am J Surg Pathol 8:655–668

332. Flynn SD, Forman BH, Stewart AF, Kinder BK (1988) Poorly differentiated ("insular") carcinoma of the thyroid gland: an aggressive subset of differentiated thyroid neoplasms. Surgery 104:963–970

333. Palestini N, Papotti M, Durando R, Fortunato MA (1993) [Poorly differentiated "insular" carcinoma of the thyroid: long-term survival]. Minerva Chir 48:1301–1305

334. Nishida T, Katayama S, Tsujimoto M, Nakamura J, Matsuda H (1999) Clinicopathological significance of poorly differentiated thyroid carcinoma. Am J Surg Pathol 23:205–211

335. Venkatesh YS, Ordonez NG, Schultz PN, Hickey RC, Goepfert H, Samaan NA (1990) Anaplastic carcinoma of the thyroid. A clinicopathologic study of 121 cases. Cancer 66:321–330

336. Dumitriu L, Stefaneanu L, Tasca C (1984) The anaplastic transformation of differentiated thyroid carcinoma. An ultrastructural study. Endocrinologie 22:91–96

337. Chang TC, Liaw KY, Kuo SH, Chang CC, Chen FW (1989) Anaplastic thyroid carcinoma: review of 24 cases, with emphasis on cytodiagnosis and leukocytosis. Taiwan Yi Xue Hui Za Zhi 88:551–556

338. LiVolsi VA, Brooks JJ, Arendash-Durand B (1987) Anaplastic thyroid tumors. Immunohistology. Am J Clin Pathol 87:434–442

339. Berry B, MacFarlane J, Chan N (1990) Osteoclastoma-like anaplastic carcinoma of the thyroid. Diagnosis by fine needle aspiration cytology. Acta Cytol 34:248–250

340. Wan SK, Chan JK, Tang SK (1996) Paucicellular variant of anaplastic thyroid carcinoma. A mimic of Riedel's thyroiditis. Am J Clin Pathol 105:388–393

341. Giuffrida D, Attard M, Marasa L, et al (2000) Thyroid carcinosarcoma, a rare and aggressive histotype: a case report. Ann Oncol 11:1497–1499

342. Donnell CA, Pollock WJ, Sybers WA (1987) Thyroid carcinosarcoma. Arch Pathol Lab Med 111:1169–1172

343. Miettinen M, Franssila KO (2000) Variable expression of keratins and nearly uniform lack of thyroid transcription factor 1 in thyroid anaplastic carcinoma. Hum Pathol 31:1139–1145

344. Neri A, Aldovini D, Leonardi E, Giampiccolo M, Pedrolli C (1990) [Primary angiosarcoma of the thyroid gland. Presentation of a clinical case]. Recenti Prog Med 81:318–321

345. Tsugawa K, Koyanagi N, Nakanishi K, et al (1999) Leiomyosarcoma of the thyroid gland with rapid growth and tracheal obstruction: a partial thyroidectomy and tracheostomy using an ultrasonically activated scalpel can be safely performed with less bleeding. Eur J Med Res 4:483–487

346. Chan YF, Ma L, Boey JH, Yeung HY (1986) Angiosarcoma of the thyroid. An immunohistochemical and ultrastructural study of a case in a Chinese patient. Cancer 57:2381–2388

347. Sahoo M, Bal CS, Bhatnagar D (2002) Primary squamous-cell carcinoma of the thyroid gland: new evidence in support of follicular epithelial cell origin. Diagn Cytopathol 27:227–231

348. Harach HR, Day ES, de Strizic NA (1986) Mucoepidermoid carcinoma of the thyroid. Report of a case with immunohistochemical studies. Medicina 46:213–216

349. Arezzo A, Patetta R, Ceppa P, Borgonovo G, Torre G, Mattioli FP (1998) Mucoepidermoid carcinoma of the thyroid gland arising from a papillary epithelial neoplasm. Am Surg 64:307–311

350. Wenig BM, Adair CF, Heffess CS (1995) Primary mucoepidermoid carcinoma of the thyroid gland: a report of six cases and a review of the literature of a follicular epithelial-derived tumor. Hum Pathol 26:1099–1108

351. Chan JK, Albores-Saavedra J, Battifora H, Carcangiu ML, Rosai J (1991) Sclerosing mucoepidermoid thyroid carcinoma with eosinophilia. A distinctive low-grade malignancy arising from the metaplastic follicles of Hashimoto's thyroiditis. Am J Surg Pathol 15:438–448

352. Chan JK, Rosai J (1991) Tumors of the neck showing thymic or related branchial pouch differentiation: a unifying concept. Hum Pathol 22:349–367

353. Iwasa K, Imai MA, Noguchi M, et al (2002) Spindle epithelial tumor with thymus-like differentiation (SETTLE) of the thyroid. Head Neck 24:888–893

354. Ahuja AT, Chan ES, Allen PW, Lau KY, King W, Metreweli C (1998) Carcinoma showing thymiclike differentiation (CASTLE tumor). AJNR Am J Neuroradiol 19:1225–1228

355. Bayer-Garner IB, Kozovska ME, Schwartz MR, Reed JA (2004) Carcinoma with thymus-like differentiation arising in the dermis of the head and neck. J Cutan Pathol 31:625–629

356. Roka S, Kornek G, Schuller J, Ortmann E, Feichtinger J, Armbruster C (2004) Carcinoma showing thymic-like elements: a rare malignancy of the thyroid gland. Br J Surg 91:142–145

357. Hazard JB, Hawk WA, Crile G (1959) Medullary (solid) carcinoma of the thyroid. A clinicopathologic entity. J Clin Endocrinol Metab 19:152–161

358. Williams ED (1965) A review of 17 cases of carcinoma of the thyroid and pheochromocytoma. J Clin Pathol 18:288–292

359. Williams ED (1966) Histogenesis of medullary carcinoma of the thyroid. J Clin Pathol 19:114–118

360. Block MA, Horn RC, Miller JM, Barrett JL, Brush BE (1967) Familial medullary carcinoma of the thyroid. Ann Surg 166:403–412

361. Albores-Saavedra J, LiVolsi VA, Williams ED (1985) Medullary carcinoma. Semin Diagn Pathol 2:137–146

362. Wolfe HJ, Melvin KE, Cervi-Skinner SJ, et al (1973) C-cell hyperplasia preceding medullary thyroid carcinoma. N Engl J Med 289:437–441

363. Mulligan LM, Kwok JB, Healey CS, et al (1993) Germ-line mutations of the RET proto-oncogene in multiple endocrine neoplasia type 2A. Nature 363:458–460

364. Hofstra RM, Landsvater RM, Ceccherini I, et al (1994) A mutation in the RET proto-oncogene associated with multiple endocrine neoplasia type 2B and sporadic medullary thyroid carcinoma [see comments]. Nature 367:375–376

365. Mulligan LM, Eng C, Healey CS, et al (1994) Specific mutations of the RET proto-oncogene are related to disease phenotype in MEN 2A and FMTC. Nat Genet 6:70–74

366. Uribe M, Fenoglio-Preiser CM, Grimes M, Feind C (1985) Medullary carcinoma of the thyroid gland. Clinical, pathological and immunohistochemical features with review of the literature. Am J Surg Pathol 9:577–594

367. Wolfe HJ, Delellis RA (1981) Familial medullary thyroid carcinoma and C cell hyperplasia. Clin Endocrinol Metab 10:351–365

368. Leboulleux S, Baudin E, Travagli JP, Schlumberger M (2004) Medullary thyroid carcinoma. Clin Endocrinol (Oxf) 61:299–310

369. Williams E, Karim S, Sandler M (1968) Prostaglandin secretion by medullary carcinoma of the thyroid: a possible cause of the associated diarrhea. Lancet 1:22–23

370. Kakudo K, Miyauchi A, Ogihara T, et al (1982) Medullary carcinoma of the thyroid with ectopic ACTH syndrome. Acta Pathol Jpn 32:793–800

371. Sipple JH (1961) The association of pheochromocytoma with carcinoma of the thyroid gland. Am J Med 31:163–166

372. Jansson S, Hansson G, Salander H, Stenstrom G, Tisell L (1984) Prevalence of C-cell hyperplasia and medullary thyroid carcinoma in a consecutive series of pheochromocytoma patients. World J Surg 8:493–500

373. Eng C (1996) RET proto-oncogene in multiple endocrine neoplasia type 2 and Hirschprung's disease. Semin Med Beth Israel Hosp, Boston 335:943–951

374. Eng C (1999) RET proto-oncogene in the development of human cancer. J Clin Oncol 17:380–393

375. Eng C, Clayton D, Schuffenecker I, et al (1996) The relationship between specific RET proto-oncogene mutations and disease phenotype in multiple endocrine neoplasia type 2. International RET mutation consortium analysis. JAMA 276:1575–1579

376. Kebebew E, Ituarte PH, Siperstein AE, Duh QY, Clark OH (2000) Medullary thyroid carcinoma: clinical characteristics, treatment, prognostic factors, and a comparison of staging systems. Cancer 88:1139–1148

377. Kambouris M, Jackson CE, Feldman GL (1996) Diagnosis of multiple endocrine neoplasia (MEN) 2A, 2B and familial medullary thyroid cancer (FMTC) by multiplex PCR and heteroduplex analyses of RET proto-oncogene mutations. Hum Mutat 8:64–70

378. Nakata S, Okugi H, Saitoh Y, Takahashi H, Shimizu K (2001) Multiple endocrine neoplasia type 2B. Int J Urol 8:398–400

379. Nguyen L, Niccoli-Sire P, Caron P, et al (2001) Pheochromocytoma in multiple endocrine neoplasia type 2: a prospective study. Eur J Endocrinol 144:37–44

380. Marsh DJ, Zheng Z, Arnold A, et al (1997) Mutation analysis of glial cell line-derived neurotrophic factor, a ligand for an RET/coreceptor complex, in multiple endocrine neoplasia type 2 and sporadic neuroendocrine tumors. J Clin Endocrinol Metab 82:3025–3028

381. Borrello MG, Smith DP, Pasini B, et al (1995) RET activation by germline MEN2A and MEN2B mutations. Oncogene 11:2419–2427

382. Eng C, Smith DP, Mulligan LM, et al (1994) Point mutation within the tyrosine kinase domain of the RET proto-oncogene in multiple endocrine neoplasia type 2B and related sporadic tumours. Hum Mol Genet 3:237–241

383. Cohen EG, Shaha AR, Rinaldo A, Devaney KO, Ferlito A (2004) Medullary thyroid carcinoma. Acta Otolaryngol 124:544–557

384. Asa SL (1997) C-cell lesions of the thyroid. Pathol Case Rev 2:210–217

385. Abrosimov A (1996) [Histologic and immunohistochemical characterization of medullary thyroid carcinoma]. Arkh Patol 58:43–48

386. Alevizaki M, Dai K, Grigorakis SI, Legon S, Souvatzoglou A (1994) Amylin/islet amyloid polypeptide expression in medullary carcinoma of the thyroid: correlation with the expression of the related calcitonin/CGRP genes. Clin Endocrinol (Oxf) 41:21–26

387. Dominguez-Malagon H, Delgado-Chavez R, Torres-Najera M, Gould E, Albores-Saavedra J (1989) Oxyphil and squamous variants of medullary thyroid carcinoma. Cancer 63:1183–1188

388. Harach HR, Williams ED (1983) Glandular (tubular and follicular) variants of medullary carcinoma of the thyroid. Histopathology 7:83–97

389. Huss LJ, Mendelsohn G (1990) Medullary carcinoma of the thyroid gland: an encapsulated variant resembling the hyalinizing trabecular (paraganglioma-like) adenoma of thyroid. Mod Pathol 3:581–585

390. Landon G, Ordonez NG (1985) Clear cell variant of medullary carcinoma of the thyroid. Hum Pathol 16:844

391. Mendelsohn G, Baylin SB, Bigner SH, Wells SA, Jr., Eggleston JC (1980) Anaplastic variants of medullary thyroid carcinoma: a light-microscopic and immunohistochemical study. Am J Surg Pathol 4:333–341

392. Kos M, Separovic V, Sarcevic B (1995) Medullary carcinoma of the thyroid: histomorphological, histochemical and immunohistochemical analysis of twenty cases. Acta Med Croatica 49:195–199

393. DeLilles RA, Rule AH, Spiler F, et al (1978) Calcitonin and carcinoembryonic antigen as tumor markers in medullary thyroid carcinoma. Am J Clin Pathol 70:587

394. Hirsch MS, Faquin WC, Krane JF (2004) Thyroid transcription factor-1, but not p53, is helpful in distinguishing moderately differentiated neuroendocrine carcinoma of the larynx from medullary carcinoma of the thyroid. Mod Pathol 17:631–636

395. Matsubayashi S, Yanaihara C, Ohkubo M, et al (1984) Gastrin-releasing peptide immunoreactivity in medullary thyroid carcinoma. Cancer 53:2472

396. Roth KA, Bensch KG, Hoffman AR (1987) Characterization of opioid peptides in human thyroid medullary carcinoma. Cancer 59:1594

397. Komminoth P, Roth J, Saremasiani P, et al (1994) Polysialic acid of the neural cell adhesion molecule in the human thyroid: a marker for medullary carcinoma and primary C-cell hyperplasia. An immunohistochemical study on 79 thyroid lesions. Am J Surg Pathol 18:399

398. Ruppert JM, Eggleston JC, deBustros A, Baylin SB (1986) Disseminated calcitonin-poor medullary thyroid carcinoma in a patient with calcitonin-rich primary tumor. Am J Surg Pathol 10:513–518

399. Randolph GW, Maniar D (2000) Medullary carcinoma of the thyroid. Cancer Control 7:253–261

400. Giuffrida D, Ferrau F, Bordonaro R, et al (2000) [Medullary carcinoma of the thyroid: diagnosis and therapy]. Clin Ter 151:29–35

401. Gimm O, Sutter T, Dralle H (2001) Diagnosis and therapy of sporadic and familial medullary thyroid carcinoma. J Cancer Res Clin Oncol 127:156–165

402. Gilliland FD, Hunt WC, Morris DM, Key CR (1997) Prognostic factors for thyroid carcinoma. A population-based study of 15,698 cases from the Surveillance, Epidemiology and End Results (SEER) program 1973–1991. Cancer 79:564–573

403. Randolph GW (1996) Medullary carcinoma of the thyroid: subtypes and current management. Compr Ther 22:203–210

404. Brierley J, Tsang R, Simpson WJ, Gospodarowicz M, Sutcliffe S, Panzarella T (1996) Medullary thyroid cancer: analyses of survival and prognostic factors and the role of radiation therapy in local control. Thyroid 6:305–310

405. Schroder S, Bocker W, Baisch H, et al (1988) Prognostic factors in medullary thyroid carcinomas. Survival in relation to age, sex, stage, histology, immunocytochemistry, and DNA content. Cancer 61:806–816

406. Albores-Saavedra J, Gorraez de la Mora T, de la Torre-Rendon F, Gould E (1990) Mixed medullary-papillary carcinoma of the thyroid: a previously unrecognized variant of thyroid carcinoma. Hum Pathol 21:1151–1155

407. Giove E, Renzulli G, Lorusso C, Merlicco D, Iacobone D (2004) [Mixed medullary and follicular carcinoma of the thyroid: report of one case]. Ann Ital Chir 75:251–256; discussion 257

408. Kashima K, Yokoyama S, Inoue S, et al (1993) Mixed medullary and follicular carcinoma of the thyroid: report of two cases with an immunohistochemical study. Acta Pathol Jpn 43:428–433

409. LiVolsi VA (2004) Mixed follicular medullary thyroid carcinoma. Diagn Cytopathol 31:434; author reply 435

410. Beressi N, Campos JM, Beressi JP, et al (1998) Sporadic medullary microcarcinoma of the thyroid: a retrospective analysis of eighty cases. Thyroid 8:1039–1044

411. Guyetant S, Dupre F, Bigorgne JC, et al (1999) Medullary thyroid microcarcinoma: a clinicopathologic retrospective study of 38 patients with no prior familial disease. Hum Pathol 30:957–963

412. Albores-Saavedra JA, Krueger JE (2001) C-cell hyperplasia and medullary thyroid microcarcinoma. Endocr Pathol 12:365–377

413. Kaserer K, Scheuba C, Neuhold N, et al (2001) Sporadic versus familial medullary thyroid microcarcinoma: a histopathologic study of 50 consecutive patients. Am J Surg Pathol 25:1245–1251

414. Mizukami Y, Kurumaya H, Nonomura A, et al (1992) Sporadic medullary microcarcinoma of the thyroid. Histopathology 21:375–377

415. Sironi M, Cozzi L, Pareschi R, Spreafico GL, Assi A (1999) Occult sporadic medullary microcarcinoma with lymph node metastases. Diagn Cytopathol 21:203–206

416. Russo F, Barone Adesi TL, Arturi A, et al (1997) [Clinico-pathological study of microcarcinoma of the thyroid]. Minerva Chir 52:891–900

417. Yamauchi A, Tomita Y, Takakuwa T, et al (2002) Polymerase chain reaction-based clonality analysis in thyroid lymphoma. Int J Mol Med 10:113–117

418. Ghazanfar S, Quraishy MS, Essa K, Muzaffar S, Saeed MU, Sultan T (2002) Mucosa associated lymphoid tissue lymphoma (MALToma) in patients with cold nodule thyroid. J Pak Med Assoc 52:131–133

419. Takano T, Miyauchi A, Matsuzuka F, Yoshida H, Kuma K, Amino N (2000) Diagnosis of thyroid malignant lymphoma by reverse transcription-polymerase chain reaction detecting the monoclonality of immunoglobulin heavy chain messenger ribonucleic acid. J Clin Endocrinol Metab 85:671–675

420. Diaz-Arias AA, Bickel JT, Loy TS, Croll GH, Puckett CL, Havey AD (1992) Follicular carcinoma with clear cell change arising in lingual thyroid. Oral Surg Oral Med Oral Pathol 74:206–211

421. LiVolsi VA, Perzin KH, Savetsky L (1974) Carcinoma arising in median ectopic thyroid (including thyroglossal duct tissue). Cancer 34:1303–1315

422. Doshi SV, Cruz RM, Hilsinger RL Jr (2001) Thyroglossal duct carcinoma: a large case series. Ann Otol Rhinol Laryngol 110:734–738

423. Cignarelli M, Ambrosi A, Marino A, Lamacchia O, Cincione R, Neri V (2002) Three cases of papillary carcinoma and three of adenoma in thyroglossal duct cysts: clinical-diagnostic comparison with benign thyroglossal duct cysts. J Endocrinol Invest 25:947–954

424. Fih J, Moore R (1963) Ectopic thyroid tissue and ectopic thyroid carcinoma. Ann Surg 157:212–222

425. Devaney K, Snyder R, Norris HJ, Tavassoli FA (1993) Proliferative and histologically malignant struma ovarii: a clinicopathologic study of 54 cases. Int J Gynecol Pathol 12:333–343

426. Kdous M, Hachicha R, Gamoudi A, et al (2003) [Struma ovarii. Analysis of a series of 7 cases and review of the literature]. Tunis Med 81:571–576

427. Rosenblum NG, LiVolsi VA, Edmonds PR, Mikuta JJ (1989) Malignant struma ovarii. Gynecol Oncol 32:224–227

428. Koo HL, Jang J, Hong SJ, Shong Y, Gong G (2004) Renal cell carcinoma metastatic to follicular adenoma of the thyroid gland. A case report. Acta Cytol 48:64–68

429. Matias-Guiu X, LaGuette J, Puras-Gil AM, Rosai J (1997) Metastatic neuroendocrine tumors to the thyroid gland mimicking medullary carcinoma: a pathologic and immunohistochemical study of six cases. Am J Surg Pathol 21:754–762

430. Baloch ZW, LiVolsi VA (1999) Tumor-to-tumor metastasis to follicular variant of papillary carcinoma of thyroid. Arch Pathol Lab Med 123:703–706

431. Bronner MP HR, LiVolsi VA (1994) Utility of frozen section analysis on follicular lesions of the thyroid. Endocr Pathol 5:154–161

432. Paessler M, LiVolsi VA, Baloch Z (2001) Role of Ultrafast Papanicolaou stained scrape preparations as an adjunct to frozen section in the surgical management of thyroid lesions. Endocr Pract 7:89–94

433. Rodriguez JM, Parrilla P, Sola J, et al (1994) Comparison between preoperative cytology and intraoperative frozen-section biopsy in the diagnosis of thyroid nodules. Br J Surg 81:1151–1154

434. Taneri F, Poyraz A, Tekin E, Ersoy E, Dursun A (1998) Accuracy and significance of fine-needle aspiration cytology and frozen section in thyroid surgery. Endocr Regul 32:187–191

435. Shaha AR, DiMaio T, Webber C, Jaffe BM (1990) Intraoperative decision making during thyroid surgery based on the results of preoperative needle biopsy and frozen section. Surgery 108:964–967; discussion 970–971

436. Shaha A, Gleich L, Di Maio T, Jaffe BM (1990) Accuracy and pitfalls of frozen section during thyroid surgery. J Surg Oncol 44:84–92

437. Basolo F, Baloch ZW, Baldanzi A, Miccoli P, LiVolsi VA (1999) Usefulness of Ultrafast Papanicolaou-stained scrape preparations in intraoperative management of thyroid lesions. Mod Pathol 12:653–657

11 Surgery for Medullary Thyroid Cancer

Oliver Gimm

CONTENTS

11.1 Introduction

Medullary thyroid cancer (MTC) is a rare type of thyroid cancer which derives from the parafollicular C cells. C cells produce calcitonin which can be used as a tumor marker. The real incidence of MTC is unknown. Based on epidemiologic studies from Scandinavia, its prevalence was estimated to be roughly 3–4% of all thyroid malignancies [9,37]. Those studies, however, analyzed data from the 1960s and 1970s, i.e., shortly after MTC was identified as a distinct entity by Hazard [32]. Hence, the real incidence of MTC was assumed to be higher. More recent studies that emphasize the need to determine calcitonin routinely in any patient with nodular thyroid disease found an unsuspected high prevalence (16–40%) of MTC [62,67,78]. This prevalence, however, appeared to be too high. Today, it is assumed that MTC accounts for 5–10% of all thyroid malignancies. MTC exists in a sporadic (about 75%) and a hereditary (about 25%) form [66] associated with several biological features that necessitate a particular surgical approach in order to offer a high chance of cure.

The management of hyperparathyroidism in patients with multiple endocrine neoplasia (MEN2A) will be discussed in Chapter 24 "Multiglandular Parathyroid Disease and MEN Syndromes."

11.2 Diagnosis

In many patients with MTC, thyroid nodules are the first clinical sign. Since MTC metastasizes early to the locoregional lymph nodes (by the time of diagnosis, more than 50% of patients with sporadic MTC have lymph node metastases), lymph node metastases may also be the first clinical sign. The parafollicular C cells synthesize and secrete calcitonin which can be used as a sensitive tumor marker. Calcitonin secretion can be stimulated by both calcium (2 mg/kg body weight of 10% Ca^{2+} injected intravenously in 1 min) and pentagastrin (0.5 µg/kg body weight, diluted in 5–10 ml sterile saline, injected intravenously in 5–15 s), the latter of which should preferably be used if available. Calcitonin levels are considered pathologic when the basal level is above normal range or when stimulation of calcitonin leads to an increase of calcitonin more than two to three times the basal level [47]. While other conditions (e.g., neuroendocrine pancreatic tumors, carcinoids, small cell lung cancers, renal or hepatic insufficiency, treatment with proton pump inhibitors) have been found to be associated with elevated basal calcitonin levels [33,46,50], an increase of at least two- to threefold after stimulation seems to be pathognomonic for both sporadic and hereditary MTC.

Routine preoperative measurement of basal calcitonin in patients with thyroid nodules has been shown to enable identification of MTC preoperatively [62,67,78]. This preoperative workup (Fig.11.1) of thyroid nodules is not recommended by all endocrinologists and endocrine surgeons but has become more and more accepted [43]. In a large recent study of more than 10,000 patients, routine measurement of calcitonin in patients with nodular thyroid disease significantly improved the 5-year (97% versus 81%) and 10-year (86% versus 43%) long-term survival of patients with MTC in comparison with historical results [19]. Of note, the routine measurement of calcitonin in patients with nodular thyroid disease has not only increased the rate of preoperatively diagnosed MTC but also may cause a diagnostic dilemma. Stimulated calcitonin levels below 100 pg/ml are rarely caused by MTC [43] but may be due to sporadic C cell hyperplasia as seen in various benign diseases of the thyroid [1,8,31]. In these patients, immediate total thyroidectomy is not advised unless the nodule is otherwise suspected to be malignant (Fig. 11.1). Instead, reevaluation after 3–6 months is recommended. In patients with stimulated calcitonin levels >100 pg/ml, total thyroidectomy is advised. In rare instances with high serum calcitonin levels, symptoms may arise from diarrhea [3] not responding well to common anti-diarrheic drugs. Since MTC may synthesize and secrete other hormones, for example corticotropin (ACTH), paraneoplastic syndromes, such as Cushing's syndrome, may occur [73].

11.2.1   Further Diagnostic Investigation

Once MTC is diagnosed, local tumor extension (primary tumor and lymph node metastases) may be assessed by ultrasonography. In particular in patients with recurrent or persistent MTC, computed tomography or magnetic resonance imaging should be per-formed. Of note, ultrasound and other imaging techniques may miss metastatic lymph nodes and small (microscopic) disease. When imaging techniques fail to distinguish between scar tissue and MTC, the use of fine-needle aspiration may be helpful. If locally advanced tumor extension (e.g., infiltration of the esophagus and/or trachea) is suspected, endoscopic examination is mandatory.

Hematogenous tumor spread occurs predominantly to the lung, liver, and bone. Various imaging techniques have been used to determine the extension of distant metastases: computed tomography, magnetic resonance imaging, octreotide scintigraphy, and positron emission tomography with various tracers (e.g., FDG, DOPA) [13,22,35,54]. In addition, selective venous catheterization has been used successfully [22]. If none of these techniques enables the localization of distant metastases but if basal calcitonin levels are above 500 pg/ml, laparoscopy is advised [77]. If laparoscopy does not reveal hepatic metastases, thoracoscopy may be helpful to assess the presence of lung metastases. Typically, multiple micrometastases can be found in these instances.

Advanced tumor stages can only be prevented by early diagnosis of MTC. Concerning sporadic MTC, this can only be achieved by routine measurement of calcitonin in patients with thyroid nodules [43]. However, routine measurement in these patients is not uniformly accepted. Regarding hereditary MTC,

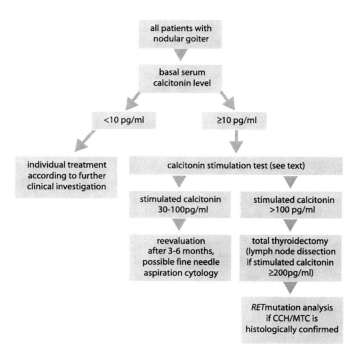

Fig. 11.1 Work-up recommendations in patients with nodular goiter. *CCH* C cell hyperplasia, *MTC* medullary thyroid carcinoma

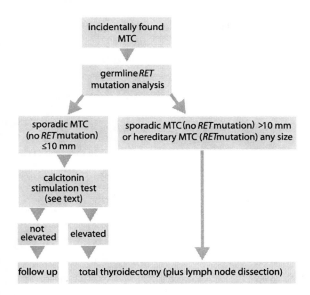

Fig. 11.2 Work-up recommendation in patients with incidentally found MTC

it can be achieved by screening at-risk family members after identification of the family-specific *RET* mutation [18,80]. Hence, once MTC is diagnosed, the patient must undergo germline *RET* mutation analysis, irrespective of his/her age [71] or the presence of any other features suggestive for hereditary MTC (Fig. 11.2).

11.2.2 The Proto-oncogene *RET*

The proto-oncogene *RET* was initially found to be rearranged during transfection of NIH 3T3 cells [75]. Later, somatic *RET* rearrangements were identified in patients with papillary thyroid carcinoma [30]. These mutations were somatic, i.e., only found in the thyroid tumor. In 1993, *RET* mutations were also found in patients with MTC [14,60]. In contrast to papillary thyroid carcinoma, these mutations were found in patients with hereditary MTC and the mutations were germline (i.e., present in every nucleus-containing cell of the human body) not somatic. The identification of *RET* as the disease-causing gene of hereditary MTC enabled identification of at-risk family members by DNA analysis of blood leukocytes. Already in 1994, the first clinical experience was reported [47,80]. For the first time, indication for surgery was solely based on the result of molecular analysis and *RET* became the paradigm of molecular medicine [18,20]. Despite the fact that *RET* is a large gene, mutation analysis is comparably simple since mutations found so far are limited to a few exons (Table 11.1).

11.3 Multiple Endocrine Neoplasia Type 2

Hereditary MTC is part of the multiple endocrine neoplasia type 2 (MEN2) syndromes. Clinically, MEN2 has been divided into three subgroups: familial MTC (FMTC), MEN2A, and MEN2B. MTC is the *conditio sine qua non* of all three subgroups (Table 11.1). In addition, patients with MEN2A may develop pheochromocytoma and/or primary hyperparathyroidism (pHPT). Primary hyperparathyroidism as part of MEN2 is usually milder than primary hyperparathyroidism as part of multiple endocrine neoplasia type 1 (MEN1) or their sporadic counterpart. Hence, routine subtotal or total parathyroidectomy plus autotransplantation as recommended in MEN1 is not necessary [12]. In the presence of MEN2-pHPT, parathyroidectomy may be limited to the enlarged parathyroid gland. Alternatively, like patients with MEN2A and in addition to MTC, patients with MEN2B may develop pheochromocytoma (Table 11.1). Further, they develop neuromas of the tongue, ganglioneuromatosis of the intestine, and/or medullated corneal nerve fibers. A marfanoid habitus may also be present. None of the latter phenotypes must be present in patients with MEN2B nor are they pathognomonic [28,29,65]. Clinically symptomatic primary hyperparathyroidism is not part of MEN2B. By definition, patients with FMTC develop MTC only (Table 11.1). Of note, there is no reliable diagnostic tool to distinguish patients with FMTC from those with MEN2A, i.e., members of families with FMTC are always at risk of developing pheochromocytoma or, even though less likely, primary hyperparathyroidism. For instance, in the past, several *RET* mutations (e.g., V804L, S891A) [36] were believed to be associated with FMTC only. However, pheochromocytomas have also been diagnosed in these patients [42,61]. It appears that the development of pheochromocytomas is rather a matter of time. Hence, no patient with an FMTC/MEN2-specific *RET* mutation should be excluded from screening for pheochromocytoma. Since FMTC is only a clinical term based on the phenotype of the patient, the use of the term FMTC/MEN2A is recommended.

MEN2 has also been named multiple endocrine adenomatosis (MEA) type 2 but this term should no longer be used. MEN2A is also known as Sipple's syndrome [72]. However, Sipple did not realize the association of pheochromocytomas and the medullary type of thyroid carcinoma. Steiner and coworkers described a kindred with pheochromocytoma, MTC, and hyperparathyroidism and proposed the term multiple endocrine neoplasia (MEN) type 2A [74].

Table 11.1 Genotype-phenotype correlation in MEN2. (– Disease/finding absent or frequency observed not higher that in the general population, + disease/finding present in most cases but neither required nor pathognomonic [28,29,65])

Exon	Codon	FMTC	MEN2A	MEN2B
8	533[a]	533		
10	609	609	609	
	611	611	611	
	618	618	618	
	620	620	620	
11	630	630		
	634	634	634	
13	768	768		
	790	790	790	
	791	791	791	
14	804	804	804[b]	804[c]
	844	844		
15	883			883
	891	891	891[d]	
16	912	912[e]		
	918			918
Mean age at diagnosis[f] (years)		45–55	25–35	10–20
Medullary thyroid carcinoma (MTC)		90–100%[g]	90–100%[g]	100%
Pheochromocytoma		–	40–60%	40–60%
Primary hyperparathyroidism		–	10–30%	–
Ganglioneuromatosis		–	–	+
Multiple mucosal neuromas		–	–	+
Marfanoid habitus		–	–	+
Thickened corneal fibers		–	–	+

[a] Based on one publication [11]

[b] Based on one report with MTC and adrenal and extra-adrenal pheochromocytoma [61]

[c] Based on several reports with additional germline *RET* mutation [44,53,55]; however, it appears that the phenotype is rather MEN2B-like than typical MEN2B

[d] Based on one report with MTC and adrenal pheochromocytoma [42]

[e] Based on one publication [41]

[f] The age at diagnosis has become younger since the identification of *RET*

[g] Since the identification of *RET*, many patients undergo surgery before MTC occurs

MEN2B has also been named MEN3 which should also no longer be used. Even less common is the term Wagenmann-Froboese syndrome [23,79].

The incidence of MEN2 is not known. About one fourth of all MTCs are thought to be hereditary [66]. Since thyroid cancer has been assumed to have an incidence of 1–3/100,000 per year, MEN2 may have an incidence of 1.25–7.5/10,000,000 per year. This would fit with its estimated prevalence of 1/35,000.

The female to male ratio is thought to be about 1:1 with a slight predominance of the female gender in some studies.

11.3.1 Diagnosis

The diagnosis of MTC in the index patients of a given family with MEN2 does not differ from that in sporadic MTC. Most patients present with either thyroid nodules or lymph node metastases or both. Hence, once MTC is diagnosed, the patient should undergo phenotype-depending *RET* mutation analysis (Table 11.1, Fig. 11.2). This can be most easily done by analyzing leukocyte DNA of a venous blood sample. If no *RET* mutation is found, the risk of these patients having MEN2 is less than 1% unless other features suggestive for MEN2 are present. In the case of a proven *RET* mutation, the mutation needs to be confirmed by analyzing a second, independently drawn blood sample. If confirmed, the patient should undergo screening for accompanying diseases of MEN2. Further, his/her at-risk family members should undergo analysis for this particular *RET* mutation. In family members with proven *RET* mutation, a thorough work-up is necessary and total (prophylactic) thyroidectomy should be advised. In rare instances (<10%), pheochromocytoma precedes the development of MTC [7]. Hence, *RET* mutation analysis is also recommended in patients with pheochromocytoma. Even less likely is the development of primary hyperparathyroidism prior to the development of MTC. Routine *RET* mutation analysis is not recommended in patients with primary hyperparathyroidism.

11.3.2 Prophylactic Thyroidectomy

In patients with hereditary MTC, biochemical penetrance, i.e., pathologic basal and/or stimulated calcitonin levels, reaches almost 100% by the age of 35 years. Based on studies in the pre-*RET* era, it is known that about 70% of patients with MEN2A develop clinically apparent MTC by the age of 70 years [64].

Since every thyroidal C cell inherits the risk of becoming malignant, total thyroidectomy is advised in any patient with FMTC/MEN2. MTC metastasizes early to locoregional lymph nodes and beyond. Once lymph node metastases are present, the chance of biochemical cure, i.e., normal basal and stimulated calcitonin levels, decreases [25]; once MTC is spread beyond the locoregional lymph nodes, biochemical cure is impossible. This is the rationale to offer timely therapy. Hence, surgery should preferably be performed before the development of MTC ("prophylactic thyroidectomy"), at the latest before the development of lymph node metastases, which means in some cases at the age of 5 years and below. It is obvious that surgery, in particular for these cases but also for MTC in general, should be performed by experienced surgeons.

Timing and extent of this prophylactic approach is based on several parameters (Fig. 11.3). First, it has

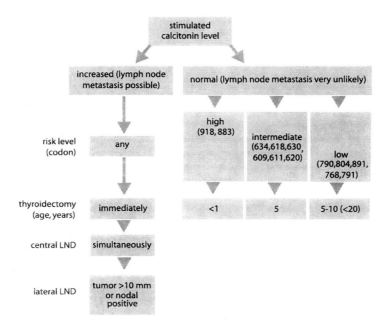

Fig. 11.3 Recommendations for timing of "prophylactic" surgery in patients with FMTC/MEN2 according to stimulated calcitonin levels and codon mutation. *LND* Lymph node dissection

been shown that a genotype-phenotype correlation exists [20,48]. Some *RET* mutations (e.g., codons 634 and 618) are associated with an early onset of the disease while others (e.g., codons 768 and 791) appear later at a greater age. Interestingly, this clinical aggressiveness somewhat correlates with the transforming activity of *RET* caused by this particular mutation [38,39]. Second, basal and stimulated calcitonin levels are helpful in assessing the extent of the disease. In the case of hereditary MTC, C cell hyperplasia [CCH; increased number of thyroidal C cells, i.e., >50 cells per low power field (×100) on histological examination] precedes the development of MTC. Soon after, lymph node metastases may occur. Actually, lymph node metastases have been found in the case of primary tumors less than 5 mm in size. While calcitonin levels can not reliably distinguish between CCH and intrathyroidal MTC, lymph node involvement can be assumed to be absent in the case of both basal and stimulated normal calcitonin levels. Third, MTC development has been shown to be age dependent [52].

11.4   Therapy

11.4.1   Surgery

Total thyroidectomy is the treatment of choice. Patients should be referred to an experienced surgeon,

in order to minimize morbidity. In patients with hereditary MTC, the coexistence of pheochromocytoma should be excluded in order to prevent intraoperative life-threatening hypertension crisis. In patients with sporadic MTC, multifocal tumors are less common (10–20%) but total thyroidectomy has also been recommended since C cells do not take up radioiodine. Nevertheless, subtotal resections have been performed successfully [56] (Fig. 11.2). However, if calcitonin remains elevated after subtotal resection, a completion (total) thyroidectomy is mandatory. Since lymphogenous spread is often (>50%) found in both patients with sporadic MTC and index patients with hereditary MTC, at least lymph node dissection of the cervicocentral compartment (C1) (Fig. 11.4a) is recommended, in particular if stimulated calcitonin level is >200 pg/ml (Fig. 11.1) [43]. Of note, lymph node metastases are often not limited to the cervicocentral compartment (Table 11.2). Hence, bilateral cervicolateral lymph node dissection (compartments C2 and C3; Fig. 11.4a) should be considered in all patients with MTC, both sporadic and hereditary [70]. The only exception may be patients who undergo prophylactic thyroidectomy (see above and Fig. 11.3). The level of basal of stimulated calcitonin level is not helpful in determining the necessary extent of lymph node dissection [26]. Primary tumor size and extrathyroidal tumor extension correlate with lymph node involvement (Table 11.3) but individually reli-

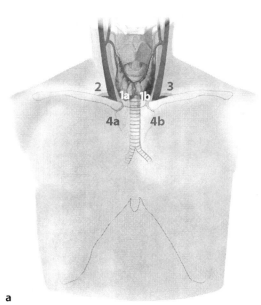 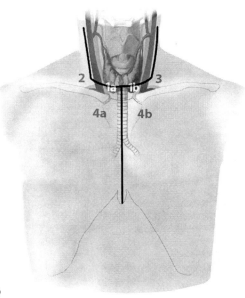

a   b

Fig. 11.4 a Compartment classification (described by Dralle et al. [16]). **b** Skin incisions according to the dissected compartment: * cervicocentral compartment (*1a* right; *1b* left), # cervicolateral compartment (*2* right; *3* left), § mediastinal compartment (*4a* right; *4b* left)

Table 11.2 Frequencies of nodal metastases (%) within different compartments in patients with primary MTC according to various references. (*n/a* Not assessed)

Reference	Patients	Lymph node compartment, node positive (%)			
		Central	Lateral		Mediastinal
			Ipsilateral	Contralateral	
Fleming et al. [21]	40	80	78	25	n/a
Moley et al. [57]	73	79	75	47	n/a
Scollo et al. [70]	101	48	49	24	n/a

Table 11.3 Frequencies of nodal metastases (%) within different compartments in patients with primary MTC according to tumor size

Tumor size	Patients	Lymph node compartment, node positive (%)				
		Ipsilateral		Contralateral		Mediastinal
		Central	Lateral	Central	Lateral	
Gimm et al. [25]						
Intrathyroidal, ≤10 mm	3	33	33	0	0	0
Intrathyroidal, >10 mm	18	56	44	17	11	0
Extrathyroidal, any size	6	83	100	17	0	50
Machens et al. [51]						
Intrathyroidal, ≤10 mm	35	14	11	3	0	0
Intrathyroidal, >10 mm	19	26	32	21	16	11
Extrathyroidal, any size	14	71	93	64	57	50

able parameters do not exist. Also, at reoperation, a tumor size-dependent approach does not seem to be justified since bilateral compartment involvement is very frequent [24]. The chance to cure the patient is unrealistic if more than two compartments contain lymph node metastases [51]. Even though mediastinal (compartment C4; Fig. 11.4a) lymph node metastases have been found quite frequently [25], prophylactic dissection of the upper mediastinum is not recommended [49]. The reason is that nodal involvement of the mediastinum is often associated with hematogenous tumor spread and, hence, "biochemical cure" is unlikely. Still, if tumor spread to the mediastinum has been proven, dissection of this compartment is advised to prevent local complications (e.g., tracheal infiltration).

11.4.2   Technique of Lymph Node Dissection

In contrast to other epithelial cancers, lymph node dissection in thyroid cancer has not been well standardized. One reason may be that lymph node metastases in papillary thyroid carcinoma, the most common type of thyroid cancer, are often believed to be of minor importance [5] even though their prognostic significance is controversial [69]. In contrast, the prognostic significance of lymph node metastases in patients with MTC is well documented [2,45] and lymphogenous spread is often found. However, MTC is rather rare (5–10% of all thyroid carcinomas) and only a few centers have experience in treating this disease. Therefore, it may not be surprising that a standardized concept of lymph node dissection for thyroid cancer is lacking. The degree of lymph node dissection varies from selective node removal ("berry picking") to radical neck dissection, a procedure originally developed for squamous cell carcinoma of the head and neck.

Lymph node metastases derived from MTC may be very small in size and neither pre- nor intraoperatively detectable. Hence, selective node dissection ("berry picking") is not recommended in patients with MTC. Instead, an en bloc systematic dissection of lymph nodes together with their surrounding adipose tissue while preserving nerves and vessels should be performed. This systematic approach achieves an improved biochemical cure rate [24,58].

The compartment-oriented approach advocated by Dralle (Fig. 11.4a) has several advantages [16]. It is based on the microdissection technique described by Tisell and Moley [59,76]. The compartments are limited by major anatomical structures, are therefore well defined, and take into account the pattern of lymphogenous spread [25].

The compartment model distinguishes four different compartments (Fig. 11.4a). The cervicocentral compartment (C1) reaches from the submandibular gland down to the brachiocephalic vein and is laterally limited by the carotid sheath. It contains the submandibular, submental, paratracheal, and paraesophageal lymph nodes (level I+VI as defined by Robbins and coworkers [68]) and is further subdivided into a right (C1a) and a left (C1b) compartment. Lateral of compartment C1 lie the cervicolateral compartments C2 (right) and C3 (left) (levels II, III, IV, and V as defined by Robbins and coworkers [68]). They reach from the mandible down to the subclavian vein and are limited medially by the carotid sheath and laterally by the trapezoid muscle. Caudal of compartment C1 lies the mediastinal compartment (C4) which reaches from the brachiocephalic vein down to the tracheal bifurcation. It is laterally limited by the pleura and, like compartment C1, is subdivided into a right (C4a) and a left (C4b) compartment. It has been shown that involvement of these compartments follows a specific pattern with the ipsilateral cervicocentral compartment and the ipsilateral cervicolateral compartment being the first regions affected [25,51].

In accordance with the various compartments, the following procedures can be distinguished [17]: cervicocentral lymph node dissection, cervicolateral lymph node dissection, and mediastinal lymph node dissection. These dissections should always be performed using ocular magnifying devices and bipolar coagulation forceps.

11.4.3   Cervicocentral Lymph Node Dissection

Dissection of the cervicocentral lymph node compartment may be performed together with total thyroidectomy. In many cases, however, cervicocentral lymph node dissection is part of completion thyroidectomy. The skin incision should be done like a Kocher incision in between the sternomastoid muscles (Fig. 11.4b). Following exposure of the first thyroid lobe (usually the dominant side), the middle thyroid vein (Kocher's vein) should be ligated. Transection of the sternothyroid muscle and sternohyoid muscle is very helpful to offer good access and should be performed without hesitation. Following identification of the inferior thyroid artery, the recurrent laryngeal nerve should be identified. The dissection in between the carotid artery (lateral border) and the trachea (medial border) may preferably be performed in a caudal-to-cranial fashion starting from the innominate artery up to the hyoid bone. The lower parathyroid glands can often not be preserved and should be autotransplanted after histologic exclusion of tumor involvement. The upper parathyroid glands should be identified and preserved or, alternatively, autotransplanted. Autotransplantation into both the right sternomastoid muscle and the forearm work well. The location should be marked with a non-absorbable suture. Preparation on the first side is completed by total mobilization of the thyroid lobe or remnant. After complete preparation on one side, the same procedure is performed on the contralateral side. Following complete mobilization on both sides, the thyroid gland and the connective adipose tissue are removed en bloc.

11.4.4   Cervicolateral Lymph Node Dissection

For technical details refer also to Chapter 9 "Modified Radical Neck Dissection." Like dissection of the cervicocentral compartment, lymph node dissection of the cervicolateral compartment is performed in a systematic way, i.e., all lymph nodes within that compartment are removed together with the connective adipose tissue while muscles, nerves, and vessels are preserved. In the case of cervicolateral lymph node dissection, the Kocher incision is extended laterally along the anterior (medial) border of the sternomastoid muscle (Fig. 11.4b). Thereafter, the carotid sheath should be identified. Separation of its content (carotid artery, internal jugular vein, vagus nerve) is not necessary, however, the vagus nerve should be identified in order to preserve function of the recurrent laryngeal nerve. General incision of the sternomastoid muscle is not necessary but may be helpful in the case of multiple lymph node involvement. If performed, the muscle should be anastomosed after completion of the dissection using absorbable sutures. Like in the cervicocentral compartment, dissection may preferably be performed in a caudal-to-cranial fashion starting at the medial border and continuing to the lateral border. Branches of the thoracic duct are ligated, and the external jugular vein should be preserved. Removal of the connective adipose tissue containing the lymph nodes should be performed en bloc preserving the nerves of the brachial plexus and cervical plexus. The accessory nerve, the phrenic nerve, and the sympathetic trunk are preserved.

11.4.5   Mediastinal Lymph Node Dissection

In the case of extended lymph node involvement, lymphogenous spread is rarely limited to the cervical compartment [51]. Actually, at reoperation, routine dissection of the upper mediastinum has identified lymph node metastases in up to 36% of cases [24]. However, biochemical cure is rare (<10%) in these instances. Currently, dissection of the upper mediastinum is recommended in the case of proven lymph node metastases using imaging techniques. Dissection of the upper mediastinum should also be considered if the presence of lymph node metastases is very likely (e.g., contralateral or bilateral cervical lymph node metastases, extrathyroidal tumor extension) [52]. Dissection of this compartment requires complete splitting of the sternum (Fig. 11.4b). Following sternotomy, the thymus and the adipose tissue surrounding the thymus are prepared in a caudal-to-cranial fashion starting down at the azygos vein and going up to the brachiocephalic vein (left side) or innominate artery (right side). Retrovascular, paratracheal, and paraesophageal lymph nodes are often involved and must be removed in the case of a mediastinal lymph node dissection. Special care should be taken to preserve the phrenic nerve.

11.4.6   Distant Metastases

The indication to resect distant metastases must be considered on an individual basis. Since these metastases are often multifocal and only a few millimeters in size, real tumor debulking is often not possible. In the case of single large metastases, most often found in the liver and lung, resection may be performed. Biochemical cure can not be achieved in these patients.

11.4.7   Non-surgical Treatment Options

Therapeutic options beyond surgery are numerous but their efficacy is limited. These include administration of somatostatin analogs (e.g., octreotide, pantreotide), radioligand therapy (e.g., iodine-131-labeled CEA, yttrium-90-labeled octreotide), conventional systemic chemotherapy, chemoembolization of liver metastases, and external radiation. External radiation to the neck should be avoided as long as possible since it causes scarring which may make both assessment of local recurrence and reoperation difficult. More recently, tyrosine kinase inhibitors have been shown to inhibit *RET* tyrosine kinase activity [6,10]. Clinical studies are underway but results have not yet been published.

11.5   Follow-up and Prognosis

The overall 5-year survival and 10-year survival rates have been reported to be 80–90% and 60–70%, respectively [2,34]. Several factors have been identified to correlate with long-term prognosis. Early postoperative normalization of calcitonin levels, i.e., normal basal and stimulated calcitonin levels ("biochemical cure") is strongly associated with a long-term disease-free survival [15,27,63]. Since the presence of lymph node metastases has been shown to lower the "cure" rate from 100% to 33% [25], lymph node metastases themselves are strong predictors of a worse long-term prognosis [2,45]. Of note, calcitonin levels may rise years after primary surgery despite initial normalization [40]. Hence, regular follow-up is necessary in all patients. Also, a subgroup of patients seem to have a delayed normalization that may take up to a few weeks [4,27]. The meaning of this phenomenon is not known.

References

1. Albores-Saavedra J, Monforte H, Nadji M, Morales AR (1988) C-cell hyperplasia in thyroid tissue adjacent to follicular cell tumors. Hum Pathol 19:795–799
2. Bergholm U, Bergstrom R, Ekbom A (1997) Long-term follow-up of patients with medullary carcinoma of the thyroid. Cancer 79:132–138
3. Bernier JJ, Rambaud JC, Cattan D, Prost A (1968) Medullary carcinoma of the thyroid associated with diarrhoea: report of five cases. Gut 9:726
4. Brauckhoff M, Gimm O, Brauckhoff K, Ukkat J, Thomusch O, Dralle H (2001) Calcitonin kinetics in the early postoperative period of medullary thyroid carcinoma. Langenbecks Arch Surg 386:434–439
5. Cady B (1991) Papillary carcinoma of the thyroid. Semin Surg Oncol 7:81–86
6. Carlomagno F, Vitagliano D, Guida T, Ciardiello F, Tortora G, Vecchio G, Ryan AJ, Fontanini G, Fusco A, Santoro M (2002) ZD6474, an orally available inhibitor of KDR tyrosine kinase activity, efficiently blocks oncogenic RET kinases. Cancer Res 62:7284–7290

7. Casanova S, Rosenberg-Bourgin M, Farkas D, Calmettes C, Feingold N, Heshmati HM, Cohen R, Conte-Devolx B, Guillausseau PJ, Houdent C, et al (1993) Phaeochromocytoma in multiple endocrine neoplasia type 2A: survey of 100 cases. Clin Endocrinol (Oxf) 38:531–537

8. Chan JK, Tse CC (1989) Solid cell nest-associated C-cells: another possible explanation for "C-cell hyperplasia" adjacent to follicular cell tumors. Hum Pathol 20:498–499

9. Christensen SB, Ljungberg O, Tibblin S (1984) A clinical epidemiologic study of thyroid carcinoma in Malmo, Sweden. Curr Probl Cancer 8:1–49

10. Cohen MS, Hussain HB, Moley JF (2002) Inhibition of medullary thyroid carcinoma cell proliferation and RET phosphorylation by tyrosine kinase inhibitors. Surgery 132:960–966; discussion 966–967

11. Da Silva AM, Maciel RM, Da Silva MR, Toledo SR, De Carvalho MB, Cerutti JM (2003) A novel germ-line point mutation in RET exon 8 (Gly(533)Cys) in a large kindred with familial medullary thyroid carcinoma. J Clin Endocrinol Metab 88:5438–5443

12. Decker RA, Geiger JD, Cox CE, Mackovjak M, Sarkar M, Peacock ML (1996) Prophylactic surgery for multiple endocrine neoplasia type IIa after genetic diagnosis: is parathyroid transplantation indicated? World J Surg 20:814–820; discussion 820–821

13. de Groot JW, Links TP, Jager PL, Kahraman T, Plukker JT (2004) Impact of 18F-fluoro-2-deoxy-D-glucose positron emission tomography (FDG-PET) in patients with biochemical evidence of recurrent or residual medullary thyroid cancer. Ann Surg Oncol 11:786–794

14. Donis-Keller H, Dou S, Chi D, Carlson KM, Toshima K, Lairmore TC, Howe JR, Moley JF, Goodfellow P, Wells SA Jr (1993) Mutations in the RET proto-oncogene are associated with MEN2A and FMTC. Hum Mol Genet 2:851–856

15. Dottorini ME, Assi A, Sironi M, Sangalli G, Spreafico G, Colombo L (1996) Multivariate analysis of patients with medullary thyroid carcinoma. Prognostic significance and impact on treatment of clinical and pathologic variables. Cancer 77:1556–1565

16. Dralle H, Damm I, Scheumann GF, Kotzerke J, Kupsch E, Geerlings H, Pichlmayr R (1994) Compartment-oriented microdissection of regional lymph nodes in medullary thyroid carcinoma. Surg Today 24:112–121

17. Dralle H, Gimm O (1996) [Lymph node excision in thyroid carcinoma]. Chirurg 67:788–806

18. Dralle H, Gimm O, Simon D, Frank-Raue K, Gortz G, Niederle B, Wahl RA, Koch B, Walgenbach S, Hampel R, Ritter MM, Spelsberg F, Heiss A, Hinze R, Hoppner W (1998) Prophylactic thyroidectomy in 75 children and adolescents with hereditary medullary thyroid carcinoma: German and Austrian experience. World J Surg 22:744–750; discussion 750–751

19. Elisei R, Bottici V, Luchetti F, Di Coscio G, Romei C, Grasso L, Miccoli P, Iacconi P, Basolo F, Pinchera A, Pacini F (2004) Impact of routine measurement of serum calcitonin on the diagnosis and outcome of medullary thyroid cancer: experience in 10,864 patients with nodular thyroid disorders. J Clin Endocrinol Metab 89:163–168

20. Eng C, Clayton D, Schuffenecker I, Lenoir G, Cote G, Gagel RF, van Amstel HK, Lips CJ, Nishisho I, Takai SI, Marsh DJ, Robinson BG, Frank-Raue K, Raue F, Xue F, Noll WW, Romei C, Pacini F, Fink M, Niederle B, Zedenius J, Nordenskjold M, Komminoth P, Hendy GN, Gharib H, Thibodeau SN, Lacroix A, Frilling A, Ponder BA, Mulligan LM (1996) The relationship between specific RET proto-oncogene mutations and disease phenotype in multiple endocrine neoplasia type 2. International RET mutation consortium analysis. JAMA 276:1575–1579

21. Fleming JB, Lee JE, Bouvet M, Schultz PN, Sherman SI, Sellin RV, Friend KE, Burgess MA, Cote GJ, Gagel RF, Evans DB (1999) Surgical strategy for the treatment of medullary thyroid carcinoma. Ann Surg 230:697–707

22. Frank-Raue K, Bihl H, Dorr U, Buhr H, Ziegler R, Raue F (1995) Somatostatin receptor imaging in persistent medullary thyroid carcinoma. Clin Endocrinol (Oxf) 42:31–37

23. Froboese C (1923) Das aus markhaltigen Nervenfasern bestehende ganlienzellenlose echte Neurom in rankenform - zugleich ein Beitrag zu den nervösen Geschwulsten der Zunge und des Augenlides. Virchows Arch Pathol Anat 240:312–327

24. Gimm O, Dralle H (1997) Reoperation in metastasizing medullary thyroid carcinoma: is a tumor stage-oriented approach justified? Surgery 122:1124–1130; discussion 1130–1131

25. Gimm O, Ukkat J, Dralle H (1998) Determinative factors of biochemical cure after primary and reoperative surgery for sporadic medullary thyroid carcinoma. World J Surg 22:562–567; discussion 567–568

26. Gimm O, Ukkat J, Niederle BE, Weber T, Thanh PN, Brauckhoff M, Niederle B, Dralle H (2004) Timing and extent of surgery in patients with familial medullary thyroid carcinoma/multiple endocrine neoplasia 2A-related RET mutations not affecting codon 634. World J Surg 28:1312–1316. Epub 2004 Nov 1304

27. Girelli ME, Dotto S, Nacamulli D, Piccolo M, De Vido D, Russo T, Bernante P, Pelizzo MR, Busnardo B (1994) Prognostic value of early postoperative calcitonin level in medullary thyroid carcinoma. Tumori 80:113–117

28. Gomez JM, Biarnes J, Volpini V, Marti T (1998) Neuromas and prominent corneal nerves without MEN2B. Ann Endocrinol (Paris) 59:492–494

29. Gordon CM, Majzoub JA, Marsh DJ, Mulliken JB, Ponder BA, Robinson BG, Eng C (1998) Four cases of mucosal neuroma syndrome: multiple endocrine neoplasm 2B or not 2B? J Clin Endocrinol Metab 83:17–20

30. Grieco M, Santoro M, Berlingieri MT, Melillo RM, Donghi R, Bongarzone I, Pierotti MA, Della Porta G, Fusco A, Vecchio G (1990) PTC is a novel rearranged form of the ret proto-oncogene and is frequently detected in vivo in human thyroid papillary carcinomas. Cell 60:557–563

31. Guyetant S, Wion-Barbot N, Rousselet MC, Franc B, Bigorgne JC, Saint-Andre JP (1994) C-cell hyperplasia associated with chronic lymphocytic thyroiditis: a retrospective quantitative study of 112 cases. Hum Pathol 25:514–521

32. Hazard JB, Hawk WA, Crile G (1959) Medullary (solid) carcinoma of the thyroid: a clinicopathologic entity. J Clin Endocrinol Metab 19:152–161

33. Henriksen JH, Schifter S, Moller S, Bendtsen F (2000) Increased circulating calcitonin in cirrhosis. Relation to severity of disease and calcitonin gene-related peptide. Metabolism 49:47–52

34. Heshmati HM, Gharib H, van Heerden JA, Sizemore GW (1997) Advances and controversies in the diagnosis and management of medullary thyroid carcinoma. Am J Med 103:60–69

35. Hoegerle S, Altehoefer C, Ghanem N, Brink I, Moser E, Nitzsche E (2001) 18F-DOPA positron emission tomography for tumour detection in patients with medullary thyroid carcinoma and elevated calcitonin levels. Eur J Nucl Med 28:64–71

36. Hofstra RM, Fattoruso O, Quadro L, Wu Y, Libroia A, Verga U, Colantuoni V, Buys CH (1997) A novel point mutation in the intracellular domain of the ret protooncogene in a family with medullary thyroid carcinoma. J Clin Endocrinol Metab 82:4176–4178

37. Hoie J, Jorgensen OG, Stenwig AE, Langmark F (1988) Medullary thyroid cancer in Norway. A 30-year experience. Acta Chir Scand 154:339–343

38. Ito S, Iwashita T, Asai N, Murakami H, Iwata Y, Sobue G, Takahashi M (1997) Biological properties of Ret with cysteine mutations correlate with multiple endocrine neoplasia type 2A, familial medullary thyroid carcinoma, and Hirschsprung's disease phenotype. Cancer Res 57:2870–2872

39. Iwashita T, Kato M, Murakami H, Asai N, Ishiguro Y, Ito S, Iwata Y, Kawai K, Asai M, Kurokawa K, Kajita H, Takahashi M (1999) Biological and biochemical properties of Ret with kinase domain mutations identified in multiple endocrine neoplasia type 2B and familial medullary thyroid carcinoma. Oncogene 18:3919–3922

40. Jackson CE, Talpos GB, Kambouris A, Yott JB, Tashjian AH Jr, Block MA (1983) The clinical course after definitive operation for medullary thyroid carcinoma. Surgery 94:995–1001

41. Jimenez C, Dang GT, Schultz PN, El-Naggar A, Shapiro S, Barnes EA, Evans DB, Vassilopoulou-Sellin R, Gagel RF, Cote GJ, Hoff AO (2004) A novel point mutation of the RET protooncogene involving the second intracellular tyrosine kinase domain in a family with medullary thyroid carcinoma. J Clin Endocrinol Metab 89:3521–3526

42. Jimenez C, Habra MA, Huang SC, El-Naggar A, Shapiro SE, Evans DB, Cote G, Gagel RF (2004) Pheochromocytoma and medullary thyroid carcinoma: a new genotype-phenotype correlation of the RET protooncogene 891 germline mutation. J Clin Endocrinol Metab 89:4142–4145

43. Karges W, Dralle H, Raue F, Mann K, Reiners C, Grussendorf M, Hufner M, Niederle B, Brabant G (2004) Calcitonin measurement to detect medullary thyroid carcinoma in nodular goiter: German evidence-based consensus recommendation. Exp Clin Endocrinol Diabetes 112:52–58

44. Kasprzak L, Nolet S, Gaboury L, Pavia C, Villabona C, Rivera-Fillat F, Oriola J, Foulkes WD (2001) Familial medullary thyroid carcinoma and prominent corneal nerves associated with the germline V804M and V778I mutations on the same allele of RET. J Med Genet 38:784–787

45. Kebebew E, Ituarte PH, Siperstein AE, Duh QY, Clark OH (2000) Medullary thyroid carcinoma: clinical characteristics, treatment, prognostic factors, and a comparison of staging systems. Cancer 88:1139–1148

46. Kotzmann H, Schmidt A, Scheuba C, Kaserer K, Watschinger B, Soregi G, Niederle B, Vierhapper H (1999) Basal calcitonin levels and the response to pentagastrin stimulation in patients after kidney transplantation or on chronic hemodialysis as indicators of medullary carcinoma. Thyroid 9:943–947

47. Lips CJM, Landsvater RM, Hoppener JWM, Geerdink RA, Blijham G, Jansen-Schillhorn van Veen JM, van Gils APG, de Witt MJ, Zewald RA, Berends MJH, Beemer FA, Brouwers-Smalbraak J, Jansen RPM, Ploos van Amstel HK, van Vroonhoven TJMV, Vroom TM (1994) Clinical screening as compared with DNA analysis in families with multiple endocrine neoplasia type 2A. N Engl J Med 331:828–835

48. Machens A, Gimm O, Hinze R, Hoppner W, Boehm BO, Dralle H (2001) Genotype-phenotype correlations in hereditary medullary thyroid carcinoma: oncological features and biochemical properties. J Clin Endocrinol Metab 86:1104–1109

49. Machens A, Gimm O, Ukkat J, Hinze R, Schneyer U, Dralle H (2000) Improved prediction of calcitonin normalization in medullary thyroid carcinoma patients by quantitative lymph node analysis. Cancer 88:1909–1915

50. Machens A, Haedecke J, Holzhausen HJ, Thomusch O, Schneyer U, Dralle H (2000) Differential diagnosis of calcitonin-secreting neuroendocrine carcinoma of the foregut by pentagastrin stimulation. Langenbecks Arch Surg 385:398–401

51. Machens A, Hinze R, Thomusch O, Dralle H (2002) Pattern of nodal metastasis for primary and reoperative thyroid cancer. World J Surg 26:22–28. Epub 2001 Nov 2022

52. Machens A, Niccoli-Sire P, Hoegel J, Frank-Raue K, van Vroonhoven TJ, Roeher HD, Wahl RA, Lamesch P, Raue F, Conte-Devolx B, Dralle H (2003) Early malignant progression of hereditary medullary thyroid cancer. N Engl J Med 349:1517–1525

53. Menko FH, van der Luijt RB, de Valk IA, Toorians AW, Sepers JM, van Diest PJ, Lips CJ (2002) Atypical MEN type 2B associated with two germline RET mutations on the same allele not involving codon 918. J Clin Endocrinol Metab 87:393–397

54. Mirallie E, Vuillez JP, Bardet S, Frampas E, Dupas B, Ferrer L, Faivre-Chauvet A, Murat A, Charbonnel B, Barbet J, Goldenberg DM, Chatal JF, Kraeber-Bodere F (2005) High frequency of bone/bone marrow involvement in advanced medullary thyroid cancer. J Clin Endocrinol Metab 90:779–788. Epub 2004 Nov 2030

55. Miyauchi A, Futami H, Hai N, Yokozawa T, Kuma K, Aoki N, Kosugi S, Sugano K, Yamaguchi K (1999) Two germline missense mutations at codons 804 and 806 of the RET proto-oncogene in the same allele in a patient with multiple endocrine neoplasia type 2B without codon 918 mutation. Jpn J Cancer Res 90:1–5

56. Miyauchi A, Matsuzuka F, Hirai K, Yokozawa T, Kobayashi K, Ito Y, Nakano K, Kuma K, Futami H, Yamaguchi K (2002) Prospective trial of unilateral surgery for nonhereditary medullary thyroid carcinoma in patients without germline RET mutations. World J Surg 26:1023–1028

57. Moley JF, DeBenedetti MK (1999) Patterns of nodal metastases in palpable medullary thyroid carcinoma: recommendations for extent of node dissection. Ann Surg 229:880–887; discussion 887–888

58. Moley JF, Dilley WG, DeBenedetti MK (1997) Improved results of cervical reoperation for medullary thyroid carcinoma. Ann Surg 225:734–740; discussion 740–743

59. Moley JF, Wells SA, Dilley WG, Tisell LE (1993) Reoperation for recurrent or persistent medullary thyroid cancer. Surgery 114:1090–1095; discussion 1095–1096

60. Mulligan LM, Kwok JBJ, Healey CS, Elsdon MJ, Eng C, Gardner E, Love DR, Mole SE, Moore JK, Papi L, Ponder MA, Telenius H, Tunnacliffe A, Ponder BAJ (1993) Germline mutations of the RET proto-oncogene in multiple endocrine neoplasia type 2A. Nature 363:458–460

61. Nilsson O, Tisell LE, Jansson S, Ahlman H, Gimm O, Eng C (1999) Adrenal and extra-adrenal pheochromocytomas in a family with germline RET V804L mutation [letter]. JAMA 281:1587–1588

62. Pacini F, Fontanelli M, Fugazzola L, Elisei R, Romei C, Di Coscio G, Miccoli P, Pinchera A (1994) Routine measurement of serum calcitonin in nodular thyroid diseases allows the preoperative diagnosis of unsuspected sporadic medullary thyroid carcinoma [see comments]. J Clin Endocrinol Metab 78:826–829

63. Pellegriti G, Leboulleux S, Baudin E, Bellon N, Scollo C, Travagli JP, Schlumberger M (2003) Long-term outcome of medullary thyroid carcinoma in patients with normal postoperative medical imaging. Br J Cancer 88:1537–1542

64. Ponder BA, Ponder MA, Coffey R, Pembrey ME, Gagel RF, Telenius-Berg M, Semple P, Easton DF (1988) Risk estimation and screening in families of patients with medullary thyroid carcinoma. Lancet 1:397–401

65. Pujol RM, Matias-Guiu X, Miralles J, Colomer A, de Moragas JM (1997) Multiple idiopathic mucosal neuromas: a minor form of multiple endocrine neoplasia type 2B or a new entity? J Am Acad Dermatol 37:349–352

66. Raue F, Kotzerke J, Reinwein D, Schroder S, Roher HD, Deckart H, Hofer R, Ritter M, Seif F, Buhr H, et al (1993) Prognostic factors in medullary thyroid carcinoma: evaluation of 741 patients from the German Medullary Thyroid Carcinoma Register. Clin Invest 71:7–12

67. Rieu M, Lame MC, Richard A, Lissak B, Sambort B, Vuong-Ngoc P, Berrod JL, Fombeur JP (1995) Prevalence of sporadic medullary thyroid carcinoma: the importance of routine measurement of serum calcitonin in the diagnostic evaluation of thyroid nodules [see comments]. Clin Endocrinol (Oxf) 42:453–460

68. Robbins KT, Medina JE, Wolfe GT, Levine PA, Sessions RB, Pruet CW (1991) Standardizing neck dissection terminology. Official report of the Academy's Committee for Head and Neck Surgery and Oncology. Arch Otolaryngol Head Neck Surg 117:601–605

69. Scheumann GF, Gimm O, Wegener G, Hundeshagen H, Dralle H (1994) Prognostic significance and surgical management of locoregional lymph node metastases in papillary thyroid cancer. World J Surg 18:559–567; discussion 567–568

70. Scollo C, Baudin E, Travagli JP, Caillou B, Bellon N, Leboulleux S, Schlumberger M (2003) Rationale for central and bilateral lymph node dissection in sporadic and hereditary medullary thyroid cancer. J Clin Endocrinol Metab 88:2070–2075

71. Shannon KE, Gimm O, Hinze R, Dralle H, Eng C (1999) Germline V804M mutation in the RET proto-oncogene in two apparently sporadic cases of FMTC presenting in the seventh decade of life. J Endocr Genet 1:39–45

72. Sipple JH (1961) The association of pheochromocytoma with carcinoma of the thyroid gland. Am J Med 31:163–166

73. Smallridge RC, Bourne K, Pearson BW, Van Heerden JA, Carpenter PC, Young WF (2003) Cushing's syndrome due to medullary thyroid carcinoma: diagnosis by proopiomelanocortin messenger ribonucleic acid in situ hybridization. J Clin Endocrinol Metab 88:4565–4568

74. Steiner AL, Goodman AD, Powers SR (1968) Study of a kindred with pheochromocytoma, medullary thyroid carcinoma, hyperparathyroidism and Cushing's disease: multiple endocrine neoplasia, type 2. Medicine (Baltimore) 47:371–409

75. Takahashi M, Ritz J, Cooper GM (1985) Activation of a novel human transforming gene, ret, by DNA rearrangement. Cell 42:581–588

76. Tisell LE, Hansson G, Jansson S, Salander H (1986) Reoperation in the treatment of asymptomatic metastasizing medullary thyroid carcinoma. Surgery 99:60–66

77. Tung WS, Vesely TM, Moley JF (1995) Laparoscopic detection of hepatic metastases in patients with residual or recurrent medullary thyroid cancer. Surgery 118:1024–1029; discussion 1029–1030

78. Vierhapper H, Raber W, Bieglmayer C, Kaserer K, Weinhausl A, Niederle B (1997) Routine measurement of plasma calcitonin in nodular thyroid diseases. J Clin Endocrinol Metab 82:1589–1593

79. Wagenmann A (1922) Multiple Neurome des Auges und der Zunge. Ber Dtsch Ophthalmol Ges 43:282–285

80. Wells SA Jr, Chi DD, Toshima K, Dehner LP, Coffin CM, Dowton SB, Ivanovich JL, DeBenedetti MK, Dilley WG, Moley JF, et al (1994) Predictive DNA testing and prophylactic thyroidectomy in patients at risk for multiple endocrine neoplasia type 2A. Ann Surg 220:237–247; discussion 247–250

12 Anaplastic Thyroid Carcinoma

Christian Passler, Reza Asari, Christian Scheuba, and Bruno Niederle

CONTENTS

12.1 Introduction

Undifferentiated (anaplastic) thyroid carcinoma (ATC) is a highly malignant tumor that histologically appears wholly or partially composed of undifferentiated cells that exhibit immunohistochemical or ultrastructural features indicative of epithelial differentiation.

In older literature, synonyms such as "spindle and giant cell carcinoma," "sarcomatoid carcinoma," "pleomorphic carcinoma," "dedifferentiated carcinoma," "metaplastic carcinoma," or "carcinosarcoma" are used to describe this very aggressive and lethal tumor, leading to death within a few months in most of the patients.

12.2 Epidemiology

Anaplastic thyroid carcinoma is a rare disease with an incidence of approximately one or two cases per million per year [1]. It accounts for 1.6% to 13% of thyroid carcinomas [2–8] but this varies geographically with a higher incidence in Europe than in the USA. A higher incidence has been reported in endemic goiter regions.

Earlier studies from the USA indicate a percentage of 20% [9]. A continuous decrease of ATC can be observed over recent decades [10–12]. One reason for this may be the introduction of iodine prophylaxis in endemic, iodine-deficient goiter regions [2,4,6,12–14]. However, other investigators could not find any influence of iodine supplementation on the incidence of ATC [15]. Nevertheless, the incidence of ATC in iodine-deficient areas, such as India, is still high (Table 12.1) [16,17]. On the other hand, through the introduction of immunohistochemical methods, many tumors formerly classified as ATC turned out to be lymphomas or medullary thyroid carcinomas [2,4,15,18,19]. As an additional explanation for the decrease of ATC, some authors postulate the more

Table 12.1 Incidence of ATC and iodine supplementation

Country	Iodine (µg/d)	Papillary (%)	Follicular (%)	Anaplastic (%)
Japan	>240	73	17	3
USA	>240	68	16	4
Switzerland	80–120	53	27	5
Germany	80–120	49	25	1
India	40–80	29	45	12

aggressive treatment of differentiated carcinomas and other thyroid pathologies preventing anaplastic transformation [1,2].

Although ATC accounts for less than 5% of clinically recognized malignant thyroid neoplasms, more than half of the 1,200 deaths attributed to thyroid cancer annually in the USA result from ATC.

Anaplastic thyroid carcinoma occurs mainly in the elderly. Only 25% of patients are younger than 60 years. The median age of onset is in the sixth to seventh decade of life [2,3,5,20–24]. There is a clear predominance of female patients (female-to-male ratio 1.5:1), as in most thyroid carcinomas [2–5, 14,18,21,23,25,26].

12.3   Etiology

There are many theories about the development of ATC, but to date, no specific etiologic agent has been identified [27]. There is clinical and pathologic evidence of ATC developing from dedifferentiation of differentiated thyroid carcinomas (DTC). The clinical evidence consists of the frequently observed longstanding history of a thyroid pathology or even forgone thyroid surgery because of DTC [27]. Foci of ATC in DTC (incidental ATC) lead to a significantly better prognosis in comparison to pure ATC [8,11,28–31]. This suggests that the tumor should be removed at an early stage of disease, before it undergoes complete transformation. Some authors found aggressive subtypes of papillary thyroid carcinomas, such as the tall cell variant, or insular thyroid carcinomas in association with ATC, leading them to the hypothesis that these subtypes represent an intermediate form in the anaplastic transformation process [8,27,32–34]. Since some authors did not find associated differentiated components in most ATCs, it remains controversial whether ATC may arise de novo or as consequence of transformation of DTC [23,27].

On the molecular level, tumor suppressor genes are thought to play an essential role in the development of ATC. The most investigated tumor suppressor gene is p53. Lack or production of abnormal p53 protein causes higher susceptibility to malignant transformation. Mutations or overexpression of p53 are frequently detected in ATC [34–38]. Other oncogenes that are believed to play a role in anaplastic transformation are bcl-2, cyclin D1, β-catenin, Met, c-myc, Nm23, and ras [27].

12.4   Clinical Presentation

The most frequent sign at presentation is a large and rapidly growing neck mass (Fig. 12.1a,b), causing local compressive symptoms such as dysphagia, dysphonia, hoarseness, stridor, dyspnea, pain, weight loss, and superior vena cava obstruction [3,4,18,22,23,30,39–41]. About 30% of patients present with a unilateral vocal cord paralysis [14]. Frequently symptoms evolve within a short time period of 1–3 months [30,40].

12.5   Macroscopy

Most of the ATCs replace the majority of the gland parenchyma. Up to 90% of patients show invasion of the tumor into adjacent structures and organs, mostly

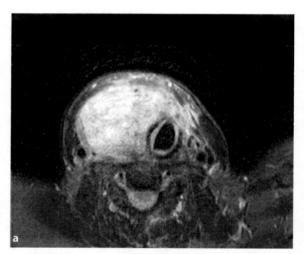

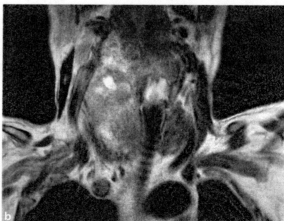

Fig. 12.1 Anaplastic (undifferentiated) thyroid cancer (ATC) in magnetic resonance imaging: partly cystic inhomogeneous 9×7×9-cm mass in the right thyroid lobe without gross infiltration of neighboring organs. **a** Axial view. **b** Coronal view

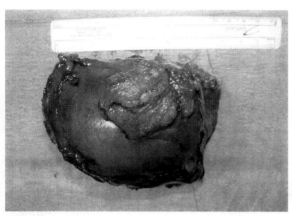

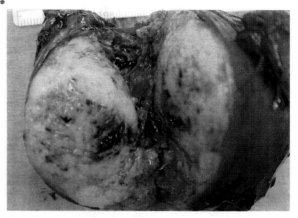

Fig. 12.2 Macroscopically radical *en bloc* thyroidectomy with adjacent strap muscles; the ATC is localized in the right thyroid lobe. The patients presented with a local recurrence (12 cm) and distant metastases (lung, pleura) 8 weeks later, and succumbed 10 weeks after primary surgery

Fig. 12.3 Macroscopic view of the opened specimen. The large tumor is fleshy, white-tan in color, and exhibits areas of necrosis and hemorrhage

in fatty tissue and muscles (Fig. 12.2), but also into the larynx, trachea, pharynx, esophagus, jugular vein, and carotid artery [4,12,14,42].

Macroscopically they are fleshy and white-tan colored tumors exhibiting areas of necrosis and hemorrhage (Fig. 12.3).

Nearly 50% of the patients present with distant metastases at diagnosis, and they may be present at any site. The most commonly involved organ is the lung (80%), followed by bone (6–15%) and brain (5–13%). Up to 75% of the patients develop distant metastases during follow-up [4,7,14,21,23,30,31,39–41].

12.6   Cytopathology

The diagnosis is often suspected through the typical clinical presentation, but nevertheless has to be ascertained by fine-needle aspiration (FNA) or core needle biopsy. Accurate diagnosis should be possible in 90% of patients [1,14,43], even though some authors report an accurate diagnosis by FNA in only 30% of cases [8]. Open biopsy should be reserved for ambiguous situations in order not to delay treatment by prolonged wound healing [44].

12.7   Fine-needle Aspiration

Aspirates are typically highly cellular [45]. The cells are presented singly or in clusters and there is a marked nuclear pleomorphism. The cell types include squamoid, giant cell and spindle cell. The nuclei are

bizarre and single or multiple. They reveal coarsely clumped chromatin and single or multiple prominent nucleoli. Mitotic figures may be numerous. Occasional osteoclast-like giant cells can be seen [45]. The background smear reveals necrotic debris often with accompanying polymorphonuclear leukocytes. Because of the presence of the latter cells care must be taken to distinguish these tumors from acute thyroiditis [45].

12.8   Histopathology

When an ATC is well sampled, it is possible to find well-differentiated or poorly differentiated thyroid carcinoma in many tumors. This finding supports the belief that ATC arises from the transformation (dedifferentiation) of a pre-existing, better differentiated carcinoma. Some cases may arise de novo [45].

The majority of ATCs are composed of an admixture of spindle cells, pleomorphic giant cells, and epithelioid cells (Fig. 12.4). The spindle cells can be slender or plump, and the giant cells may contain single or multiple, bizarre nuclei. About 20–30% of the tumors can present frankly epithelioid areas, sometimes exhibiting squamoid features. Mitotic figures are a very frequent finding [45].

Some tumors may be highly vascularized and the neoplastic cells can be arranged in a hemangiopericytic-like pattern or may form irregular anastomosing tumor cell-lined clefts mimicking an angiosarcoma [45].

It is of the utmost importance to rule out lymphomas and medullary thyroid carcinomas. This can be done by immunohistochemical staining for calcitonin, carcinoembryonic antigen, and chromogranin A

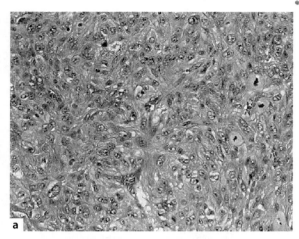

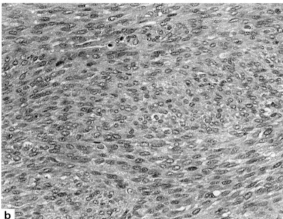

Fig. 12.4 The thyroid mass, classified as undifferentiated thyroid cancer, shows two cell populations histologically, giant cells (**a**) and spindle cells (**b**)

in the case of medullary thyroid carcinoma, and for leukocyte common antigen (LCA), CD 79a, and CD 3 in the case of lymphoma. In addition, the diagnosis of ATC can immunohistochemically be confirmed by coexpression of mesenchymal (vimentin) and epithelial (CAM 5.2) markers [12].

In order to determine the extent of local tumor growth and the presence of distant metastases, it is helpful to perform pretherapeutic computed tomography or magnetic resonance imaging of the neck and chest [41].

12.9   Pathologic Staging

All ATC are considered to be T4 tumors (T4a: ATC within the thyroid gland; T4b: ATC infiltrating beyond the thyroid gland). All are staged as "stage 4" (stage IVA: T4a, N0 or N1, M0; stage IVB: T4b, N0 or N1, M0; stage IVC: every T, No or N1, M1) [46].

12.10   Prognostic Factors and Outcome

As stated above, ATC is one of the most lethal carcinomas. Median survival ranges from 2.5 to 12 months [2–4,21,22,24,42,47,48]. Long-term survival or cure is reserved to very few, mostly young patients without distant metastases at presentation and with a completely resectable tumor responding to additional radiotherapy and chemotherapy.

Multiple studies have analyzed prognostic factors for survival in ATC. A reliable factor predicting death within a short time period is distant metastases at time of presentation [5,19,21,40,42,49]. Other inconsistently found favorable prognostic factors are young age [21,24,40], small tumor size (<5 cm) [2,4,30,40,47,49], focal anaplastic transformation in DTC [8,30,32,40,50], and completeness of tumor resection [4,12,22,29,47,51]—all predict improved survival. Other series reported the same fatal outcome in patients with or without associated DTC (Fig. 12.5) [12,20,21,25,51].

Sugitani et al. [30] developed a prognostic index (PI) for patients with ATC based on four independent prognostic factors identified by multivariate analysis. The factors were acute onset of symptoms (within 1 month), tumor diameter >5 cm, white blood cell (WBC) count ≥10,000/mm³, and distant metastases at presentation. For every present factor one point was given resulting in five different patient groups from P0 to P4. The difference in survival between the different groups was statistically significant. They resolved to perform multimodal therapy with a combination of surgery, radiotherapy, and chemotherapy in patients with a low PI, and palliative therapy in patients with a high PI.

12.11   Treatment

In many patients is it impossible to radically remove the primary tumor because of its early invasive growth. Thus the main goal of therapy is control of local disease in order to avoid death from suffocation. Surgery, radiotherapy, or chemotherapy alone is seldom sufficient to control the disease [21,52,53]. At the present time there is no known curative treatment in case of distant metastases. Multimodal treatment using hyperfractionated radiotherapy, chemotherapy, and surgery seems to be the best way to achieve this goal and is thus the treatment of choice [7,21,51,54,55].

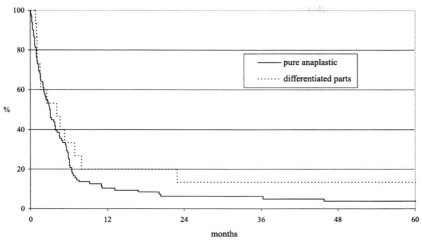

Fig. 12.5 Estimated survival according to Kaplan-Meier in 120 patients with ATC comparing pure ATCs and ATCs with differentiated parts; $P=0.334$ [12]

12.11.1 Surgery

The role of surgery is controversial. On the one hand, surgery seems indicated only for open biopsy when needle biopsy fails to obtain enough tissue to differentiate ATC from thyroid lymphoma. Surgery seems ineffective in achieving local tumor control, but it is indicated for securing the airway, via tracheostomy when necessary, in individual patients [39]. On the other hand, extended surgery, including partial resection of vital organs, has been recommended, since long-term survival has been reported with low morbidity through the use of this procedure [56,57]. Other authors described a high rate of complications in extended surgery for ATC [20,21,58]. The main role of surgery concerns debulking of tumor masses that facilitates radiotherapy and chemotherapy for local tumor control [4,21,59,60]. It seems to be useful to do primary, preoperative hyperfractionated radiotherapy in combination with chemotherapy in order to enhance resectability [7,55]. Whereas Tennvall et al. [55] reported local tumor control in 60% of the patients but no impact on survival using this treatment protocol including surgery, Sugino et al. [31] have observed a significantly better survival rate in patients undergoing debulking surgery followed by radiation in comparison to patients who did not undergo surgery (1-year survival 60% versus 20%, respectively). Other authors also reported prolonged survival in patients in whom complete surgical resection in combination with radiotherapy and/or chemotherapy was performed [22,30,40,51]. A recent report showed no impact on survival, either by the extent or the achieved completeness of resection [23]. Our own experience shows a statistically significant higher survival rate in patients where complete microscopic tumor resection (R0) can be achieved. R0-resected patients had a median survival of 6.1 months compared to 2.2 months in patients with micro- or macroscopic (R1/R2) tumor residues ($P<0.001$) (Fig. 12.6) [12].

Complete tumor resection can be achieved mainly in incidental ATCs limited to the thyroid [40], and therefore only in a small number of patients and at the expense of a higher morbidity, especially vocal cord paralysis [12]. Because of the high incidence of complications and the questionable impact on survival we do not see any justification for an ultraradical surgical approach involving segmental resections of esophagus, larynx, and trachea, except in very special cases (young patient with limited infiltration without distant metastases). However, we are consistent in removing infiltrated neck muscles and in performing (partial) sleeve resections of the laryngeal, tracheal, and esophageal wall, if macroscopic tumor resection seems possible (restricted radical approach) [12]. This aggressive surgical management with organ preservation (without ultraradical en bloc resections of esophagus, trachea, or larynx) is considered the preferred surgical approach, as is the case in other centers [51]. According to a recently published consensus on the treatment of ATC, total thyroidectomy is justified if cervical and mediastinal disease can be resected with limited morbidity [41].

Apart from emergency situations (intratracheal hemorrhage, acute dyspnea, bilateral vocal cord paralysis) a primary tracheostomy should be avoided [61]. Nevertheless in our own experience a tracheostomy became inevitable in 9% of R0 resections and in 23% of R1/R2 resections [12].

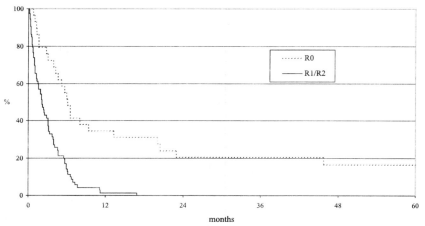

Fig. 12.6 Estimated survival according to Kaplan-Meier of 120 patients with ATC, comparing R0 and R1/R2 resections; $P<0.001$ [12]

12.11.2 Radiotherapy

Radiotherapy plays an important role in achieving local tumor control. A minimum radiation dose of >30 Gy seems necessary [19]. Pierie et al. [40] showed a better outcome in patients who received a total dose of >45 Gy than in those who received ≤45 Gy. In order to reduce toxicity and allow a high total radiation dose, hyperfractionation is useful [59]. Additionally, acceleration of radiotherapy seems to improve local tumor control [55]. Tennvall et al. [55] report on three protocols combining doxorubicin, hyperfractionated radiotherapy, and surgery in 55 patients with ATC. In protocol A a target dose of 30 Gy was administered preoperatively for a period of 3 weeks and an additional 16 Gy postoperatively for 1.5 weeks. The radiation dose was administered twice daily with a target dose of 1 Gy per fraction. In protocol B radiotherapy was accelerated by administering 1.3 Gy per fraction twice daily to the same total doses pre- and postoperatively. The total treatment time was shortened from 70 to 50 days by acceleration. In protocol C radiotherapy was further accelerated by increasing the target dose to 1.6 Gy per fraction twice daily and administering the radiation only preoperatively to a total dose of 46 Gy in 29 fractions within 3 weeks. Radiation therapy was combined with weekly administration of doxorubicin at 20 mg i.v., and was continued after the completion of local treatment for a maximum of 3 months. A strong correlation between local tumor control and acceleration of radiotherapy could be found. Additional surgery was, however, a prerequisite for eradication of local disease. Among patients undergoing surgery, 83% showed no signs of local recurrence. No significant improvement of sur-

vival could be reached, since there was no observed response in distant metastases. Nevertheless 5 patients (9%) survived for longer than 2 years and seem to be cured.

Other investigators also find improved local control using a combination of radiotherapy and chemotherapy, but no or only little improvement of survival [54,59].

12.11.3 Chemotherapy

According to Ain [14] successful systemic chemotherapy is of major importance for survival because of the high incidence of patients with distant metastases at presentation. Unfortunately, no chemotherapeutic agent has yet been found that leads to improved survival or that has an effect on present distant metastases [40,41,55,62].

Doxorubicin is the most commonly used drug, showing no evidence of complete response when used as monotherapy [53,63]. Addition of other chemotherapeutic agents such as cisplatin and/or bleomycin did not show an improvement in survival [53,62,64,65]. The main limitation is high drug toxicity. Chemotherapy has its role for local tumor control in combination with radiotherapy, since doxorubicin is successfully used as a radiosensitizer [40,55].

Schlumberger et al. [54] reported on 20 patients who had been treated with radiotherapy and, age-dependent, received chemotherapy with a combination of doxorubicin and cisplatin (<65 years) or mitoxantrone. Although local tumor control was achieved, occurrence and continuing existence of distant metastases could not be influenced.

Kober et al. [66] reported on the results of combination chemotherapy using cisplatin, vincristine, and mitoxantrone. Out of 15 patients, 10 who responded, completely (4 patients) or partially (6 patients), were compared with non-responders, and these patients demonstrated a markedly prolonged median survival (20.8 months versus 4.5 months, respectively).

Ain et al. [67] reported on the good results with reduced cell counts of all ATC cell lines in vivo and on diminishing size of xenograft tumors using paclitaxel. A subsequent phase II study showed a 53% response rate using paclitaxel. Patients who demonstrated a therapeutic response showed a significantly improved survival of 32 weeks, compared to 7 weeks in non-responding patients [68]. Further studies are necessary to eventually confirm an impact on survival by using paclitaxel.

Controversies remain about the optimal sequence of treatment modalities in ATC. Some centers use surgery as the first-line therapy in ATC with postoperative chemo- and radiotherapy [40,54], whereas others prefer primary chemo- and radiotherapy, followed by surgery, if feasible [7,55]. Potential disadvantages of the latter approach may be a delay in securing the airway and a possible delay in surgery because of the toxicity of combined radiotherapy/chemotherapy [69]. The decision about the sequence must finally be an individual one, based on patients' conditions and tumor characteristics.

12.12   Future Therapeutic Aspects

Tumor suppressor gene therapy is a promising future directive. In vitro analysis showed inhibition of growth and dedifferentiation of ATC cell lines by reintroduction of p53 wild-type [70–72]. In vivo studies followed. After subcutaneous injection of anaplastic tumor cells in nude mice adenovirus-mediated tumor suppressor p53 gene therapy led to near complete inhibition of tumor growth, and tumor regression was observed with the addition of doxorubicin [73]. Histone deacetylase (HDAC) inhibitors promote apoptosis and differential cell cycle arrest in anaplastic cancer cell lines [74]. Clinical trials using HDAC inhibitors to treat ATC have not yet been carried out [27]. Angiogenesis inhibitors are additional substances showing some effect against human ATC xenografts in nude mice [75]. A further therapeutic directive is to use bone morphogenic proteins as negative regulators to thyroid carcinoma growth. Franzen and Heldin [76] showed cell cycle arrest of anaplastic carcinoma cells in the G1-phase by using bone morphogenic protein

(BMP-7). Injection of bovine seminal ribonuclease resulted in complete regression of in vivo established anaplastic thyroid cancer in nude mice by inducing apoptosis [77].

As shown recently [78], lovastatin, a 3-hydroxy-3-methylglutaryl coenzyme A reductase inhibitor, induces a dose-dependent apoptosis and differentiation in ATC cells.

12.13   Conclusion

Multimodal treatment using hyperfractionated radiotherapy, chemotherapy, and surgery may be the treatment of choice for ATC. Surgery plays an important role because local tumor control cannot be achieved without debulking of large tumor masses.

Current evidence indicates that undifferentiated thyroid carcinoma originates from follicular cells. Therefore prognostic factors are related primarily to the extent of the disease at presentation. A small number of patients with completely resectable tumors (mainly as incidental ATC in the form of small foci of ATC in differentiated carcinomas) may be cured by aggressive surgery in combination with radiotherapy and chemotherapy. Nevertheless, in most patients death from ATC cannot be avoided, since multimodal treatment does not have much influence on distant metastases and thus on the survival rate. However, quality of life can be improved. It is probably less severe to die from distant metastases, than from suffocation due to failure of local tumor control. Although future therapeutic aspects are promising, clinical trials showing their impact on survival are still lacking.

References

1. Ain KB (1999) Anaplastic thyroid carcinoma: a therapeutic challenge. Semin Surg Oncol 16:64–69
2. Demeter JG, De Jong SA, Lawrence AM, Paloyan E (1991) Anaplastic thyroid carcinoma: risk factors and outcome. Surgery 110:956–961; discussion 961–963
3. Hadar T, Mor C, Shvero J, Levy R, Segal K (1993) Anaplastic carcinoma of the thyroid. Eur J Surg Oncol 19:511–516
4. Tan RK, Finley RK 3rd, Driscoll D, Bakamjian V, Hicks WL Jr, Shedd DP (1995) Anaplastic carcinoma of the thyroid: a 24-year experience. Head Neck 17:41–47; discussion 47–48

5. Gilliland FD, Hunt WC, Morris DM, Key CR (1997) Prognostic factors for thyroid carcinoma. A population-based study of 15,698 cases from the Surveillance, Epidemiology and End Results (SEER) program 1973–1991. Cancer 79:564–573

6. Bakiri F, Djemli FK, Mokrane LA, Djidel FK (1998) The relative roles of endemic goiter and socioeconomic development status in the prognosis of thyroid carcinoma. Cancer 82:1146–1153

7. Besic N, Auersperg M, Us-Krasovec M, Golouh R, Frkovic-Grazio S, Vodnik A (2001) Effect of primary treatment on survival in anaplastic thyroid carcinoma. Eur J Surg Oncol 27:260–264

8. Rodriguez JM, Pinero A, Ortiz S, Moreno A, Sola J, Soria T, Robles R, Parrilla P (2000) Clinical and histological differences in anaplastic thyroid carcinoma. Eur J Surg 166:34–38

9. Thomas GG Jr, Buckwalter JA (1973) Poorly differentiated neoplasms of the thyroid gland. Ann Surg 177:632–642

10. Demeure MJ, Clark OH (1990) Surgery in the treatment of thyroid cancer. Endocrinol Metab Clin North Am 19:663–683

11. Schmid KW, Gerber M, Tötsch M, Sandbichler P, Ladurner D (1990) Zur Inzidenz anaplastischer Schilddrüsenkarzinome und dem prognostischen Aussagewert differenzierter Anteile beim anaplastischen Karzinom. Wien Klin Wochenschr 102:4

12. Passler C, Scheuba C, Prager G, Kaserer K, Flores JA, Vierhapper H, Niederle B (1999) Anaplastic (undifferentiated) thyroid carcinoma (ATC). A retrospective analysis. Langenbecks Arch Surg 384:284–293

13. Bacher-Stier C, Riccabona G, Totsch M, Kemmler G, Oberaigner W, Moncayo R (1997) Incidence and clinical characteristics of thyroid carcinoma after iodine prophylaxis in an endemic goiter country. Thyroid 7:733–741

14. Ain KB (1998) Anaplastic thyroid carcinoma: behavior, biology, and therapeutic approaches. Thyroid 8:715–726

15. Pettersson B, Coleman MP, Ron E, Adami HO (1996) Iodine supplementation in Sweden and regional trends in thyroid cancer incidence by histopathologic type. Int J Cancer 65:13–19

16. Franceschi S, Boyle P, Maisonneuve P, La Vecchia C, Burt AD, Kerr DJ, MacFarlane GJ (1993) The epidemiology of thyroid carcinoma. Crit Rev Oncog 4:25–52

17. Hellman P, Goretzki P, Witte J, Röher HD (2001) Follicular thyroid carcinoma. Lippincott Williams and Wilkins, Philadelphia

18. Holting T, Moller P, Tschahargane C, Meybier H, Buhr H, Herfarth C (1990) Immunohistochemical reclassification of anaplastic carcinoma reveals small and giant cell lymphoma. World J Surg 14:291–294; discussion 295

19. Levendag PC, De Porre PM, van Putten WL (1993) Anaplastic carcinoma of the thyroid gland treated by radiation therapy. Int J Radiat Oncol Biol Phys 26:125–128

20. Nel CJ, van Heerden JA, Goellner JR, Gharib H, McConahey WM, Taylor WF, Grant CS (1985) Anaplastic carcinoma of the thyroid: a clinicopathologic study of 82 cases. Mayo Clin Proc 60:51–58

21. Venkatesh YS, Ordonez NG, Schultz PN, Hickey RC, Goepfert H, Samaan NA (1990) Anaplastic carcinoma of the thyroid. A clinicopathologic study of 121 cases. Cancer 66:321–330

22. Junor EJ, Paul J, Reed NS (1992) Anaplastic thyroid carcinoma: 91 patients treated by surgery and radiotherapy. Eur J Surg Oncol 18:83–88

23. McIver B, Hay ID, Giuffrida DF, Dvorak CE, Grant CS, Thompson GB, van Heerden JA, Goellner JR (2001) Anaplastic thyroid carcinoma: a 50-year experience at a single institution. Surgery 130:1028–1034

24. Lu WT, Lin JD, Huang HS, Chao TC (1998) Does surgery improve the survival of patients with advanced anaplastic thyroid carcinoma? Otolaryngol Head Neck Surg 118:728–731

25. Carcangiu ML, Steeper T, Zampi G, Rosai J (1985) Anaplastic thyroid carcinoma. A study of 70 cases. Am J Clin Pathol 83:135–158

26. Agrawal S, Rao RS, Parikh EM, Parikh HK, Borges AM, Sampat MB (1996) Histologic trends in thyroid cancer 1969–1993: a clinico-pathologic analysis of the relative proportion of anaplastic carcinoma of the thyroid. J Surg Oncol 63:251–255

27. Wiseman SM, Loree TR, Rigual NR, Hicks WL Jr, Douglas WG, Anderson GR, Stoler DL (2003) Anaplastic transformation of thyroid cancer: review of clinical, pathologic, and molecular evidence provides new insights into disease biology and future therapy. Head Neck 25:662–670

28. Nishiyama RH, Dunn EL, Thompson NW (1972) Anaplastic spindle-cell and giant-cell tumors of the thyroid gland. Cancer 30:113–127

29. Hollinsky C, Kober F, Hermann M, Loicht U, Keminger K (1990) [Prognostic factors in highly malignant thyroid tumors]. Wien Klin Wochenschr 102:249–253

30. Sugitani I, Kasai N, Fujimoto Y, Yanagisawa A (2001) Prognostic factors and therapeutic strategy for anaplastic carcinoma of the thyroid. World J Surg 25:617–622

31. Sugino K, Ito K, Mimura T, Nagahama M, Fukunari N, Kubo A, Iwasaki H (2002) The important role of operations in the management of anaplastic thyroid carcinoma. Surgery 131:245–248

32. Moreno A, Rodriguez JM, Sola J, Soria T, Parrilla P (1993) Prognostic value of the tall call variety of papillary cancer of the thyroid. Eur J Surg Oncol 19:517–521

33. Saunders CA, Nayar R (1999) Anaplastic spindle-cell squamous carcinoma arising in association with tall-cell papillary cancer of the thyroid: a potential pitfall. Diagn Cytopathol 21:413–418

34. Lam KY, Lo CY, Chan KW, Wan KY (2000) Insular and anaplastic carcinoma of the thyroid: a 45-year comparative study at a single institution and a review of the significance of p53 and p21. Ann Surg 231:329–338

35. Ito T, Seyama T, Mizuno T, Tsuyama N, Hayashi T, Hayashi Y, Dohi K, Nakamura N, Akiyama M (1992) Unique association of p53 mutations with undifferentiated but not with differentiated carcinomas of the thyroid gland. Cancer Res 52:1369–1371

36. Donghi R, Longoni A, Pilotti S, Michieli P, Della Porta G, Pierotti MA (1993) Gene p53 mutations are restricted to poorly differentiated and undifferentiated carcinomas of the thyroid gland. J Clin Invest 91:1753–1760

37. Fagin JA, Matsuo K, Karmakar A, Chen DL, Tang SH, Koeffler HP (1993) High prevalence of mutations of the p53 gene in poorly differentiated human thyroid carcinomas. J Clin Invest 91:179–184

38. Farid NR (2001) P53 mutations in thyroid carcinoma: tidings from an old foe. J Endocrinol Invest 24:536–545

39. Carty S (2001) Anaplastic thyroid carcinoma, thyroid metastases and lymphoma. Lippincott Williams and Wilkins, Philadelphia

40. Pierie JP, Muzikansky A, Gaz RD, Faquin WC, Ott MJ (2002) The effect of surgery and radiotherapy on outcome of anaplastic thyroid carcinoma. Ann Surg Oncol 9:57–64

41. Pasieka JL (2003) Anaplastic thyroid cancer. Curr Opin Oncol 15:78–83

42. Voutilainen PE, Multanen M, Haapiainen RK, Leppaniemi AK, Sivula AH (1999) Anaplastic thyroid carcinoma survival. World J Surg 23:975–978; discussion 978–979

43. Us-Krasovec M, Golouh R, Auersperg M, Besic N, Ruparcic-Oblak L (1996) Anaplastic thyroid carcinoma in fine needle aspirates. Acta Cytol 40:953–958

44. Besic N (2003) The role of initial debulking surgery in the management of anaplastic thyroid carcinoma. Surgery 133:453–454; author reply 454–455

45. Ordonez N, Balogh Z, Matias-Gulu X, Evans H, Farid NR, Fagin JA, Kitamura Y, Taillini G, Eng C, Haigh PI, Faquin WC, Sugitani I, Gluffrida D, Boerner S (2004) Undifferentiated (anaplastic) carcinoma. In: Delellis RA, Lloyd RV, Heitz PU (eds) Pathology and genetics of tumours of the endocrine organs. Eng Charis, Lyon, pp 77–80

46. DeLellis RA, Williams ED (2004) Thyroid and parathyroid tumours: introduction. In: Delellis RA, Lloyd RV, Heitz PU (eds) Pathology and genetics of tumours of the endocrine organs. Eng Charis, Lyon, pp 51–56

47. Kobayashi T, Asakawa H, Umeshita K, Takeda T, Maruyama H, Matsuzuka F, Monden M (1996) Treatment of 37 patients with anaplastic carcinoma of the thyroid. Head Neck 18:36–41

48. Nilsson O, Lindeberg J, Zedenius J, Ekman E, Tennvall J, Blomgren H, Grimelius L, Lundell G, Wallin G (1998) Anaplastic giant cell carcinoma of the thyroid gland: treatment and survival over a 25-year period. World J Surg 22:725–730

49. Staunton MD (1994) Thyroid cancer: a multivariate analysis on influence of treatment on long-term survival. Eur J Surg Oncol 20:613–621

50. Pacheco-Ojeda LA, Martinez AL, Alvarez M (2001) Anaplastic thyroid carcinoma in Ecuador: analysis of prognostic factors. Int Surg 86:117–121

51. Haigh PI, Ituarte PH, Wu HS, Treseler PA, Posner MD, Quivey JM, Duh QY, Clark OH (2001) Completely resected anaplastic thyroid carcinoma combined with adjuvant chemotherapy and irradiation is associated with prolonged survival. Cancer 91:2335–2342

52. Aldinger KA, Samaan NA, Ibanez M, Hill CS Jr (1978) Anaplastic carcinoma of the thyroid: a review of 84 cases of spindle and giant cell carcinoma of the thyroid. Cancer 41:2267–2275

53. Shimaoka K, Schoenfeld DA, DeWys WD, Creech RH, DeConti R (1985) A randomized trial of doxorubicin versus doxorubicin plus cisplatin in patients with advanced thyroid carcinoma. Cancer 56:2155–2160

54. Schlumberger M, Parmentier C, Delisle MJ, Couette JE, Droz JP, Sarrazin D (1991) Combination therapy for anaplastic giant cell thyroid carcinoma. Cancer 67:564–566

55. Tennvall J, Lundell G, Wahlberg P, Bergenfelz A, Grimelius L, Akerman M, Hjelm Skog AL, Wallin G (2002) Anaplastic thyroid carcinoma: three protocols combining doxorubicin, hyperfractionated radiotherapy and surgery. Br J Cancer 86:1848–1853

56. Goldman JM, Goren EN, Cohen MH, Webber BL, Brennan MF, Robbins J (1980) Anaplastic thyroid carcinoma: long-term survival after radical surgery. J Surg Oncol 14:389–394

57. Machens A, Hinze R, Lautenschlager C, Thomusch O, Dunst J, Dralle H (2001) Extended surgery and early postoperative radiotherapy for undifferentiated thyroid carcinoma. Thyroid 11:373–380

58. Zimmermann G, Hermann M, Kober F, Ladurner D, Pimpl W (1990) Intra- und postoperative Komplikationen in der Chirurgie hochmaligner Schilddrüsentumore. Wien Klin Wochenschr 102:10–11

59. Kim JH, Leeper RD (1987) Treatment of locally advanced thyroid carcinoma with combination doxorubicin and radiation therapy. Cancer 60:2372–2375

60. Tallroth E, Wallin G, Lundell G, Lowhagen T, Einhorn J (1987) Multimodality treatment in anaplastic giant cell thyroid carcinoma. Cancer 60:1428–1431

61. Hölting T, Meybier H, Buhr H (1990) Stellenwert der Tracheotomie in der Behandlung des respiratorischen Notfalls beim anaplastischen Schilddrüsenkarzinom. Wien Klin Wochenschr 102:264–266

62. Asakawa H, Kobayashi T, Komoike Y, Maruyama H, Nakano Y, Tamaki Y, Matsuzawa Y, Monden M (1997) Chemosensitivity of anaplastic thyroid carcinoma and poorly differentiated thyroid carcinoma. Anticancer Res 17:2757–2762

63. Ahuja S, Ernst H (1987) Chemotherapy of thyroid carcinoma. J Endocrinol Invest 10:303–310

64. Williams SD, Birch R, Einhorn LH (1986) Phase II evaluation of doxorubicin plus cisplatin in advanced thyroid cancer: a Southeastern Cancer Study Group Trial. Cancer Treat Rep 70:405–407

65. De Besi P, Busnardo B, Toso S, Girelli ME, Nacamulli D, Simioni N, Casara D, Zorat P, Fiorentino MV (1991) Combined chemotherapy with bleomycin, adriamycin, and platinum in advanced thyroid cancer. J Endocrinol Invest 14:475–480

66. Kober F, Heiss A, Keminger K, Depisch D (1990) [Chemotherapy of highly malignant thyroid tumors]. Wien Klin Wochenschr 102:274–276

67. Ain KB, Tofiq S, Taylor KD (1996) Antineoplastic activity of taxol against human anaplastic thyroid carcinoma cell lines in vitro and in vivo. J Clin Endocrinol Metab 81:3650–3653

68. Ain KB, Egorin MJ, DeSimone PA (2000) Treatment of anaplastic thyroid carcinoma with paclitaxel: phase 2 trial using ninety-six-hour infusion. Collaborative Anaplastic Thyroid Cancer Health Intervention Trials (CATCHIT) Group. Thyroid 10:587–594

69. Veness MJ, Porter GS, Morgan GJ (2004) Anaplastic thyroid carcinoma: dismal outcome despite current treatment approach. Aust N Z J Surg 74:559–562

70. Fagin JA, Tang SH, Zeki K, Di Lauro R, Fusco A, Gonsky R (1996) Reexpression of thyroid peroxidase in a derivative of an undifferentiated thyroid carcinoma cell line by introduction of wild-type p53. Cancer Res 56:765–771

71. Moretti F, Farsetti A, Soddu S, Misiti S, Crescenzi M, Filetti S, Andreoli M, Sacchi A, Pontecorvi A (1997) p53 re-expression inhibits proliferation and restores differentiation of human thyroid anaplastic carcinoma cells. Oncogene 14:729–740

72. Nagayama Y, Shigematsu K, Namba H, Zeki K, Yamashita S, Niwa M (2000) Inhibition of angiogenesis and tumorigenesis, and induction of dormancy by p53 in a p53-null thyroid carcinoma cell line in vivo. Anticancer Res 20:2723–2728

73. Nagayama Y, Yokoi H, Takeda K, Hasegawa M, Nishihara E, Namba H, Yamashita S, Niwa M (2000) Adenovirus-mediated tumor suppressor p53 gene therapy for anaplastic thyroid carcinoma in vitro and in vivo. J Clin Endocrinol Metab 85:4081–4086

74. Greenberg VL, Williams JM, Cogswell JP, Mendenhall M, Zimmer SG (2001) Histone deacetylase inhibitors promote apoptosis and differential cell cycle arrest in anaplastic thyroid cancer cells. Thyroid 11:315–325

75. Hama Y, Shimizu T, Hosaka S, Sugenoya A, Usuda N (1997) Therapeutic efficacy of the angiogenesis inhibitor O-(chloroacetyl-carbamoyl) fumagillol (TNP-470; AGM-1470) for human anaplastic thyroid carcinoma in nude mice. Exp Toxicol Pathol 49:239–247

76. Franzen A, Heldin NE (2001) BMP-7-induced cell cycle arrest of anaplastic thyroid carcinoma cells via p21(CIP1) and p27(KIP1). Biochem Biophys Res Commun 285:773–781

77. Kotchetkov R, Cinatl J, Krivtchik AA, Vogel JU, Matousek J, Pouckova P, Kornhuber B, Schwabe D, Cinatl J Jr (2001) Selective activity of BS-RNase against anaplastic thyroid cancer. Anticancer Res 21:1035–1042

78. Wang CY, Zhomg WB, Chang TC, Lai SM, Tsai YF (2003) Lovastatin, a 3-hydroxy-3-methylglutaryl coenzyme A reductase inhibitor, induces apoptosis and differentiation in human anaplastic thyroid carcinoma cells. J Clin Endocrinol Metab 88:3021–3026

13 Thyroid Lymphoma and Other Metastatic Lesions

Rebecca S. Sippel and Herbert Chen

CONTENTS

13.1   Thyroid Lymphoma

13.1.1   Clinical Presentation

Malignant tumors of the thyroid are rare, with an incidence of 1–2 cases per 100,000 people [1]. Thyroid lymphomas comprise less than 5% of thyroid malignancies and 2% of all malignant lymphomas [2–4]. The majority of thyroid lymphomas are non-Hodgkin's lymphomas of B cell origin, although a variety of histologic subtypes are seen [3,5,6].

Thyroid lymphomas frequently arise within a background of lymphocytic thyroiditis (Hashimoto's), which is the only known risk factor [7,8]. The presence of Hashimoto's thyroiditis can increase the risk of developing thyroid lymphoma by up to 60 times [9]. Unlike other thyroid cancers, head and neck radiation has not been shown to be a risk factor for the development of thyroid lymphoma.

Thyroid lymphoma typically presents as a rapidly enlarging neck mass, frequently causing obstructive symptoms. The diagnosis of primary lymphoma of the thyroid is usually made between the ages of 50 and 80, with a peak incidence in the sixth decade [10]. It occurs more than twice as frequently in women [5,6]. The most common symptom is a rapidly growing thyroid mass with an acute worsening within the last 2 months. The mass may cause symptoms due to compression and/or infiltration of the surrounding neck organs. The most commonly reported symptoms are dyspnea, dysphagia, choking, and pain. Symptoms resulting in airway and/or esophageal obstruction occur in approximately 30% of all cases [5]. While symptoms are usually only present for a few months, up to 20% of patients have a history of a longstanding goiter. The classic "B" symptoms of lymphoma (fever, night sweats, weight loss) are present in only 10% of patients. Because of the association with Hashimoto's thyroiditis, a history of hypothyroidism is not uncommon, occurring in approximately 15% of patients [10]. Hyperthyroidism is rare. In addition, synchronous/metachronous gastrointestinal lymphomas occur in 10–60% of patients with thyroid lymphoma [11]. Laboratory abnormalities can exist, but are not specific to thyroid lymphoma. Up to two thirds of patients will have positive serum antimicrosomal antibody titers and one third will have positive thyroglobulin antibody titers [10].

During a physical examination, the thyroid can be palpated as a hard, smooth, rubbery mass, which can be either bilateral or unilateral [6]. The thyroid may be slightly tender and is often fixed to adjacent structures. Up to 50% will have palpable nodal involvement on physical examination [12].

Using the National Cancer Institute Working Formulation [13] to classify lymphomas, the majority of thyroid lymphomas are classified as intermediate grade (approximately 70%) [14]. The REAL classification system [15], developed in recent years, has led to the identification of a new subgroup of lymphomas. A subset of small lymphocytic tumors has been identified that are called low-grade B cell lymphomas of mucosa-associated lymphoid tissue (MALT)-type. MALT tumors are frequently associated with predisposing inflammatory conditions, such as Hashimoto's thyroiditis, and may serve as a precursor to higher-grade lesions.

An important clinical distinction is to distinguish between anaplastic thyroid carcinoma and thyroid lymphoma. Anaplastic thyroid carcinoma is rapidly progressive and has a 2-year survival approaching 0% compared to 80% for thyroid lymphoma [16].

The diagnosis of lymphoma is typically made by fine-needle aspiration (FNA). In the past making a

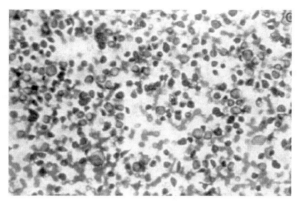

Fig. 13.1 Fine-needle aspiration sample diagnostic of thyroid lymphoma. A highly cellular aspirate containing numerous large, neoplastic lymphocytes

Table 13.1 Staging of thyroid lymphoma. (*E* Extranodal lymphoma)

Stage IE	Disease confined to the thyroid gland
Stage IIE	Disease confined to the thyroid gland and locoregional lymph nodes
Stage IIIE	Disease on both sides of the diaphragm
Stage IV	Diffuse disease

diagnosis of lymphoma using FNA was difficult due to the limitations of the small sample size obtained, however advances in FNA technology have now made FNA diagnosis possible in most patients (Fig. 13.1). In a series of 83 patients, Matsuzuka and colleagues found that FNA accurately diagnosed lymphoma in 78% of cases [10]. It is important to notify the cytopathologist that a thyroid lymphoma is suspected and thereby anticipate the need to obtain flow cytomorphology on the FNA specimen.

Ultrasound for lymphoma usually shows an asymmetric pseudocystic pattern in 93% of cases. This pattern is only seen in 11% of patients with pure Hashimoto's thyroiditis. While this ultrasound finding can help to make the diagnosis of lymphoma, it can be frequently mistaken for simple cysts and interpreted as benign [10]. The local extent of the tumor can be evaluated using either magnetic resonance imaging or computed tomography (CT), which can look for tracheal invasion or substernal extension. The tumor characteristics of lymphoma seen on CT scans may be useful in distinguishing it from an anaplastic thyroid cancer. Lymphomas appear homogeneous with little to no calcifications or necrosis present, while anaplastic cancers tend to be more heterogeneous with prominent calcifications and necrosis [16]. Nuclear imaging plays no role in the diagnosis of thyroid lymphoma.

13.1.2   Adjuvant Measures

Thyroid lymphomas are very sensitive to both radiation and chemotherapy. For localized disease, radiation is the primary therapy. Radiation fields include the neck and upper mediastinum and have local

response rates up to 75% [2,17]. The response to induction radiation therapy is often dramatic and can lead to rapid shrinking of the tumor. Unfortunately, approximately 30% of patients with stage IE or IIE (see Table 13.1) or localized disease develop distant relapses [2]. This fact suggests the need for adjuvant chemotherapy even in patients who appear to have localized disease.

Chemotherapy can be used as an adjunct to radiation in localized disease or as the primary therapy in advanced lymphomas. The standard chemotherapy for the treatment of patients with diffuse large B cell lymphoma is chemotherapy consisting of cyclophosphamide, doxorubicin, vincristine, and prednisone (CHOP) [6,18]. Several different regimens have been used to treat thyroid lymphoma, but due to the small number of patients treated, no single combination has been proven to be superior.

Since a high percentage of patients present with what appears to be localized disease, but then go onto develop distant disease, combined modality therapy has become the standard of care. Doria et al. [2] found that distant and overall relapse rates were significantly lower in those patients who received combined modality therapy in comparison to either chemotherapy or radiation therapy individually. DiBiase and colleagues [19] found in a series of 27 patients treated with either radiation alone or radiation with chemotherapy that the relapse rate was only 12% in the combination treatment in comparison to 47% in the radiation alone group. Similarly Ha and associates [20] reported in their series of 51 patients, a 5-year failure-free survival of 50% for chemotherapy and 76% for radiation alone, but as high as 91% for those treated with combined modality therapy.

13.1.3   Indication for Surgery

The role of surgery in the treatment of malignant lymphoma of the thyroid has evolved significantly over the last 20 years. While surgery previously was considered the primary treatment, the current standard of care consists of chemotherapy and external beam radiation [2,19,21].

Open surgical biopsy has traditionally been required in order to diagnose thyroid lymphoma. However, FNA combined with modern immunophenotypic analysis has greatly increased the ability to diagnose lymphoma [22]. FNA can now eliminate the need for surgical intervention for diagnosis in most patients.

Today, the role of surgical intervention for treatment of thyroid lymphoma is controversial. While some earlier series have shown a survival advantage to surgical debulking [12,23], this finding has not been consistently reproduced. More recently, several studies have shown that there is no advantage to surgical resection in comparison to radiation or combined modality therapy [24,25]. Pyke and colleagues [24] analyzed 62 patients and found that the addition of surgical debulking to adjuvant therapy led to a remission rate of 85% in comparison to 88% in the group of patients treated with adjuvant therapy alone. Another argument given against surgical therapy is the perceived higher complication rate compared with thyroid surgery for benign diseases. The infiltrative nature of the disease can make the dissection of the recurrent nerve and parathyroid glands more difficult leading to a potentially higher morbidity [14,24]. However, in our multicenter series we found that the complication rate in surgery for thyroid lymphoma was no higher when performed by an experienced endocrine surgeon [26].

Occasionally surgical intervention is needed on an urgent basis in order to decompress the airway or to place a tracheostomy. Because surgical intervention can be done with minimal delay and has an immediate effect on symptoms, some surgeons advocate surgical decompression in the highly symptomatic patient [14,24,26,27]. The need for a tracheostomy should always be anticipated in patients with thyroid lymphoma, as up to 25% of patients will ultimately require one during the course of their treatment.

13.1.4   Outcomes

The staging system for thyroid lymphoma is shown in Table 13.1. About 50% of patients with thyroid lymphoma present with disease limited to the thyroid gland (stage IE). Forty-five percent of patients present with locoregional nodes (stage IIE), while only 5% have involvement on both sides of the diaphragm or diffuse involvement [12,17,28]. Up to 85% of patients

with localized disease achieve an initial remission of their disease, however, half have been shown to go onto relapse within 10 years [20]. Most deaths due to disease occur within the first 3 years of diagnosis [5].

Combination therapy with radiation and chemotherapy without extensive surgery has been shown in several studies to have equal or superior 5-year survival rates while avoiding the inherent risks of thyroid surgery [25]. The 5-year survival from surgical series ranges from 42% to 88%, in comparison to the combined modality therapy series with 5-year survival rates of 77–85% [5]. Patients with stage IE disease tend to have a better prognosis with 5-year survivals of 80%, compared to stage IIE disease in which the 5-year survival is closer to 50% [20].

Most authors agree that bulky tumors, extension outside of the gland, and the presence of lymph node metastasis are associated with a worse prognosis [19,29]. As in other thyroid cancers, age is a significant prognostic factor. Patients under the age of 65 have a substantially better prognosis. Dibiase et al. [19] demonstrated a 5-year overall survival of 81% in those patients under age 65 in comparison to a 5-year survival of only 37% in those patients older than 65.

Histologic subtype can also help to define the prognosis for a given patient (Fig. 13.2). The most common histologic subtype is diffuse large B cell lymphoma, which accounts for greater than 50% of patients and is associated with a high incidence of disseminated disease and subsequent poor prognosis [8,19]. CD20 antibody staining is classic for lymphomas of B cell origin (Fig. 13.3). MALT lymphomas, which are usually associated with Hashimoto's thyroiditis, tend to be localized. Thieblemont and colleagues report 6 patients with localized MALT lymphoma of the thyroid who were treated successfully with surgery alone with a 100% disease-free and overall survival at 5 years [8]. In a larger series by Laing et al. [30] patients with MALT lymphoma had a 5-year survival of 90% in comparison to those without a MALT origin who had a 55% 5-year survival.

Due to the rare nature of these tumors, prospective randomized studies will likely never be performed. A number of retrospective series have been reported and for most patients the prognosis appears to be relatively good. For low-grade lesions, local therapy with surgery or radiation therapy may be adequate. For intermediate grade tumors, even if the disease appears to be localized, the treatment should consist of combined modality therapy (chemotherapy and radiation). For high-grade lesions the mainstay of therapy is chemotherapy with or without radiation as a local control adjuvant.

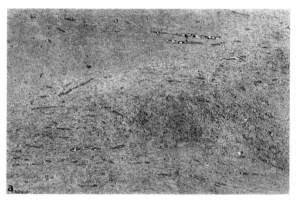
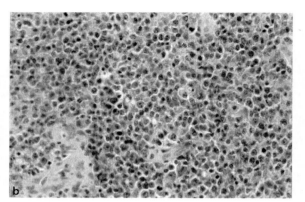

Fig. 13.2 Permanent histology analysis of a thyroid lymphoma. **a** Note the entire gland is replaced with lymphocytes. Areas of central necrosis can often be seen (4× magnification). **b** 40× magnification

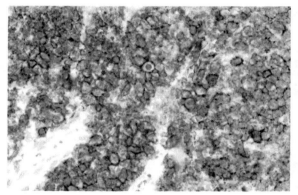

Fig. 13.3 CD20 antibody staining indicating that the thyroid lymphoma is of B cell origin (40× magnification)

13.2 Metastatic Lesions to the Thyroid

13.2.1 Clinical Presentation

Autopsy series suggest that as many as 22% of patients with generalized malignancies will have identifiable thyroid metastasis [31]. However, the number of tumors that are clinically detected is substantially smaller. Metastatic lesions account for 1–7% of all thyroid malignancies identified during the workup of a thyroid nodule [32,33]. Among patients with a known history of malignancy, the incidence of thyroid metastasis in a thyroid nodule can be as high as 20–66% [34,35].

The majority of patients with a thyroid metastasis present with an asymptomatic thyroid nodule. Occasionally patients complain of symptoms related to their thyroid enlargement, including dysphagia, stridor, or hoarseness. Patients most commonly are in their sixth or seventh decades of life [36].

In autopsy studies, the most common locations of the primary tumor are breast and lung, but in these patients the thyroid metastasis is usually part of a widely metastatic picture and is not clinically relevant. In clinical series, renal cell carcinoma is the most common tumor to metastasize to the thyroid [37,38]. Other tumors that have been shown to metastasize to the thyroid include melanoma and those from esophagus, stomach, pancreas, colon, rectum, uterus, and larynx. Thyroid metastasis can be the first manifestation of disease or can occur as late as 19 years after the primary tumor is resected [39]. In renal cell carcinoma, the first sign of disease is a thyroid metastasis in up to 30% of patients [40]. The majority of patients with a thyroid metastasis present within 3 years of the diagnosis of their primary tumor [37].

Fine-needle aspiration is able to make a diagnosis of malignancy in up to 100% of metastatic lesions [35,41]. However, several studies have shown that FNA is less accurate in distinguishing between a primary thyroid malignancy and a metastatic lesion, with accuracy rates of only 50% [32,36,42]. It becomes especially difficult for the cytologist to distinguish between an anaplastic thyroid cancer and a high-grade metastatic lesion. However, if an FNA is positive for metastatic disease it can help direct the patient to the appropriate therapy and avoid any unnecessary surgical intervention. Despite the potential limitations, FNA should be the diagnostic procedure of choice for any patient with a new thyroid nodule and a history of malignancy.

13.2.2 Indication for Surgery

Surgery may play a role in the diagnosis of metastatic disease to the thyroid or in its treatment. FNA is very accurate at diagnosing malignancy, but it is limited in its ability to distinguish between a metastatic lesion and a primary thyroid cancer. Hence, surgical intervention may be indicated in order to determine the diagnosis.

The role of surgery in the treatment of a known metastatic lesion is less clear. Since thyroid metastases are frequently only one manifestation of a widely metastatic disease, surgical resection plays no role in the management of this process. Occasionally patients may present with isolated thyroid metastasis with a substantial disease-free interval, and surgical intervention may provide some survival advantage and assist in local disease control. However, given the rarity of isolated thyroid metastasis there are no solid data to support this practice.

13.2.3   Adjuvant Measures

Since thyroid metastases are frequently part of a widely metastatic picture, the treatment of choice is systemic therapy for the primary tumor.

13.2.4   Outcomes

The outcomes for patients with thyroid metastasis are dependent upon many factors. The most important factor affecting outcome is whether the disease is limited to the thyroid or is part of a diffuse metastatic process. When a thyroid metastasis is part of a widely metastatic disease, the prognosis is poor with a survival of less than 2 years [42]. When the thyroid is the only identified site of metastatic disease the prognosis appears to be better and there may be a benefit to surgical excision. In our series of 10 patients with isolated disease we had 100% local control at 5 years with a 60% 5-year survival [37]. While isolated metastasis is most common in renal cell carcinoma, successful treatment of isolated metastasis has been reported in other tumors, such as rectal cancer [43].

The second factor affecting prognosis is the source of the primary tumor. Breast and lung cancer tend to have the worst prognosis, with the identification of a thyroid metastasis considered to be a preterminal event in most patients. In a series of 79 Chinese patients, in which the majority had metastasis from either a breast or lung primary, the mean survival was only 3 months [36]. The best prognosis exists for renal cell carcinoma. In our series, 4 of 5 patients who underwent resection for renal cell carcinoma were still alive after 5 years [37]. In a series of 36 patients with metastatic renal cell carcinoma, Heffess and colleagues [40] found that 36% were alive or died without evidence of disease with a mean follow-up of 9.1 years.

The third factor that alters prognosis is the disease-free interval. When a metastatic thyroid lesion is the initial presentation of a tumor, the disease tends to be widespread, and the prognosis is worse [40]. The best outcomes have been reported in patients with indolent tumors who present with long disease-free intervals.

Additional factors affecting outcomes are the ability to perform a complete surgical resection and the effectiveness of adjuvant therapy for the tumor type. In 1996, Nakhjavani and associates [41] reported their experience with 43 patients with thyroid metastasis who were treated with a combination of surgery, radiation, and chemotherapy. When they compared the patients who had surgery as part of their therapy to those who were treated non-surgically, they had a mean survival of 34 months in comparison to only 25 months.

Clinically relevant thyroid metastases are rare. In most cases the disease in the thyroid is only part of a diffusely metastatic process and the treatment of choice remains chemotherapy for the primary tumor. However, there are exceptions and some patients present with an isolated metastasis, an indolent tumor, or a long disease-free interval and clearly may benefit from surgical excision. Due the rarity of these lesions we will never have a definitive study to determine the true survival advantage of surgical intervention for these patients, but clearly consideration for surgical intervention should be performed.

Acknowledgements

We would like to thank Dr. Josephine Harter from the Department of Pathology at the University of Wisconsin for obtaining the histology figures.

References

1. Roeher HD, Simon D (1999) Surgical therapy of thyroid cancer. G Chir 20:5–8

2. Doria R, Jekel JF, Cooper DL (1994) Thyroid lymphoma. The case for combined modality therapy. Cancer 73:200–206

3. Compagno J, Oertel JE (1980) Malignant lymphoma and other lymphoproliferative disorders of the thyroid gland. A clinicopathologic study of 245 cases. Am J Clin Pathol 74:1–11

4. Samaan NA, Ordonez NG (1990) Uncommon types of thyroid cancer. Endocrinol Metab Clin North Am 19:637–648

5. Derringer GA, Thompson LD, Frommelt RA, Bijwaard KE, Heffess CS, Abbondanzo SL (2000) Malignant lymphoma of the thyroid gland: a clinicopathologic study of 108 cases. Am J Surg Pathol 24:623–639

6. Ansell SM, Grant CS, Habermann TM (1999) Primary thyroid lymphoma. Semin Oncol 26:316–323

7. Pasieka JL (2000) Hashimoto's disease and thyroid lymphoma: role of the surgeon. World J Surg 24:966–970

8. Thieblemont C, Mayer A, Dumontet C, Barbier Y, Callet-Bauchu E, Felman P, Berger F, Ducottet X, Martin C, Salles G, Orgiazzi J, Coiffier B (2002) Primary thyroid lymphoma is a heterogeneous disease. J Clin Endocrinol Metab 87:105–111

9. Holm LE, Blomgren H, Lowhagen T (1985) Cancer risks in patients with chronic lymphocytic thyroiditis. N Engl J Med 312:601–604

10. Matsuzuka F, Miyauchi A, Katayama S, Narabayashi I, Ikeda H, Kuma K, Sugawara M (1993) Clinical aspects of primary thyroid lymphoma: diagnosis and treatment based on our experience of 119 cases. Thyroid 3:93–99

11. Herrmann R, Panahon AM, Barcos MP, Walsh D, Stutzman L (1980) Gastrointestinal involvement in non-Hodgkin's lymphoma. Cancer 46:215–222

12. Tupchong L, Hughes F, Harmer CL (1986) Primary lymphoma of the thyroid: clinical features, prognostic factors, and results of treatment. Int J Radiat Oncol Biol Phys 12:1813–1821

13. Krueger GR, Medina JR, Klein HO, Konrads A, Zach J, Rister M, Janik G, Evers KG, Hirano T, Kitamura H, Bedoya VA (1983) A new working formulation of non-Hodgkin's lymphomas. A retrospective study of the new NCI classification proposal in comparison to the Rappaport and Kiel classifications. Cancer 52:833–840

14. Skarsgard ED, Connors JM, Robins RE (1991) A current analysis of primary lymphoma of the thyroid. Arch Surg 126:1199–1203

15. Harris NL, Jaffe E, Stein H, et al (1994) A revised European-American classification of lymphoid neoplasms: a proposal from the International Lymphoma Study Group. Blood 84:1361–1392

16. Ishikawa H, Tamaki Y, Takahashi M, Higuchi K, Sakaino K, Nonaka T, Shioya M, Mitsuhashi N, Niibe H (2002) Comparison of primary thyroid lymphoma with anaplastic thyroid carcinoma on computed tomographic imaging. Radiat Med 9–15

17. Tsang RW, Gospodarowicz MK, Sutcliffe SB, Sturgeon JF, Panzarella T, Patterson BJ (1993) Non-Hodgkin's lymphoma of the thyroid gland: prognostic factors and treatment outcome. The Princess Margaret Hospital Lymphoma Group. Int J Radiat Oncol Biol Phys 27:599–604

18. Fisher RI, Gaynor ER, Dahlberg S, Oken MM, Grogan TM, Mize EM, Glick JH, Coltman CA Jr, Miller TP (1993) Comparison of a standard regimen (CHOP) with three intensive chemotherapy regimens for advanced non-Hodgkin's lymphoma. N Engl J Med 328:1002–1006

19. DiBiase SJ, Grigsby PW, Guo C, Lin HS, Wasserman TH (2004) Outcome analysis for stage IE and IIE thyroid lymphoma. Am J Clin Oncol 27:178–184

20. Ha CS, Shadle KM, Medeiros LJ, Wilder RB, Hess MA, Cabanillas F, Cox JD (2001) Localized non-Hodgkin lymphoma involving the thyroid gland. Cancer 91:629–635

21. Udelsman R, Chen H (1999) The current management of thyroid cancer. Adv Surg 33:1–27

22. Cha C, Chen H, Westra W, Udelsman R (2002) Primary thyroid lymphoma: can the diagnosis be made solely by fine-needle aspiration? Ann Surg Oncol 9:298–302

23. Rosen IB, Sutcliffe SB, Gospodarowicz MK, Chua T, Simpson WJ (1988) The role of surgery in the management of thyroid lymphoma. Surgery 104:1095–1099

24. Pyke CM, Grant CS, Habermann TM, Kurtin PJ, van Heerden JA, Bergstralh EJ, Kunselman A, Hay ID (1992) Non-Hodgkin's lymphoma of the thyroid: is more than biopsy necessary? World J Surg 16:604–609

25. Klyachkin ML, Schwartz RW, Cibull M, Munn RK, Regine WF, Kenady DE, McGrath PC, Sloan DA (1998) Thyroid lymphoma: is there a role for surgery? Am Surg 64:234–238

26. Sippel RS, Gauger PG, Angelos P, Thompson NW, Mack E, Chen H (2002) Palliative thyroidectomy for malignant lymphoma of the thyroid. Ann Surg Oncol 9:907–911

27. Wirtzfeld DA, Winston JS, Hicks WL Jr, Loree TR (2001) Clinical presentation and treatment of non-Hodgkin's lymphoma of the thyroid gland. Ann Surg Oncol 8:338–341

28. Pedersen RK, Pedersen NT (1996) Primary non-Hodgkin's lymphoma of the thyroid gland: a population based study. Histopathology 28:25–32

29. Belal AA, Allam A, Kandil A, El Husseiny G, Khafaga Y, Al Rajhi N, Ahmed G, Gray A, Ajarim D, Schultz H, Ezzat A (2001) Primary thyroid lymphoma: a retrospective analysis of prognostic factors and treatment outcome for localized intermediate and high grade lymphoma. Am J Clin Oncol 24:299–305

30. Laing RW, Hoskin P, Hudson BV, Hudson GV, Harmer C, Bennett MH, MacLennan KA (1994) The significance of MALT histology in thyroid lymphoma: a review of patients from the BNLI and Royal Marsden Hospital. Clin Oncol (R Coll Radiol) 6:300–304

31. Willis RA (1931) Metastatic tumors in the thyroid gland. Am J Pathol 7:187–208

32. Lin JD, Weng HF, Ho YS (1998) Clinical and pathological characteristics of secondary thyroid cancer. Thyroid 8:149–153

33. Michelow PM, Leiman G (1995) Metastases to the thyroid gland: diagnosis by aspiration cytology [see comment]. Diagn Cytopathol 13:209–213

34. Lin SY, Sheu WH, Chang MC, Tang KT, Lee TI, Lin HD (2002) Diagnosis of thyroid metastasis in cancer patients with thyroid mass by fine needle aspiration cytology and ultrasonography. Chung Hua I Hsueh Tsa Chih 65:101–105

35. Watts NB (1987) Carcinoma metastatic to the thyroid: prevalence and diagnosis by fine-needle aspiration cytology. Am J Med Sci 293:13–17

36. Lam KY, Lo CY (1998) Metastatic tumors of the thyroid gland: a study of 79 cases in Chinese patients. Arch Pathol Lab Med 122:37–41

37. Chen H, Nicol TL, Udelsman R (1999) Clinically significant, isolated metastatic disease to the thyroid gland. World J Surg 23:177–180; discussion 181

38. Wood K, Vini L, Harmer C (2004) Metastases to the thyroid gland: the Royal Marsden experience. Eur J Surg Oncol 30:583–588

39. Kihara M, Yokomise H, Yamauchi A (2004) Metastasis of renal cell carcinoma to the thyroid gland 19 years after nephrectomy: a case report. Auris Nasus Larynx 31:95–100

40. Heffess CS, Wenig BM, Thompson LD (2002) Metastatic renal cell carcinoma to the thyroid gland: a clinicopathologic study of 36 cases. Cancer 95:1869–1878

41. Nakhjavani MK, Gharib H, Goellner JR, van Heerden JA (1997) Metastasis to the thyroid gland. A report of 43 cases. Cancer 79:574–578

42. Rosen IB, Walfish PG, Bain J, Bedard YC (1995) Secondary malignancy of the thyroid gland and its management. Ann Surg Oncol 2:252–256

43. Hacker U, Lenz G, Brehm G, Muller-Hocker J, Schalhorn A, Hiddemann W (2003) Metastasis of a rectal adenocarcinoma to the thyroid gland: diagnostic and therapeutic implications. Anticancer Res 23:4973–4976

14 Multinodular and Retrosternal Goiter

Rachel Rosenthal and Daniel Oertli

CONTENTS

14.1 Introduction

Multinodular goiter is a quite common condition with a marked female preponderance and it affects about 13% of the world population. Large differences in goiter prevalence have been found in different regions: 32% in the Eastern Mediterranean area, 20% in Africa, 15% in Europe, 12% in Southeast Asia, 8% in the Western Pacific, and 5% in the Americas [27]. The cause of multinodular goiter remains unclear, but is probably multifactorial. Iodine deficiency, naturally occurring goitrogens, thyroid growth factors, and heredity have been postulated as possible contributors to goiter development [13].

14.2 World Health Organization (WHO) Definitions

The WHO originally developed the criteria for the clinical evaluation of the size of the thyroid gland (Table 14.1) [9]. More recently, in 1993, the WHO proposed a modified classification system in which the former grades Ia and Ib are combined and the former grades II and III are combined (Table 14.2) [69].

The minimum criterion for the presence of goiter is thyroid lobes larger than the terminal phalanges of the thumb of the examined person. However, the clinical examination tends to overestimate thyroid size, especially in children [33,49].

In addition to the clinical classification of the thyroid gland, the WHO published a histological classification in 1974, which was substantially reworked in 1988 (Table 14.3) [23].

Table 14.1 Clinical evaluation of thyroid size

0	No goiter
Ia	Goiter palpable, no enlargement visible
Ib	Goiter palpable and visible with head reclination
II	Goiter palpable and visible with normal head position
III	Goiter palpable and visible from a distance with signs of local compression

Table 14.2 Clinical evaluation of thyroid size, modified classification

Grade 1	No palpable or visible goiter
Grade 2	Goiter palpable but not visible in normal head position
Grade 3	Goiter palpable and visible in normal head position

14.3   Other Classifications

Goiter is a clinical finding and it describes an enlarged thyroid gland. Various classifications are in use. The clinical assessment enables classification of the thyroid according to its size represented by the above-mentioned WHO classifications of clinical evaluation and to distinguish diffuse enlargement from a single nodule or multinodular goiter. The hormonal status can be euthyroid, hypothyroid, or hyperthyroid. Histologically, the enlarged thyroid may be benign or malignant. The classification according to the pathogenesis is given in Table 14.4.

14.4   Pathogenesis

The pathogenesis of multinodular goiter mainly describes two concepts: the iodine-deficiency goiters

Table 14.3 Histological classification of thyroid tumors

Epithelial tumors

- Benign: follicular adenoma, others
- Malignant: follicular carcinoma, papillary carcinoma, medullary carcinoma (C cell carcinoma), undifferentiated (anaplastic) carcinoma, others

Non-epithelial tumors

Malignant lymphomas

Miscellaneous tumors

Secondary tumors

Unclassified tumors

Tumor-like lesions

Table 14.4 Pathogenetic mechanisms of goiter

Iodine deficiency

Autonomy

Immunological thyropathy

Thyroiditis

Cyst formation, hematoma, trauma

Tumors

Neoplastic production of thyroid-stimulating hormone (TSH) or TSH analog

Acromegaly

Hormonal resistance

Enzyme deficiency

Involvement of thyroid gland in extrathyroid/systemic diseases

Goitrogenic substances

with chronic stimulation by a trophic hormone (endemic goiters) and the non-iodine-deficiency goiters (sporadic goiters) [14].

One hundred and fifty years ago, the role of iodine in goitrogenesis was first described and iodine was first administered for the prevention of goiter. Iodine supplementation using salt as the usual vehicle has substantially decreased the goiter rate. In China, for instance, iodine deficiency disorders can be considered to have been eliminated [10]. In iodine deficiency less thyroid hormones are produced. A feedback mechanism involving the hypothalamus and hypophysis leads to increased thyroid-stimulating hormone (TSH) production and consequently to proliferation of thyroid follicles [30]. The stimulation leads to hypertrophy and hyperplasia of the thyroid gland [62]. When iodine deficiency is severe (<25 μg I/g creatinine) more than 30% of the population is affected by goiters [14].

In goitrogenesis due to iodine deficiency, all follicular cells are exposed to the same environment. Therefore, hyperplastic follicles with little colloid content in a diffuse and homogenous enlarged thyroid would be expected. In contrast, in nodular goiter, nodules are surrounded by normal as well as connective tissue suggesting that they result from heterogeneity of growth. Functional heterogeneity is suggested by a patchy pattern of iodide isotope distribution on scintigraphs of nodular goiters. Cellular and molecular biological investigations have shown the nodular goiter growth to consist of three different parts: clonal nodules, polyclonal nodules, and pseudonodules. Pseudonodules are diffusely expanding follicles forced to grow in a network of connective tissue (hyperplastic micronodular thyroid tissue); polyclonal and clonal nodules are encapsulated nodules of polyclonal or clonal origin and are true benign neoplasias [14]. Multiple clonal nodules of different origin may coexist with polyclonal nodules. Clonal nodules may overgrow from primarily polyclonal ones; clonal growth does not necessarily implicate mutations or aberrations [63]. Autonomous growth may occur in toxic as well as in euthyroid nodular goiter depending on whether the gland produces excessive amounts of hormones or not [15]. From the histological point of view, an adenoma is a solitary tumor surrounded by a well-defined intact fibrous capsule, and molecular biological methods are used to confirm its clonal origin [24]. In a clinical setting, the term adenoma is frequently used to refer to a toxic or autonomous adenoma with higher uptake in technetium or radioiodine scintigraphy [16].

Iodine shortage may induce diffuse hyperplasia, enhancing genetic and chromosomal aberrations, and leading to intercellular heterogeneity. In the development of multinodular goiter, the genetic background is also relevant [5]. A study of over 5,000 pairs of twins described a heritability of the predisposition to develop nodular goiters of 82%. Low intrathyroidal iodine concentration may also be present in sporadic goiter and could be a consequence rather than a cause of nodular goiter [14]. In summary, iodine shortage enhances the incidence of multinodular goiter by adding a growth factor, but the fundamental process of goitrogenesis is independent of iodine deficiency.

Other possible factors leading to thyroid proliferation are the epidermal growth factor and the insulin-like growth factor I [30]. Nodules may develop under the influence of growth factors even in the absence of iodine deficiency. Iodine deficiency alone may not explain either the nodularity nor the heterogeneity of most goiters. Several characteristics have not been explained, such as heterogeneity of growth and function and clonality/polyclonality of goiter nodules [14]. Iodine-independent mechanisms have been attributed to the evolution of thyrotoxicosis and to the poor response of nodular goiters to TSH-suppressive therapy, in contrast to diffuse iodine-deficiency goiters, which respond well to iodine or T_4 treatment [12,14].

14.5   Iodine Prophylaxis

For prophylaxis of endemic goiter in iodine-deficient areas, a supplementation with 150 μg iodine a day is recommended for adults, and in case of pregnancy with 200 μg iodine a day. This recommended daily iodine intake should be adjusted for children to 50 μg for the first year of life, 90 μg for ages 1–6, and 120 μg for ages 7–12 [16,17].

14.6   Preoperative Assessment

14.6.1   Patient's History

The patient's history may be without complaint or may, apart from an awareness of the goiter size, include a globus sensation, dysphagia, choking, stridor, or dyspnea. The tendency to growth over time must be evaluated as well as symptoms of hypo- or hyperthyrosis. Symptoms of hyperthyrosis are increased appetite, weight loss, heat intolerance, nervousness, agitation, palpitation, diarrhea, muscular weakness (thyrotoxic myopathia) as well as oligo-/dysmenorrhea. Elderly patients frequently present with tachyarrhythmia only [16]. Symptoms of hypothyrosis are

weight gain (myxedema), depression, concentration weakness, cold intolerance, fatigue, constipation, and oligo-/amenorrhea.

14.6.2   Clinical Presentation

The WHO criteria for clinical evaluation of the size of the thyroid gland have been mentioned above. Retrosternal goiter may not be visible on clinical examination and may be unrecognized for many years. It may cause superior vena caval obstruction. The palpation is performed from the back of the patient, asking them to swallow. The size of the gland is evaluated, nodules are palpated, and signs of local compression are assessed (Fig. 14.1a,b). Additionally, lymph nodes are evaluated for enlargement, which may indicate malignancy.

Signs of hyperthyrosis may be tachycardia, tachyarrhythmia absoluta, hyperreflexia, an enhanced physiological tremor, warm and moist hands, soft and fine hair as well as hair loss. Thyrotoxic crisis/coma is a severe condition of untreated exacerbated hyperthyrosis in the presence of Graves' disease, autonomous adenoma, or multinodular toxic goiter. This is frequently induced by iodine (e.g. contrast product), severe general disease such as sepsis, general surgery, or thyroid surgery in hyperthyrosis. It presents with tachycardia, tachyarrhythmia, hyperthermia, diarrhea, vomiting, dehydration, muscular weakness, excitation (grade 1), disorientation, hallucination, somnolence (grade 2), and coma (grade 3).

Signs of hypothyrosis are bradycardia, hypotension, cardiac insufficiency, slow tendon reflexes, dry, pale, cold, rough and doughy skin (myxedema), rough hair, and a hoarse voice. Myxedema coma is a severe condition that frequently occurs after chronic untreated hypothyrosis with acute exacerbation due to infection, operation, severe general disease, cold, or sedative presenting with somnolence, severe hypothermia, hypotension, bradycardia, hypoventilation, hyponatremia, hypoglycemia, and possible pericardial and pleural effusion.

14.6.3   Radiological Findings

14.6.3.1   Sonography

Sonography is the most precise tool for evaluating the organ size (see also Chapter 4) [30]. The normal volume of the thyroid is 7–20 ml [4]. Besides the size, echogenicity gives further information. All patients scheduled for thyroid or parathyroid surgery should

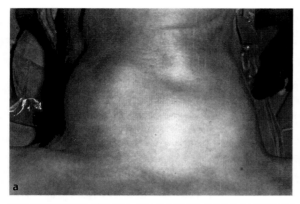

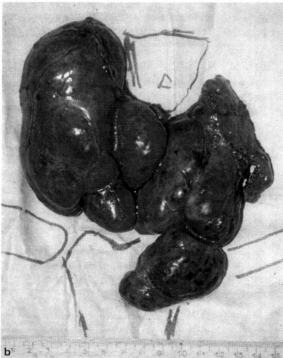

Fig. 14.1 Clinical presentation of a multinodular grade III goiter (**a**) with corresponding resected thyroid gland (**b**)

pathological findings. Ultrasound-guided fine-needle aspiration may, therefore, be helpful. In the case of follicular neoplasms, cytopathology may not discriminate between an adenoma and a follicular carcinoma. Ultrasound allows differentiation between solid nodules and simple or complex cysts, and may give information on regional lymphadenopathy [25].

14.6.3.2 Scintigraphy

Scintigraphy has become rare as a result of progress in ultrasound techniques. It should be performed only if it implicates a therapeutic consequence, for instance in a young patient with a solitary nodule, possibly a carcinoma, or in case of hyperthyrosis [30]. Scintigraphy provides an image of the spatial distribution of thyroid functional attributes. Thyroid nodules may be hot in the presence of autonomously functioning thyroid tissue, and are then rarely malignant; alternatively they may be cold in which case the incidence of malignancy is 10–20% [66].

14.6.3.3 Radiography and Tomography

Substernal goiter may be visible on plain chest X-rays (Fig. 14.2). X-ray examination of the trachea or a radiographic swallow study of the esophagus may give further information [16]. Computed tomography and magnetic resonance tomography are indicated for large tumors extending to adjacent structures such as the mediastinum or the retropharyngeal region [66] (Figs. 14.3, 14.4). It should be considered that goiter and malignancies may develop in ectopic thyroid tissue, which is found between the posterior tongue and the isthmus of the thyroid gland, in the region of the lateral neck, the mediastinum, and the oral cavity [66].

14.6.4   Fine-needle Aspiration

For evaluation of the potential malignancy of a nodule, ultrasound-guided aspiration cytology may give further information. Indications are suspected malignancy with the following findings: young patient, hypoechogenic in ultrasound, cold in scintigraphy, >1 cm diameter nodule, rapid growth, ill-defined nodule, solitary nodule in a goiter, and previous radiation exposure of the neck [16].

undergo a preoperative ultrasound (as opposed to scintigraphy). The ultrasound examination is combined with a cytological sample in cases of suspected malignancy.

Sonographically, the normal thyroid is isoechogenic or slightly hyperechogenic. Nodules larger than 2 mm in diameter may be identified [4]. Ultrasound may differentiate extrathyroidal structures from the thyroid gland. Color-flow Doppler ultrasonography gives further information on vascular flow and velocity. Ultrasound does not correlate with histo-

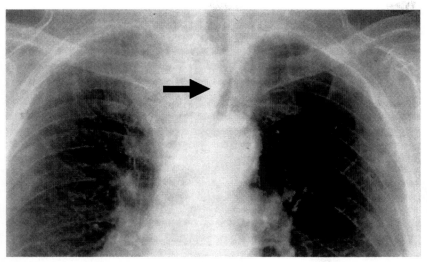

Fig. 14.2 Chest X-ray: left tracheal deviation (*arrow*) by a retrosternal goiter

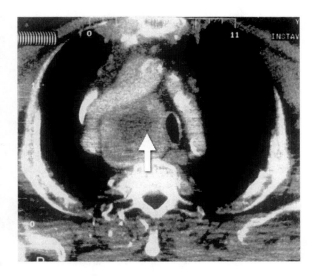

Fig. 14.3 Computed tomography: retrosternal goiter (*arrow*)

14.6.5   Laboratory Findings

The most important parameter is the basal TSH serum level. If it is within the normal range, euthyroid metabolism is present. If it is not within the normal range, more laboratory parameters should be tested, including fT_4 and fT_3. If an autoimmune process is suspected, thyroid autoantibodies should be tested [e.g. those against thyroperoxidase (formerly microsomal antibody) and TSH receptor] bearing in mind the fact that they may also be positive in healthy individuals or patients with goiter or autonomy [30].

The thyrotropin-releasing hormone (TRH) stimulation test measures the basal TSH level and the TSH level after an i.v. TRH bolus. Hyperthyroidism leads to a blunted response whereas primary hypothyroidism leads to an exaggerated TSH response. If the hypothalamic-pituitary axis is intact this test offers no advantage over measuring the basal TSH value [60].

14.6.6   Airway Assessment

In head and neck surgery, airway management depends on evidence of a compromised airway. The patient's history may reveal respiratory difficulties such as positional dyspnea, in some cases associated with dysphagia [18]. Signs of significant airway obstruction are stridor, labored breathing, intercostal retractions, and agitation in case of retrosternal goiter vena caval

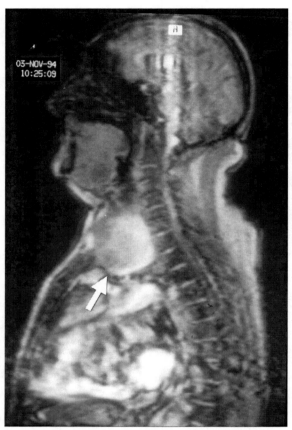

Fig. 14.4 Magnetic resonance imaging: retrosternal goiter (*arrow*)

laryngoscopy after application of topical anesthesia and oxygen. If the presence of a compromised airway is excluded, routine tracheal intubation may be performed. In all other cases, oral or nasal intubation while the patient is awake may be necessary [2]. Adjuncts to intubation are fiberoptic-guided intubation, retrograde intubation with a guide wire passed through the cricothyroid membrane into the nasal or oral cavity, or the transillumination technique with the use of a lightwand device [26]. In acute respiratory distress, tracheotomy, transtracheal jet ventilation, or cricothyroidotomy may be mandatory. If neither intubation, nor surgical airway control are possible, femoral–femoral cardiopulmonary bypass under local anesthesia, followed by a formal tracheotomy, is the ultimate option [2].

14.7   Non-operative Treatment

The conservative therapy of multinodular goiter with iodine and levothyroxine may be effective or partially effective, especially in reducing the volume of relatively small, benign, solitary, solid thyroid nodules and the combined nodular volume of multinodular goiter [7,20,32,44,67]. Low- and high-level TSH suppression are equally effective in reducing nodule volume [31]. Therefore, considering potential complications from high-level TSH suppression, low-level TSH suppression is recommended to reduce the size of thyroid nodules. However, some authors found a volume reduction without treatment, probably due to spontaneous regression [8,20]. Even if shrinkage of the majority of nodules may not be expected, some authors propose a treatment trial for a year, since the subgroup of responders may not be identified through baseline hormonal or imaging studies [44].

Alternatively, euthyroid multinodular goiters may be treated by TSH suppression therapy or radioiodine therapy; the latter is used particularly in elderly patients or those with contraindications for surgery [35]. The lifetime risk of cancer due to radioiodine is negligible in patients over 65 years old.

In Graves' disease, surgery, radiotherapy, and medical thyrostatic treatment are possible, whereas autonomy is a classical indication for radiotherapy except in solitary autonomous nodules where surgery is equally effective. Thyroid neoplasms are an indication for surgery as are iodine-induced hyperthyroidism and hyperthyroidism that cannot be managed conservatively [30].

obstruction [2]. Airway assessment includes distance between incisors, the thyromental distance, the degree of protrusion of the lower teeth, neck mobility, and the visualization of the hypopharynx [29,54]. Indirect laryngoscopy may be helpful and should be a routine examination in repeat surgery for recurrent goiter or if there are signs and symptoms of recurrent laryngeal nerve dysfunction. Some authors recommend routine preoperative laryngoscopy for all patients [55]; we do not. A chest X-ray is evaluated for tracheal deviation and compression [18] (Fig. 14.2). Other examinations, such as computed tomography and magnetic resonance imaging, are not routinely performed, but may give additional information especially in cases of retrosternal goiter [18] (Figs. 14.3, 14.4). Respiratory function tests are debatable. In 153 consecutive patients presenting with thyroid enlargement, upper airway obstruction was found in 33% [22].

If there is no evidence of a compromised airway, general anesthesia via inhalation or intravenous routes followed by paralysis and intubation is recommended [2]. In patients with evidence of a compromised airway, the airway is assessed using fiberoptic

14.8   Surgical Approach

14.8.1   Indications for and Extent of Surgery

Indications for surgery of the thyroid gland vary depending on the pathology: in euthyroid goiter the main indications are goiter size, compression symptoms, and suspected malignancy. In contrast to thyroid neoplasms and Graves' disease, where radical surgical principles are precisely defined, in euthyroid goiter and thyroid autonomy various surgical options exist: excision—ideally with a margin of normal tissue for easier histological evaluation—or enucleation of a solitary nodule, subtotal thyroidectomy, hemithyroidectomy (lobectomy), near-total thyroidectomy, or total thyroidectomy.

Today, functional and morphologically orientated thyroidectomy is generally performed, resecting pathological tissue as completely as possible and leaving normal thyroid parenchyma in place [51,65] (Fig. 14.5a,b). If the thyroid gland contains nodules throughout, complete thyroidectomy is necessary [6]. Because of a reportedly high frequency of complications in some series, controversy exists about the routine use of total thyroidectomy for the management of benign multinodular goiter [3,19,21]. When performed by experienced hands, total thyroidectomy, compared with subtotal resection, does not increase morbidity in benign pathologies [34,37,40,41,50,58]. In cases of substernal goiter, total thyroidectomy is preferred for reasons of malignant potential and to reduce recurrence rate [43]. It is of the utmost importance to emphasize that proper training and individual surgeon experience are significantly associated with low complication rates in thyroid surgery [38,59].

14.8.2   Approach to Retrosternal Goiter

Most retrosternal goiters can be resected through a standard cervical approach [43,68,72]. The head is reclined and the patient positioned in anti-Trendelenburg of about 15–20 degrees. Retrosternal goiters frequently compress veins, which may complicate surgery. By adopting this position, venous pressure may be reduced. The standard incision is the Kocher's incision, which is planned and marked with an insoluble pen before surgery on the reclining awake patient following the line of the wrinkles. Alternatively, the incision is marked with a thread once the patient is on the operation table. In order to gain good access to the retrosternal gland, the incision should be placed 1–2 cm higher than usual [68]. The skin platysma flap is prepared as usual, the superficial and middle neck fascia are separated at the midline, and the muscles held aside. In the case of a very large goiter, the muscles are incised laterally.

First, the upper pole is prepared and resected under ligation of the superior thyroid artery and vein. It is essential not to deliver the retrosternal component until these vessels have been ligated. By this procedure, the upper pole of the thyroid gland is mobilized, which will be important in the subsequent upward movement of the thyroid gland from the retrosternal to a cervical position. Attention must be paid to the external branch of the superior laryngeal nerve close to the superior thyroid artery. The cervical gland is further prepared and the superior parathyroid gland and the recurrent laryngeal nerve are routinely identified [64]. As the inferior parathyroids may be more difficult to find in retrosternal goiter, special care must be taken to identify the superior glands.

The next step is the delivery of the thyroid gland by blunt dissection with the finger inferiorly, completed by sharp dissection under vision. If the gland extends to the aortic arch and, therefore, may not be fully accessible with the finger, a sterile soup spoon can be slipped along the anterolateral aspect of the thyroid, breaking the negative intrathoracic pressure [1,68]. After elevating the gland from the mediastinum, the inferior vascular structures are ligated as near as possible to the gland [43]. When carrying out a near-total thyroidec-

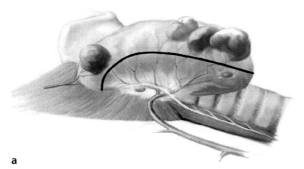
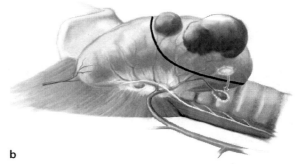

a   b

Fig. 14.5 Morphologically orientated thyroidectomy. **a** Subtotal resection with dorsal remnant. **b** Atypical subtotal resection

tomy or hemithyroidectomy and to maintain adequate vascularization of the parathyroid gland, the inferior thyroid artery should not be ligated at the main stem [16,65]. The branches at the level of the thyroid capsule are ligated selectively. Traction on the recurrent nerve must be carefully avoided during this maneuver and the capsule of the gland should not be opened due to the possibility of unsuspected malignancy. If the thyroid lobe cannot be brought to a cervical position, a possibility to provide more room is to remove the opposite thyroid lobe in its cervical position.

Hemostasis control is performed meticulously and no drainage is used. Two randomized trials did not show any advantage of drainage [57,70]. The muscles are sutured continuously with a 3-0 absorbable thread, the platysma with a 4-0 thread, and the skin intradermally with a 5-0 absorbable thread. A smooth collar may be used for the first 24 hours and anti-Trendelenburg positioning of about 30 degrees is advisable.

In cases of very large intrathoracic goiters, invasive tumors, dense adhesions from prior surgery, uncontrollable bleeding, or with the rare truly ectopic intrathoracic gland with its major blood supply from intrathoracic vessels, a mediastinal approach is required. In such cases sternotomy is performed [43,68]. As an alternative to complete sternotomy, a partial upper sternal split (manubriotomy) is possible in most cases [72]. Division of the manubrium to below the manubriosternal junction is performed (Fig. 14.6a). The suprasternal notch is prepared and the innominate vein and the pleura freed from the back of the manubrium. The manubrium and the upper sternum are divided in the middle and gently spread with a right-angled retractor (Fig. 14.6b). For better visualization, the thyroid gland is subluxated and the esophagotracheal groove and the angle formed by the arch of the aorta and the innominate artery are carefully prepared. Sternotomy is closed using sternal wires. In the case of complete sternotomy, the skin incision is extended to just above the xiphoid process and the pericardial and diaphragmatic attachments are freed from the back of the sternum before its division.

For resection of a crossed substernal goiter with extension from a left-side gland to the right mediastinum, right anterolateral thoracotomy can be helpful [68].

14.9   Complications of Retrosternal Goiter Surgery

As with cervical goiter, the main complications of retrosternal goiter surgery are hemorrhage, recurrent nerve injury, and hypoparathyroidism.

An intrathoracic goiter was found to be an independent risk factor for postoperative complications [50]. In a prospective study of 2,235 thyroid resections, 312 were performed for retrosternal goiter [61]. At surgery for retrosternal goiter, the complication rate was significantly elevated, for example secondary hemorrhage (3.2%), wound infections (2.2%), hypocalcemia for less than 6 months (24.7%), and transient recurrent nerve paresis (6.4%). However, persistent hypocalcemia (1.3%) or permanent recurrent nerve palsy (1.0%) were not significantly elevated as compared to the entire patient population.

Additionally, because of the surgical access, mediastinal injuries may occur. If mediastinal hemorrhage occurs, immediate surgical revision is indicated in order to avoid tracheal compression with consequent intubation problems or asphyxia. In the case of sternotomy, lesion of the innominate vein may cause major hemorrhage. To gain control of the hemorrhage, the vein is compressed against the back of the sternum, the ends are identified, and the vein is sutured. Mostly complete sternotomy is necessary in this case.

Pneumothorax after pleural injury is treated with insertion of a chest tube. More rare complications are infections (mostly due to an infected hematoma), injury of the pharynx, the trachea, or the sympathicus with resultant Horner's syndrome, accessory nerve paresis, lesions of the neck vessels, or tracheomalacia. Sternal infection may manifest late and is treated with a surgical debridement.

14.10   Results of Surgical Treatment of Multinodular Goiter

The rate of secondary hemorrhage is about 1%, whereas the rate of persistent recurrent nerve paresis and of hypoparathyroidism has dropped to below 1% in the last 20 years [6,52].

Adequate surgery is part of the prophylaxis of recurrence [65]. The incidence of nodular tissue correlates with the remnant thyroid volume and is around 50% at >5 ml remnant thyroid volume [36].

An analysis of histopathological findings after bilateral near-total thyroidectomy for multinodular goiter with suspected malignancy in 7.7.% of the cases showed malignant final pathological findings in 12.2% [48].

In a case-control study, young age and multiple nodules at initial surgery have been identified as independent risk factors for recurrence [21]. Despite suppressive postoperative thyroxin treatment, 14% of patients after subtotal thyroidectomy will develop

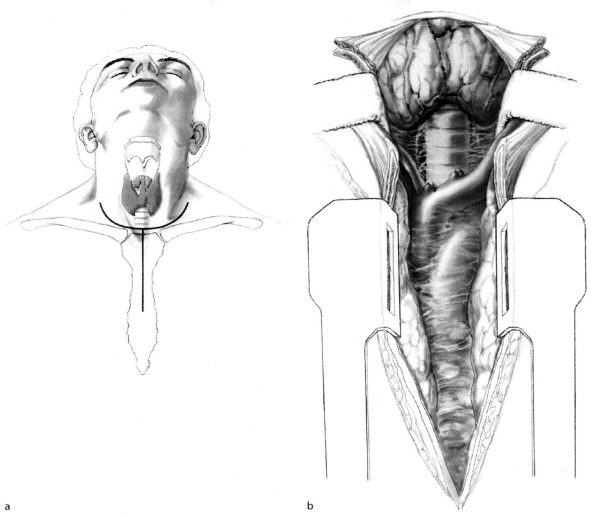

a   b

Fig. 14.6 Upper sternotomy. **a** Kocher's incision with additional inferior incision from the midpoint of the collar incision to below the manubriosternal junction. **b** Manubrial and partial sternal division with insertion of a sternal spreader

recurrent goiter after a median follow-up time of 14.5 years [45]. Without suppressive therapy the rate of recurrences rises to 41% of cases [47,53]. Since total thyroidectomy can be performed with a minimal complication rate, this option is increasingly being accepted and recommended for the treatment of benign nodular thyroid disease [11,40].

14.11   Prophylaxis of Recurrence

In addition to surgical care, postoperative substitution of iodine and thyroxine is important [65]. Iodine and the synthetic hormones are identical to the iodine in food and the endogenously produced hormones and therefore do not have side effects even after life-

long treatment, provided a correctly individualized dosage is used, with no hypo- or hyperthyroidism [16,28,46,56]. In iodine-deficiency goiter with no substitution, every fourth patient will have a recurrence. For an iodine-deficiency goiter with adequate remaining postoperative volume (>16 ml nodule-free thyroid), iodine substitution of 100–200 µg per day is sufficient. In the case of a nodule-free thyroid of an 8- to 16-ml volume, TSH must be assessed 4 weeks after surgery and the initial iodine substitution has to be completed with 50–100 µg levothyroxine in some cases. With <8 ml thyroid, 75–125 µg levothyroxine is given postoperatively with a TSH control 4–6 weeks postoperatively accompanied by 100–150 µg iodine per day unless the thyroid gland is smaller than 2 ml (4 ml in Graves' disease), when thyroxine is given

Table 14.5 Prophylaxis of recurrence

Nodule-free residual thyroid (ml)	Iodine 100–200 µg/d	Thyroxin 75–125 µg/d
>16	+	–
8–16	+	(+)
2–8	+	+
<2	–	+

without iodine [65]. Malignancy has to be excluded prior to postoperative thyroxine substitution. Table 14.5 gives an overview of the prophylaxis of recurrence. The aim is a TSH in the lower normal range (0.3–1 mU/l), in contrast with malignancies where the TSH should be suppressed. Strong TSH suppression increases the risk of cardiac complications and accelerates osteoporosis [28,56].

14.12   Recurrent Goiter

Surgery for recurrent goiter has a higher complication rate than in the primary setting [39,71]. Temporary laryngeal nerve palsy was found in 5% and permanent in 3%, both significantly higher than at primary operation [42]. Therefore, the indication is restricted to third-degree goiters or suspicion of malignancy. Preoperatively, laryngoscopy for documentation of the recurrent nerve function is mandatory. Intraoperative recurrent nerve monitoring may be helpful. If preoperative unilateral recurrent nerve paresis is present, if possible, only ipsilateral hemithyroidectomy should be considered. If extensive adhesions are present, it may be helpful to perform an incision on the longitudinal neck muscles [65]. The position of the recurrent nerve may be altered [16]. Rarely, lateral incision on the medial border of the sternocleidoid muscle below the lateral neck lodge is necessary in order to look for the passage of the recurrent nerve through the thoracic opening [65].

References

1. Allo MD, Thompson NW (1983) Rationale for the operative management of substernal goiters. Surgery 94:969–977
2. Belmont MJ, Wax MK, DeSouza FN (1998) The difficult airway: cardiopulmonary bypass—the ultimate solution. Head Neck 20:266–269
3. Bergamaschi R, Becouarn G, Ronceray J, Arnaud JP (1998) Morbidity of thyroid surgery. Am J Surg 176:71–75
4. Bischof P (2004) Update endocrinology: thyroid sonography. Schweiz Rundsch Med Prax 93:695–700
5. Brix TH, Kyvik KO, Hegedus L (1999) Major role of genes in the etiology of simple goiter in females: a population-based twin study. J Clin Endocrinol Metab 84:3071–3075
6. Buhr HJ, Mann B (1999) Thyroidectomy and lymphadenectomy. Chirurg 70:987–998
7. Celani MF (1993) Levothyroxine suppressive therapy in the medical management of nontoxic benign multinodular goiter. Exp Clin Endocrinol 101:326–332
8. Cheung PS, Lee JM, Boey JH (1989) Thyroxine suppressive therapy of benign solitary thyroid nodules: a prospective randomized study. World J Surg 13:818–821
9. Delange F, Bastani S, Benmiloud M, et al (1986) Definitions of endemic goiter and cretinism, classification of goiter size and severity of endemias, and survey techniques. In: Dunn JT, Pretell A, Daza CH, et al (eds) Towards the eradication of endemic goiter, cretinism, and iodine deficiency. Pan American Health Organization, World Health Organization, Washington, pp 373–376
10. Delange F, Burgi H, Chen ZP, et al (2002) World status of monitoring iodine deficiency disorders control programs. Thyroid 12:915–924
11. Delbridge L, Guinea AI, Reeve TS (1999) Total thyroidectomy for bilateral benign multinodular goiter: effect of changing practice. Arch Surg 134:1389–1393
12. Derwahl M, Studer H (1998) Pathogenesis and treatment of multinodular goiter. In: Fagin JA (ed) Thyroid cancer. Kluwer Academic, Boston, pp 155–186
13. Derwahl M, Studer H (2000) Multinodular goiter: much more than simply iodine deficiency. Baillieres Best Pract Res Clin Endocrinol Metabol 14:577–600
14. Derwahl M, Studer H (2001) Nodular goiter and goiter nodules: where iodine deficiency falls short of explaining the facts. Exp Clin Endocrinol Diabetes 109:250–260
15. Derwahl M, Studer H (2002) Hyperplasia versus adenoma in endocrine tissues: are they different? Trends Endocrinol Metab 13:23–28
16. Derwahl KM, Zielke A, Rothmund M (2000) Euthyreote Knotenstruma. In: Siewert JR, Harder F, Rothmund M (eds) Endokrine Chirurgie. Springer, Berlin Heidelberg New York, pp 63–88
17. Dunn JT, Semigran MJ, Delange F (1998) The prevention and management of iodine-induced hyperthyroidism and its cardiac features. Thyroid 8:101–106
18. Farling PA (2000) Thyroid disease. Br J Anaesth 85:15–28
19. Gardiner KR, Russell CF (1995) Thyroidectomy for large multinodular colloid goitre. J R Coll Surg Edinb 40:367–370
20. Gharib H, James EM, Charboneau JW, et al (1987) Suppressive therapy with levothyroxine for solitary thyroid nodules. A double-blind controlled clinical study. N Engl J Med 317:70–75

21. Gibelin H, Sierra M, Mothes D, Ingrand P, Levillain P, Jones C, Hadjadj S, Torremocha F, Marechaud R, Barbier J, Kraimps JL (2004) Risk factors for recurrent nodular goiter after thyroidectomy for benign disease: case-control study of 244 patients. World J Surg 28:1079–1082

22. Gittoes NJ, Miller MR, Daykin J, et al (1996) Upper airways obstruction in 153 consecutive patients presenting with thyroid enlargement. BMJ 312:484

23. Hedinger C, Williams ED, Sobin LH (1988) World Health Organization (ed) International histological classification of tumours. Histological typing of thyroid tumours. Springer, Berlin Heidelberg New York

24. Hedinger C, Williams ED, Sobin LH (1989) The WHO histological classification of thyroid tumors: a commentary on the second edition. Cancer 63:908–911

25. Hegedus L (2001) Thyroid ultrasound. Endocrinol Metab Clin North Am 30:339–360

26. Hung OR, Stewart RD (1996) Illuminating stylet (light wand). In: Benumhof JL (ed) Airway management. Principles and practice. Mosby, St Louis, pp 342–352

27. ICCIDD, UN Children's Fund, and WHO (2001) Assessment of iodine deficiency disorders and monitoring their elimination. http://www.who.int/nutrition/publications/en/idd_assessment_monitoring_elimination.pdf

28. Kann P, Jocham A, Beyer J (1997) Hypothyroidism, hyperthyroidism and therapy with thyroid hormones: effect on the skeletal system. Dtsch Med Wochenschr 122:1392–1397

29. Karkouti K, Rose DK, Wigglesworth D, et al (2000) Predicting difficult intubation: a multivariable analysis. Can J Anaesth 47:730–739

30. Kobberling J, Hintze G (1999) [Differential indications for thyroid gland operation]. Chirurg 70:971–979

31. Koc M, Ersoz HO, Akpinar I, Gogas-Yavuz D, Deyneli O, Akalin S (2002) Effect of low- and high-dose levothyroxine on thyroid nodule volume: a crossover placebo-controlled trial. Clin Endocrinol 57:621–628

32. Lima N, Knobel M, Cavaliere H, et al (1997) Levothyroxine suppressive therapy is partially effective in treating patients with benign, solid thyroid nodules and multinodular goiters. Thyroid 7:691–697

33. Lisboa HR, Gross JL, Orsolin A, et al (1996) Clinical examination is not an accurate method of defining the presence of goitre in schoolchildren. Clin Endocrinol (Oxf) 45:471–475

34. Liu Q, Djuricin G, Prinz RA (1998) Total thyroidectomy for benign thyroid disease. Surgery 123:2–7

35. Manders JMB, Corstens FHM (2002) Radioiodine therapy of euthyroid multinodular goiters. Eur J Nucl Med 29: S466–S470

36. Mann B, Schmale P, Stremmel W (1996) Thyroid morphology and function after surgical treatment of thyroid diseases. Exp Clin Endocrinol Diabetes 104:271–277

37. Marchesi M, Biffoni M, Tartaglia F, et al (1998) Total versus subtotal thyroidectomy in the management of multinodular goiter. Int Surg 83:202–204

38. Martin L, Delbridge L, Martin J, Poole A, Crummer P, Reeve TS (1989) Trainee surgery in teaching hospitals: is there a cost ? Aust N Z J Surg 59:257–260

39. Ménegaux F, Turpin G, Dahman M, Leenhardt L, Chadarevian R, Aurengo A, du Pasquier L, Chigot JP (1999) Secondary thyroidectomy in patients with prior thyroid surgery for benign disease: a study of 203 cases. Surgery 126:479–483

40. Mishra A, Agarwal A, Agarwal G, Mishra SK (2001) Total thyroidectomy for benign thyroid disorders in an endemic region. World J Surg 25:307–310

41. Muller PE, Schmid T, Spelsberg F (1998) Total thyroidectomy in iodine-deficient goiter: an effective treatment alternative? Zentralbl Chir 123:39–41

42. Muller PE, Jakoby R, Heinert G, et al (2001) Surgery for recurrent goitre: its complications and their risk factors. Eur J Surg 167:816–821

43. Netterville JL, Coleman SC, Smith JC, et al (1998) Management of substernal goiter. Laryngoscope 108:1611–1617

44. Papini E, Bacci V, Panunzi C, et al (1993) A prospective randomized trial of levothyroxine suppressive therapy for solitary thyroid nodules. Clin Endocrinol (Oxf) 38:507–513

45. Pappalardo G, Guadalaxara A, Frattaroli FM, Illomei G, Falaschi P (1998) Total compared with subtotal thyroidectomy in benign nodular disease: personal series and review of published reports. Eur J Surg 164:501–506

46. Peters H, Hackel D, Schleusener H (1996) The prevention of the recurrence of endemic goiter. The efficacy of a once-a-week dose of 1.53 mg iodide. Dtsch Med Wochenschr 121:752–756

47. Piraneo S, Vitri P, Galimberti A, Guzzetti S, Salvaggio A, Bastagli A (1994) Recurrence of goitre after operation in euthyroid patients. Eur J Surg 160:351–356

48. Prades JM, Dumollard JM, Timoshenko A, et al (2002) Multinodular goiter: surgical management and histopathological findings. Eur Arch Otorhinolaryngol 259:217–221

49. Rasmussen SN, Hjorth L (1974) Determination of thyroid volume by ultrasonic scanning. J Clin Ultrasound 2:143–147

50. Rios-Zambudio A, Rodriguez J, Riquelme J, Soria T, Canteras M, Parrilla P (2004) Prospective study of postoperative complications after total thyroidectomy for multinodular goiters by surgeons with experience in endocrine surgery. Ann Surg 240:18–25

51. Röher HD (1999) Surgical technique: thyroid gland surgery 1999. Current challenges of problem-oriented thyroid gland surgery. Chirurg 70:969–970

52. Röher HD, Goretzki PE, Hellmann P, et al (1999) Complications in thyroid surgery. Incidence and therapy. Chirurg 70:999–1010

53. Rojdmark J, Jarhult J (1995) High long term recurrence rate after subtotal thyroidectomy for nodular goitre. Eur J Surg 161:725–727

54. Rose DK, Cohen MM (1994) The airway: problems and predictions in 18,500 patients. Can J Anaesth 41:372–383

55. Rowe-Jones JM, Rosswick RP, Leighton SE (1993) Benign thyroid disease and vocal cord palsy. Ann R Coll Surg Engl 75:241–244

56. Sawin CT, Geller A, Wolf PA, et al (1994) Low serum thyrotropin concentrations as a risk factor for atrial fibrillation in older persons. N Engl J Med 331:1249–1252

57. Schoretsanitis G, Melissas J, Sanidas E, et al (1998) Does draining the neck affect morbidity following thyroid surgery? Am Surg 64:778–780

58. Siragusa G, Lanzara P, Di Pace G (1998) [Subtotal thyroidectomy or total thyroidectomy in the treatment of benign thyroid disease. Our experience]. Minerva Chir 53:233–238

59. Sosa JA, Bowman HM, Tielsch JM, Powe NR, Gordon TA, Udelsman R (1998) The importance of surgeon experience for clinical and economic outcomes from thyroidectomy. Ann Surg 228:320–330

60. Spencer CA, Schwarzbein D, Guttler RB, et al (1993) Thyrotropin (TSH)-releasing hormone stimulation test responses employing third and fourth generation TSH assays. J Clin Endocrinol Metab 76:494–498

61. Steinmuller T, Ulrich F, Rayes N, et al (2001) [Surgical procedures and risk factors in therapy of benign multinodular goiter. A statistical comparison of the incidence of complications]. Chirurg 72:1453–1457

62. Stubner D, Gartner R, Greil W, et al (1987) Hypertrophy and hyperplasia during goitre growth and involution in rats: separate bioeffects of TSH and iodine. Acta Endocrinol (Copenh) 116:537–548

63. Studer H, Derwahl M (1995) Mechanisms of nonneoplastic endocrine hyperplasia—a changing concept: a review focused on the thyroid gland. Endocr Rev 16:411–426

64. Thomusch O, Machens A, Sekulla C, Ukkat J, Lippert H, Gastinger I, Dralle H (2000) Multivariate analysis of risk factors for postoperative complications in benign goiter surgery: prospective multicenter study in Germany. World J Surg 24:1335–1341

65. Wagner PK (1999) Surgical techniques for benign goiter. Chirurg 70:980–986

66. Weber AL, Randolph G, Aksoy FG (2000) The thyroid and parathyroid glands. CT and MR imaging and correlation with pathology and clinical findings. Radiol Clin North Am 38:1105–1129

67. Wémeau JL, Caron P, Schvartz C, Schlienger JL, Orgiazzi J, Cousty C, Vlaeminck-Guillem V (2002) Effects of thyroid-stimulating hormone suppression with levothyroxine in reducing the volume of solitary thyroid nodules and improving extranodular nonpalpable changes. J Clin Endocrinol Metab 87:4928–4934

68. Wheeler MH (1999) Clinical dilemma. Retrosternal goitre. Br J Surg 86:1235–1236

69. WHO, UNICEF, and ICCIDD (1993) Indicators for assessing iodine deficiency disorders and their control programmes. http://whqlibdoc.who.int/hq/1993/WHO_NUT_93.1.pdf

70. Wihlborg O, Bergljung L, Martensson H (1988) To drain or not to drain in thyroid surgery. A controlled clinical study. Arch Surg 123:40–41

71. Wilson DB, Staren ED, Prinz RA (1998) Thyroid reoperations: indications and risks. Am Surg 64:674–678

72. Wright CD, Mathisen DJ (2001) Mediastinal tumors: diagnosis and treatment. World J Surg 25:204–209

15 Surgery for Hyperthyroidism

Peter E. Goretzki and Bernhard J. Lammers

CONTENTS

15.1 Definition and Epidemiology

Hyperthyroidism is defined by inappropriate high peripheral serum thyroid hormone levels of free thyroxine (fT4) and free tri-iodothyronine (fT3). Distinct metabolic changes in various nonthyroidal tissues in hyperthyroid patients cause a complex picture of neurological, cardiac, metabolic, and mental disturbances [1–8]. Hyperthyroidism occurs in approximately 0.2% of women and 0.02% of men. The predominant two entities (more than 90%) leading to hyperthyroidism are the immunologic activation of follicular thyroid cells by stimulating antibodies (thyroid-stimulating immunoglobulin, TSI) to the receptor for thyroid-stimulating hormone (TSH-R), known as Graves' disease (GD), and the nonimmunologic hyperthyroidism caused by autonomously functioning thyroid tissue (AFTT). The latter may express different forms: (1) isolated single nodule (autonomous adenoma), (2) multifocal autonomy (multinodular goiter), and (3) disseminated AFTT in diffusely enlarged but also normal-sized thyroid glands. Therefore, the diagnosis of hyperthyroidism requires clarification of the underlying pathophysiological mechanism of the disease. Measurements of serum thyroidal antibodies, ultrasonography, and scintigraphy of the thyroid gland (Fig. 15.1) with thyroidal uptake of radioiodine (RI) or technetium pertechnetate are often necessary in the diagnosis of the disease [1,9,10]. In two investigations, pathologically high TSIs were found in 2.6% of unselected women and 1.1% of men, sometimes even compatible with GD [11,12].

Besides GD and primary functional thyroid autonomy, various other causes for hyperthyroidism exist, including thyroid stimulation by pituitary adenomas that secrete thyroid stimulating hormone (TSH), stimulation of thyroid gland by human chorionic gonadotropin (hCG), produced in pregnancy and or by in rare placental, ovarian, and testicular tumors. In addition, hyperthyroidism has been described in patients with differentiated thyroid cancer and distant metastases, in patients with ovarian thyroid tissues and GD (hCG), in patients under alpha-interferon therapy and with other forms of thyroiditis (Hashimoto's and postpartum thyroiditis, thyroiditis De Quervain, and type 2 hyperthyroidism after amiodarone, which has a high iodine content), [1,2,13–19]. Moreover, some patients taking prescribed thyroid hormones (i.e., after thyroidectomy for thyroid cancer) may become

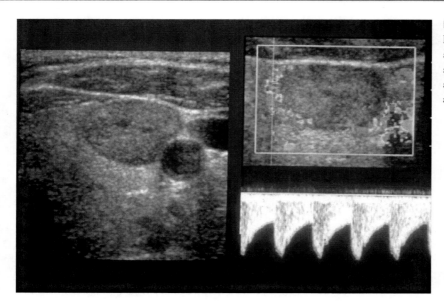

Fig. 15.1 Colour Doppler-enhanced ultrasonography of an autonomous functioning adenoma shows a typical low echogeneity and increased blood supply of an autonomous adenoma

Table 15.1 Different forms of hyperthyroidism. *TSH* Thyroid-stimulating hormone, *fT3* free tri-iodothyronine, *fT4* free thyroxine, *TPO* thyroid peroxidase, *Ab* antibody, *TSI* thyroid-stimulating immunoglobulin, *BSS* blood sedimentation speed, *AFTT* autonomously functioning thyroid tissue, *hCG* human chorionic gonadotropin, *TG* thyroglobulin, *TcTU* technetium thyroid uptake, *US* ultrasound

Hyperthyroidism	Measurement	Symptoms
Subclinical	TSH suppressed fT3,fT4 normal	None
Clinical	TSH suppressed; fT3,fT4 elevated	Neurovegetative, metabolic, cardiac
Diagnosis	Additional measurements	Illness
Immunologic	TSI elevated TPO-Ab; TG-Ab normal/elevated	Graves' disease
	TSI normal; TPO-Ab; TG-Ab elevated	Hashimoto's thyroiditis; postpartum thyroiditis
	TSI; TPO-Ab normal; pain+BSS elevated	Thyroiditis de Quervain
Non-immunologic	TcTU elevated; US-nodular; TSI negative	AFTT
	TSH elevated; hCG elevated	TSH-oma; paraneoplastic hormonal stimulation (hCG)
	TG negative	Hyperthyroidism factitia (T3/T4) ingestion medication/ or other reasons

hyperthyroid. Finally, some patients take thyroid hormones for intended weight loss or because of psychological problems (e.g., Münchhausen's syndrome; Table 15.1).

The often-addressed iodine intake as reason for an acute hyperthyroidism only dismantles an underlying thyroid disease, leading to hyperthyroidism. In normally functioning thyroid tissue an iodine intake would induce hypothyroidism rather hyperthyroidism. This can be explained by the Wolff-Chaikoff effect (enzyme suppression by substrate overload). Iodine intake may cause hyperthyroidism only in patients with AFTT or with GD [12].

Hyperthyroid children, adults, and elderly patients present with a different clinical picture, even though neurovegetative, cardiac, and metabolic symptoms increase parallel to the increase in serum thyroid hormone levels. In the vast majority of all patients (70–95%), tachycardia, goiter, and weight loss can be found, independent of age (Fig. 15.2) [20–25].

Besides tachycardia, growing goiter, and weight loss, hyperthyroid children often present with school problems, anxiety, nervousness, and enuresis nocturna. Older people are often oligosymptomatic and may present with cardiac (atrial) arrhythmia, weight loss, and diarrhea. Infiltrative dermopathy (localized

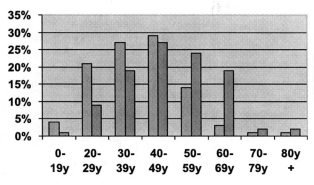

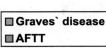

Fig. 15.2 Age distribution of Graves' disease (GD) and autonomously functioning thyroid tissue (*AFTT*) patients undergoing surgery between 1992 and 1999 in the University Hospital, Duesseldorf, Germany

Table 15.2 Symptoms in different age groups in a low-iodine area

	Children (<14 years)	Adults	Older patients (>65 years)
Symptoms	85/15%	45/55%	10/90%
Main Symptoms (as a percentage of all patients proven)			
Tachycardia	90%	95%	70%
Growing goiter	95%	70%	50%
Weight loss	90%	75%	75%
Other Symptoms			
Fatigue, tiredness			
Tremor	30–80%	60–70%	50–70%
Muscle weakness			
Anxiety, sleeping problem			
Diarrhea	20%	20%	20%
Age-specific symptoms			
Atrial fibrillation	–	10%	40%
Enuresis nocturna	65%	–	–
School problems	90%	–	–

myxedema) is the least common manifestation of GD (Fig. 15.3). It occurs in at most 5% of patients with GD, most of whom are older and nearly all of who have had both hyperthyroidism and ophthalmopathy (Table 15.2).

The prevalence, clinical picture, and probability of hyperthyroidism in patients with GD and with AFTT, respectively are summarized in Table 15.3.

15.2 Biochemical and Morphological Investigation in Hyperthyroid Patients

In addition to serum TSH, fT3, and fT4 levels, measurement of thyroid-specific serum antibodies is important in patients with hyperthyroidism and questionable immunologic thyroid stimulation. Thus, highly sensitive stimulating TSH-receptor antibodies (TRAK; TSI) differentiate GD from disseminated primary thyroid autonomy. In patients with Hashimoto's thyroiditis and postpartum thyroiditis, antibodies against thyroid peroxidase (TPO) are predominantly elevated, but not stimulating TSH-receptor antibodies. Antibodies against thyroglobulin can be detected in almost all patients with immunologic thyroid diseases. Antibody patterns are usually specific for different immunologic thyroid diseases, but there may be some overlap. Thus, patients with GD, Hashimoto's thyroiditis, and postpartum thyroiditis may present with some similar features and findings (e.g., hypothyroidism in long-term follow up; Table 15.4) [10,20,26–28].

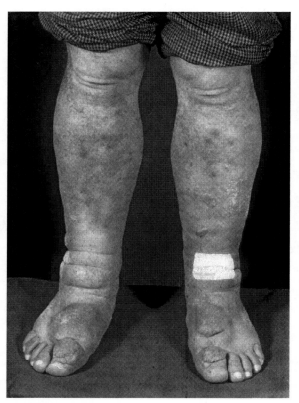

Fig. 15.3 Infiltrative dermopathy in a patient with GD showing bilateral involvement of the lower legs and feet with multiple localized livid efflorescenses of orange-peel appearance

15.3   Pathophysiology-Directed Treatment of Hyperthyroidism

The distinct pathophysiological differences between GD and AFTT have therapeutic implications. In AFTT patients, TSH-R and Gs mutations consistently cause an overactive thyroid tissue, rendering patients hyperthyroid. Thyreocytes with these mutations are refractory to antithyroid drug (ATD) therapy. Therefore, effective treatment requires excision or radioactive ablation of the AFTT [6,7]. The inappropriate antibody production stimulating the thyroid gland in patients with GD may decrease over time. While antithyroid drugs in AFTT patients are only used to render them euthyroid in preparation for a definitive therapy, antithyroid drugs in GD patients may lead to a continuous euthyroid state, even after discontinuance of the therapy (up to 50% of all GD patients) [4,23–25,29,30].

Antithyroid drug treatment is the first-line treatment of choice in GD patients (Table 15.5). In the USA, most endocrinologists favor early RI treatment [20]. Ablative thyroid therapy is usually reserved as primary treatment for patients with questionable malignancy, large goiters, and if patients desire a fast treatment effect. Ablative therapies (i.e., RI or surgery) are indicated as second-line options for patients with recurrent hyperthyroidism, allergic reactions

Table 15.3   Graves' disease (*GD*) versus AFTT. *TSH-R* Receptor for TSH, *Stim.* stimulated

Factors	GD*	AFTT
Local distribution		
Prevalence and	Small difference	High in iodine depleted areas
Iodine intake	Iodine rich–iodine depleted	Low in iodine-rich areas
Age and sex distribution		
Men/women	1–2/10	2–3/10
Age	Maximum 20–40 years	Increases with age
Diagnosis		
Goiter	Diffuse/nodular 9/1	Diffuse/nodular 1/9
Endocrine orbitopathy	up to 80%	No
Stim. TSH-R Ab (TSI)*	95%	2–5%
Diagnosis after iodine load	approximately 35%	approximately 85%
Probability of hyperthyroidism		
Hyperthyroidism	High TSI titers	AFTT mass and iodine intake dependent
Critical mass	2–4 ml thyroid tissue	10–13 ml AFTT in low iodine area
		5–10 ml AFTT in iodine rich area
Critical TcTU	Unpredictable	2.5–5% (under suppressed TSH!)

*New sensitive assays with TSH-R in Chinese hamster ovary cells

Table 15.4 Biochemical definition and clinical symptoms of hyperthyroidism. *sTSH* Serum TSH

Biochemical diagnosis of hyperthyroidism	
Subclinical	sTSH < 0.4 mIU/l; fT3 + fT4 normal
Clinical	sTSH < 0.4 mIU/l; fT3 and/or fT4 elevated

Clinical signs of hyperthyroidism	
Former preclinical	No typical signs
Clinical	Neurovegetative hyperactivity:
	nervousness, anxiety, tremor, hyperreflexia, psychic instability, sleep loss, restlessness
	Metabolic hyperactivity:
	sweating, heat intolerance, tachycardia, early exhaustion, increased oxygen consumption, osteoporosis
	Cardiac hyperactivity:
	cardiac-atrial arrhythmia, soft and frequent peripheral pulse, low diastolic pressure, increased cardiac output

to antithyroid drugs, and with high probability of permanent or recurrent hyperthyroidism. Increased risks for hyperthyroid recurrences have been shown for young individuals, patients with large goiters, with recurrent GD, with persistently high TSIs after reaching euthyroidism by antithyroid drug treatment, and for smokers (Table 15.6) [4,19,29,23]. The incidence of hyperthyroid recurrence is up to 60–80% in these patients and this supports an early ablative treatment. Furthermore, ablative therapy is indicated in patients with nodular goiter and GD (i.e., Marine-Lenhart syndrome) [29]. The coexistence of GD with strongly positive antithyroid antibodies with multifocal autonomous nodules that often develop after adequate treatment of GD is a phenomenon associated with Marine-Lenhart syndrome.

15.4 Therapy Indications for Patients with Different Severities of Hyperthyroidism

Primarily, the diagnosis of hyperthyroidism is based on biochemical findings, with a decreased serum TSH level (0.4 mU/l) and high normal or elevated

Table 15.5 Primary (first- and second-line, *1* and *2*, respectively) treatment options for patients with GD and AFTT. *RI* Radioactive iodine, *ATD* antithyroid drug, *Surg* surgery

Factors affecting primary treatment	GD		AFTT	
	1	2	1	2
Goiter size				
(25–50 ml)	ATD	RI	RI	Surg
(above 55 ml)	Surg	RI	Surg	RI
Multinodular goiter	Surg	RI	Surg	RI
Questionable malignancy	Surg		Surg	
Children (<14 years of age)	ATD	Surg	Surg	
Pregnancy	ATD	(Surg)	ATD	(Surg)
Smokers	RI/Surg	ATD	RI/Surg	Surg/RI
Iodine-induced thyrotoxicosis	ATD	Surg	Surg	ATD
Elderly patients in poor general condition	Extremely rare	Extremely rare	RI	ATD

Table 15.6 Typical findings in immunologic-induced hyperthyroidism. *Inhib* Inhibition, *CRP* C-reactive protein

Thyroiditis type	Specific clinical picture	TSI	Inhib TSH-R Ab	TPO-Ab	TG-Ab
Graves' disease	Orbitopathy	High	Negative – low	Enlarged	Enlarged
Hashimoto's		Negative	High	High	High
Postpartum		Negative	High	High	High
De Quervain's	Pain, CRP elevation	Negative	Negative – low	Enlarged	Enlarged

serum levels of fT3 and fT4. "Subclinical hyperthyroidism" describes the scenario in which serum TSH is decreased while fT3 and fT4 are normal and the patient is asymptomatic. Long-term studies have shown that 3–10% of patients with subclinical hyperthyroidism will develop clinical signs of hyperthyroidism over time, such as osteoporosis and atrial fibrillation (three times greater risk compared with euthyreotic patients). These patients may even die prematurely from acute heart failure. Therefore, patients with subclinical hyperthyroidism should be treated effectively [21,26,27,31–36].

Treatment is unquestionably necessary in all patients with biochemically proven hyperthyroidism and/or symptoms of hyperthyroidism. Patients experiencing hyperthyroidism symptoms are referred to having an overt hyperthyroidism, clinical hyperthyroidism, or thyrotoxicosis (these terms are used synonymously). A gradual parallel increase in symptoms and pathologic laboratory tests will lead to the stage of severe thyrotoxicosis.

A culmination of hyperthyroid symptoms is referred to as thyrotoxic crisis, a definition that is based primarily on clinical symptoms. The severity of thyrotoxic crisis is subdivided into three stages. Patients with life-threatening tachycardia, arrhythmia, hyperthermia, dehydration, tremor, and nervousness are defined as suffering from stage 1 thyrotoxic crisis. Further mental deterioration with stupor, somnolence, signs of disorientation, and psychotic symptoms describe stage 2 thyrotoxic crisis, which may lead finally to coma. The latter situation is defined as severity stage 3 thyrotoxic crisis. The percentage of fatal outcomes in patients with thyrotoxic crisis is considerable (30–50%). Death due to thyrotoxic crisis parallels the grade of mental deterioration, which is hence used to define the different stages (Table 15.7) [37–45].

15.5 Treatment Options in Hyperthyroidism: History, Advantages, and Disadvantages

15.5.1 History

In 1914, E. Waller from Birmingham, controlled hyperthyroidism with high-dose iodine tinctura. This was confirmed by Plummer and Boothby in 1923 in 600 patients [46]. High doses of iodine, given orally (Plummer's solution) or by intravenous administration, reduces thyroid enzyme activity by substrate in-

Table 15.7 Clinical classification and severity of hyperthyroidism

Preclinical hyperthyroidism	Biochemical proof of hyperthyroidism without clinical signs
Overt hyperthyroidism	Biochemical proof and clinical signs of hyperthyroidism
Thyrotoxic crisis	Life threatening: tachycardia, arrhythmia, hyperthermia, dehydration, tremor, nervousness
Stage one	Nervousness, anxiety
Stage two	Stupor, somnolence, disorientation, psychotic symptoms
Stage three	Coma

hibition (the Wolff-Chaikoff effect) and may lead to euthyroidism for 10–14 days. This effect is time limited, however, and hyperthyroidism may recur. During this time period, perfusion velocity of the thyroid vessels is reduced. The metabolic and local effects of iodine have been adopted in preparing patients for thyroid surgery, especially in times when only surgery was available for the treatment of hyperthyroidism and neither antithyroid drugs nor RI treatment were established. Nowadays, the time limitation of high-dose iodine treatment is feared, especially in non-compliant patients, and antithyroid drug treatment is thus the predominantly used procedure for preparing patients for thyroid surgery or RI treatment [2–6,44].

15.5.2 Antithyroid Drugs

Treatment with thionamides was started in 1943 by E. Astwood from Boston, USA. The two clinically used compounds are propylthiouracil (6-propyl-2-thiouracil) and methimazole (1-methyl-2-mercaptoimidazole), which inhibit the iodination of tyrosine by inhibiting TPO. In addition, propylthiouracil partially blocks the conversion of T4 to T3 in peripheral tissues. Both drugs are used to normalize thyroid function in severely hyperthyroid patients before a definite treatment (e.g., RI or surgical treatment; Table 15.8) [4,20,30]. In older patients with severe comorbidity (e.g., cardiovascular disease) a medication for unlimited time can be applied. In hyperthyroid pregnant women, propylthiouracil is preferred over methimazole, since it only minimally crosses the placenta boundary [45,47,48]. In these patients a high-dose antithyroid drug medication with addition of thyroxin is contraindicated, since all antithyroid

Table 15.8 ATD treatment and preparation of patients for surgery or RI therapy

High-dose iodine (Lugol's solution)		
3 × 30 drops per day for up to 14 days		
ATD therapy		
Compound	Starting daily dosage (mg)	Long-term daily dosage (mg)
Thiamazole	10–30	2.5–10
Methimazole	15–30	5–15
Propylthiouracil	150–300	50–200
Preventing hyperthyroidism before iodine contamination		
Potassium perchlorate	3 × 30 drops per day for up to 1 week	
Methimazole	15–30 mg per day for up to 3 weeks	

drugs do cross the placental boundary more easily than thyroid hormones and thus would render the fetus hypothyroid, even if the mother is euthyroid [47].

ATDs have a variety of side effects, such as skin rash (4–6%), arthralgias (1–5%), nausea (1–5%) and polyarthritis (1–2%). Severe allergic reactions such as agranulocytosis, immunohepatitis, and pancreatitis occur in only 0.1–0.2% of cases, but may be life threatening. These side effects show some dose dependency and occur mainly in the first months of treatment. Therefore, low-dose ATD treatment has been accepted as the treatment of choice and seems to be superior to high-dose ATD treatment with addition of thyroxin (combination therapy) [4,49]. Long-term treatment with ATDs has the disadvantage of increased thyroid growth in most patients, due to elevated serum TSH levels. For preoperative preparation of hyperthyroid patients using ATDs, serum TSH levels should be rendered normal. Elevated serum TSH levels induce increased thyroid perfusion and tissue softness, which makes the operation more difficult.

Patients with severe thyrotoxicosis or thyrotoxic crisis need a fast clinical relief from their symptoms and therefore a high-dose ATD treatment. The triple combination therapy of potassium perchlorate with methimazole or propylthiouracil, and lithium is useful. This also makes sense from a biochemical point of view, since potassium perchlorate inhibits iodine uptake into thyroid cells, ATDs reduce the iodination of thyroglobulin by inhibition of TPO, and lithium prevents the excretion of already produced thyroid hormones [40,50,51]. In addition, glucocorticoids inhibit the conversion of T4 to T3. The other supplementary measures for thyrotoxic patients are beta-adrenergic blocking agents, tranquilizers, and chemical and physical temperature reduction. They only relieve symptoms, and have no effect on thyroid activity.

15.5.3 RI Treatment

RI therapy was introduced by S. Hertz and A. Roberts in Boston, 1942, and has now reached worldwide acceptance for the treatment of thyroid cancer and hyperthyroidism. Patients have to be euthyroid prior to RI treatment as it has been described for surgery, since RI uptake into the thyroid gland could aggravate hyperthyroidism before thyreocytes could be destroyed. Some centers estimate the needed dosages prior to the effective I^{131} treatment, whereas others primarily give a large therapeutic I^{131} dose (200–300 Gy). In both cases a comparable primary success rate of 80–95% for GD patients and 60–80% for AFTT patients, after 6 months, have been described [11,12]. Patients with AFTT and a large goiter may require higher doses of ^{131}I of up to 600 Gy. RI in patients with thyroid autonomy (AFTT) is always administered for TSH suppression, which leads to specific I^{131} enrichment exclusively in AFTT, resulting in a high percentage of posttherapeutic euthyroid patients [11,12]. With regard to cost effectiveness, RI treatment has been proved advantageous compared with ATD treatment and surgery in patients younger than 50 years of age and with goiters of less than 50 ml total volume. Therefore, RI treatment is the accepted primary treatment for these patients [1].

The disadvantage of RI therapy is related to its time lag to effectiveness in comparison to thyroid surgery. While thyroid surgery leaves patients directly euthyroid or hypothyroid after the operation, it takes approximately 4 months for RI. Moreover, some patients will become increasingly hypothyroid during the years following RI treatment and continuous laboratory and clinical controls are necessary. RI is contraindicated in pregnancy and is not used in patients below 14 years of age in most European countries. In the USA, even children are treated with RI, which may be without harm. Nevertheless, sufficient data to prove the security of RI in children are still lacking [52].

15.5.4 Surgery

Surgical treatment is the oldest treatment modality for hyperthyroidism and was first evaluated by Rehn,

Kocher, Halsted, and Mayo in the late 19th century. The operative mortality rate was 3–5% and dropped to approximately 1% after Plummer introduced preoperative therapy with Lugol's solution [53]. Surgery directly relieves hyperthyroidism by resection of AFTT or most of the thyroid gland in the case of GD patients. The extent of resection remains a matter of debate. Nowadays, most authors regard total thyroidectomy being superior to less radical resections in the treatment of GD [54–61], while selective surgery is preferred by others, especially in patients with localized or circumscribed AFTTs [7,8]. For these patients postoperative euthyroidism may be reached, comparable to the results of RI treatment.

The disadvantages of thyroid surgery include intraoperative and postoperative hemorrhage, temporary or permanent recurrent laryngeal nerve paralysis, temporary or permanent hypocalcemia in connection to postoperative hypoparathyroidism, and a very low (below 1/1000) perioperative mortality rate (see also section 15.6.4).

15.6   Surgical Therapy

Since thyroid surgery in low-iodine areas is a frequently performed operation, most general surgeons treat patients with thyroid diseases. This surely includes patients with autonomously functioning multinodular goiter and patients with single autonomously functioning thyroid adenomas, but should be questioned for patients with an increased risk of local and general complications. Thus, patients with GD and with disseminated thyroid autonomy require total or near-total thyroidectomy, which has an increased complication rate in nonspecified surgical units, when compared to less radical thyroid resec-

tions [50,62–66]. We therefore advocate the referral of these specifically challenging thyroid patients to specialized endocrine surgeons.

15.6.1   Preoperative Treatment

Severely hyperthyroid patients with clinically evident preoperative hyperthyroidism are routinely treated medically (ATDs and/or Lugol's solution) to reach a stable peripheral euthyroid metabolism. In most cases ATDs (i.e., methimazole, thiamazole, or propylthiouracil) are chosen in defined dosages until euthyroidism has been achieved, and then medication is reduced to keep the euthyroid metabolic state (normal serum levels of fT3/fT4 and TSH) for at least 4–6 weeks. High-dose iodine can be administered as per-oral Lugol's solution or intravenously as potassium iodine solution preoperatively. In patients suffering from severe nervousness and tachycardia, tranquilizers and beta-adrenergic blocking agents can be administered. Propranolol was proven to mitigate the symptoms of hyperthyroidism but does not change hormone production or secretion in the given dosages [7,40]. Some US American endocrinologists advocate iopanoic acid as an alternative therapeutic agent [44,47,67].

The maintenance of a euthyroid metabolism for a certain preoperative time period (3–6 weeks) is reasonable, since the accelerated bone turnover due to hyperthyroidism persists for some time. This may result in early postoperative hypocalcemia, the major current postoperative problem in patients with GD (Table 15.9) [51,66,68,69]. Some authors, however, still prefer fast preoperative treatment of GD patients with Lugol's solution, which has been proven to reduce the blood perfusion of thyroid gland (decreased

Table 15.9 Early postoperative hypocalcemia after surgery for benign thyroid diseases. *sTX* Subtotal thyroidectomy, *TX* complete thyroidectomy, *Ca* calcium, *postop* postoperative

Serum Ca levels after thyroid operation (sTX/TX)							
Patients with GD (n = 21)				Patients with nodular goiter (n = 41)			
Time postop (h)	serum Ca mean ± sd (mmol/l)	Hypocalcemia < 2.0 mmol/l/total n/N	(%)	Time postop (h)	Serum Ca mean ± sd (mmol/l)	Hypocalcemia < 2.0 mmol/l/ total n/N	(%)
0	2.44 ± 0.20	0 / 21	0	0	2.42 ± 0.1	0 / 41	0
6	2.26 ± 0.22	1 / 21	5	6	2.27 ± 0.10	0 / 41	0
24	2.17 ± 0.23	7 / 21	33	24	2.20 ± 0.11	1 / 41	2
48	2.13 ± 0.28	4 / 21	24	48	2.20 ± 0.16	9 / 41	7
Total 7/21 (33%)				Total 4/41 (19%)			

vascular velocity) making thyroid surgery perhaps more easy and may decrease intraoperative blood loss [62].

In our experience, however, a clear operative strategy and technically meticulous thyroid resection are more important than specific preoperative therapeutic regimens.

15.6.2 Special Technique and Operative Strategy

As a prerequisite of thyroid surgery we recommend the routine use of surgical loupes (enlarging the operative field 2.4–4.8 times) or of an endoscopic camera (enlarging the visual field approximately 20 times). For dissection we use pediatric surgical instruments (Halsted clamps). Although neuromonitoring of the recurrent laryngeal nerve (RLN) is not generally accepted as standard of care, we routinely use this intraoperative method with the exception of single nodules that are anteriorly located [69].

After a small Kocher's incision (3–5 cm) the midline of strap muscles is divided longitudinally and the thyroid capsule is totally freed. In the case of GD, this procedure requires precise (bipolar) coagulation of small vessels, while it can be performed by blunt dissection in patients with normal multinodular goiters with and without autonomy. After pushing the muscle aside, the middle thyroid vein (Kocher's vein) is dissected. Soft and well-perfused thyroid tissue in GD with additionally enlarged lymphatic vessels and lymph nodes around the thyroid gland make this operation different and technically more demanding than a "routine" thyroid operation.

In a second step, the almost avascular area between the laryngeal muscles and the medial lower part of the upper pole is cleared. It is important to preserve a low-running upper laryngeal nerve. Then the upper pole can be dissected in separate steps until the upper parathyroid gland is visualized. Next, the trachea below the isthmus is freed and the search starts for the RLN lateral to and below the lower thyroid pole. On the left side the RLN most frequently lies close to the trachea, whereas it can often be found under the middle part of the lower pole on the right side. After the RLN is visualized (if intraoperative monitoring is applied), dissection of the nerve leads to ligation of small branches of the inferior thyroid artery up to the ligament of Berry.

In the case of a large goiter, the vascular supply of the lower parathyroid glands, lying anterior to the RLN may be harmed. It may thus be advantageous to excise them, cut them into small pieces of less than 1 mm^3, and transplant them into the sternocleidomastoid muscle rather than hoping for questionable perfusion recovery.

After this extensive dissection, the thyroid is only fixed to the trachea, but still has a sufficient blood supply. In the case of partial resection, ligature stitches surrounding the preserved tissue (in former times vascular clamps) are applied or the tissue is dissected with a dissection-free vessel-sealing device (LigaSure, Ultracision). In both cases we then close the dissection area with a running atraumatic resorbable suture (for example 3.0 Vicryl). In the case of total lobectomy the lower lateral thyroid is freed and often only one crossing central vein and artery (just below the ligament of Berry) has to be closed using an atraumatic, monofil suture (for example 5.0 Prolene or 4.0 PDS). This prevents unnecessary hemorrhage and attempts to cauterize near the RLN, which may be harmful even when using bipolar cauters.

Using this technical procedure we never need to dissect and ligate thyroid arteries centrally. This carries the risk of damaging the upper laryngeal nerve by ligating the superior thyroid artery or damaging the lower parathyroid gland supply by tying the inferior thyroid artery at de Quervain's point. The latter procedure has been described to endanger even the sympathetic nerve in some rare cases, which definitely can be prevented.

15.6.3 Operative Radicality with Specific Problems in Surgery for GD

When defining the necessary radicality of surgery to treat GD the potential persistent and recurrent hyperthyroidism has to be weighted against potential surgical complications and the ability to reach long-term euthyroidism by less radical procedures. A remnant volume of more than 4 ml definitely increases the risk of persistent or recurrent hyperthyroidism above 5% and should be prevented. Smaller remnants will, however, lead to persistent hypothyroidism and the need for thyroxine substitution in over 80% of patients [7]. In the treatment of patients with GD, less radical procedures are therefore dismissed and a near total or total thyroidectomy is advocated by most authors.

Whether total thyroidectomy has a more pronounced positive effect on antibody reduction and on Graves' ophthalmopathy compared to subtotal resection has not been proven so far [55–58,62–66,70–72]. Since more radical surgery increases the risk of RLN paralysis and postoperative hypoparathyroidism in nonspecialized general surgery but not in specialized centers, it can be assumed that the outcome difference is due to the case load and the experience of the surgeon [69].

15.6.4   Postoperative Complications

The frequency of postoperative bleeding of 0.5–2% is not different between high- and low-volume series, which draws our attention particularly to the procedure of dissecting the RLNs and the parathyroid glands (see 15.6.2). Magnifying glasses, careful dissection in a bloodless field, and early autotransplantation of all devitalized parathyroid tissue into the muscle pockets of the neck should be used routinely. Under these conditions, radical thyroid surgery increases only the incidence of early postoperative hypocalcemia and has no effect on the frequency of either RLN paralysis or permanent hypoparathyroidism [7,30,58,66].

Since nonspecialized general surgeons experience more complications after total thyroidectomy than do endocrine surgeons, we advocate that only the latter should perform surgery for GD [55,65,69]. We have investigated the occurrence of early postoperative hypocalcemia and hyperreflexia (potential hypoparathyroidism) and showed that the tendency of GD patients to experience hyperreflexia and paresthesia increases (21–44% and 7–38 % of cases, respectively), findings that are exacerbated by thyroidectomy. This may be due to parathyroid gland injury, persistent hyperthyroid symptoms even after reaching an euthyrotic

state, and an increased bone turnover (elevated serum osteocalcin), and results in symptoms in 20–35% of all patients. We therefore advocate supplementation with calcium and vitamin D for 1–2 weeks in these patients [54,60,61,69,73].

The frequency of postoperative RLN paralysis for GD is higher than after surgery for other benign thyroid diseases and should be prevented in the future using the aforementioned equipment and techniques (Table 15.10) [50,55,57,64–65,74].

15.7   Endocrine Orbitopathy in the Postoperative Course

Endocrine orbitopathy (EO) occurs in up to 80% of all patients with GD and may be the most important associated clinical finding (Fig. 15.4). EO is of minor prevalence and severity in children compared to

Table 15.10 Recurrent laryngeal nerve paralysis (*RLNP*) after thyroidectomy in GD

Procedure	Patients (*n*)	Early postop RLNP	Permanent RLNP
Lobectomy	317	9.5%	1.4%
Subtotal resection	633	4.4%	1.0%
Near-total/total	295	3.4%	0.7%

Results from non specialized general surgeons* and in HHU-D 1986–1999

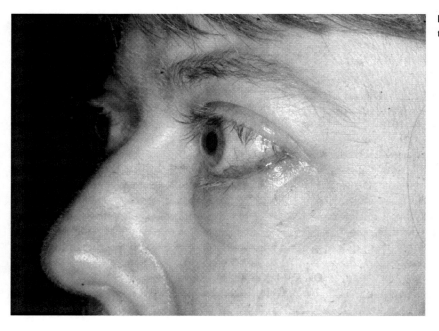

Fig. 15.4 Clinical picture of exophthalmos in a patient with GD

adults with GD. The acute inflammatory symptoms of EO, such as redness, tearing of the eyes, and local pain, should be distinguished from the bulbous protrusion of the eyes and possible optic nerve compression. In addition to bilateral protrusion of the eyes, single eye protrusion has been observed in GD patients. In this situation, tumor growth must be excluded by computed tomography (Fig. 15.5) or magnetic resonance imaging. Within the 1st year of clinically proven EO, surgery improves the condition in approximately two-thirds of cases and less than 5–10% of patients demonstrate a worsening. However, the morphologic changes resulting in increased orbital tissue mass is not resolved by thyroid surgery [30,39,75–80]. Severe local symptoms and optical compression warrant local and systemic antiinflammatory therapy with glucocorticoids and somatostatin receptor antagonists as well as local radiation therapy (20 Gy). Some patients need surgical decompression of the orbita in order to save their vision.

In contrast to the beneficial effects of thyroid surgery (Fig. 15.6), RI rather worsens concomitant EO. This can be prevented, however, by administering glucocorticoids during RI therapy. In surgical patients only perioperative glucocorticoids are used (1 mg prednisolone equivalent/kg body weight/day for 1 week) in patients with a severe and acute orbital inflammation.

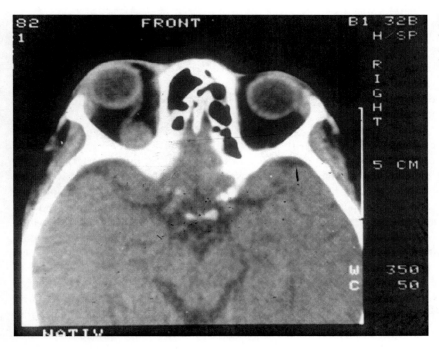

Fig. 15.5 Computed tomography of a patient with GD depicting an asymmetric increase of the retrobulbar soft tissue

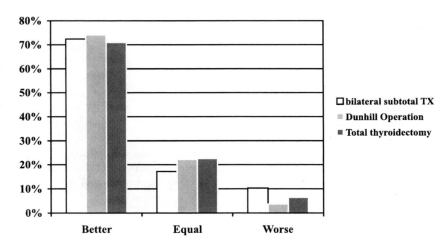

Fig. 15.6 Incidences of endocrine orbitopathy after different resection types; results 6 months postoperatively, after Witte et al. [30]. *TX* Thyroidectomy

□ bilateral subtotal TX
▨ Dunhill Operation
■ Total thyroidectomy

The question arises as to whether total thyroidectomy improves EO more than subtotal thyroid resections. In our experience the effect on antithyroid antibodies and EO is not different in patients with almost no remnant and remnants of up to 4 ml [30]. This is in contrast to results from other authors who reported differences in postoperative antibody titers 6 months after thyroid surgery, depending on the degree of radicality [34,37,48,81]. Further randomized trials are needed to demonstrate whether total thyroidectomy is the treatment of choice in all GD patients with significant EO.

15.8   Operative Radicality and Specific Problems Associated with Surgery for AFTT

In contrast to surgery for GD, therapy in patients with AFTT allows one to resect only the pathologic nodular tissue and to leave normal thyroid tissue behind. Whether this is useful and beneficial for the patient was debated by Kocher and von Miculicz in the late 19th century; the debate is still ongoing.

Following the principle of resecting only pathological thyroid tissue, 46% of patients had normal postoperative thyroid function, 23% of patients had increased serum TSH (above 2.5 mIU/l) but normal fT3 and fT4, and 13% of patients had hypothyroidism after surgery [6,8]. In 5% of all patients, persistent nodules could be demonstrated after less than near total thyroid resection. Long-term investigations will show whether the outcome is less favorable due to unnecessary hypothyroidism (63% versus 13%) or due to preventable goiter recurrence and the need to repeat operations.

15.9   Minimally Invasive Thyroid Surgery for Autonomous Adenomas and for Small Goiters in GD

Minimally invasive thyroid surgery has been introduced by Asian surgeons and by an Italian group. Under the prerequisites of circumscript pathologies and total thyroid volumes of less than 30 ml, minimally invasive techniques have proved to be as safe and useful as conventional thyroid procedures. The difference lies mainly in the skin incision, which can be reduced by using video-assisted devices from 3–4 cm in normal thyroid surgery to 1.5–2 cm. Some patients seem to have less pain, which can also be prevented in open surgery, when overextension of the neck is avoided and perioperative pain medications are commenced prior to surgery [73,74,82–86]. While minimally invasive surgery has revolutionized adrenal and parathyroid surgery, it is of limited importance in thyroid surgery, especially in patients with hyperthyroidism.

Another minimally invasive ablative therapy for solitary autonomous adenomas is the injection of 98% ethanol. This can be used only in selected patients on an outpatient basis [37,38]. Outpatient management of patients is not indicated for thyroid surgery, since even a small volume of postoperative bleeding may lead to dramatic consequences as a result of reactive laryngeal swelling and airway obstruction [8,66].

15.10   Special Aspects

15.10.1   Thyrotoxicosis

The majority of patients with acute thyrotoxicosis and thyrotoxic crisis have proven AFTT, which is activated by a significant iodine load. In the past, radiological contrast dye has been the most important source for this iodine load. In recent years, however, amiodarone therapy has been shown to initiate the thyrotoxicosis with increasing frequency. While iodine originating from amiodarone increases thyroid hormone production, in some of these patients (e.g., those with type 1 disease), it may also induce thyrocyte destruction with acute thyroid hormone efflux. The latter situation can be treated with glucocorticoids; the former requires ATD medication and sometimes even an early thyroidectomy.

Thus, the combination therapy of potassium chlorate (to prevent further iodine intake into thyrocytes), ATDs (methimazole or propylthiouracil to prevent iodination by TPO inhibition), and lithium (to inhibit thyroid hormone excretion) represents the first-line treatment together with symptomatic therapy in comatose patients (e.g., antipyretic drugs, antibiotics, glucocorticoids, oxygen, sufficient fluid substitution, high caloric parenteral/enteral nutrition, beta-adrenergic blocking drugs, antiarrhythmia therapy, and sedatives). Thyroidectomy is indicated if conservative therapy fails or hyperdynamic heart insufficiency emerges. Under these circumstances the expected mortality rate of 30–50% can be reduced to 10–20% (Table 15.11).

Table 15.11 Surgically treated patients with iodine-induced thyrotoxicosis and thyrotoxic crisis

Author	Year	N total	N iodine	Crisis stage 3	Death
Köbberling	1985	16	16	3	1
Dralle	1985	8	8	2	0
Frilling	1990	5	4	5	0
Hintze	1992	40	40	7	4
Houghton	2004	34	34	8	3
LukasNeuss	2005	14	10	11	3
Total		117	112	36	11

Table 15.12 Prevalence of thyroid malignancy in GD and in goiters with AFTT. *TC* Thyroid cancer

Author	Year	GD			AFTT		
		Total (N)	With TC (n)	(%)	Total (N)	With TC (n)	(%)
Wahl	1982	176	2	(1.1%)	534	16	(3.1%)
Haid	1989	183	2	(1.1%)	567	12	(2.1%)
Belfiore	1990	132	13	(9.8%)	227	9	(8.0%)
Zanella	1998	38	2	(5.3%))	164	10	(6.1%)
Kraimps	2000	557	21	(3.8%)	–	–	
Goretzki	2001	150	1	(0.7%)	127	5	(3.9%)
Gabriele	2003	64	0	(–)	361	7	(1.7%)
Total		1300	39	(3.0)	1980	59	(3.0%)

15.10.2 Postoperative Diagnosis of Thyroid Cancer

Postoperative histology reveals an unexpected differentiated thyroid cancer in 1–10% and 2–8% of patients with GD and hyperthyroid multinodular goiter, respectively (Table 15.12) [76–80,87,88]. The prognosis of these cancers is not different from that in patients with euthyroid goiters. Small-sized, differentiated thyroid cancers of papillary or follicular origin under 1 cm require no further treatment than suppressive thyroxine therapy, whereas larger tumors indicate the need of complete total thyroidectomy and RI treatment.

15.11 Postoperative Management

Postoperative treatment of patients with thyrotoxicosis includes therapy for potential postoperative hypoparathyroidism using calcium and vitamin D substitution, and for RLN paralysis with logopedic treatment. Depending on the size of the remnant thyroid tissue, hormone substitution (remnants of less than 9–6 ml) or iodine supplementation (larger remnants in low-iodine areas) may be required [6,7,88]. In patients with GD, postoperative hypothyroidism should be prevented to minimize the risk of endocrine orbitopathy deterioration, which seems to parallel the increase in serum TSH levels [21,34,89].

Weight gain after surgery for hyperthyroidism represents a problem for some patients. It is related to the changed body metabolism, often due to inadequate thyroxine substitution, and is related to central and peripheral changes in leptin levels [73,90,91]. Postoperative weight gain can be best prevented through a close follow up within the first 2 years.

References

1. Paschke R, Ludgate M (1997) The thyrotropin receptor in thyroid diseases. N Engl J Med 337:1675–1681
2. Krohn K, Paschke R (2001) Clinical review 133. Progress in understanding the etiology of thyroid autonomy. J Clin Endocrinol Metab 86:3336–3345

3. Führer D, Mix M, Willegerodt H, Holzapfel HP, von Pet-rykowski W, Wonerow P, Paschke R̃ (1998) Autosomal dominant nonautoimmune hyperthyroidism. Clinical features – diagnosis – therapy. Exp Clin Endocrinol Diabetes 106:10–15

4. Cooper DC (2003) Hyperthyroidism. Lancet 362:459–468

5. Davison S, Lennard TWJ, Davison J, Kendall-Taylor P, Perros P (2001) Management of a pregnant patient with Graves' disease complicated by thionamide-induced neutropenia in the first trimester. Clin Endocrinol 54:559–561

6. Röher HD, Horster FA, Frilling A, Goretzki PE (1991) Morphologie und funktionsgerechte Chirurgie verschiedener Hyperthyreoseformen. Chirurg 62:176–181

7. Goretzki PE, Dotzenrath C, Witte J, Schulte KM, Röher HD (2000) Chirurgie des Morbus Basedow. Viszeralchirurgie 35:117–123

8. Dralle H, Sekulla C, Lorenz K, Grond S, Irmscher B (2004) Ambulante und kurzstationäre Schilddrüsen- und Nebenschilddrüsenchirurgie. Chirurg 75:131–143

9. Demers LM, Spencer CA (2003) Laboratory medicine practice guidelines: diagnosis and management of thyroid disease. Thyroid 13:45–56

10. Meller J, Jauho A, Hüfner M (2000) Disseminated thyroid autonomy or Graves' disease: reevaluation by a second-generation TSH receptor antibody assay. Thyroid 10:1073–1079

11. Meller J, Wisheu S, Munzel U, et al (2000) 99mTcTU-based radio-iodine therapy of Plummer's disease. Eur J Nucl Med 27:1286–1291

12. Bartalena L, Brogioni S, Grasso L, et al (1996) Treatment of amiodarone induced thyrotoxicosis, a difficult challenge: results of a prospective study. J Clin Endocrinol Metab 81:2930–2933

13. Gerstein HC (1990) How common is postpartum thyroiditis? Arch Intern Med 150:1397–1400

14. Beckers A, Abs R, Mahler C, et al (1991) Thyrotropin-secreting pituitary adenomas: report of seven cases. J Clin Endocrinol Metab 72:477–483

15. Desai RK, Norman RJ, Jialol I, et al (1988) Spectrum of thyroid function abnormalities in gestational trophoblastic neoplasia. Clin Endocrinol (Oxf) 29:583–592

16. Hershman JM (1992) Role of human CG as a thyroid stimulator. J Clin Endocrinol Metab 74:258–259

17. Judd ES, Buie LA Jr (1962) Hyperthyroidism associated with struma ovarii. A rare surgical challenge. Arch Surg 84:692–697

18. King AWC, Ma JTC, Wang C, et al (1990) Hyperthyroidism during pregnancy due to coexistence of struma ovarii and Graves' disease. Postgrad Med J 66:132–133

19. Grüters A (2004) Besonderheiten von Autoimmunerkrankungen der Schilddrüse bei Kindern. Z Arztl Fortbild Qualitatssich 98:67–71

20. Ginsberg J (2003) Diagnosis and management of Graves' disease. CMAJ 168:575–585

21. Trivalle C, Doucet J, Chassague P, et al (1996) Differences in the signs and symptoms of hyperthyroidism in older and younger patients. J Am Geriatr Soc 44:50–53

22. Lahey FH (1931) Non-activated (apathic) type of hyperthyroidism. N Engl J Med 204:747–748

23. Mokshaguidam AD, Wong NCW (1994) Age-related changes in thyroid hormone action. Eur J Endocrinol 131:451–461

24. Meng W (1992) Medikamentöse Therapie des Morbus Basedow: Langzeitergebnisse. Akt Endokrinol Stoffw 13:9–15

25. Quadbeck B, Janssen OE, Mann K (2004) Therapie des Mb.Basedow: Probleme und neue Entwicklungen: medikamentöse Therapie. Z Arztl Fortbild Qualitatssich 98:37–44

26. Schaaf L, Pohl T, Schmidt R, et al (1993) Screening for thyroid disease in a working population. Clin Investig 71:126–131

27. Vanderpump MPJ, Tunbridge WMG, French JW, Appleton D, Bates D, Rodgers H, Evans JG, Clark F, Tunbridge F, Young ET (1995) The incidence of thyroid disorders in the community: a twenty-year follow up of the Wickham survey. Clin Endocrinol 43:55–68

28. Yunta PJ, Ponce JL, Prieto M, Lopez-Aznar D, Sancho-Fornos S (2001) Solitary adrenal gland metastasis of a follicular thyroid carcinoma presenting with hyperthyroidism. Ann Endocrinol (Paris) 62:226–229

29. Nordyke RA, Gilbert FI, Harada AS (1998) Graves' disease. Influence of age on clinical findings. Arch Intern Med 148:626–631

30. Witte J, Goretzki PE, Dotzenrath C, Simon D, Röher HD (2000) Surgery for Graves' disease: total versus subtotal thyroidectomy – results of a prospective randomized trial. World J Surg 24:1303–1311

31. Parle JV, Maisonneuve P, Sheppard MC, Boyle P, Franklyn JA (2001) Prediction of all-cause and cardiovascular mortality in elderly people from one low serum thyrotropin result: a 10-year cohort study. Lancet 358:861–865

32. Canaris GJ, Manowik NR, Mayor G, Ridgway EC (2000) The Colorado thyroid disease prevalence study. Arch Intern Med 160:526–534

33. Mishra A, Agarwal A, Agarwal G, Mishra SK (2001) Total thyroidectomy for benign thyroid disorders in an endemic region. World J Surg 25:307–310

34. Momotani N, Noh J, Oyanagi H, et al (1986) Antithyroid drug therapy in Graves' disease during pregnancy. N Engl J Med 315:24–28

35. Sawin CT (2002) Subclinical hyperthyroidism and atrial fibrillation. Thyroid 12:501–503

36. Kreuzberg U, Theissen P, Schicha H (2000) Single-channel activity and expression in atrial l-type Ca (2+) channels in patients with latent hyperthyroidism. Am J Physiol Heart Circ Physiol 278:723–730

37. Seminara SB, Daniels GH (1998) Amiodarone and the thyroid. Endocr Pract 4:48–57

38. Williams M, Lo Gerfo P (2002) Thyroidectomy using local anesthesia in critically ill patients amiodarone-induced thyrotoxicosis: a review and description of the technique. Thyroid 12:523–525

39. Bogazzi F, Miccoli P, Berti P, Cosci C, Brogioni S, Aghini-Lombard, Materazzi G, Bartalena L, Pinchera A, Bravermann LE, Martino E (2002) Preparation with iopanoic acid rapidly controls thyrotoxic patients with amiodarone-induced thyrotoxicosis before thyroidectomy. Surgery 132:1114–1117

40. Pruijm MT, Pereira AM (2004) Thyrotoxic crisis in patient with Graves' disease. Ned Tijdschr Geneeskd 148:1691–1694

41. Klein I, Ojamaa K (2001) Thyroid hormone and the cardiovascular system. N Engl J Med 344:501–509

42. Pruijm MT, Pereira AM. Thyrotoxic crisis in an patient with Graves' disease. Ned Tijdschr Geneeskd (2004) 148:1691–1694

43. Caparros-Lefebvre D, Benabdallah S, Bertagna X, Ekindi N (2003) Subacute motor neuropathy induced by T3 hyperthyroidism. Ann Med Interne (Paris) 154:475–478

44. Fazio S, Palmieri EA, Lombardi G, Biondi B (2004) Effects of thyroid hormone on the cardiovascular system. Recent Prog Horm Res 59:31–50

45. Goretzki PE, Dotzenrath C, Witte J, Schulte KM, Roher HD (2000) Chirurgie des Morbus Basedow. Viszeralchirurgie 35:117–123

46. Plummer S, Boothby WM (1923) The value of iodine in exophthalmic goitre. Coll Pap Mayo Clin Mayo Found 69:565–576

47. Atkins P, Cohen SB, Phillips BJ (2000) Drug therapy for hyperthyroidism in pregnancy: safety issues for mother and fetus. Drug Saf 23:229–244

48. Miehle K, Paschke R (2003) Therapy of hyperthyroidism. Exp Clin Endocrinol Diabetes 111:305–311

49. Davidson S, Lennard TW, Davison J, Kendall-Taylor P, Perros P (2001) Management of a pregnant patient with Graves' disease complicated by thionamide-induced neutropenia in the first trimester. Clin Endocrinol (Oxf) 2001 54:559–561

50. Al-Fakhri N, Schwartz A, Runkel N, Buhr HJ (1998) Rate of complications with systemic exposure of the recurrent laryngeal nerve and parathyroid glands in operations for benign thyroid gland disease. Zentralbl Chir 123:21–24

51. Röher HD, Goretzki PE, Hellmann P, Witte J (1999) Risiken und Komplikationen der Schilddrüsenchirurgie. Chirurg 70:999–1010

52. Kahaly G, Kampmann C, Mohr-Kahaly S (2002) Cardiovascular hemodynamic and exercise tolerance in thyroid disease. Thyroid 12:473–481

53. Bilosi M, Binquet C, Goudet P, Lalanne-Mistrih ML, Brun JM, Cougard P (2002) Is subtotal thyroidectomy still indicated in patients with Graves' disease? Ann Chir 127:115–120

54. Goretzki PE, Dotzenrath C, Witt J, Schulte KM, Röher HD (2000) Chirurgie des Morbus Basedow. Viszeralchirurgie 35:1–8

55. de Ronde W, ten Have SM, van Daele PL, Feelders RA, van der Lely (2004) Hungry bone syndrome, characterized by prolonged symptomatic hypocalcemia, as a complication of the treatment hyperthyroidism. Ned Tijdschr Geneeskd 148:231–234

56. Kurihara H (2002) Total thyroidectomy for the treatment of hyperthyroidism in patients with ophthalmopathy. Thyroid 12:265–267

57. Werga-Kjellman P, Zedenius J, Tallstedt L, Traisk F, Lundell G, Wallin G (2001) Surgical treatment of hyperthyroidism: a ten-year experience. Thyroid 11:187–192

58. Rosato L, Avenia N, Bernante P, De Palma M, Gulino G, Nasi PG, Pelizzo MR, Pezzullo L (2004) Complications of thyroid surgery: analysis of a multicentric study on 14,934 patients operated on in Italy over 5 years. World J Surg 28:271–276.

59. Mittendorf EA, McHenry CR (2001) Thyroidectomy for selected patients with thyrotoxicosis. Arch Otolaryngol Head Neck Surg 127:61–65

60. Robert J, Mariethoz S, Pache JC, Bertin D, Caulfield A, Murith N, Peytremann A, Goumaz M, Garcia B, Martin-Du Pan R, Jacot-des-Combes B, Burger A, Spiliopoulos A (2001) Short- and long-term results of total vs subtotal thyroidectomy in the surgical treatment of Graves' disease. Swiss Surg 7:20–24

61. Yamashita H, Noguchi S, Murakami T, Uchino S, Watanabe S, Ohshima A, Toda M, Yamashita H, Kawamoto H (2001) Predictive risk factors for postoperative tetany in female patients with Graves' disease. J Am Coll Surg 192:465–468

62. Schneider P, Biko J, Demidchik YE, Drozd VM, Capozza RF, Cointry GR, Frreti JL (2004) Impact of parathyroid status and Ca and Vitamin-D supplementation on bone mass and muscle-bone relationship in 208 Belarussian children after thyroidectomy because of thyroid carcinoma. Exp Clin Endocrinol Diabetes 112:444–450

63. Thomusch O, Sekulla C, Machens A, Neumann HJ, Timmermann W, Dralle H (2004) Validity of intra-operative neuromonitoring signals in thyroid surgery. Langenbecks Arch Surg 389:499–503

64. Acun Z, Cihan A, Ulukent SC, Comert M, Ucan B, Cakmak GK, Cesur A (2004) A randomized prospective study of complications between general surgery residents and attending surgeons in near-total thyroidectomies. Surg Today 34:997–1001

65. Pelizzo MR, Toniato A, Piotto A, Bernante P, Pagetta C, Bernandi C (2001) Prevention and treatment of intra-post-operative complications in thyroid surgery. Ann Ital Chir 72:723–726

66. Rosato L, Avenia N, Bernante P, De Palma M, Gulino G, Nasi PG, Pelizzo MR, Pezzullo L (2004) Complications of thyroid surgery: analysis of a multicentric study on 14,934 patients operated on in Italy over 5 years. World J Surg 28:271–276

67. Panzer C, Beazley R, Bravermann L (2004) Rapid preoperative preparation for severe hyperthyroid Graves' disease. J Clin Endocrinol Metab 89:5866–5867

68. Dumont JE, Jauniaux JC, Roger PP, et al (1989) The cyclic AMP-mediated stimulation of cell proliferation. Trends Biochem Sci 14:67–71

69. Dralle H, Sekulla C (2004) Morbidität nach subtotaler und totaler Thyreoidektomie beim Morbus Basedow: Entscheidungsgrundlage für Operationsindikation und Resektionsausmaß. Z Arztl Fortbild Qualitatssich 98:45–53

70. Chi SY, Hsei KC, Sheen-Chen SM, Chou FF (2005) A Prospective randomized comparison of bilateral subtotal thyroidectomy versus unilateral total and contralateral subtotal thyroidectomy for Graves' disease. World J Surg 29:160–163

71. Gemsenjäger E, Valko P, Schweizer I (2002) Basedow disease. From subtotal to total thyroidectomy. Schweiz Rundsch Med Prax 91:206–215

72. Bilosi M, Binquet C, Goudet P, Lalanne-Mistrih ML, Brun JM, Cougard P (2002) Is subtotal thyroidectomy still indicated in patients with Graves' disease? Ann Chir 127:115–120

73. Brunova J, Bruna J, Joubert G, Koning M (2003) Weight gain in patients after therapy for hyperthyroidism. S Afr Med J 93:529–531

74. Yamashita H, Noguchi S, Murakami T, Uchino S, Watanabe S, Ohshima A, Kawamoto H, Toda M, Yamashita H (2000) Calcium and its regulating hormones in patients with Graves' disease: sex differences and relation to postoperative tetany. Eur J Surg 166:924–928

75. Claret-Gardette M, Lalanne-Mistrih ML, Verges B, Goudet P, Brun Cougard P (2003) Does thyroidectomy worsen Graves' ophthalmopathy? Ann Chir 128:88–93

76. Miccoli P, Bellantone R, Mourad M, Walz M, Rafaelli M, Berti P. Minimally invasive video-assisted thyroidectomy: multiinstitutional experience. World J Surg 26:972–975

77. Gabriele R, Letizia C, Borghese M, De Toma G, Celi M, Izzo L, Cavallaro A (2003) Thyroid cancer in patients with hyperthyroidism. Horm Res 60:79–83

78. Lian X, Bai Y, Tang W, Dai W, Guo Z (2000) A clinical study on coincidence with hyperthyroidism and thyroid carcinoma. Zhongguo Yi Xue Ke Xue Yuan Xue Bao 22:273–275

79. Lin CH, Chiang FY, Wang LF (2003) Prevalence of thyroid cancer in hyperthyroidism treated by surgery. Kaohsiung J Med Sci 19:379–384

80. Bitton RN, Sachmechi I, Tabriz MS, Murphy L, Wassermann P (2001) Papillary carcinoma of the thyroid with manifestations resembling Graves' disease. Endocr Pract 7:106–109

81. Moleti M, Mattina F, Salamone I, Violi MA, Nucera C, Baldari SL, Schiavo MG, Regalbuto C, Trimarchi F, Vermiglio F (2003) Effects of thyroidectomy alone or followed by radio-iodine ablation of thyroid remnants on the outcome of Graves' ophthalmopathy. Thyroid 13:653–658

82. Takamia H, Ikeda Y (2003) Total endoscopic thyroidectomy. Asian J Surg 26:82–85

83. Shimizu K, Tanaka S (2003) Asian perspective on endoscopic thyroidectomy – a review of 193 cases. Asian J Surg 26:92–100

84. Berti P, Materazzi G, Galleri D, Donatini G, Minuto M, Micolli P (2004) Video-assisted thyroidectomy for Graves' disease: report of a preliminary experience. Surg Endosc 18:1208–1210

85. Yamamoto M, Sasaki A, Asahi H, Shimada Y, Sato N, Nakajima J, Mashima R, Saito K (2001) Endoscopic subtotal thyroidectomy for patients with Graves' disease. Surg Today 31:1–4

86. Schabram J, Vorländer C, Wahl RA (2004) Differentiated operative strategy in minimally invasive, video-assisted thyroid surgery. Results in 196 patients. World J Surg 28:1282–1286

87. Kraimps JL, Bouin-Pineau MH, Mathonnet M, De Calan L, Roncer Visset J, Marechaud R, Barbier J (2001) Multicentre study of thyroid nodules in patients with Graves' disease. Br J Surg 87:1111–1113

88. Suzuki K, Nakagawa O, Aizawa Y (2001) A case of pulmonary metastatic thyroid cancer complicated Graves' disease. Endocr J 48:175–179

89. Badenhoop K, Usadel KH (1994) Therapie der Hyperthyreose. In: Reinwein D, Weinheimer B (eds) Schilddrüse 1993. de Gruyter Berlin-New York, pp 352–359

90. Sivanandan R, Ng LG, Khin LW, Lim TH, Soo KC (2004) Postoperative endocrine function in patients with surgically treated thyrotoxicosis. Head Neck 26:331–337

91. Tigas S, Idiculla J, Beckett G, Toft A (2000) Is excessive weight gain after ablative treatment of hyperthyroidism due to inadequate thyroid hormone therapy. Thyroid 10:1107–1111

16 Thyroiditis

Michel Adamina and Daniel Oertli

16.1 Introduction

Thyroiditides make up approximately 20% of all thyroid diseases [1] and are caused by multiple factors (Table 16.1). Autoimmune diseases represent the most common etiologies. According to the clinical course, thyroiditides have been subdivided into acute, subacute, and chronic forms. Once a suppurative inflammation has been ruled out, most other types of thyroiditis have either a definitive autoimmune etiology or are possibly autoimmune in nature [2].

In life, one out of 100 individuals will develop an overt autoimmune thyroiditis. Thyroid autoantibodies may be found in up to 10% of the general population [3,4]. These autoantibodies are mainly directed against thyroid peroxidase or thyroglobulin. They are not the cause of the disease, but the consequence of a lost immune tolerance to the thyroid gland. Autoantibodies may promote thyroid hormone dysfunctions (stimulating thyroid autoantibodies, blocking thyroid autoantibodies). An association of autoimmune thyroiditis with defined HLA haplotypes implies a genetic predisposition [5]. Iodine therapy, viral infections, pregnancy and menopause, stress [6], and immuno-modulating drugs (interferon-α, interleukin-2) have also been linked to autoimmune thyroiditis. Except for Graves' disease, most autoimmune thyroiditides initially present with a limited hyperthyroid state, and thereafter return to euthyroidism or definitively fall to permanent (subclinical or overt) hypothyroidism. Thus, over 90% of cases of clinical hypothyroidism are caused by an autoimmune thyroiditis. Conversely, about 1–10% of cases of hyperthyroidism are related to a thyroiditis. Clinically, patients may present either with an acute illness with severe thyroid pain (e.g., subacute de Quervain's thyroiditis, acute suppurative thyroiditis, radiation thyroiditis, traumatic thyroiditis) or without evident inflammation but with thyroid dysfunction or a goiter (e.g., silent thyroiditis, Hashimoto's or Riedel's thyroiditis).

Table 16.1 Etiologies of thyroiditis

Autoimmune thyroiditis	Chronic lymphocytic thyroiditis (Hashimoto's)
	Fibrotic variant of Hashimoto's thyroiditis
	Atrophic thyroiditis (primary myxedema)
Variants of autoimmune thyroiditis	Postpartum thyroiditis
	Silent or painless thyroiditis
	Subacute de Quervain's thyroiditis
	Fibrotic Riedel's thyroiditis
Non-immune thyroiditis	Acute infectious thyroiditis
	Radiation thyroiditis
	Palpation/trauma-induced thyroiditis
	Sarcoidosis
	Vasculitis
	Postoperative necrotizing thyroiditis
	Drug-induced thyroiditis
	Carcinoma-associated thyroiditis

16.2   Autoimmune Thyroiditis

The largest community study published so far on autoimmune thyroiditis revealed elevated thyroid autoantibodies against thyroid peroxidase and thyroglobulin in more than 10% of a British community (Whickham study) [3]. On the one hand, in 7.5% of this community, elevated TSH together with a euthyroid state indicated a subclinical hypothyroidism, which became overt hypothyroidism in 1.9% of the study's population. On the other hand, subclinical or overt hyperthyroidism was shown in 2% of people in the Whickham community. Women showed a 10 times higher prevalence of autoimmune thyroiditis, but this gender difference declined with age so that, for people over 75 years of age, 16% of the men and 20% of the women showed subclinical hypothyroidism.

16.2.1   Hashimoto's Thyroiditis

Synonyms: chronic lymphocytic thyroiditis, struma lymphomatosa

Hashimoto's thyroiditis is the most frequent autoimmune thyroiditis and is the archetypic example of organ-specific autoimmune disease. With a prevalence of about 3% it represents the most common cause of hypothyroidism in the general population [1]. In regions where iodine intake is adequate, Hashimoto's thyroiditis also represents the most common cause of goiter. The peak incidence culminates in the fifth decade of life and the prevalence increases with age. Women are 10–20 times more affected than men. A genetic association with the haplotypes HLA-DR3, -DR4, and -DR5 is found. Many other autoimmune diseases are associated with Hashimoto's thyroiditis: Graves' disease, juvenile diabetes, Addison's disease, pernicious anemia, rheumatoid arthritis, Sjögren's syndrome, and systemic lupus erythematosus. Hashimoto's thyroiditis mostly presents with an oligosymptomatic clinical course, a painless homogeneous goiter, and with signs of hypothyroidism. Low concentrations of thyroid hormones with high TSH and circulating thyroid autoantibodies (against peroxidase in 70–90% of cases and against thyroglobulin in 40–70% of cases) confirm the diagnosis [1]. Occasionally, a transient hyperthyroidism state may be noted, up to a marked hyperthyroidism or hashitoxicosis, associated with the presence of anti-TSH receptor antibodies. Like all autoimmune diseases, the clinical picture is one of relapsing episodes, with up to one quarter of the patients showing a spontaneous recovery. Hashimoto's thyroiditis is probably related to an acquired defect of the thyroid's specific T suppressor lymphocytes, resulting in the emergence of helper T lymphocytes directed against the gland, and the production of autoantibodies against various components of the thyroid. The binding of these autoantibodies to the thyrocytes accounts for complement and T lymphocyte-mediated lysis of the thyrocytes and non-regulated release of thyroxine and triiodothyronine, resulting in the transient hyperthyroidism occasionally noted. Later, the destruction of thyroid parenchyma may lead to permanent hypothyroidism.

A causal treatment is unknown and substitutive thyroid hormone therapy is indicated when overt hypothyroidism (i.e., in about 20% of patients) is identified. Most patients require lifelong replacement therapy.

On fine-needle biopsy, Hürthle cells or oncocytes are frequently seen. Hashimoto's thyroiditis may at times be difficult to distinguish on a fine-needle aspiration biopsy from a follicular neoplasm, papillary carcinoma, or low-grade MALT lymphoma. Immunohistochemistry studies may help to clear the differential diagnosis.

16.2.1.1   Fibrotic Hashimoto's Thyroiditis

A fibrotic variant of Hashimoto's thyroiditis accounts for up to 10% of the clinical presentations, predominantly in elderly patients with preexisting goiter. The disease is characterized by a rapid increase of goiter size, which may lead to the suspicion of malignancy and to subsequent surgery. Nevertheless, the extensive fibrotic changes and metaplasia noted on specimen or biopsies are always limited to the gland, in contrast to the invasive Riedel's fibrosing thyroiditis.

16.2.1.2   Atrophic Autoimmune Thyroiditis

Synonyms: primary myxedema, idiopathic myxedema, atrophic Hashimoto's thyroiditis

The atrophic autoimmune thyroiditis is the cause of primary myxedema and should not be confused with endstage fibrotic Hashimoto's thyroiditis. Most of the cases proceed over years without overt signs or symptoms. The related hypothyroidism then becomes clinically obvious around the fourth to sixth decade of life. Women are 5 times more affected than men. On histologic specimen, the thyroid gland weighs less than 5 g, whereas in some milder asymptomatic cases, the thyroid gland weighs around 10 g (reference weights: male 20 g, female 17 g [7]).

16.2.2 Focal Lymphocytic Thyroiditis

Synonyms: focal autoimmune thyroiditis, chronic unspecific thyroiditis

Focal lymphocytic thyroiditis is a coincidental finding in 50% of women's and 25% of men's autopsies, without clinical relevance. This low-grade autoimmune thyroiditis is characterized by focal lymphocytic infiltrates of less than 5% of the thyroid gland.

16.2.3 Postpartum Thyroiditis

A postpartum thyroiditis occurs in 2–16% of women 4–6 months following delivery (by definition within one year after parturition or abortion) [8,9]. The disease represents an exacerbation of a preceding (undiagnosed) autoimmune thyroiditis and is classically linked to the haplotypes HLA-DR3, -DR4, and -DR5. It may be interpreted as rebound autoimmunity after the pregnancy-associated immunosuppression. Eighty-five percent of these patients develop autoantibodies against thyroid peroxidase and thyroglobulin, which may vanish over time. Clinically, women may show a transient hyperthyroidism state, which rapidly converts to hypothyroidism, and then to euthyroidism within 12 months. Treatment consists of thyroid hormone substitution when required. Thyreostatic medication, occasionally β-blockers, may be needed in the presence of exacerbated hyperthyroidism. Neither prophylaxis nor predicting marker have been identified so far and women affected once have a higher probability of relapse following further pregnancies.

Women with a known autoimmune thyroiditis prior to pregnancy and an elevated titer of autoantibodies against thyroglobulin during pregnancy nearly always suffer from a postpartum exacerbation of their autoimmune thyroiditis.

16.2.4 Subacute de Quervain's Thyroiditis

Synonyms: granulomatous thyroiditis, pseudotuberculous thyroiditis, giant cell thyroiditis

Subacute de Quervain's thyroiditis is a self-limiting disease accounting for 0.5–3% of all thyroid pathologies and lasts a few weeks to 2 months [10]. Women are 3–6 times more affected than men. The peak incidence is between the second and fifth decade of life. Patients complain of moderate to severe pain in the neck of sudden onset that irradiates to the jaw, ear, face, and down to the thorax; they present with fever, lassitude, and a feeling of illness. The thyroid is exquisitely tender and enlarged to palpation. The erythrocyte sedimentation rate is markedly elevated. Initially, the local inflammation process leads to a destruction of thyroid follicles with a transient hyperthyroidism, due to the breakdown of stored thyroglobulin. Later on, hypothyroidism emerges as the thyroid is not able to cope with the body's demand for thyroid hormones. Finally, as the subacute thyroiditis heals, euthyroidism returns. Subacute de Quervain's thyroiditis tends to recur, although at a low rate of 4% [11]. Permanent hypothyroidism requiring substitutive therapy is then noted in 15% of the patients [11].

The etiology of subacute de Quervain's thyroiditis remains uncertain, but evidence implicates viral infection. A postviral cytokine-mediated inflammation of the thyroid is suspected because a seasonal frequency and an association with upper respiratory tract infection is noted. In half of the patients antibodies against mumps, measles, influenza, adenovirus, coxsackievirus, or echovirus are found. Furthermore, a genetic predisposition exists with the haplotype HLA-Bw35.

The differential diagnosis encompasses acute suppurative thyroiditis. In contrast to acute suppurative thyroiditis, the gland sonographically reveals irregular hypoperfused areas instead of hyperperfused tissue. On fine-needle biopsy, the differential diagnosis further includes palpation thyroiditis, as well as other granulomatous diseases such as sarcoidosis, tuberculosis, and rheumatoid diseases.

Treatment is supportive with non-steroidal antiinflammatory agents (NSAR) and β-blockers in severe cases with hyperthyroidism. Corticosteroids are useful (about 40 mg hydrocortisone equivalents daily) when the NSAR medication is not successful. Symptoms usually improve within 2–3 days after the initiation of corticosteroid treatment. However, it may take about 4 weeks for the disappearance of the thyroid mass.

16.2.5 Painless Thyroiditis

Synonym: subacute lymphocytic thyroiditis

Patients present with a diffuse but modest enlargement of the thyroid and function tests reveal a transient hyperthyroidism, followed by hypothyroidism. The painless thyroiditis is self-limited and rarely necessitates thyroid hormone substitution therapy. Women are again more often affected than men with a peak of incidence in middle life and in the postpartum period. Autoantibodies against thyroid peroxidase and thyroglobulin are found, as well as an association with HLA-DR3 and -DR5 haplotypes. Histologic examination of a specimen reveals a lymphocytic infiltration with destruction of follicles; this is in contrast to Hashimoto's thyroiditis. Neither giant cell granulomas (typical for a subacute thyroiditis) nor an association with a viral infection are present.

16.2.6   Riedel's Fibrosing Thyroiditis

Riedel's thyroiditis is a rare chronic thyroiditis in which the thyroid gland is replaced by fibrous tissue. The underlying etiologic mechanisms are unclear. An autoimmune component is suspected, due to elevated titers of thyroid autoantibodies. The prevailing view is that Riedel's thyroiditis is part of a multifocal fibroinflammatory process also involving other tissues (mediastinum, liver, lung, retroperitoneum, orbital). Women in middle to advanced ages are more affected than men. The clinical manifestations of Riedel's thyroiditis are protean, often resembling malignancy due to a goiter of remarkably hard consistency. Patients complain of a rapid indolent enlargement of the thyroid that becomes very hard on palpation and difficult to delineate. Neck discomfort and dysphagia are frequently reported. Thirty to 40% of these patients develop overt hypothyroidism. Hoarseness and hypoparathyroidism may also appear due to involvement of the recurrent laryngeal nerve and/or the parathyroid glands. Physical examination, laboratory analysis, cytology, and imaging features are not useful for differentiating between Riedel's thyroiditis and neoplastic diseases or the fibrotic variant of Hashimoto's thyroiditis [12]. Histologic examination is necessary to establish the final diagnosis and surgical biopsy is mandatory. The differential diagnosis further encompasses anaplastic carcinoma and sarcoma of the thyroid. In contrast to the fibrotic variant of Hashimoto's thyroiditis where fibrosis is strictly limited to the gland, Riedel's thyroiditis displays a dense fibrotic replacement of thyroid parenchyma that penetrates the capsule and extends into contiguous neck structures. Once the diagnosis is confirmed, treatment is supportive with thyroid hormone substitution, when required.

16.3   Acute Infectious Thyroiditis

Synonym: acute suppurative thyroiditis

Infectious thyroiditis is a rare disease of the thyroid. A bacterial or a fungal infection is the main cause, though only a few hundred cases are reported worldwide. Mycobacterial, parasitic, and viral forms of thyroiditis have also been described, predominantly in immunodepressed hosts. The thyroid gland appears to be relatively resistant to infection. A rich vascular supply and an extended lymphatic drainage, as well as a fibrous capsule and an anatomic separation from the other structures of the neck by fascial planes, represent protective mechanisms. The high iodine content of the gland may account for some bactericidal effect. Infection of the gland occurs either through hematogenous spread from a primary focus or by direct extension from adjacent neck structures such as infected tonsil, pharynx, thyroglossal duct cyst, or through a pyriform sinus fistula, especially in children [13].

Other less common sources of infection include neck trauma or lymphatic spread; surgical site infections are extremely rare [14]. The most common predisposing factor for suppurative thyroiditis is immunodepression in association with HIV, tuberculosis, old age, or debilitation. Other predisposing factors include preexisting thyroid diseases, such as multinodular goiter, autoimmune thyroiditis, and thyroid cancers [14–16].

Patients are febrile with a sudden onset of disease, a painful, mostly unilateral enlargement of the thyroid, and local inflammatory signs (Fig. 16.1). The thyroid hormone tests are usually normal, but a slight hyper- or hypothyroidism may appear. The erythrocyte sedimentation rate and acute phase proteins are elevated, and leucocytosis is present. Neck sonography reveals patchy hyperperfused areas in the thyroid with liquid content when an abscess is present. A fine-needle biopsy and cultures allow for pathogen identification and guide the antibiotic treatment. Depending on the clinical context, dedicated stainings and/or immunohistochemistry or in situ hybridization techniques may be necessary to identify the causative pathogen. Immunodepressed patients tend to present with more chronic thyroid infections, bilateral disease, and less prominent signs and symptoms: a high index of suspicion and aspiration biopsy are invaluable to pose the correct diagnosis and initiate correct treatment.

The differential diagnosis of a painful anterior neck mass with febrile status encompasses subacute de Quervain's thyroiditis, hemorrhage into a thyroid nodule, an infected thyroglossal or branchial cleft cyst, an infected cystic hygroma, and cervical adenitis. In addition to fine-needle biopsy, sonography helps to establish the correct diagnosis: acute suppurative thyroiditis usually shows hyperperfused areas (Fig. 16.2). In contrast, sonography in de Quervain's thyroiditis depicts only microabscesses and no hyperperfused areas. Computed tomography (CT) and/or contrast oesography may further refine the diagnosis

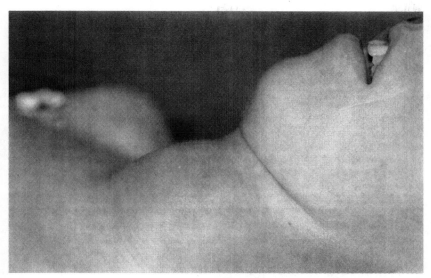

Fig. 16.1 Clinical picture of a 31-year-old female with acute infectious thyroiditis. Steroid therapy was initiated for a subacute de Quervain's thyroiditis. Six weeks later, the patient developed a unilateral painful neck mass, dysphagia, and fever. Surgical incision and drainage was necessary to cure this condition

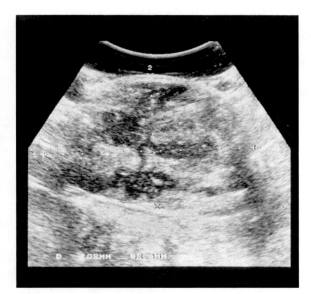

Fig. 16.2 Thyroid sonography in acute infectious thyroiditis of the patient shown in Fig. 16.1. Hyperperfused areas and a liquid collection in the left thyroid lobe are shown. Fine-needle biopsy revealed *Streptococcus constellatus, Peptostreptococcus,* and fusobacteria

(Fig. 16.3) and help to delineate the extent of surgical treatment, particularly in the case of an infected pyriform sinus fistula.

16.3.1   Etiologies of Infectious Thyroiditis

A bacterial infection (mainly gram-positive bacteria) contracted through hematogenous spread or neck trauma is the most common cause of acute thyroiditis in the immunocompetent patient. Viral, fungal,

or parasitic infections occur preferentially in immunodepressed patients. Dedicated stainings and a high index of suspicion may be necessary to identify atypical pathogens, such as *Pneumocystis carinii* and mycobacteria. Table 16.2 lists the pathogens commonly involved in acute thyroiditis. In children, an acute suppurative thyroiditis is caused in up to 90% of the cases by a pyriform sinus fistula [17].

16.3.2   Surgical Treatment

When an abscess is identified, surgical drainage is mandatory. Surgical incision and drainage of the abscess are curative only in patients whose acute thyroiditis is unrelated to a pyriform sinus fistula or thyroglossal duct fistula. Sometimes an affected thyroid lobe needs complete resection (Fig. 16.4a–c). In patients with recurrent acute thyroiditis, an undetected fistula must be postulated. Complete removal of the infected fistula is therefore required to prevent recurrence. Injection of 0.5% methylene blue solution through a Nélaton's catheter into the fistula usually enables the complete resection of the fistula tract. When the origin of the fistula is difficult to identify, transection of the inferior pharyngeal constrictor muscle makes intervention easier.

16.4   Non-autoimmune Thyroiditis

Non-immune thyroiditis consist of a heterogeneous and rare group of thyroid inflammatory diseases. Some of them are clearly iatrogenic, such as drug-induced thyroiditis, postoperative necrotizing

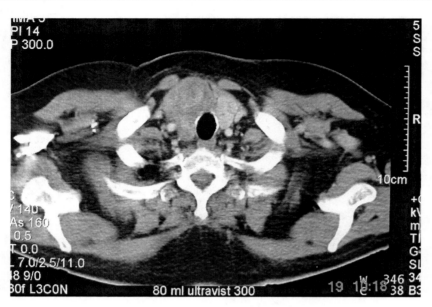

Fig. 16.3 Thyroid aspergilloma in an immunodepressed kidney transplant patient. CT scan of the neck reveals a diffuse enlargement of the right thyroid gland with abscess formation

Table 16.2 Pathogens involved in acute thyroiditis

Bacteria	*Staphylococcus aureus* (30%)
	Staphylococcus pyogenes
	Staphylococcus pneumoniae
	Streptococcus
	Enterobacteria
Fungi	Aspergillus
	Pneumocystis carinii
	Cryptococcus
	Candida
Virus	EBV
	CMV
	Measles
	Adenovirus
	Echovirus
	Mumps
Parasites	Echinococcus
	Strongyloides
	Taenia

thyroiditis, and radiation thyroiditis. Other causes are related to a local process, such as an acute hemorrhage into a thyroid cyst or nodule.

Palpation thyroiditis refers to a mild, self-limited thyroiditis occurring after physical examination, surgery, or trauma to the thyroid. It is not associated with any thyroid disease.

Finally, a few thyroiditides are caused by systemic diseases, such as a vasculitis-associated thyroiditis (phenytoin therapy may precipitate a hypersensitive thyroid vasculitis), a sarcoidosis (the thyroid is involved in up to 6% of sarcoidoses [18]), metastatic cancer, or a globus hystericus.

16.4.1   Drug-induced Thyroiditis

Chronic iodine therapy may cause a drug-induced thyroiditis with follicular hyperplasia. Likewise, lithium therapy may cause a goiter with or without hypothyroidism in 5–15% of patients under long-term lithium therapy [1]. Anticonvulsants (phenytoin, carbamazepine) may cause unspecific thyroiditis with subclinical or clinical hypothyroidism. Patients with chronic hepatitis or with cancer treated using interferon-α will develop a painless thyroiditis in about 1–5% of cases [19]. Elevated antithyroid antibodies are noted in a higher percentage in these patients and permanent hypothyroidism as well as Grave's disease may appear [20]. Prior interferon-α therapy in the presence of antithyroid antibodies is associated with a higher probability of a subsequent antibody titer elevation and thyroid dysfunction [21]. These changes usually occur within 3 months of interferon-α therapy and seldom thereafter. As a practical matter, TSH should be measured prior to initiation of interferon-α therapy and periodically during treatment.

For immunomodulation, interleukin-2 is also used in malignant melanoma, renal cell cancer, and leuke-

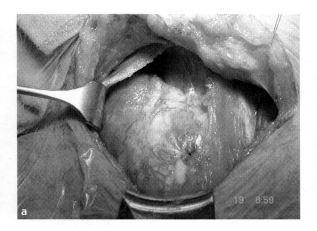

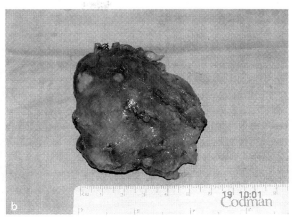

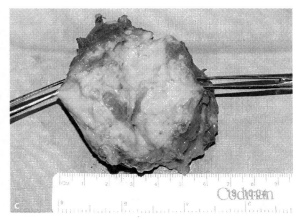

Fig. 16.4 a Intraoperative finding of the patient depicted in Fig. 16.3 showing inflammatory swelling of the right thyroid lobe with aspergilloma. **b** Removed lobe after right hemithyroidectomy. **c** Opened specimen presenting abscess with aspergilloma

mia, alone or in combination with chemotherapy. In several studies, interleukin-2 therapy has been linked to the development of a painless thyroiditis in about 2% of the patients treated [22].

Finally, the antiarrhythmic drug amiodarone contains 35% iodine and may cause thyroid dysfunctions in several different ways [23]. Amiodarone may cause a thyrotoxic crisis, due to its high iodine content (usually in patients with preexisting nodular goiter). Conversely, amiodarone may cause hypothyroidism via the antithyroid action of iodine, especially in patients with preexisting thyroid disease. Amiodarone decreases the conversion of T_4 to the biologically active T_3. It is worth noting that if the decision is taken to cease amiodarone therapy, the drug is not eliminated for months due to a very long half-life.

16.4.2 Postoperative Necrotizing Thyroiditis

Postoperative necrotizing thyroiditis is a rare surgical complication [24,25]. No predictive marker or factor has been identified and the very rich vascular supply of the thyroid usually prevents this rarest complication. On histologic examination, the specimen typically shows postoperative granulomas, as found in other organs (bladder, prostate) following surgery.

Postoperative necrotizing thyroiditis is related to a trauma of the thyroid, through vigorous manipulation of the gland at surgery or through repeated fine-needle aspiration [26]. Such manipulation could induce an acute thyroiditis, which in turn may lead to thyrotoxicosis or to a necrotizing thyroiditis.

16.4.3 Radiation Thyroiditis

Radiation thyroiditis occurs in a dose-related fashion after radioiodine or external beam radiation therapy. Follicle destruction due to radiation injury may cause a transient hyperthyroidism, followed eventually by hypothyroidism. Neck pain and tenderness usually develop 5–10 days following treatment. Symptoms are mild and subside spontaneously in a week.

16.5   Indications for Surgery

Surgical interventions are exceptionally indicated for the management of a thyroiditis, accounting for less than 1% of all thyroid procedures [27]. Patients with autoimmune thyroiditis may pose significant technical challenges to the endocrine surgeon. The glands are firm, rigid, and highly vascular. The tissues surrounding the thyroid are inflamed with lymphadenopathy. This makes preservation of the parathyroids and recurrent nerves a highly demanding task. However, it is rather the exception than the rule to pose a surgical indication for an autoimmune thyroiditis, as most patients are effectively managed with thyroid hormone replacement therapy.

In the rare instance where a large Hashimoto's goiter may develop and become symptomatic, near-total thyroidectomy is an option [2,27,28]. Moreover, as thyroiditis patients bear a higher risk of developing thyroid carcinoma, a cold nodule suspicious on fine-needle biopsy may indicate a thyroid lobectomy. Similarly, the rapid growth of a chronic lymphocytic thyroid gland is suggestive of non-Hodgkin's lymphoma. While total thyroidectomy may surgically cure a stage I lymphoma (i.e., confined to the thyroid), most thyroid lymphomas involve regional lymph nodes and distant sites and require multimodal systemic therapy. Open biopsy or thyroid lobectomy is sufficient in these cases to establish the definitive diagnosis.

A subacute de Quervain's thyroiditis exceptionally deserves surgical consideration. This indication is given when intractable neck pain is present in spite of a consequent analgesic and substitution therapy with thyroxin over 6 months. Thyroidectomy may then be indicated for definitive cure [27].

Riedel's fibrosing thyroiditis often requires an open biopsy to confirm the diagnosis and rule out an anaplastic carcinoma (or the fibrotic variant of Hashimoto's thyroiditis). However, thyroidectomy can be highly demanding because of the dense fibrotic reaction extending beyond the thyroid that puts the surrounding structures at risk for injury. Surgery is therefore confined to diagnosis of thyroiditis and exclusion of malignancy or to decompression of the trachea and the esophagus by isthmectomy and/or lobectomy.

The fibrotic variant of Hashimoto's thyroiditis is characterized by a rapid enlargement of a preexisting goiter that may lead to the suspicion of a thyroid cancer and to surgical resection.

Amiodarone-induced thyrotoxicosis in the setting of a rare patient with otherwise intractable arrhythmia is an indication for thyroidectomy.

Finally, the acute suppurative thyroiditis is a classic indication for surgical drainage followed by antibiotic therapy. Rarely lobectomy is necessary when the suppurative process is necrotizing. An underlying thyroglossal (pyriform) fistula should be excluded by the time of surgical exploration.

References

1. Sheu SY, Schmid KW (2003) Entzündliche Schilddrüsenerkrankungen. Pathologe 24:339–347

2. Khan A, Nosé V (2004) Pathology of the thyroid gland. In: Lloyd RV (ed) Endocrine pathology. Humana, Totowa, New Jersey, pp 153–189

3. Tunbridge WM, Evered DC, Hall R, et al (1977) The spectrum of thyroid diseases in a community: the Whickham survey. Clin Endocrinol 7:481–493

4. Weetman AP (2001) Determinants of autoimmune thyroid disease. Nat Immunol 2:769–770

5. Weetman AP (2000) Chronic autoimmune thyroiditis. In: Braverman LE, Utiger RD (eds) Werner & Ingbar's the thyroid. Williams & Wilkins, Lippincott, Philadelphia, pp 721–732

6. Mizokami T, Wu Li A, El-Kaissi S, et al (2004) Stress and thyroid autoimmunity. Thyroid 14:1047–1055

7. Pankow BG, Michalak J, McGee MK (1985) Adult human thyroid weight. Health Phys 49:1097–1103

8. Amino N, Tada H, Hidaka Y (1999) Postpartum autoimmune thyroid syndrome: a model of aggravation of autoimmune disease. Thyroid 9:705–713

9. Stagnaro-Green A (2002) Clinical review 152: postpartum thyroiditis. J Clin Endocrinol Metab 87:4042–4047

10. Volpe R (1993) The management of subacute (de Quervain) thyroiditis. Thyroid 3:253–255

11. Fatourechi V, Aniszewski JP, Fatourechi GZ, et al (2003) Clinical features and outcome of subacute thyroiditis in an incidence cohort: Olmsted County, Minnesota, study. J Clin Endocrinol Metab 88:2100–2105

12. Papi G, LiVolsi VA (2004) Current concepts on Riedel thyroiditis. Am J Clin Pathol 121:S50–S63

13. Gan YU, Lam SL (2004) Imaging findings in acute neck infections due to pyriform sinus fistula. Ann Acad Med Singapore 33:636–640

14. Farwell AP (2000) Infectious thyroiditis. In: Braverman LE, Utiger RD (eds) Werner & Ingbar's the thyroid: a fundamental and clinical text. Williams & Wilkins, Lippincott, Philadelphia, pp 1044–1050

15. Miyauchi A, Matsuzuku F, Kuma K, et al (1990) Piriform sinus fistula: an underlying abnormality common in patients with acute suppurative thyroiditis. World J Surg 14:400–405

16. Jeng LB, Lin JD, Chen MF (1994) Acute suppurative thyroiditis: a ten-year review in a Taiwanese hospital. Scand J Infect Dis 26:297–300

17. Rich EJ, Mendelmann PM (1987) Acute suppurative thyroiditis in pediatric patients. Pediatr Infect Dis J 6:936–940

18. Porter N, Beynon HL, Randeva HS (2003) Endocrine and reproductive manifestations of sarcoidosis. QJM 96:553–561

19. Preziati D, La Rosa L, Covini G, et al (1995) Autoimmunity and thyroid function in patients with chronic active hepatitis treated with recombinant interferon alpha-2a. Eur J Endocrinol 132: 587–593

20. Roti E, Minelli R, Giuberti T, et al (1996) Multiple changes in thyroid function in patients with chronic active HCV hepatitis treated with recombinant interferon-alpha. Am J Med 172:482–487

21. Deutsch M, Dourakis S, Manesis EK, et al (1997) Thyroid abnormalities in chronic viral hepatitis and their relationship to interferon alfa therapy. Hepatology 26:206–210

22. Schwartzentruber DJ, White DE, Zweig MH, et al (1991) Thyroid dysfunction associated with immunotherapy for patients with cancer. Cancer 68:2384–2390

23. Harjai KJ, Licata AA (1997) Effects of amiodarone on thyroid function. Ann Intern Med 126:63–73

24. McDermott A, Onyeaka CV, Macnamara M (2002) Surgery-induced thyroiditis: fact or fiction? Ear Nose Throat J 81:408–410

25. Manson CM, Cross P, De Sousa B (1992) Post-operative necrotizing granulomas of the thyroid. Histopathology 21:392–393

26. Kobayashi A, Kuma K, Matsuzuka F, et al (1992) Thyrotoxicosis after needle aspiration of thyroid cyst. J Clin Endocrinol Metab 75:21–24

27. Röher HD, Schulte KM (2000) Operative Therapie bei Thyreoiditis. In: Rothmund M, Harder F, Siewert JR (eds) Praxis der Viszeralchirurgie: Endokrine Chirurgie. Springer, Berlin Heidelberg New York, pp 199–202

28. Kon YC, DeGroot LJ (2003) Painful Hashimoto's thyroiditis as an indication for thyroidectomy: clinical characteristics and outcome in seven patients. J Clin Endocrinol Metab 88:2667–2672

17 Complications in Thyroid and Parathyroid Surgery

Andrea Frilling and Frank Weber

17.1   Introduction

Mortality from thyroid and parathyroid surgery is virtually disregarded nowadays. During the eighteenth century, however, the mortality rate of thyroid surgery was as high as 40% from bleeding and sepsis [1]. As a consequence, in 1850 the French Academy of Medicine recommended its routine use be abandoned, and many leading surgeons would not perform it. The greatest advance in thyroid surgery is to be credited to Theodor Kocher who first recognized the importance of anti- and aseptic handling, hemostasis, and precise operative technique. Within a decade, his overall operative mortality decreased from 15% to 2.4%. With the exclusion of complicated cases, in 1898 he reported a mortality rate of only 0.18%. Following Kocher's principles, William Halsted, Charles Mayo, George Crile, and others contributed further to the development of thyroid surgery.

Once death from thyroid operation became an exception, specific pitfalls of the procedure, namely, injuries to the laryngeal nerves and damage to the parathyroid glands, became obvious. While some surgeons, including Kocher, tried to prevent recurrent laryngeal nerve injuries by avoiding any contact with the region of the nerve, others advocated routine identification and dissection of the nerve. The importance of the external branch of the superior laryngeal nerve was not appreciated until decades later. Halsted is credited for his studies of surgical anatomy and blood supply of the parathyroid glands and the introduction of the technique of capsular dissection that implemented preservation of the vascular pedicle of a parathyroid gland and led to a safer approach to thyroid and parathyroid surgery. Today morbidity remains a subject of concern for surgeons performing thyroid and parathyroid procedures. Injury of the recurrent laryngeal nerve and hypoparathyroidism are the most frequent complications. The key issue of an effective and safe surgical approach is a profound knowledge of specific anatomy and pathophysiology in combination with meticulous handling and dissection of tissue. The overall permanent complication rate should not exceed 1% in centers providing expertise [2–4]. The relationship between volume of operations and outcome has been extensively examined by Sosa et al. in the State of Maryland [2]. They demonstrated a significant inverse relationship between the volume of thyroidectomies performed by individual surgeons and complication rates, postoperative length of stay, and hospital charges. Surgeons who performed more than 100 thyroidectomies over a 6-year period had the lowest hospital charges, compared with those performing 30–100 cases, 10–29 cases, and between one and nine cases.

17.2   General Complications

Endocrine neck surgery is associated with general non-surgical morbidity in less than 1.5% of patients, corresponding to respiratory (1.5%), urologic (0.9%), gastrointestinal (0.8%), and cardiac (0.5%) complications. In addition, allergy, drug, or other abnormal reactions are reported in 0.4% of patients [2].

17.3   General Surgical Complications

17.3.1   Wound Infection

Wound infections, usually caused by *Staphylococcus* or *Streptococcus* species are considered to be rare events, occurring in 0.3% [5] to 0.8% [2] of cases. Antibiotic prophylaxis is recommended only in immunocompromised patients or in those with valvular cardiac disorders. While mild neck cellulitis frequently regresses under conservative treatment, abscesses require rapid incision and evacuation. Delay of invasive treatment can result in devastating mediastinitis. Clinically evident seromas respond well to percutaneous aspiration.

17.3.2   Edema

Laryngotracheal edema can be a cause of respiratory obstruction after extensive thyroid surgery. After bilateral lymphadenectomy, disturbances of lymphatic flow may be the cause of edema. Pharyngolaryngeal edema, in addition, is a well-recognized complication caused by the endotracheal tube or laryngeal mask and can also occur in association with an anaphylactoid reaction [6]. Steroid therapy, occasionally in combination with temporary reintubation, leads to rapid relief.

17.3.3   Bleeding

The incidence of symptomatic hemorrhage requiring reintervention amounts to 0.1–1.5% [5–9]. Postoperative bleeding will characteristically be prefaced by respiratory distress, pain, or cervical pressure, dysphagia, and increased blood drainage. No specific perioperative risk factors that would allow identification of the high-risk patient population for this potentially lethal complication are known. High surgical volume does not reduce the incidence of hematoma formation. Consequently, the key issue of prevention is attention to anatomic detail and careful hemostasis during surgery. If the surgeon is uncertain about the dryness of the operative field, a Valsalva maneuver, which elevates the intrapulmonary pressure to 40 cm H_2O and facilitates recognition of bleeding vessels, can be performed prior to wound closure. Routine use of suction drains does not prevent postoperative cervical bleeding.

In the majority of patients, symptomatic hemorrhage occurs between 6 and 12 hours after the initial operation. Since in approximately 20% of cases the onset of hematoma symptoms is reported beyond 24 hours postoperatively, ambulatory surgery with a 4- to 8-hour observation period might harbor risk of delayed intervention [7]. Once recognized, the wound should be deliberately reopened and the hematoma evacuated. In case of significant respiratory distress emergency bedside hematoma evacuation, if necessary in combination with endotracheal intubation, is required. The requirement for tracheotomy either in the emergency setting or due to persisting airway obstruction after hematoma removal is generally a rare event.

17.3.4   Malpositioning

The brachial plexus and ulnar nerve may be at risk when a patient is malpositioned on the operating table. In order to avoid nerve paralysis both arms should be adducted and secured. Hyperextension of the head causes nausea and headache during the early postoperative course.

17.4   Specific Surgical Complications

17.4.1   Unilateral Injury to the Recurrent Laryngeal Nerve

Recurrent laryngeal nerve (RLN) injury is one of the most serious complications in endocrine surgery. It is related to significant morbidity and frequent malpractice litigation [10]. The recurrent laryngeal nerve originates from the trunk of the vagus nerve. Upon reaching the larynx, it is renamed the inferior laryngeal nerve. It innervates all the intrinsic muscles of the same side with the exception of the cricothyroid muscles, and supplies sensory innervation to the laryngeal mucosa below the true vocal folds. While ascending, the nerve on the right and on the left side delivers branches that supply the trachea and the esophagus. The morphologic appearance and course of the recurrent laryngeal nerve are subject to great anatomic variability. In addition, it may often be overlooked that the nerve most frequently does not consist only of a single trunk but exhibits a network of smaller branches. On the right side it usually loops around and behind the subclavian artery and then ascends into the neck in the tracheoesophageal groove to enter the larynx distal to the inferior cornu of the thyroid cartilage. In instances of embryologic malformation of the aortic arch in terms of retroesophageal right subclavian artery, the nerve passes with a more median course directly to the larynx (non-recurrent laryngeal nerve) (Fig. 7.4). Although the reported incidence of non-recurrent laryngeal nerve is less than 1%, the surgeon has to be aware of the existence of this rare anatomic condition [11,12]. The left recurrent laryngeal nerve courses upward around the ligamentum arteriosum and the aortic arch and runs vertically toward the tracheoesophageal groove. On their way to the cricothyroid muscle where they enter the larynx, both nerves run close to the capsule of the lateral aspect of the thyroid and cross the inferior thyroid artery. Several variations of the relationship between the nerve and the artery, particularly on the right side, can be observed. The nerve may pass superficially to the artery, deep to it, or between the branches of the vessel (Fig. 17.1). After running into the laryngeal wall the nerve separates into two branches that supply the innervation of various laryngeal muscles, and a third branch that serves as a connection with the superior laryngeal nerve.

During cervical exploration the recurrent laryngeal nerve can be exposed at different levels; caudally, at the crossing with the common carotid artery, in the neighborhood of the inferior thyroid artery, and cranially, at Berry's ligament, a dense condensation of the posterior thyroid capsule near the cricoid cartilage and upper tracheal rings. In addition to visual identification, the nerve can be located by direct palpation of the tracheal wall below the lower thyroid pole. Considerable debate has long existed concerning the necessity of deliberate exposure of the recurrent laryngeal nerve during thyroid surgery. Kocher commented on postoperative hoarseness and stated that, following his technique of thyroid dissection, injury to the nerve can with certainty be avoided without the direct exposure. The first surgeon who advocated routine dissection and demonstration of the nerves in 1911 was August Bier of Berlin; he was followed by Frank Lahey of Boston in 1938 [13]. Others advocated that exposure itself is a risk due to potential induction of local edema by dissection of adjacent tissues and hemorrhage. Following these initial experiences, several studies revealed that depending upon the skill of an individual surgeon principal identification of the nerve reduces the risk of permanent laryngeal nerve injuries from over 5% to less than 1% (Table 17.1) [2,5,14–18]. Nowadays, the practice of visual identification of the nerve represents the gold standard.

To alleviate the visual identification of the nerve and to provide an intraoperative tool to prove its functional integrity, diverse monitoring methods, i.e., intramuscular vocal cord electrodes inserted either through the cricothyroid membrane or placed endoscopically, endotracheal tube surface electrodes, endoscopic visualization of the vocal cords in combination with nerve stimulation [19], and palpation of

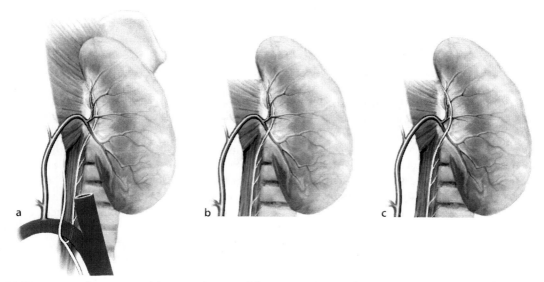

Fig. 17.1 Variations in the anatomy of the cervical course of the recurrent laryngeal nerve. **a** The nerve runs dorsally to the thyroid artery. **b** The nerve passes the vessel between its branches. **c** The nerve passes the vessel superficially to the thyroid artery. With permission of A. Zielke and M. Rothmund, Praxis der Viszeralchirurgie. Endokrine Chirurgie, Springer, 2000

Table 17.1 Incidence of transient and permanent recurrent laryngeal nerve palsy after thyroidectomy in large series. (*RLN* Recurrent laryngeal nerve, *N.R.* not reported)

Author	Publication year	Period	Number of patients	Transient RLN palsy (%)	Permanent RLN palsy (%)
Jatzko [15]	1994	1984–1991	803	3.6	0.5
Wagner [16]	1994	1983–1991	1,026	5.9	2.4
Sosa [2]	1998	1991–1996	5,860	N.R.	0.8
Hermann [14]	2002	1979–1990	9,385	N.R.	3.0
		1991–1998	6,128	N.R.	2.0
		1991	651	N.R.	1.3
Rosato [5]	2004	1995–2000	14,934	2.0	1.0
Goncalves [17]	2005	1990–2000	1,020	1.4	0.4

the cricoarytenoid muscle with simultaneous neural stimulation [20], have been developed. Although intraoperative neuromonitoring might be of use in the presence of extended thyroid surgery, particularly in a patient with a preoperatively documented vocal cord paralysis or in difficult anatomic situations, it does not further reduce the low risk of permanent recurrent nerve lesions and it fails to reliably predict the outcome [21–23]. This experience has been found not only in primary but also in reoperative thyroid and parathyroid procedures [24].

Damage to the recurrent laryngeal nerve may be caused by different mechanisms: cutting, clamping, or stretching of the nerve, nerve skeletonization, local compression of the nerve due to edema or hematoma, or thermal injury by electrocoagulation. Transient cord paresis, which is often caused by edema or axon damage by excessive nerve stretching, seldom lasts more than 4–6 weeks. When no restitution of function is notable within 6–12 months postoperatively, permanent damage should be assumed. Accidental injury to the recurrent laryngeal nerve is not recognized during surgery in most of the cases. If the surgeon is aware of this complication intraoperatively, primarily repair of the nerve using microsurgical techniques and epineural sutures or a cable graft from the greater auricular nerve can be attempted. Even if the nerve is reanastomosed, the dysfunctioning vocal cord will probably never completely recover. Delayed nerve repairs are virtually always ineffective in restoring cord function. When a paralyzed vocal cord stays in the paramedian position the patients frequently remain asymptomatic. This phenomenon is due to compensatory overadduction of the intact cord and consecutive constriction of the glottic chink. The majority of asymptomatic patients need no special treatment but close observation. Unless

routine indirect laryngoscopy or videostroboscopy is performed, many cases of vocal cord paresis will remain unrecognized. The authors recommend preoperative and postoperative laryngoscopic examination of the vocal cord function, not only for medicolegal reasons but also to document potential preexisting pathologies and consecutively adapt the surgical approach. If the paretic cord moves to the lateralized position, hoarseness or aspiration can occur. The prognosis considering gain of normal function is favorable in cases of delayed onset of symptoms. In symptomatic patients either treatment by a speech and language pathologist or invasive interventions such as injection laryngoplasty or medialization laryngoplasty are necessary.

17.4.2 Bilateral Recurrent Laryngeal Nerve Injury

This serious complication results in a near midline position of the vocal cords and variable degrees of airway obstruction. As reported by Rosato et al., diplegia may occur in 0.4% of bilateral thyroidectomies [5]. Commonly, it will be diagnosed directly after extubation or during the early postoperative phase. The patient should be reintubated without delay and treated systemically with corticosteroids. In the presence of reversible nerve injury, extubation under controlled conditions is feasible in most cases after 24–72 hours and no further treatment is necessary. In case of persisting respiratory obstruction, reintubation and a tracheostomy must be carried out immediately. If the vocal cords fail to recuperate after a waiting period of 9–12 months, tracheostomy remains as a permanent solution or transverse laser cordotomy is performed [25].

17.4.3 Injury to the Superior Laryngeal Nerve

Although the risk of injury to the superior laryngeal nerve during thyroid surgery is significant, this complication is less reported, probably because of the difficulty to asses its manifestation [26]. Laryngeal electromyography provides the most accurate diagnosis. The superior laryngeal nerve separates from the main trunk of the vagus nerve outside the jugular foramen. It passes anteromedially on the thyrohyoid membrane where it is joined by the superior thyroid artery and vein. At about the level of the hyoid bone it divides into two branches. The external laryngeal nerve innervates the cricothyroid muscle and the internal branch provides sensory innervation of the supraglottic larynx. The internal laryngeal nerve separates into three branches that communicate with the recurrent laryngeal nerve posterior to the cricoid cartilage. Injuries to the internal branch are rare during thyroid or parathyroid surgery. The most common position of the external branch in relation to the superior thyroid artery is medial to it (Fig. 17.2). In about 20–30% of cases the nerve crosses the upper thyroid vessels below the upper border of the superior thyroid pole. This condition places the nerve at high risk of damage during mobilization and division of the superior thyroid vessels [27]. In order to avoid damage during ligation of the superior thyroid pedicle, meticulous dissection of the adventitial tissue between the upper thyroid pole, which should be retracted laterally, and the laryngeal wall is necessary. Electrocautery should be omitted if bleeding within the cricothyroid muscle occurs. Neuromonitoring may facilitate the identification of the nerve. Since the cricothyroid muscle is a tensor of the vocal cord, injury to the external branch of the superior laryngeal nerve often results in detrimental voice changes and inability to perform high-pitch phonation. For those patients who rely on their voice quality professionally this may be of essential consequence.

It should be pointed out that not every vocal cord dysfunction following thyroid or parathyroid surgery is caused by the surgical procedure itself. Most probably, 0.3% of patients exhibit laryngeal injury as a result of the intubation technique or use of the laryngeal mask [28].

17.4.4 Rare Neural, Vascular, and Visceral Lesions

The cervical sympathetic trunk is injured on rare occasions (1:5,000 cases) when for instance a retroesophageal extension of a goiter is being dissected [29]. Therefore, care should be taken over the prespinal surface when mobilizing the carotid sheath. Injury to the cervical sympathetic trunk causes Horner's syndrome, characterized by a constricted pupil, drooping eyelid, and facial dryness.

Damage to the phrenic nerves, inducing hemidiaphragmatic elevation, or to the spinal accessory nerve, causing dropping of the shoulder, muscle atrophy, and weakened or limited elevation of the arm and shoulder, can occur during lymph node dissection for thyroid carcinoma. These rare injuries may especially occur after extensive cervical lymphadenectomy. In the presence of a large substernal goiter or mediastinal lymph node metastases which necessitate dissection toward the upper thoracic aperture,

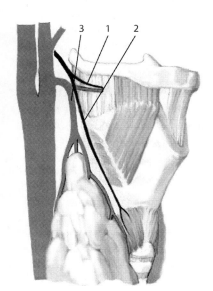 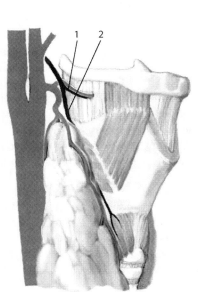

Fig. 17.2 Most common variations of the external branch of the superior laryngeal nerve. *1* Internal branch of the superior laryngeal nerve, *2* external branch of the superior laryngeal nerve, *3* superior thyroid artery. With permission of A. Zielke and M. Rothmund, Praxis der Viszeralchirurgie. Endokrine Chirurgie, Springer, 2000

complications such as pneumothorax or transection of the subclavian artery or vein can occur. Clinically significant pneumothoraces require air evacuation via an inserted needle or placement of a thoracic drain.

The carotid artery is rarely at risk during thyroidectomy, although excessive lateral retraction of a diseased artery with arteriosclerosis during mobilization of an enlarged thyroid gland may injure the vessel wall or damage the blood flow to the cerebrum. This complication is avoidable if assistants are carefully instructed by the surgeon with regard to the handling of retractors. Arteriovenous fistula may occur at superior pole vessels. This complication can be prevented by ligating the superior pole vessels at the end of the surgery and by isolating arteries and veins and ligating them independently. This maneuver also helps in the prevention of injury to the external branch of the superior laryngeal nerve.

In the course of surgery for extended thyroid disease, injury to the anterolateral esophageal wall can be observed occasionally. This risk is greater if the surgeon has difficulty locating the recurrent laryngeal nerve in the presence of an altered anatomy which can occur in large multinodular goiters. The management of this rare condition includes direct suturing and total parenteral nutrition (TPN) for 2–3 days.

17.4.5   Tracheal Instability

Tracheomalacia resulting in tracheal collapse rarely occurs after removal of a large goiter. In such an event, endoluminal stenting in order to regain tracheal stability may be necessary. External splinting by custommade rings or Marlex mesh has also been tried. However, tracheostomy remains the ultimate treatment if the above-mentioned measures fail.

17.4.6   Injury to the Lymphatic Structures

Patients in whom lymph node dissection is a component of thyroid surgery are at risk for injury to the thoracic duct on the left side and to the lymphatic duct on the right side. Development of chyloma is the hallmark of this complication. If the injury is evident during surgery, ligation of the duct should be performed. In cases of delayed diagnosis a conservative management by continuous drainage and reduction of chyle production by TPN or by oral administration of a low fat, high carbohydrate, and high protein diet may be carried out. In our experience additional systemic administration of somatostatin proved extremely efficient. If the chyle leak persists, surgical correction with an aim to ligate the fistula should be considered.

17.4.7   Hypoparathyroidism

The reported rate of hypocalcemia after thyroid surgery varies from 1% to over 50% [29–31]. While the majority of instances of postoperative hypocalcemia are transient, permanent hypoparathyroidism is decidedly unusual and should amount to less than 1%. Although the pathogenesis of postthyroidectomy hypocalcemia is multifactorial, damage to the parathyroid glands in the form of direct injury, unrecognized inadvertent removal, or indirectly by devascularization of the gland are the most common causes. Other causative factors are negative calcium balance due to calcium absorption by bones in repair of osteodystrophy in hyperthyroid patients, decreased serum albumin levels caused by hemodilution, increased secretion of calcitonin during thyroid mobilization, or conditions associated with increased renal excretion of calcium [32].

Knowledge of the specific anatomic details and meticulous surgical technique are prerequisite conditions for successful restriction of the risk of hypocalcemia. The superior parathyroid glands are derived from the fourth branchial pouch and descend along the posterior surface of the upper thyroid pole toward the inferior thyroid artery. Usually, the gland lies laterally to the recurrent laryngeal nerve. The inferior parathyroid glands, derived from the third branchial pouch, migrate along the lower thyroid pole toward the mediastinum in close relation to the thyrothymic pole. In the majority of cases they can be found superficially to the recurrent laryngeal nerve below the crossing of the nerve with the inferior thyroid artery. Although the number and localization of the parathyroid glands may vary, symmetric position, particularly of the superior glands, can be expected in the majority of patients. The arterial blood supply to the parathyroid glands is provided by a single terminal artery in 80% of cases. In 20%, two to four separate arteries can be found. Most frequently superior and inferior glands are supplied by the inferior thyroid artery. To preserve the blood supply to the parathyroid glands during thyroid resection, the technique of individual ligation of peripheral branches of the inferior thyroid artery rather than ligation of the main trunk of the vessel should be followed. In 15% of patients, the superior parathyroid gland may receive its blood from the superior thyroid artery and in 10% an anastomotic communication of both systems can be found.

A controversial debate exists about the number of parathyroid glands that should be identified and preserved during thyroid surgery in order to avoid postoperative hypocalcemia. While some argue that preservation of a singular intact parathyroid gland is sufficient for normal homeostasis, others recommend the identification and in situ preservation of at least three glands [33]. If it becomes evident that a safe dissection of a parathyroid gland is technically not feasible or that its viability has been compromised, the gland should be removed from the thyroid capsule, cut into small fragments, and implanted into a muscle pocket in the sternocleidomastoid muscle (orthotopic autotransplantation). The site of autotransplantation should be marked in case the tissue transplanted subsequently becomes pathologic. With an exception of one older report [34], several studies reported a decrease of the risk of permanent hypoparathyroidism to less than 1% when this approach is practiced [35,36]. Biopsies of normal parathyroid glands should be omitted during thyroid procedures since they contribute significantly to postoperative parathyroid dysfunction.

A mild case of postoperative hypocalcemia is self-limiting and may not be recognized unless routine calcium determination is carried out. Nevertheless we would recommend measurement of serum calcium levels routinely in every patient prior to and after bilateral thyroid surgery. After an uncomplicated unilateral thyroid resection, hypocalcemia will virtually never be observed. Recently it was shown that intraoperative parathyroid hormone (PTH) determination allows prediction of postoperative hypocalcemia (PTH <10 pg/ml) and the necessity of early vitamin D supplementation in order to reduce the risk of postoperative symptomatic hypocalcemia [37]. Intraoperative PTH monitoring facilitates early discharge and reduces the costs of following up postoperative serum calcium levels. Patients exhibiting clinical signs of hypocalcemia, such as circumoral or acral paresthesia, muscle cramps, or numbness of the hands and feet, may be orally treated with calcium carbonate or calcium lactate in divided doses to a total of 2–8 g per day. Additionally, calciferol or dihydrotachysterol may be required in order to enhance calcium absorption. After normalization of serum calcium levels, oral calcium therapy is continued until stabilization of calcium homeostasis is achieved. Severe symptoms require immediate intravenous therapy with 10 ml 10% calcium gluconate over 3–5 minutes and subsequent continuous infusion of 0.9% saline containing 30–40 ml 10% calcium gluconate per 24 hours. Permanent hypocalcemia (more than 6 months postoperatively) is a major concern since it may be associated with significant impairment of life quality, chronic gastrointestinal discomfort, changes in bone metabolism, and development of cataracts. Single reports on heterologous transplantation of parathyroid tissue after microencapsulation with amitogenic alginate exist, however, reliable clinical systems are not yet widely available [38].

17.4.8 Thyroid Storm

Postoperative thyroid crisis as a complication of thyroidectomy was once fairly common, but is now rarely seen. At the beginning of this century, the mortality from thyroidectomy in patients with toxic goiter was at least 5% due to the frequent occurrence of thyroid crisis after goiter resection. The symptoms that may be seen are tachycardia, fever, nausea and vomiting, restlessness, mental stimulation, and frequently coma. Today, no patient should be subjected to elective thyroid surgery if not euthyroid, either as a result of his or her own thyroid function or after appropriate preoperative medical treatment. Medical therapy includes antithyroid drugs (propylthiouracil, metimazole), β-adrenergic blockers (propranolol), and administration of iodine (saturated solution of potassium iodide).

References

1. Becker WF (1977) Pioneers in thyroid surgery. Ann Surg 185:493–504
2. Sosa JA, et al (1998) The importance of surgeon experience for clinical and economic outcomes from thyroidectomy. Ann Surg 228:320–330
3. Rios-Zambudio A, et al (2004) Prospective study of postoperative complications after total thyroidectomy for multinodular goiters by surgeons with experience in endocrine surgery. Ann Surg 240:18–27
4. Udelsman R, et al (2004) Experience counts. Ann Surg 240:26–27
5. Rosato L, et al (2004) Complications of thyroid surgery: analysis of a multicentric study on 14,934 patients operated on in Italy over 5 years. World J Surg 28:271–276
6. Lacoste L, et al (1993) Airway complications in thyroid surgery. Ann Otol Rhinol Laryngol 102:441–446
7. Burkey SH, et al (2001) Reexploration for symptomatic hematomas after cervical exploration. Surgery 130:914–920
8. Shaha AR (1994) Practical management of postthyroidectomy hematoma. J Surg Oncol 57:235–238
9. Bergamaschi R (1998) Morbidity of thyroid surgery. Am J Surg 176:71–75

10. Kern KA (1993) Medicolegal analysis of errors in diagnosis and treatment of surgical endocrine disease. Surgery 114:1167–1173

11. Mra Z, Wax MK (1999) Nonrecurrent laryngeal nerves: anatomic considerations during thyroid and parathyroid surgery. Am J Otolarnyngol 20:91–95

12. Henry JF, Audiffret J, Denizot A (1988) The non recurrent inferior laryngeal nerve: review of 33 cases including two on the left side. Surgery 104:977–984

13. Lahey FH (1958) Routine dissection and demonstration of the recurrent laryngeal nerve in subtotal thyroidectomy. Surg Gynecol Obstet 66:775–777

14. Hermann M, et al (2002) Laryngeal recurrent nerve injury in surgery for benign thyroid diseases: effect of nerve dissection and impact of individual surgeon in more than 27,000 nerves at risk. Ann Surg 235:261–268

15. Jatzko GR, et al (1994) Recurrent nerve palsy after thyroid operations: principal nerve identification and a literature review. Surgery 115:139–144

16. Wagner HE, Seiler C (1994) Recurrent laryngeal nerve palsy after thyroid gland surgery.Br J Surg 81:226–228

17. Goncalves Filho J, Kowalski LP (2005) Surgical complications after thyroid surgery performed in a cancer hospital. Otolaryngol Head Neck Surg 132:490–494

18. Steurer M, et al (2002) Advantages of recurrent laryngeal nerve identification in thyroidectomy and parathyroidectomy and the importance of preoperative and postoperative laryngoscopic examination in more than 1000 nerves at risk. Laryngoscope 112:124–133

19. Hillermann CL, Tarpey J, Phillips DE (2003) Laryngeal nerve identification during thyroid surgery: feasibility of a novel approach. Can J Anaesth 50:189–192

20. Randolph GW, et al (2004) Recurrent laryngeal nerve identification and assessment during thyroid surgery: laryngeal palpation. World J Surg 28:755–760

21. Beldi G, Kinsbergen T, Schlumpf R (2004) Evaluation of intraoperative recurrent nerve monitoring in thyroid surgery. World J Surg 28:589–591

22. Hermann M, Hellebart C, Freissmuth M (2004) Neuromonitoring in thyroid surgery: prospective evaluation of intraoperative electrophysiological responses for the prediction of recurrent laryngeal nerve injury. Ann Surg 240:9–17

23. Dralle H, et al (2004) Risk factors of paralysis and functional outcome after recurrent laryngeal nerve monitoring in thyroid surgery. Surgery 136:1310–1322

24. Yarbrough DE, et al (2004) Intraoperative electromyographic monitoring of the recurrent laryngeal nerve in reoperative thyroid and parathyroid surgery. Surgery 136:1107–1115

25. Fewins J, Simpson CB, Miller FR (2003) Complications of thyroid and parathyroid surgery. Otolarnygol Clin N Am 36:189–206

26. Friedman M, LoSavio P, Ibrahim H (2002) Superior laryngeal nerve identification and preservation in thyroidectomy. Arch Otolaryngol Head Neck Surg 128:296–303

27. Cernea CR, et al (1992) Surgical anatomy of the external branch of the superior laryngeal nerve. Head Neck 14:380–383

28. Peppard SB, Dickens JH (1983) Laryngeal injury following short-term intubation. Ann Otol Rhinol Laryngol 92:327–330

29. Reeve T, Thompson NW (2000) Complications of thyroid surgery: how to avoid them, how to manage them, and observations of their possible effect on the whole patient. World J Surg 24:971–975

30. Harness JK, et al (2000) Future of thyroid surgery and training surgeons to meet the expectations of 2000 and beyond. World J Surg 24:976–982

31. Ozbas S, et al (2005) Comparison of the complications of subtotal, near total and total thyroidectomy in the surgical management of multinodular goitre. Endocr J 52:199–205

32. McHenry CR, et al (1994) Risk factors for postthyroidectomy hypocalcemia. Surgery 116:641–648

33. Pattou F, et al (1998) Hypocalcemia following thyroid surgery: incidence and prediction of outcome. World J Surg 22:718–724

34. Öhman U, et al (1978) Function of the parathyroid glands after total thyroidectomy. Surg Gynecol Obstet 146:773–778

35. Shaha AR, et al (1991) Parathyroid autotransplantation during thyroid surgery. J Surg Oncol 46:21–24

36. Olson JA, et al (1996) Parathyroid autotransplantation during thyroidectomy. Results of long-term follow-up. Ann Surg 223:472–480

37. Quiros RM, et al (2005) Intraoperative parathyroid hormone levels in thyroid surgery are predictive of postoperative hypoparathyroidism and need for vitamin D supplementation. Am J Surg 189:306–309

38. Hasse C, et al (2000) Parathyroid xenotransplantation without immunosuppression in experimental hypoparathyroidism: long-term in vivo function following microencapsulation with clinically suitable alginate. World J Surg 24:1361–1366

18 Outcomes Analysis in Thyroid Surgery: A Review of Patient and Provider Predictors

Kate V. Viola and Julie Ann Sosa

CONTENTS

18.1   Introduction

There has been a litany of large, population-based studies over the last decade demonstrating in a consistent fashion that clinical and economic outcomes from a number of surgical procedures are superior at hospitals that perform these procedures in high volumes [1,2,3]. This "volume-outcomes" relationship is most compelling for cardiovascular operations [e.g., coronary artery bypass graft surgery (CABG), abdominal aortic aneurysm repair] and major cancer resections (e.g., pancreatic cancer resection, esophagectomy). In a 2002 study that captured 2.5 million procedures over a six-year period using the Nationwide Inpatient Sample and the Medicare claims database, operative mortality decreased as hospital volume increased for 14 types of procedures; absolute differences in adjusted mortality rates between very low volume and very high volume hospitals ranged from over 12% for pancreatic resection to 0.2% for carotid endarterectomy [4].

These kinds of reviews suggest that thousands of preventable surgical deaths occur each year in the USA because elective surgery is performed in hospitals that have inadequate experience. As a result, efforts are underway to concentrate certain high-risk operations in centers likely to have better results. The most visible employer-led endeavor has been the Leapfrog Group, a coalition of more than 150 public and private health care purchasers representing over 40 million people, which in 2001 began "value-based purchasing"; that is, leveraging large payers to encourage improvements in surgical quality by directing patient referrals to hospitals that meet minimum-volume standards. Birkmeyer et al. assessed the potential benefits of utilizing the Leapfrog initiative and concluded that institution of these initiatives by employers and healthcare purchasers could prevent many surgical deaths by requiring hospital volume standards for high-risk procedures [5,6].

There is a paucity of objective evidence outside of clinical series published by endocrine surgeons to support a consistent association between surgeon or hospital experience and patient outcomes from thyroidectomy. Unlike pancreatic resections and other high-risk operations on older patients with mortal diseases and multiple comorbidities, thyroidectomy is rarely associated with mortality, and the incidence of complications such as recurrent laryngeal nerve injury, hypoparathyroidism, and neck hematoma is low. Patients with thyroid disease are generally young and middle-aged women with few other medical problems that might increase the risk of poor outcomes. The diagnosis of postoperative complications is often delayed until after discharge, and can therefore not be ascertained from most administrative databases as they capture inpatient data only. There is no benchmark for comparison that represents the outcomes of thyroid patients operated on by community surgeons. In addition, much of the evidence is contradictory; some small series have suggested that low-volume surgeons, well-supervised surgical trainees, and surgeons at community hospitals can obtain excellent clinical outcomes [7].

18.2   History

Theodor Billroth (1829–1894) is considered the premier surgeon of the nineteenth century having performed the first laryngectomy, the first total esophagectomy, the first gastrectomy, and the first pancreatectomy for cancer. He was also one of the most prolific medical authors of his time [8]. Billroth performed his first 20 thyroidectomies at the University of Zurich, a highly endemic goiter region. Without adequate hemostats, artery forceps, antiseptics, and minimal anesthesia, Billroth's mortality rate was 40%. Billroth was discouraged by these early outcomes and abandoned thyroid surgery for over a decade. With the development of anesthesia, antisepsis, and artery forceps, Billroth performed a subsequent 48 thyroidectomies with a mortality rate of 8.3%. Perhaps the best evidence to date for an association between provider volume and patient outcomes is over 150 years old.

Theodor Kocher (1841–1917) was the first high-volume thyroid surgeon, and his career provided early evidence supporting a relation between surgeon experience and clinical outcomes from thyroidectomy. Kocher was the "Father of Thyroid Surgery," and he was the first surgeon to receive the Nobel Prize in Medicine in 1909 for "his work in physiology, pathology, and surgery on the thyroid gland." In an era when the mortality rate for thyroid surgery was approximately 40%, Kocher was able to reduce his mortality rate from 12.8% after his first 101 thyroidectomies to 0.5% after 5,000 operations (Fig. 18.1).

Charles Mayo (1863–1939) is referred to as the "Father of American Thyroid Surgery" and probably represents the first high-volume American endocrine surgeon. He was the first to use the term "hyperthyroidism," and he improved outcomes from thyroidectomy by teaching preservation of the parathyroid glands and division of the strap muscles to afford better exposure of neck anatomy. George Crile (1864–1943) in Cleveland improved outcomes by performing the first subtotal thyroidectomy, by which he left a margin of thyroid behind in order to protect the recurrent laryngeal nerve and parathyroid glands and preserve enough native thyroid function to avoid myxedema [9]. Crile performed over 5,000 thyroid surgeries with a 1% mortality rate. The last turn of the century high-volume American thyroid surgeon was Frank Lahey (1880–1953), who pioneered use of the basal metabolic rate (BMR) as a criterion for surgery for hyperthyroidism and meticulous preservation of the recurrent laryngeal nerve.

18.3   Clinical Outcomes from Thyroidectomy

In the modern era, mortality is an extremely rare outcome following thyroidectomy; it approaches 0% in the largest clinical series. Rare sequelae following thyroidectomy include recurrent or superior laryngeal

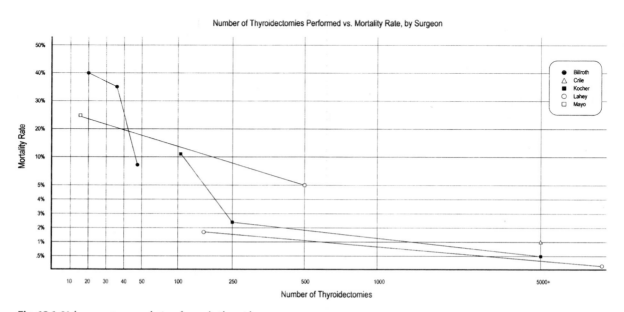

Fig. 18.1 Volume outcome relation for early thyroid surgeons

nerve injury, hypoparathyroidism, thyroid storm, hemorrhage, wound complications, and more generic complications, such as urinary tract infection or upper respiratory tract infection.

Early vocal changes following thyroidectomy are common. In a 2002 study presented at the American Head and Neck Society annual meeting, Stojadinovic et al. demonstrated that 30% of patients are likely to report early subjective voice changes, while 14% reported late (3-month) subjective voice changes [10]. Voice changes following thyroidectomy were also demonstrated in cases where the laryngeal nerves were preserved; surgical trauma and/or laryngotracheal fixation of the prelaryngeal strap musculature produced voice disturbances. Unilateral injury to the recurrent laryngeal nerve results in hoarseness and is diagnosed with indirect laryngoscopy; bilateral injury leads to airway compromise requiring reintubation and temporary versus permanent tracheostomy. Neurapraxia resolves in weeks to months, while paralysis is permanent.

A recent comprehensive study of thyroid surgery complications was completed by Rosato et al. [11]. It analyzed complications following 14,934 thyroid surgeries over a five-year period (1995–2000). Recurrent laryngeal nerve injury occurred in 3.4% of all patients undergoing thyroid surgery (22% of total complications), with a 4.3% incidence of unilateral injury and 0.6% incidence of bilateral nerve injury in total thyroidectomies, 2.0% in lobectomy, 3.0% of subtotal thyroidectomies with a unilateral remnant, and 2.0% of subtotal thyroidectomies with bilateral remnants. Among patients with thyroid cancer undergoing thyroidectomy, the incidence of recurrent laryngeal nerve injury was 5.7%. Routine identification of the recurrent laryngeal nerve during thyroidectomy markedly reduces the incidence of permanent injury. Superior laryngeal nerve injury (0.4–3.7%) is difficult to diagnose and is probably reported less frequently, as change in pitch after surgery can be subtle. Injury manifests as a lowered voice tone, vocal fatigue, and difficult singing note intonation. Seventy years ago, the famous opera singer Amelita Galli-Curci underwent thyroid surgery for a goiter; she sustained a superior laryngeal nerve injury, which led to the demise of her career. Recently, several instrumental set-ups (e.g., Neurosign; Indomed, Teningen, Germany) have become commercially available, and neuromonitoring has gained some popularity. However, in a recent series of 328 patients reported by Hermann et al., the utility of neuromonitoring in the setting of difficult surgery when the device would be most useful was shown to be lacking. In reoperations, the sensitivity of

the Neurosign device dropped to less than 60% even in benign disease (and 25% in malignant disease), and the negative predictive value of 95.9% to 91.9% in high-risk groups instilled a false sense of security [12]. This adjunct is not a substitute for surgical experience and routine identification of the recurrent laryngeal nerves.

Hypoparathyroidism resulting in hypocalcemia, the most frequent complication of thyroidectomy, may be permanent or transient. It arises when the parathyroids are removed or the vascular supply (inferior thyroid artery) is disrupted. Rosato et al. reported that symptomatic hypocalcemia represented 63% of all complications in the study [11]. It occurred in 10.0% (8.3% transient, 1.7% definitive) of patients following thyroid surgery; its incidence was 0.4% following lobectomy, 14.0% after total thyroidectomy (2.2% permanent), and 5.0% following subtotal thyroidectomy. The incidence of permanent hypocalcemia in thyroid cancer surgery is considerably higher (3.3%) compared with operations for benign disease, as total thyroidectomy is usually required with or without central compartment lymphadenectomy. Treatment includes calcium supplements (temporary or permanent), with or without vitamin D supplementation.

Thyroid storm is a very rare but potentially fatal complication of thyroid surgery. Medical treatment with thionamides and beta-blockers prior to surgery in patients with thyrotoxicosis has dramatically decreased the incidence of perioperative thyroid storm. Thyroid storm is treated with high-dose thioureas (propylthiouracil 200 mg every 6 hours) and aggressive supportive care. Heart rate should be closely monitored, and beta-blockers may be administered. In addition, prednisone, which inhibits conversion of thyroxine, may be given.

Wound complications including neck hematoma, infection, seroma, and necrosis of skin flaps are rare. Careful planning of skin incisions and wound closure, occasional use of prophylactic antibiotics in high-risk patients, and suction drainage in cases of increased vascularity (Graves' disease) decreases the probability of wound complications. If necessary, emergency evacuation of hematoma or aspiration of seroma must be performed.

18.4 Economic Outcomes from Thyroidectomy

Data about economic outcomes from thyroidectomy, including length of hospital stay (LOS) and cost, are scarce. Over the last decade, payers have pressed thyroid surgeons to reduce routine hospitalization following thyroidectomy from 72 to 48 hours to the ambulatory setting or a 23-hour observation period with an overnight hospital stay and early morning discharge. A longer LOS had been advocated to monitor the neck for postoperative bleeding and serum calcium levels in order to diagnose and treat hypocalcemia and prevent potential life-threatening sequelae such as tetany, seizures, and laryngospasm. However, more recent data have shown that "same-day" thyroid surgery can be safe and cost-effective. In a retrospective review of 71 patients over a four-year period that underwent thyroidectomy for nodular thyroid disease, McHenry showed a 1.2% incidence of neck hematoma which is comparable to the 0.4% to 3.0% incidence reported in the literature [13]. There was a 10% incidence of transient symptomatic hypocalcemia in the series, but it was effectively treated on an outpatient basis with no adverse sequelae. The net cost savings was an estimated $79,000 to $108,500 for the 71 patients who underwent same-day thyroid surgery [13]. Lo Gerfo from Columbia University concurred that outpatient surgery for thyroidectomy is medically safe and well-accepted by patients but requires surgical expertise, close supervision, open communication, and an educated patient [14]. In spite of these data, one can challenge the true cost savings if even 1% of patients develop a neck hematoma and a compromised airway that could be managed far more expeditiously in the hospitalized patient.

18.5 Patient Characteristics Predictive of Outcome

18.5.1 Demographic Characteristics

Prevalence of thyroid disease increases significantly with age. In particular, the incidence of poorly differentiated and undifferentiated (i.e., anaplastic) thyroid cancers rises among the elderly. In addition, the prognosis of well-differentiated thyroid cancers (i.e. papillary and follicular malignancies) is worse in elderly patients; according to the AGES (Age, Grade, Extent, Size) or AMES (Age, Metastases, Extent, Size) classification systems, women older than 50 years and men older than 40 years are at higher long-term risk of disease recurrence and death from their thyroid cancer.

Although age alone is rarely a contraindication for major surgery if adjustment is made for comorbid conditions, the willingness of physicians to refer patients for elective surgery diminishes with increasing patient age [15]. With increasing age, morbidity and mortality after surgery also increase. The 30-day mortality rates following elective general surgical and orthopedic procedures are between 5.8 and 9%. [15]. However, in the short term, age alone should not be used as a contraindication to elective thyroid surgery, as a large body of data suggest that patients 75 years or older can tolerate surgery with low morbidity [16,17]. In a large retrospective analysis of 738 patients who underwent thyroid surgery over a five-year period at a busy university hospital center, the mortality rates for patients ≥75 years and <75 years were the same, 0%. The frequency of early, postoperative complications was also similar in the two age groups (21.8% in younger patients, 25.5% in the geriatric group); the rates of permanent complications were statistically similar as well (1.9% and 3.6%, respectively).

18.5.2 Clinical Characteristics

New procedural approaches to improve the outcome of thyroidectomy have included the use of loupe magnification and utilization of local/regional anesthesia as an alternative to general anesthesia. Testini et al. studied a group of 97 patients to substantiate the use of loupe magnification in improving outcomes after total thyroidectomy by allowing for careful isolation of recurrent laryngeal nerves, parathyroid glands, and branches of the thyroid artery [18]. The patients were randomly assigned to two groups, with one group having thyroidectomy by a surgeon utilizing 2.5× magnification and microsurgical instruments in the procedure, and the other group undergoing thyroidectomy by the same surgeon utilizing no magnification. Total clinical complications (transient and permanent hypoparathyroidism, transient and permanent recurrent laryngeal nerve lesions, hematoma) in patients following thyroidectomy in the group utilizing loupe magnification was 4.3%, while the group utilizing no magnification was 24%, a statistically significant and clinically relevant difference. Additionally, the researchers noted a significant reduction in operative time while using loupe magnification for the identification of the recurrent laryngeal nerves.

The principle advantage of regional anesthesia is avoidance of nausea, vomiting, and postoperative disorientation that is commonly associated with general anesthesia. Patients' desire to avoid general anesthesia and economic pressures have sparked a renewed interest in performing thyroid operations under regional anesthesia. Specht et al. studied 58 patients who underwent thyroid surgery under local anesthesia and compared outcomes with 116 who had thyroid-ectomy under general anesthesia [19]. Characteristics including patient age, gender, tumor pathology, and anesthesia were analyzed. Rates of complications were similar for local anesthesia and general endotracheal intubation groups. Results indicated that local anesthesia was a safe alternative to general endotracheal intubation. Additionally, regional anesthesia resulted in a decreased length of hospital stay, in that 19% of patients given local anesthesia were discharged the day of the operation, compared with only 2% of patients undergoing general anesthesia. It is important to note that the study concluded that obese patients [defined as body mass index (BMI) greater than 27 for men and 30 for women] were not ideal candidates for local anesthesia because difficulty breathing and lower back pain were exacerbated while they were supine. In addition, operative time is longer in obese patients because the dissection of the thyroid is a greater challenge. The mean total operative time (± standard deviation) in an obese patient was 242 minutes ± 64 minutes, while in non-obese patients the mean operative time was 200 minutes ± 54 minutes ($P<0.001$).

Lo Gerfo evaluated 203 patients during a nine-year period that underwent thyroid surgery with regional anesthesia [20]. Surprisingly, he demonstrated that operative times increased 25% with the use of regional anesthesia. It is possible that surgeons were more cautious in their operative approach because of concerns about inducing pain, particularly during the mobilization of the superior pole vessels. However, Lo Gerfo also noted that the number of patients choosing local anesthesia increased during the study period; both confidence of the endocrine surgeon in using regional anesthesia and patient preference, primarily though referral patterns, played a role in the choice of anesthesia. Ninety-five percent of patients rated the level of pain equivalent or less severe than dental procedures, and 100% of patients reported they would choose regional anesthesia again. Lo Gerfo, who performed over 2,500 thyroid/parathyroid procedures over a 20-year period, also noted that the key to providing a good anesthetic block by the surgeon was to give the regional block before scrubbing for the procedure, thus allowing approximately 10 minutes for it to take effect. These data suggest that thyroidectomy can be performed with local or regional anesthesia, and this is associated with low morbidity, high patient satisfaction, and a shorter discharge time.

18.6 Provider Characteristics Predictive of Outcome

18.6.1 Surgeon Experience

The relationship between volume of operations performed by surgeons and outcomes has been examined for thyroid surgery, but not to the extent of some other operations. Sosa et al. demonstrated a significant inverse relationship between the volume of thyroidectomies performed by individual surgeons in Maryland and complication rates, postoperative length of stay, and hospital charges [21]. In this cross-sectional analysis of all patients who underwent thyroidectomy in Maryland between 1991 and 1996, the experiences of 5,860 patients and 658 surgeons were analyzed in 52 non-federal acute care hospitals. Surgeons included in the study performed a median of 25 thyroidectomies (range, 4–98), but nearly two thirds of the surgeons performed less than one thyroidectomy, on average, per year.

Surgeons performing 100 or more thyroidectomies over a six-year period had the lowest complication rate, the shortest hospital stay, and the lowest hospital charges compared with surgeons performing 30–100 cases, 10–29 cases, and between one and nine cases (Table 18.1). Hospital volume, in contrast to surgeon volume, had no consistent association with patient outcomes. A subgroup analysis of the surgeons with operating privileges at more than one hospital demonstrated that patients' length of stay was associated with the volume of the surgeon's thyroid practice rather than the number of procedures done at the hospital where the procedure was performed; as volume increased among surgeons operating at multiple hospitals, length of stay decreased, controlling for hospital volume. The results of the study suggested that more than 20% of the complications and 1,700 hospital days could have been saved if high-volume surgeons performed all thyroidectomies. Directing more patients toward high-volume thyroid surgeons should result in fewer adverse surgical outcomes.

In addition to surgeon caseload, patient diagnosis and procedure were associated with clinical and economic outcomes. Patients with thyroid cancer and patients who underwent total or substernal thyroidectomy also had worse outcomes than similar patients with benign diagnoses who underwent less extensive operations; recurrent laryngeal nerve injury was most common in thyroid cancer patients after substernal thyroidectomy (4.6%) and total thyroidectomy (1.1%). The high-volume surgeons had one third fewer complications from thyroidectomy performed for benign disease, and two thirds fewer complications from thyroid surgery performed for cancer, than surgeons who performed between one and nine thyroidectomies during the study period (Table 18.2). Sosa et al. provided compelling evidence for a significant association between increased surgeon volume and improved patient outcomes following surgical procedures for both benign and malignant thyroid disease [21]. The referral of patients for thyroidectomy to high-volume surgeons is especially convincing for patients with known or suspected thyroid cancer or patients for whom a near-total or total thyroidectomy is the procedure of choice. This is consistent with many other reports providing evidence that regionalization is particularly beneficial for high-risk operations. In a recent editorial, Udelsman reinforced the clear association between surgeon experience and the decrease in complication rates following thyroidectomy; the author stressed that judgment, meticulous technique, and adequate training are the hallmarks required for success [22].

Table 18.1 Unadjusted and adjusted clinical and economic outcomes from thyroidectomy by surgeon volume (number of cases). Adjusted for patient age, race, comorbidities, insurance status, diagnosis, procedure, hospital volume, and time period using the Charlson comorbidity index

	Number of cases			
	1–9	10–29	30–100	>100
Complication rate				
Unadjusted (%)	10.1 *	6.7 *	6.9 *	5.9
Adjusted (%)	8.6 *	6.1 *	6.1 *	5.1
Length of stay				
Unadjusted (days)	2.8 **	2.1 **	2.2 **	1.7
Adjusted (days)	1.9 **	1.7 **	1.7 **	1.4
Hospital charges				
Unadjusted ($)	5,078 *	4,084 *	4,016 *	4,777
Adjusted ($)	3,901	3,693 *	3,585 *	3,950

* $P<0.001$ compared to group with >100 cases
** $P<0.05$ compared to group with >100 cases

Table 18.2 Factors associated with outcomes from thyroidectomy

Factor	Complication rate[a] (%)	Length of stay (days)	Charges ($)
Patient age			
<70 years	6.3	1.7	3,697
≥70 years	10.3	2.0	4,195
Diagnosis			
Adenoma	4.8	1.6	3,496
Other benign	6.6	1.7	3,733
Cancer	8.1	1.9	4,029
Procedure			
Lobectomy	5.8	1.6	3,503
Other subtotal	6.0	1.7	3,597
Total thyroidectomy	8.4	2.0	4,534
Substernal thyroidectomy	10.8	2.2	4,461

[a] Complications included all medical and surgical problems occurring in hospital after surgery (i.e., hypoparathyroidism, nerve injury, wound infection and hematoma, cardiac, respiratory, and urologic morbidity)

18.6.2   Surgeon Training and Specialty

Other studies have provided contradictory evidence assessing factors related to surgeon experience and thyroidectomy volume, including surgical training and specialty. Certainly, there is a great deal of variation in experience with thyroidectomy among graduating chief residents in accredited general surgery programs in the USA. In accordance with the Accreditation Council for Graduate Medical Education, there is no specific minimum number of thyroidectomies required to graduate from a general surgery residency program. In the 2004 academic year, the national average of endocrine cases completed by graduating categorical general surgery chief residents was 29.4, of which 19 on average were thyroid procedures. In 1993–1994, six graduating chief residents had zero experience with thyroidectomy, whereas one resident performed a maximum of 48 thyroidectomies. Altogether, 516 (52%) residents performed 11 or fewer thyroidectomies, and 769 (77%) performed 16 or fewer thyroid operations. These data raise the question of whether the majority of chief residents in general surgery are competent at graduation to perform thyroidectomy safely.

Traditionally, both general surgeons and otolaryngologists have performed thyroidectomies. Although there are data to suggest that otolaryngology residents can perform thyroidectomies safely when supervised by experienced faculty, there is also evidence suggesting that otolaryngologists have higher rates of permanent postoperative hypoparathyroidism than their general surgery colleagues. In a retrospective review by Shindo et al., 186 thyroidectomy cases performed by otolaryngology residents were analyzed [23]. Transient hypocalcemia of less than 2 weeks duration occurred in 26% of patients, while the incidence of permanent hypocalcemia requiring replacement therapy occurred in 5% of patients.

Mishra et al. showed in a series of 232 patients who underwent total thyroidectomy that patients operated on by attending/consultant surgeons had rates of hypoparathyroidism, recurrent laryngeal nerve injury, and hemorrhage (0.8%, 0.8%, and 1.6%, respectively) that were not significantly different from similar patients who had their surgery by experienced, supervised surgical trainees (1.9%, 0.9%, and 3.8%, respectively) [7]. In a retrospective study of 142 patients who underwent total or subtotal thyroidectomy over an eight-year period in New Mexico, Burge et al. reported that 29% of patients who had surgery by otolaryngologists met criteria for permanent postoperative hypoparathyroidism, while only 5% of patients of general surgeons developed this complication ($P<0.001$) [24]. Adjustment for other factors such as stage of disease did not eliminate this effect of surgical specialty on clinical outcomes.

18.7   Conclusions

In summary, outcomes from thyroidectomy have improved dramatically since Theodor Billroth published his first series of 20 thyroidectomies with a corresponding mortality rate of 40%. In large part, this historical trend toward excellence has been the result of improvements in surgical technique and increasing specialization among surgeons with experience and excellence in thyroidectomy.

When nine internationally recognized endocrine surgeons were asked to find consensus on shaping the future of thyroid surgery in the new millennium, they suggested that outcomes from thyroid surgery might be improved by organizing teams of specialists into thyroid centers (centers of excellence), which could:

- Increase efficiency
- Increase quality of care
- Encourage a more individualized approach to surgery
- Lower complication rates
- Foster innovation in technology and thyroid disease management [25]

Standardization of health care has been shown to increase quality while reducing cost. Clinical pathways have long been used to guide the delivery of care in a variety of practice settings. Even though hospitalization from thyroidectomy is short, standardization of postoperative care has been shown to effectively reduce variation in practice and, in so doing, LOS and cost. When a clinical pathway for thyroidectomy was implemented at the University of Virginia health system between 1997 and 1999, average LOS decreased from 1.4 to 1.2 days (14%). The most striking reductions in costs were in laboratory (44%) and pharmacy costs (54%) [26].

Endocrine centers of excellence would not only help to improve patient outcomes from thyroidectomy in the present, but they might also facilitate the training of future thyroid surgeons. One- and two-year fellowship programs in endocrine surgery are rare, but increasing in number. With the goal of improving patient outcomes from thyroidectomy, the creation of such programs and (potentially) formal certification of endocrine surgery fellowship graduates might help to assure that there will be high-volume specialists with experience and expertise in this area.

A number of challenges lie ahead for students of outcomes from thyroidectomy. We need to place a higher priority on measuring patient-centered outcomes. To date, quality improvement initiatives have focused on measures of morbidity at the expense of health-related quality of life measures. Regionalization and centralization of excellence in thyroid surgery raises questions about access to care, particularly for patients with thyroid disease who live in isolated rural areas. These include unreasonable travel burdens, problems with continuity of care after surgery, and underutilization of some procedures. Losing surgical volume, since thyroidectomy is the most commonly performed endocrine operation in the United States, could threaten financial viability of local hospitals or their ability to recruit and retain surgeons, with attendant effects on patient access to routine surgical care.

Recently, public awareness may have additionally played a significant role in determining patient outcomes. One particular organization, the Light of Life Foundation for Thyroid Cancer (www.checkyourneck. com), led the first nationwide media project dedicated to thyroid cancer awareness that was featured in magazines throughout the world (Fig. 18.2). Such organizations are driven to improving the quality of life of the thyroid cancer patient and their families

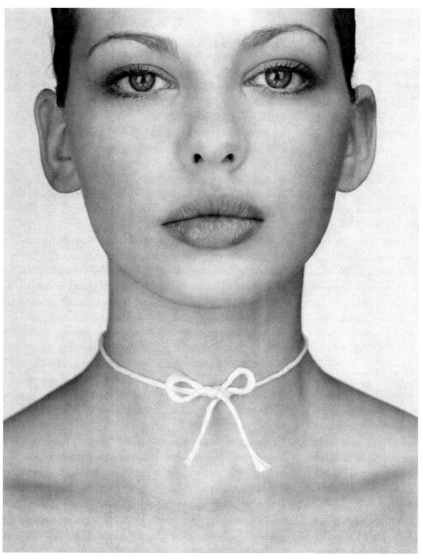

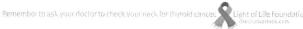

Fig. 18.2 Public health advertising campaign to increase awareness of thyroid cancer

through hospital support networks, educating the lay public and medical community, and supporting the advancement of research and development in thyroid cancer treatment. In particular, patient education and better surveillance with regard to thyroid nodules by patients and their physicians might lead to an earlier diagnosis with optimal treatment and improved outcomes.

It has yet to be seen whether Leapfrog and payer-driven initiatives like it will eventually direct referrals for thyroidectomy in the same way that they are already affecting referrals for cardiovascular and oncologic surgery. As endocrine surgeons, it will be important to work together with patients, referring doctors, payers, and policy makers to collect evidence and anticipate essential changes in policy sooner, rather than later.

References

1. Luft HS, Bunker JP, Enthoven AC (1979) Should operations be regionalized? The empirical relation between surgical volume and mortality. N Engl J Med 301:1364–1369
2. Hannan EL, O'Donnell JF, Kilburn H Jr, Bernard HR, Yazici A (1989) Investigation of the relationship between volume and mortality for surgical procedures performed in New York State hospitals. JAMA 262:503–510
3. Begg CB, Cramer LD, Hoskins WJ, Brennan MF (1998) Impact of hospital volume on operative mortality for major cancer surgery. JAMA 280:1747–1751
4. Birkmeyer JD, Siewers AE, Finlayson EV, Stukel TA, Lucas FL, Batista I, Welch, HG, Wennberg DE (2002) Hospital volume and surgical mortality in the United States. N Engl J Med 346:1128–1137
5. Birkmeyer JD, Finlayson EV, Birkmeyer BS (2001) Volume standards for high-risk surgical procedures: potential benefits of the Leapfrog initiative. Surgery 130:415–422
6. Birkmeyer JD, Dimick JB (2004) Potential benefits of the new Leapfrog standards: effect of process and outcome measures. Surgery 135:569–575
7. Mishra A, Agarwal G, Agarwal A, Mishra S (1999) Safety and efficacy of total thyroidectomy in hands of endocrine surgery trainees. Am J Surg 178:377–380
8. Becker WF (1977) Presidential address: pioneers in thyroid surgery. Ann Surg 185:493–504
9. Colcock BP (1968) Lest we forget: a story of five surgeons. Surgery 64:1162–1172
10. Stojadinovic A, Shaha A, Orlikoff R, Nissan A, Kornak MF, Singh B, Boyle J, Shah J, Brennan M, Kraus D (2002) Prospective functional voice assessment in patients undergoing thyroid surgery. Ann Surg 236:823–832
11. Rosato L, Avenia N, Bernante P, De Palma M, Gulino G, Nasi PG, Pelizzo MR, Pezzullo L (2004) Complications of thyroid surgery: analysis of a multicentric study on 14,934 patients operated on in Italy over 5 years. World J Surg 28:271–276
12. Hermann M, Hellebart C, Freissmuth M (2004) Neuromonitoring in thyroid surgery. Prospective evaluation of intraoperative electrophysiological responses for the prediction of recurrent laryngeal nerve injury. Ann Surg 240:9–17
13. McHenry CR (1997) "Same-day" thyroid surgery: an analysis of safety, cost savings, and outcome. Am Surg 67:586–590
14. Schwartz AE, Clark OH, Ituarte P, Lo Gerfo P (1998) Thyroid surgery: the choice. J Clin Endocrinol Metab 83:1097–1100
15. Hosking M, Warner M, Lobdell C, Offord K, Melton L (1989) Outcomes of surgery in patients 90 years of age and older. JAMA 261:1909–1915
16. Bliss R, Patel N, Guinea A, Thomas R, Delbridge L (1999) Age is no contraindication to thyroid surgery. Age Ageing 28:363–366
17. Passler C, Avanessian R, Kaczirek K, Prager G, Scheuba C, Niederle B (2002) Thyroid surgery in the geriatric patient. Arch Surg 137:1243–1248
18. Testini M, Nacchiero M, Piccinni G, Portincasa P, Di Venere B, Lissidini G, Bonomo GM (2004) Total thyroidectomy is improved by loupe magnification. Microsurgery 24:39–42
19. Specht M, Romero M, Barden C, Esposito C, Fahey T (2001) Characteristics of patients having thyroid surgery under regional anesthesia. J Am Coll Surg 193:367–372
20. Lo Gerfo P (1998) Local/regional anesthesia for thyroidectomy: evaluation as an outpatient procedure. Surgery 124:975–979
21. Sosa J, Bowman H, Tielsch J, Powe N, Gordon T, Udelsman R (1998) The importance of surgeon experience for clinical and economic outcomes from thyroidectomy. Ann Surg 228:320–330
22. Udelsman R (2004) Experience counts. Ann Surg 240:26–27
23. Shindo M, Sinha U, Rice D (1995) Safety of thyroidectomy in residency: a review of 186 consecutive cases. Laryngoscope 105:1173–1175
24. Burge M, Zeise TM, Johnsen M, Conway M, Qualls C (1998) Risks of complication following thyroidectomy. J Gen Intern Med 13:24–31
25. Harness J, van Heerden J, Lennquist S, Rothmund M, Barraclough B, Goode A, Rosen I, Fujimoto Y, Proye C (2000) Future of thyroid surgery and training surgeons to meet the expectations of 2000 and beyond. World J Surg 24:976–982
26. Markey D, McGowan J, Hanks, J (2000) The effect of clinical pathway implementation on total hospital costs for thyroidectomy and parathyroidectomy patients. Am Surg 66:533–539

19 Physiology and Pathophysiology of the Parathyroid Glands and Preoperative Evaluation

Elizabeth H. Holt and Silvio E. Inzucchi

CONTENTS

19.1   Introduction

Calcium is essential to the functioning of a variety of processes throughout the body, including the contraction of the heart and other muscles, the conduction of nervous impulses and other intracellular signals, the clotting of blood, and the secretion of glandular tissues. Precise maintenance of calcium concentration within a very narrow range in extracellular fluids is therefore critically important.

Maintenance of calcium homeostasis requires a complex interplay of dietary intake, intestinal absorption, skeletal remodeling, and urinary excretion. The key organs involved in the changes in calcium metabolism include the intestine, the bone, and the kidney. The parathyroid gland plays an essential role in monitoring extracellular calcium levels and maintaining them within the necessary precise range for physiologic functions to proceed [1].

19.2   Calcium

Most clinical laboratories identify a normal range for serum total calcium concentration between approximately 8.8 and 10.5 mg/dl. Of this total calcium, 50% to 60% is bound to circulating proteins or is complexed with anions such as citrate and phosphate. The remaining ionized (unbound or "free") calcium is the portion responsible for controlling the physiologic processes listed above [2].

19.2.1   Measurement of Calcium

Recognition of a disorder of calcium metabolism requires accurate measurement of serum calcium or ionized calcium. Total serum calcium measurements are performed in most clinical laboratories by spectrophotometry; atomic absorption spectrophotometry is a more costly method but may be used for greater accuracy. Awareness of sources of error in calcium measurements is important. Elevations in albumin or other serum proteins may allow a larger amount of calcium to be carried in the serum in the bound form, thus giving the impression of an abnormally elevated total serum calcium level. An elevated calcium level may also occur with prolonged placement of the phlebotomist's tourniquet before the blood is drawn, which can elevate serum calcium values by up to 1 mg/dl. Dilution of blood when samples are taken from central venous catheters is a common error, leading to low calcium readings. Ionized calcium determinations are accurate only when the blood is collected anaerobically (i.e., into a blood gas syringe), placed on ice, and analyzed within minutes. Since this method of measuring ionized calcium is cumbersome, it may only be necessary occasionally for a given patient, to confirm an elevation in ionized calcium; thereafter the total serum calcium should be a reasonable parameter to follow.

19.2.2   Calcium Regulation

19.2.2.1   Parathyroid hormone

Parathyroid hormone (PTH) is a key regulator of calcium homeostasis. PTH is secreted by the parathyroid glands as an 84-amino acid peptide with a brief plasma half-life (2–4 minutes). The short half-life of PTH allows the parathyroids to respond to minute-to-minute changes in extracellular calcium, thus maintaining the calcium level within the narrow range needed for optimal physiologic function of tissues throughout the body. The parathyroid chief cells constantly monitor extracellular ionized calcium concentration through their cell surface calcium-sensing receptor (CaSR) [3]. Interaction of calcium ions with the extracellular domain of the CaSR triggers a series of intracellular signals, which controls PTH release. As circulating concentrations of calcium fall, the CaSR mediates an increase in PTH secretion; elevations in serum calcium result in decreased PTH release.

19.2.2.2   Calcitriol

The other essential mediator of calcium homeostasis is the sterol 1,25-dihydroxyvitamin D (1,25-$(OH)_2D$) or calcitriol. Synthesis of calcitriol is a complex process controlled by PTH. Calcitriol production begins when cholecalciferol (vitamin D) is generated in skin exposed to ultraviolet light. Vitamin D may also be supplied by dietary sources (mainly fortified milk and cereals). In the liver, vitamin D is readily hydroxylated to 25-(OH)D. PTH controls the tightly regulated final step of calcitriol production in the kidney, where 25-(OH)D is hydroxylated to the potent 1,25-$(OH)_2D_3$ (calcitriol) [4].

19.2.2.3   Maintenance of Calcium Homeostasis

Parathyroid hormone and calcitriol act at the level of the gastrointestinal tract, bone, and the kidney to maintain circulating ionized calcium concentrations under extremely tight control, with a variation of <0.1 mg/dl, despite variations in calcium supply. Calcium consumption ranges from 400 to 2,000 mg daily [5]. Due to the actions of calcitriol on the gut, net calcium absorption from the GI tract averages about 150 to 200 mg daily. At equilibrium, under the control of PTH and calcitriol, an equivalent amount of calcium is excreted by the kidneys. Calcium homeostasis in bone is regulated by PTH. PTH increases serum calcium by acting indirectly on the osteoclasts in the skeleton to promote bone resorption and thus release of calcium into extracellular fluid. Bone remodeling consumes and releases approximately 500 mg of calcium a day. If calcium intake or absorption is insufficient to meet demands, the large calcium reservoir in bone can be accessed to maintain extracellular calcium levels in a narrow range despite increased physiologic need or decreased intake. PTH also enhances calcium resorption at the distal nephron of the kidney. In the kidney, PTH triggers production of calcitriol, which in turn increases fractional calcium absorption in the gut. If calcium intake increases beyond the body's needs, PTH secretion decreases, leading to decreased calcitriol production and decreased calcium absorption by the gut. If calcium is absorbed in excess of requirements, it will be promptly excreted. Through this series of checks and balances, extracellular fluid ionized calcium concentration is carefully maintained, sometimes at the expense of skeletal calcium stores (Fig. 19.1). Disturbances of PTH or vitamin D will result in altered serum calcium concentration. Examples of such pathologic processes will be discussed in the following sections.

19.3   Hypercalcemia and Hyperparathyroidism

Primary hyperparathyroidism is one of the most common metabolic conditions requiring surgical intervention. Today, with automated blood chemistry panels having become a routine part of medical care, the most typical presentation is that of asymptomatic hypercalcemia. The individual found to have an elevated serum calcium level may have one of several conditions, however, and other potential causes must be carefully excluded before making a diagnosis of hyperparathyroidism and proceeding to any consideration of operative intervention.

19.3.1   Differential Diagnosis

The diagnostic workup of hypercalcemia is relatively straightforward; the clinician can usually quickly distinguish its cause, after a good clinical evaluation and review of a few selected laboratory tests. The measurement of the serum PTH concentration has a critical place in this evaluation, with causes of hypercalcemia divided into those that are "parathyroid-mediated" (when PTH levels are elevated or inappropriately normal) and those that are "non-parathyroid mediated" (when PTH levels are secondarily suppressed) (see Table 19.1). It is important to underscore that

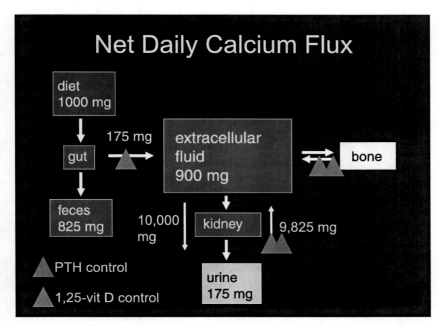

Fig. 19.1 Control of daily calcium flux. This summary shows the tissues involved in calcium metabolism. Points of regulation by PTH and calcitriol are indicated

Table 19.1 Differential diagnosis of hypercalcemia

Parathyroid-mediated	Non-parathyroid-mediated
1. Primary hyperparathyroidism	1. Malignancy-associated hypercalcemia
a. Parathyroid adenoma(ta)	a. Humoral hypercalcemia of malignancy (PTHrP, calcitriol)
b. Parathyroid hyperplasia	b. Local osteolytic hypercalcemia
c. Parathyroid carcinoma	
2. Tertiary hyperparathyroidism	2. Granulomatous diseases (e.g. sarcoid, TB)
3. Familial hypocalciuric hypocalcemia (FHH)	3. Endocrinopathies (e.g., hyperthyroidism, adrenal insufficiency)
4. Lithium therapy	4. Drugs (thiazides, calcium supplements, vitamin D)
	5. Immobilization
	6. Other

normally functioning parathyroid cells will abruptly cease hormone release when the ambient extracellular fluid calcium concentration is elevated. Therefore, in all cases in which hypercalcemia is resulting from a condition unrelated to abnormal parathyroid gland function, PTH levels will be suppressed, i.e., near or below the lower limit of the normal range in most assays (Fig. 19.2).

19.3.1.1 Parathyroid Hormone-mediated Hypercalcemia

Most PTH-mediated forms of hypercalcemia fall into the category of *hyperparathyroidism* (HPTH). *Primary*

HPTH is the most common form and is the most frequent explanation for hypercalcemia in the outpatient arena. Population-based estimates reveal an overall incidence of primary HPTH of approximately 4 per 100,000/year [6]. The peak incidence is in the fifth to sixth decade of life, with a female to male ratio of approximately 3:2. As a result, some surveys place the overall prevalence of HPTH in the elderly at 2–3% [7]. The most common clinical presentation is that of asymptomatic mild hypercalcemia, although a variety of other symptoms may occur, which generally track in severity to the degree of serum calcium elevation [8]. Primary HPTH is caused by a solitary, benign parathyroid adenoma in roughly 80–85% of patients. In approximately 5%, two distinct adenomas ("double

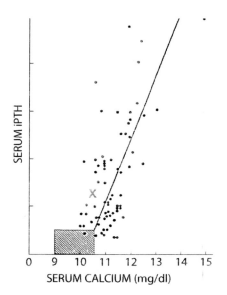

Fig. 19.2 Typical laboratory nomogram of the relationship between serum calcium and PTH levels. The patient marked by an "X" (who had normal renal function) has obvious primary hyperparathyroidism. Normal patients will have results in the *shaded area*. *Black dots* indicate patients with primary hyperparathyroidism

adenoma") are found, a frequency which may actually be higher in the elderly. Multigland parathyroid hyperplasia is present in 15–20%, usually in familial syndromes, such as multiple endocrine neoplasia (MEN) type 1 (Wermer syndrome) and type 2A (Sipple syndrome) [9]. Parathyroid carcinoma occurs in less than 1% of cases [10]. A very rare familial syndrome, the hyperparathyroidism–jaw tumor syndrome (HPTH-JT) is another autosomal dominant inherited condition presenting with early-onset primary HPTH and fibro-osseous, cystic jaw neoplasms [11]. Several kindreds with familial isolated primary HPTH have also been described, outside of MEN1, MEN2A, and HPTH-JT syndromes [12].

Secondary HPTH occurs when decreased circulating calcium concentrations stimulate the increased secretion of PTH, most commonly in patients with chronic renal insufficiency (associated with renal osteodystrophy) or in patients with gastrointestinal calcium malabsorption [13]. As such, the stimulus for PTH hypersecretion is a reduced extracellular calcium concentration, and, therefore, hypercalcemia is *not* present and secondary HPTH is *never* a consideration in the differential diagnosis of hypercalcemia. Conversely, however, certain patients with secondary HPTH may, over time, develop one or more enlarged parathyroid glands (hyperplasia) or a more generalized dysregulation of parathyroid func-

tion that actually progresses to hypercalcemia. It is not uncommon in this setting for patients to develop multigland disease, although marked asymmetry is typical. This condition, *tertiary HPTH*, does lead to hypercalcemia, often severe and frequently requiring parathyroid resection [14]. It is typically encountered in patients with end-stage renal disease on dialysis. Optimization of serum calcium and phosphate levels and vitamin D status in patients with chronic kidney disease is necessary to avoid this complication.

Familial hypocalciuric hypercalcemia (FHH), once referred to as "benign familial hypercalcemia," is an inherited autosomal dominant condition due to a deactivating mutation in the extracellular CaSR [15]. In this condition, the receptor is subnormally activated by the extracellular calcium concentration. As a result, PTH levels are inappropriately normal or slightly elevated, in the face of mild elevation of serum calcium. However, and in contrast to what occurs in primary HPTH (see below), urinary calcium excretion is reduced, due to the same defective CaSRs in the nephron, with consequent increased urinary calcium reabsorption. Although FHH is generally classified in the "parathyroid mediated" category of hypercalcemia since parathyroid hormone secretion is abnormal, it is clearly a unique disease and distinct from primary HPTH. It does *not* require surgical intervention. Indeed, parathyroidectomy will not cure the condition. Finally, chronic *lithium therapy* may increase serum calcium levels with inappropriately normal or mildly elevated PTH concentrations. Lithium appears to alter the sensitivity of the CaSR [16]. As a result, the extracellular calcium set-point for PTH release is increased. Parathyroid adenomas have also been described in patients chronically treated with lithium. Distinguishing those patients with drug-induced hypercalcemia from those with mild primary HPTH can be challenging.

19.3.1.2 Non-parathyroid Hormone-mediated Hypercalcemia

This category encompasses those conditions in which hypercalcemia results from anything *other* than abnormal parathyroid function. As its name implies, this group of diseases is associated with PTH levels that are appropriately suppressed, as the parathyroid cells perceive excess extracellular calcium concentrations, and markedly reduce their hormonal release. Cancer is the most frequently diagnosed cause of non-PTH-mediated hypercalcemia, especially in hospitalized patients. So-called *malignancy-associated hypercalcemia* is classified into two main forms, distinguished by pathogenesis [17]. *Humoral hypercalcemia of malignancy (HHM)* results from the systemic effect of a circulating factor produced by the neoplasm. Most commonly, the factor involved is the peptide, parathyroid hormone-related protein (PTHrP). The N-terminal fragment of PTHrP is largely homologous with PTH itself, and has been shown to recapitulate most of the metabolic effects of PTH, including the stimulation of bone turnover and the alteration in renal handling of both calcium and phosphate. Normally, in humans, PTHrP serves as an important paracrine factor in many tissues, including skin, bone, breast, the gravid uterus, and the vasculature [18]. Neoplasms that produce PTHrP are usually squamous cell carcinomas (nasopharynx, oropharynx, larynx, lung, esophagus, and cervix). Tumors of other cell types may also elaborate PTHrP, including adenocarcinoma of the breast and ovary, renal cell carcinoma, transitional cell carcinoma of bladder, carcinoids and other neuroendocrine neoplasms, and T cell lymphomas. It should be noted that, typically, these cancers produce PTHrP in minute quantities. As a result, any patient presenting with hypercalcemia due to PTHrP usually have significant tumor burden. It is therefore quite unusual for HHM to be the presenting feature of malignancy. The other form of HHM is much less common: that caused by the uncontrolled production of 1,25-vitamin D (calcitriol), usually by B cell lymphomas.

The second form of malignancy-associated hypercalcemia is known as *local osteolytic hypercalcemia (LOH)*. As its name implies, LOH occurs when a neoplasm directly invades the skeleton, leading to its localized destruction and release of calcium. This appears to result from the production or local stimulation of bone-active cytokines and/or other osteoclast-activating factors. In contrast to HHM, LOH does not involve the elaboration of systemically active products. The classic tumor leading to LOH is multiple myeloma, although other tumors, including a variety of adenocarcinomas (especially breast) and certain lymphomas, may also be to blame. Recent investigations suggest that local bone-derived factors further enhance the growth potential of some of these tumors, resulting in cycles of bone resorption leading to further tumor growth leading to more bone resorption [19].

There are many non-PTH-mediated causes of hypercalcemia encountered in clinical medicine. Included are various medications/supplements, such as thiazide diuretics, vitamin D and its analogues, excess calcium, especially when consumed with alkali ("milk-alkali syndrome"), and excess vitamin A. Other conditions include granulomatous diseases (sarcoidosis, tuberculosis), through the direct production of calcitriol, and several endocrinopathies,

hyperthyroidism (augmented bone turnover), adrenal failure (decreased calcium clearance), and pheochromocytoma (PTHrP production). Rarely, hypercalcemia may result from immobilization, especially when bone turnover is already stimulated as in growing adolescents or adults with Paget's disease, a condition marked by abnormal bone formation.

19.3.2 Signs, Symptoms, and Laboratory Findings

In general, the clinical manifestations of hypercalcemia relate to both the degree and rapidity of the serum calcium elevation. Mild hypercalcemia (serum calcium levels <11.0 mg/dl) usually results in few symptoms. Polyuria and polydipsia may occur, due to nephrogenic diabetes insipidus because of a reduction in renal concentrating ability. Dyspepsia may result from calcium-mediated increase in gastrin secretion. Mild cognitive impairment and vague neuromuscular symptoms, including difficulty concentrating, depression, fatigue, and muscle weakness, may also be encountered. In general, symptoms become more striking as the calcium levels progress into the moderately elevated range (11.0–13 mg/dl). Manifestations here include fatigue, muscle weakness, anorexia, nausea, and constipation. Severe hypercalcemia (i.e., serum calcium >13 mg/dl) leads to further progression of the above, accompanied by dehydration, abdominal pain, vomiting, lethargy, obtundation, and even coma. Other clinical manifestations may include pancreatitis, and, depending on the etiology of the hypercalcemia, osteopenia/osteoporosis, azotemia, nephrolithiasis, nephrocalcinosis, and other soft tissue calcification such as chondrocalcinosis and corneal deposition ("band keratopathy"). On the electrocardiogram, moderate-severe hypercalcemia can shorten the QT interval.

Due to the typical chronicity of primary HPTH, however, even patients with advanced disease may be surprisingly asymptomatic [20]. PTH, when chronically elevated, stimulates bone turnover. In adults who have achieved peak bone mass (in the early to mid-third decade of life), osteoclastic bone resorption is activated out of proportion to osteoblastic bone formation. This results in net bone loss, leading to osteopenia or osteoporosis [21]. Mineral is lost preferentially at sites rich in cortical bone, such as the distal radius and proximal femur, as opposed to those predominately composed of cancellous bone (e.g., the lumbar spine). Therefore, the classic pattern of bone loss in HPTH patients on dual energy X-ray absorptiometry (DEXA) is for more severe deficits (i.e., lower

T scores) at the wrist and hip than at the spine. In contradistinction, in routine menopausal bone loss, mineral is preferentially lost from cancellous sites. More advanced forms of hyperparathyroid bone disease, such as *osteitis fibrosa cystica*, are no longer encountered with any frequency. Decades ago, however, prior to the development of routine blood chemistry analyzers, it was the presenting feature in many patients. Radiographic manifestations of *osteitis fibrosa cystica* include irregular demineralization of the skull (leading to a "salt-and-pepper" appearance on plain films), periosteal resorption at the phalanges, and Brown tumors (lucent areas of intense osteoclastic resorption).

Patients with HPTH are frequently hypercalciuric (urinary calcium output >4 mg/kg per day). This occurs despite the tendency of PTH to increase renal tubular calcium reabsorption, because the filtered load of calcium is increased, overwhelming the reclamation capacity of the nephron. Hypercalciuria increases the risk of nephrolithiasis, another prime manifestation of this disorder [22]. Urinary tract stones in HPTH consist of mainly calcium oxalate. In HPTH patients with severe hypercalcemia and/or in those who develop superimposed dehydration, nephrocalcinosis, azotemia, or acute renal failure may be the result. Other symptoms which are related to HPTH include hypertension and peptic ulcer disease, although a cause-and-effect relationships have not been convincingly demonstrated.

Other laboratory manifestations of primary HPTH include mild-moderate hypophosphatemia, since the hormone lowers the renal threshold for phosphate clearance. Because PTH additionally increases renal bicarbonate output, a mild hyperchloremic metabolic acidosis is also frequently present. Urine calcium excretion is either normal or elevated, a feature which in part reflects the degree of hypercalcemia, total daily calcium intake, as well as circulating concentrations of 1,25-vitamin D (calcitriol) [23]. Because calcitriol enhances calcium and phosphate transport by the gut, those with the highest levels have the greatest degree of hypercalciuria, an indirect reflection of gastrointestinal calcium absorption. If measured, calcitriol levels, which are under the direct control of PTH, are high-normal, if not frankly elevated. Conversely, 25-vitamin D levels, which reflect total body vitamin stores (i.e., dietary vitamin D and daily ultraviolet light exposure), are usually normal. Finally, since PTH activates osteoclast and osteoblast activity, serum and urine bone turnover markers, such as pyridinoline crosslinks, N-telopeptide, bone alkaline phosphatase, and osteocalcin, are increased. In patients being con-

sidered for one of the familial syndromes, measurement of serum prolactin (or other pituitary markers, based on the clinical scenario) and/or calcitonin levels are/is indicated.

19.3.3   Diagnostic Evaluation

19.3.3.1   *History and Physical Examination*

The history in the patient being evaluated for primary HPTH should focus on symptoms of hypercalcemia, such as fatigue, weakness, cognitive impairment, and polyuria, as well as those that might be specifically associated with hyperparathyroidism (HPTH), such as bone discomfort or evidence of bone loss (i.e., previous DEXA study reports or personal history of fragility fractures) or renal tract stones (abdominal, back, or flank pain, hematuria). If medical records are available, it is also vital to assess the chronicity of the hypercalcemia, since primary HPTH typically presents as mild, stable, or, at most, slowly progressive serum calcium elevation over years. If the patient has an elevated calcium level but the diagnosis of primary HPTH is not yet established, then evidence of other conditions associated with hypercalcemia should be sought, including malignancy, granulomatous, and other endocrine diseases. A complete medication list should be examined for any potential offending agents, including thiazides, calcium supplements, and vitamin D. It is additionally important to explore the family history for disorders of calcium metabolism as well as related endocrinopathies, such as pituitary, adrenal, pancreatic, and thyroid neoplasms, as might be seen in kindreds with MEN syndromes. A history of multiple family members having mild hypercalcemia, particularly if resistant to parathyroidectomy, would suggest the possibility of FHH.

The physical examination in patients with HPTH is usually non-specific. Cautious cognitive testing may uncover subtle abnormalities, but this may be difficult to discern in most patients. Occasionally, mild tenderness over bony prominences, such as the anterior tibia may be encountered in patients with very active bone turnover. Patients with moderate-severe hypercalcemia may have more prominent neurologic findings such as muscle weakness or memory deficits. A neck mass is rarely palpable, unless a parathyroid carcinoma is present. In patients with MEN1 syndrome, other associated features, such as evidence of visual field deficits or clinical evidence of hypopituitarism should be pursued. In those MEN1 patients whose pituitary tumor is a prolactinoma, galactorrhea may be detected. Less commonly, features of Cushing's syndrome or acromegaly may be present if the pituitary tumor secretes ACTH or growth hormone, respectively. In MEN2A patients, HPTH is accompanied by medullary carcinoma of the thyroid and pheochromocytoma. As a result a thyroid mass may be palpated and paroxysmal or sustained hypertension may complete the clinical picture.

19.3.3.2 Laboratory Testing

In the patient with newly recognized hypercalcemia, it is first important to rule out factitious hypercalcemia, due to elevated concentration of plasma proteins, as may be seen in patients with myeloma. Fifty to sixty percent of total circulating calcium is bound to plasma proteins, mostly albumin. In situations where plasma proteins are elevated, a correction must be made, with the serum calcium lowered by 0.8 mg/dl for every 1.0 mg of albumin or total protein above the normal range. Alternatively, one can measure the ionized calcium level. Next, the serum PTH concentration (drawn simultaneously with serum calcium) is measured. Several PTH assays are available, including a C-terminal radioimmunoassay (RIA) and the more popular two-site immunochemiluminometric assay (ICMA) or "bio-intact" PTH [24]. Whereas the C-terminal assay measures not only PTH but other fragments of the molecule that circulate in increased concentrations in renal failure, PTH ICMAs have the advantage of measuring only the intact PTH molecule. It is therefore the preferred test in patients with serum creatinine >2.0 mg/dl. We feel it is also important for clinicians to become familiar with the quality of locally available assays so that the appropriate choices can be made. At our institution, for instance, we have diagnosed several patients with mild hyper-

parathyroidism based on clearly elevated PTH levels in a local, highly sensitive mid-molecule PTH RIA, whereas the commercially available bio-intact PTH assay yielded low-normal results.

If the PTH level is high or inappropriately normal, the patient has primary hyperparathyroidism, unless proven otherwise. Serum phosphorous, electrolytes, BUN, creatinine, and the 24-hour urine calcium excretion should also be measured at this juncture. The urine test is important to rule out FHH. As mentioned, HPTH patients usually have normal to elevated urinary calcium output, whereas, FHH patients, by definition, have low urinary calcium. A renal calcium:creatinine clearance ratio <0.01 suggests this diagnosis. If FHH diagnosis appears likely, parathyroid resection is not indicated. Confirmation of the mutation in the gene coding for the CaSR can be obtained through specific research laboratories.

Once the diagnosis of primary HPTH is confirmed, the symptomatic patient should proceed to a localization study, preferably with a technetium 99m sestamibi scan. All symptomatic patients should be referred to an experienced parathyroid surgeon. In the asymptomatic patient, guidelines from the 2002 National Institutes of Health Workshop on Asymptomatic Primary Hyperparathyroidism should be employed (see Table 19.2) [25]. Patients meeting criteria should also proceed to parathyroid surgery. Accordingly, asymptomatic patients should undergo bone density measurement using DEXA, and, if not already performed, a 24-hour urine calcium and an assessment of renal function.

Those patients with mild hypercalcemia who are truly asymptomatic and do not meet surgical indication may be followed clinically, with intervention in those patients whose condition worsens (i.e., progressive rise in serum calcium, diminution in bone density, deterioration of renal function, etc.). The major-

Table 19.2 Surgical indications in patients with primary hyperparathyroidism. (From the 2002 National Institutes of Health Workshop)

1. Significant bone, renal, gastrointestinal, or neuromuscular symptoms typical of primary hyperparathyroidism

In otherwise asymptomatic patients:

2. Elevation of serum calcium by 1 mg/dl or more above the normal range (i.e., ≥11.5 mg/dl in most laboratories)

3. Marked elevation of 24-hour urine calcium excretion (e.g., >400 mg)

4. Decreased creatinine clearance (e.g., reduced by ≥30% compared with age-matched normal persons)

5. Significant reduction in bone density of more than 2.5 standard deviations below peak bone mass at any measured site (hip, lumbar spine, wrist; i.e., "T score" approximately <2.5 at any of these sites)

6. Consistent follow-up is not possible or is undesirable because of coexisting medical conditions

7. Age younger than 50 years

ity of patients will, however, remain asymptomatic and may not require intervention [26].

Additionally, consideration should be given to the possibility of one of the MEN syndromes, especially if the patient is young (<30 years) or has a personal or family history of a related endocrinopathy. If the diagnosis of MEN is suspected, depending on the type, measurements of prolactin (or other markers of pituitary function, based on the clinical assessment), calcitonin, and plasma, and/or urinary catecholamine metabolites are required. DNA diagnostic testing is now available for genetic mutations associated with MEN1 and MEN2A [27]. This information will be useful preoperatively, since patients with MEN frequently have four-gland parathyroid hyperplasia and a subtotal parathyroidectomy or total cervical parathyroidectomy with heterotopic parathyroid transplant may be necessary. Certainly, failure to consider a pheochromocytoma (in MEN2A) would be a serious omission in the preoperative evaluation of such a patient.

If the PTH level is low or entirely unmeasurable, the patient by definition has non-PTH-mediated hypercalcemia, and further evaluation by an endocrinologist will be necessary.

19.4   Summary

Calcium homeostasis is of critical importance to living organisms. In man, a complex hormonal system exists to finely regulate the extracellular calcium concentration. A common aberration of this system is primary hyperparathyroidism, the leading cause of chronic hypercalcemia. While usually presenting with few symptoms, this disease is a frequent explanation for osteoporosis and nephrolithiasis. If undiagnosed, it may progress with severe sequelae. It is therefore useful for the surgeon to have a general understanding of the regulation of calcium metabolism as well as the clinical features, diagnostic strategies, and the accepted surgical indications for this common endocrine condition.

References

1. Bringhurst FR (1989) Calcium and phosphate distribution, turnover and metabolic actions. In: DeGroot LJ (ed) Endocrinology, 2nd edn, vol 2. Saunders, Philadelphia, pp 805–843

2. Broadus AE (1999) Mineral balance and homeostasis. In: Favus MJ (ed) Primer on the metabolic bone diseases and disorders of mineral metabolism, 4th edn. Lippincott Williams & Wilkins, Philadelphia, pp 74–80

3. Brown EM (1999) Physiology and pathophysiology of the extracellular calcium-sensing receptor. Am J Med 106:238

4. Norman AW, Roth J, Orci L (1982) The vitamin D endocrine system: steroid metabolism, hormone receptors and biologic response. Endocr Rev 3:331–366

5. Dietary Reference Intakes (DRI) and Recommended Dietary Allowances (RDA) (2002) Food and Nutrition Information Center, USDA/ARS/National Agriculture Library, Beltsville, MD. http://www.nal.usda.gov/fnic/etext/000105.html

6. Wermers RA, Khosla S, Atkinson EJ, Hodgson SF, O'Fallon WM, Melton LJ 3rd (1997) The rise and fall of primary hyperparathyroidism: a population-based study in Rochester, Minnesota, 1965–1992. Ann Intern Med 126:433–440

7. Akerstrom G, Ljunghall S, Lundgren E (1997) Natural history of untreated primary hyperparathyroidism. In: Clark OH, Duh QY (eds) Textbook of endocrine surgery. Saunders, Philadelphia, pp 303–310

8. Silverberg SJ, Bilezikian JP, Bone HG, Talpos GB, Horwitz MJ, Stewart AF (1999) Therapeutic controversies in primary hyperparathyroidism. J Clin Endocrinol Metab 84:2275–2285

9. Brandi ML, Gagel RF, Angeli A, Bilezikian JP, Beck-Peccoz P, Bordi C, Conte-Devolx B, Falchetti A, Gheri RG, Libroia A, Lips CJ, Lombardi G, Mannelli M, Pacini F, Ponder BA, Raue F, Skogseid B, Tamburrano G, Thakker RV, Thompson NW, Tomassetti P, Tonelli F, Wells SA Jr, Marx SJ (2001) Guidelines for diagnosis and therapy of MEN type 1 and type 2. J Clin Endocrinol Metab 86:5658–5671

10. Clayman GL, Gonzalez HE, El-Naggar A, Vassilopoulou-Sellin R (2004) Parathyroid carcinoma: evaluation and interdisciplinary management. Cancer 100:900–905

11. Chen JD, Morrison C, Zhang C, Kahnoski K, Carpten JD, Teh BT (2003) Hyperparathyroidism-jaw tumour syndrome. J Intern Med 253:634–642

12. Simonds WF, James-Newton LA, Agarwal SK, Yang B, Skarulis MC, Hendy GN, Marx SJ (2002) Familial isolated hyperparathyroidism: clinical and genetic characteristics of 36 kindreds. Medicine 81:1–26

13. Yudd M, Llach F (2000) Current medical management of secondary hyperparathyroidism. Am J Med Sci 320:100–106

14. Imanishi Y, Tahara H, Palanisamy N, Spitalny S, Salusky IB, Goodman W, Brandi ML, Drueke TB, Sarfati E, Urena P, Chaganti RS, Arnold A (2002) Clonal chromosomal defects in the molecular pathogenesis of refractory hyperparathyroidism of uremia. J Am Soc Nephrol 13:1490–1498

15. Brown EM (2000) Familial hypocalciuric hypercalcemia and other disorders with resistance to extracellular calcium. Endocrinol Clin North Am 29:503–522
16. Bendz H, Sjodin I, Toss G, Berglund K (1996) Hyperparathyroidism and long-term lithium therapy: a cross-sectional study and the effect of lithium withdrawal. J Intern Med 240:357–365
17. Stewart AF (2005) Clinical practice. Hypercalcemia associated with cancer. N Engl J Med 352:373–379
18. Strewler GJ (2000) The physiology of parathyroid hormone-related protein. N Engl J Med 342:177–185
19. Goltzman D, Karaplis AC, Kremer R, Rabbani SA (2000) Molecular basis of the spectrum of skeletal complications of neoplasia. Cancer 88(12 suppl):2903–2908
20. Bilezikian JP, Silverberg SJ (2004) Clinical practice. Asymptomatic primary hyperparathyroidism. N Engl J Med 350:1746–1751
21. Khan A, Bilezikian J (2000) Primary hyperparathyroidism: pathophysiology and impact on bone. Can Med Assoc J 163:184–187
22. Rodman JS, Mahler RJ (2000) Kidney stones as a manifestation of hypercalcemic disorders. Hyperparathyroidism and sarcoidosis. Urol Clin North Am 27:275–285
23. Beckerman P, Silver J (1999) Vitamin D and the parathyroid. Am J Med Sci 317:363–369
24. Yamashita H, Gao P, Cantor T, Noguchi S, Uchino S, Watanabe S, Ogawa T, Kawamoto H, Fukagawa M (2004) Comparison of parathyroid hormone levels from the intact and whole parathyroid hormone assays after parathyroidectomy for primary and secondary hyperparathyroidism. Surgery 135:149–156
25. Bilezikian JP, Potts JT Jr, Fuleihan G-H, Kleerekoper M, Neer R, Peacock M, Rastad J, Silverberg SJ, Udelsman R, Wells SA (2002) Summary statement from a workshop on asymptomatic primary hyperparathyroidism: a perspective for the 21st century. J Clin Endocrinol Metab 87:5353–5361
26. Silverberg SJ, Shane E, Jacobs TP, et al (1999) A 10-year prospective study of primary hyperparathyroidism with or without parathyroid surgery. N Engl J Med 341:1249
27. Marx SJ, Simonds WF, Agarwal SK, Burns AL, Weinstein LS, Cochran C, Skarulis MC, Spiegel AM, Libutti SK, Alexander HR Jr, Chen CC, Chang R, Chandrasekharappa SC, Collins FS (2002) Hyperparathyroidism in hereditary syndromes: special expressions and special managements. J Bone Miner Res 17(suppl 2):N37–N43

20 Parathyroid Imaging

David Cheng, Ludwig A. Jacob, and Leslie Scoutt

20.1   Introduction

The role of preoperative imaging in the evaluation of patients with primary hyperparathyroidism (HPTH) depends upon the surgical approach. The choice of modality further depends on what instrumentation is available, the experience of both the examiners and the interpreters of the examinations, and where the lesion is most likely to be. It also depends on the setting when localization tests are performed for primary or reoperative cases.

Traditionally, the standard surgical approach consisted of a bilateral neck exploration with direct visualization of all four parathyroid glands. If this is done by an experienced parathyroid surgeon, parathyroidectomy may be curative in over 95% of cases [1]. For many decades, routine preoperative localization was not regarded as standard of care for primary HPTH. As radiologist Dr. John Doppman wrote in 1968, "the only localizing study indicated in a patient with untreated primary HPTH is to localize an experienced parathyroid surgeon." [2,3] Currently, however, mini-mally invasive surgical techniques are advocated for patients with primary HPTH, allowing a targeted excision of a single parathyroid adenoma [4], resulting a smaller incision, shorter surgical time often performed as an outpatient employing the use of local rather than general anesthesia, and substantially reducing the risk of damage to the recurrent laryngeal nerve. However, accurate preoperative localization of the parathyroid adenoma must be provided for this approach to be successful. While most cases (80–85%) of primary HPTH are caused by a single parathyroid adenoma, multiple adenomas account for approximately 5% of cases and parathyroid hyperplasia for approximately 12% of cases [5–7]. Parathyroid carcinomas are extremely rare and account for <1% of all cases primary HPTH [4–7]. Hence, another role of preoperative localization is to distinguish between a single parathyroid adenoma and multiple gland disease.

Over the last decade, considerable efforts have been devoted to improving parathyroid imaging. New radionucleotide agents and scanning procedures have markedly increased the success rate of localization studies. Parathyroid imaging focuses on the detection of adenomas in patients with primary HPTH scheduled for minimally invasive parathyroidectomy and plays an important role in the preoperative assessment of patients with persistent or recurrent HPTH. Ultrasound (US) is ideal for eutopic lesions nearby the thyroid gland, whereas computed tomography (CT) and magnetic resonance imaging (MRI) are more effective in detecting ectopic parathyroid glands. Sestamibi scintigraphy has emerged as the single most sensitive study for both perithyroidal and ectopic glands, detecting most of the adenomas and a large proportion of hyperplastic glands.

20.2   Nuclear Imaging

While there is a variety of nuclear imaging techniques aimed at identifying a parathyroid adenoma from the thyroid gland, we prefer single-radioisotope scintigraphy using technetium-99m (^{99m}Tc) sestamibi. A still popular choice used by many nuclear medicine physicians is a dual-radioisotope combination using thallium-201 (^{201}Tl) and ^{99m}Tc pertechnetate (^{201}Tl/^{99m}Tc) with the aid of a subtraction program. The premise of this combination imaging is that thallium (a potassium analogue) is taken up by both the thyroid and the parathyroid glands, whereas the pertechnetate is taken up only by the thyroid gland. Taking advantage of the built-in multichannel analyzers of present-day gamma cameras, photons from the decays of both isotopes can be registered simultaneously using different energy windows for each of the radioisotopes. However, the photo peak from ^{201}Tl (69–83 keV) is much lower than that from ^{99m}Tc (140 keV), which will result in "spill down" phenomenon from ^{99m}Tc photons into the energy window used for ^{201}Tl centered at 80 keV. Another technical obstacle is that due to the relatively long physical half-life of ^{201}Tl at 73 h, the typical dose used is 2–4 mCi (equivalent to 74–148 MBq), which will not afford any opportunities for quality tomographic imaging. Hence, this combination imaging is limited to the use of planar views using a converging or a pinhole collimator. Due to the low dose of ^{201}Tl used, imaging time is often long and increases the risk for patient movement artifacts, which can severely compromise the quality of the images. In addition to the simultaneous acquisition using multiple energy windows, a subtraction program will also need to be implemented to demonstrate differential accumulation of both radiotracers. Although the technique provides useful information, without tomographic imaging, the precise location of the adenoma cannot be obtained. While sensitivities of 85–95% have been reported [8], many practitioners concede that the sensitivity is much lower for hyperplastic glands as compared to primary adenomas as well as for glands under 300 mg in weight [9,10]. While the most common false-positive finding is solid thyroid nodule(s), whether solitary or multinodular in nature, other medical conditions such as sarcoidosis [11], thyroid carcinoma [12], and lymphoma [13] have also been described.

Sestamibi is a lipophilic cationic complex that is sequestered primarily within the mitochondria [14] and was developed for myocardial perfusion studies. With the attachment of a ^{99m}Tc radionuclide, ^{99m}Tc sestamibi has the ability to yield good-quality planar as well as tomographic images in a reasonable imaging time. With a physical half-life of only 6 h, a typical dose for cardiac studies is in the range of 15–35 mCi (555–1295 MBq). However, for parathyroid imaging aiming at a smaller target organ, a smaller dose of 20–25 mCi (740–925 MBq) is typically sufficient. By taking advantage of the differential clearance between parathyroid and thyroid tissues, delayed imaging at 1–3 h can yield a good signal (parathyroid) to background (thyroid) ratio. While some nuclear medicine physicians prefer to get early images at 10–15 min followed by delayed images at 2–3 h, we have the opinion that the early images often add very little to the final interpretation of a study, while it adds to the burden of camera time in a busy nuclear medicine practice.

The large number of mitochondria within parathyroid adenomas compared with normal thyroid tissue may be responsible for a differential sestamibi clearance [15]. Due to the small size of normal parathyroid glands, they are below the resolution of gamma cameras, and hence will not interfere with imaging as a false-positive finding. However, since sestamibi can be considered as a tumor-seeking agent, additions to our list of false-positive differential findings would include parathyroid carcinoma (versus benign parathyroid adenoma), parathyroid metastases, and brown tumors [16]. From our experience, 1- to 1.5-h postinjection yields a good balance between retention within a parathyroid adenoma and clearance from the thyroid gland (Fig. 20.1). Using a parallel-hole collimator, our field of view includes the mediastinum for detection of ectopic parathyroid adenomas as well as enabling us to perform single-photon-emission tomography (SPECT) imaging, both of which improve the chances of success in a surgical cure. Although the literature may not decisively demonstrate an improvement in the sensitivity of detection using SPECT over planar imaging, the information it yields on anatomic

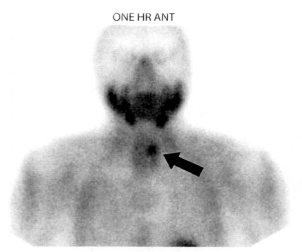

ONE HR ANT

Fig. 20.1 Scintigraphic image from Yale's ^{99m}Tc-sestamibi parathyroid protocol depicting a left lower parathyroid adenoma (*arrow*)

localization allows greater precision, regardless of whether it is located within the neck or in the mediastinum, which is especially critical in a minimally invasive surgical approach (Fig. 20.2). From a recent publication, we report a definite advantage in localization using SPECT images [17].

Still popular among many nuclear medicine practitioners is combination imaging using ^{99m}Tc sestamibi and ^{123}I sodium iodide. Dual energy windows are again used with ^{123}I photo peak centered at 159 keV. With the aid of a subtraction computer program, this technique can enhance the contrast between a parathyroid adenoma and the thyroid gland. Compensation for "spill down" interference of the more energetic ^{123}I photons into the ^{99m}Tc energy window should be performed for optimal contrast. Logistically, there are limitations with this technique that precluded us from adopting it into our practice. Firstly, it is a 2-day protocol, with the ^{123}I sodium iodide capsule given on day 1 and the patient returning for imaging on day 2, which will add to the complexity as well as reduce the flexibility in scheduling. Secondly, ^{123}I is produced

from a cyclotron with an approximately 13-h physical half-life has to be ordered in advance at a much higher cost than ^{99m}Tc pertechnetate for a similar purpose. However, since both the sestamibi and the pertechnetate share a common radionuclide (^{99m}Tc), dual-energy window imaging cannot be employed. Thirdly, with a small dose of ^{123}I used, typically less than 1 mCi (<37 MBq) partly due to the high cost of the isotope, imaging is often performed using a pinhole collimator for planar imaging. A disadvantage is that SPECT imaging may be hampered by patient movement artifacts due to the long imaging time it will require.

Promising experimental nuclear imaging techniques employing new radiotracers include parathyroid-specific antibodies (used in animal models) [18,19] and ^{131}I-toluidine blue [20]. While there is more work to be done with these radiotracers, the incorporation of radioactive iodine may yield a higher background from the uptake of metabolized free iodine by the thyroid gland. Depending on the dose of the radiotracer employed, patients may need to take

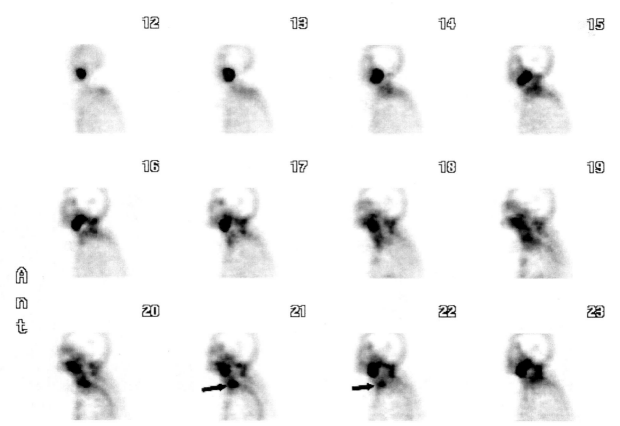

Fig. 20.2 Scintigraphic images from sestamibi single-photon-emission tomography of the same patient presented in Fig. 20.1 depicting multiple sagittal tomographic planes. The parathyroid adenoma is marked with *arrows*. *Ant* Anterior

a supersaturated cold iodine solution (such as Lugol's solution) for protection from the metabolized free radioactive iodine (especially ^{131}I). Efforts have also been undertaken incorporating positron emission tomography (PET) imaging using ^{18}F-fluoro-2-deoxy-d-glucose with mixed results [21,22] and ^{11}C-methionine [23], both of which will require more work. PET imaging has the advantages of greater spatial resolution and shorter-lived isotopes, which will enable the administration of higher doses of radiotracer for better signals. However, in the absence of reimbursements for parathyroid imaging using PET, the cost of the isotope and equipment make this modality unaffordable for many patients.

20.3　　Ultrasound

US plays a complementary role to ^{99m}Tc sestamibi, angiographic venous sampling, CT, and MRI in the preoperative localization of parathyroid adenomas in patients with primary HPTH. In addition, US plays a unique role in preoperative fine-needle aspiration (FNA) of extrathyroidal masses to confirm the diagnosis of a parathyroid adenoma, particularly in patients with recurrent HPTH following a failed neck exploration.

Although ^{99m}Tc sestamibi imaging is generally considered the most specific preoperative imaging modality, US has an important complimentary role. US provides much more detailed anatomic information than nuclear medicine imaging in the neck, is able to assess concurrent thyroid disease, which is estimated to be present in approximately 40% of patients, and is able to guide percutaneous FNA to confirm the diagnosis. In addition US, is less expensive, move readily available, and does not expose the patient to ionizing radiation. However, US examination is quite operator dependent and the reported sensitivities of US for accurately localizing parathyroid adenomas have ranged from 34 to 92% (averaging in the 60–80% range) [24–29]. US is of less value in identifying ectopic parathyroid glands outside of the neck, particularly in the mediastinum and retrotracheal or retroesophageal areas [30], The reported specificity of US examination is higher, ranging from 92 to 97% [29,31]. To achieve sensitivities and specificities in the higher range, the ultrasonographer must recognize the typical appearance and location of adenomas on US examination and pay careful attention to technique.

The normal parathyroid gland is generally too small to be visualized on US examination. The most classic appearance of an adenoma on US examination is of a homogeneously hypoechoic extrathyroidal oval mass ranging in size from 0.8 to 1.5 cm in length with a clear fat plane separating the adenoma from the thyroid gland (Fig. 20.3). However, the larger a parathyroid adenoma grows, the more irregular the shape will become. Cystic degeneration and calcification are uncommon findings. Adenomas are typically quite vascular with a very specific pattern of blood flow. A feeding artery, usually a branch of the inferior or superior thyroid artery, can often be followed directly into either the upper or lower pole of the adenoma, so

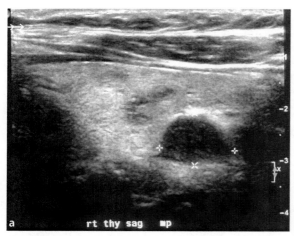
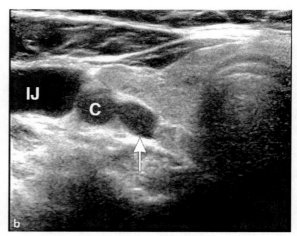

Fig. 20.3 Sagittal (**a**) and transverse (**b**) images of a parathyroid adenoma posterior to the inferior pole of the right lobe of the thyroid gland in a 56-year-old woman with newly diagnosed hypercalcemia. The parathyroid adenoma is uniform in echotexture and less echogenic than the adjacent thyroid tissue. Note the echogenic fat plane clearly separating the parathyroid adenoma from the thyroid gland. Parathyroid adenoma (*calipers* on **a** and *arrow* in **b**). *C* Carotid artery, *IJ* internal jugular vein

called polar distribution (Fig. 20.4a) [32]. Typically, a prominent peripheral rim of vascularity is present (Fig. 20.4b) [33]. Asymmetrically increased blood flow in the adjacent thyroid tissue has also been described [3,32,34]. Patients with multiple gland disease can either have multiple adenomas or diffuse parathyroid hyperplasia. A hyperplastic parathyroid gland is indistinguishable on US from an adenoma. If all four parathyroid glands are enlarged, the diagnosis is probably parathyroid hyperplasia (Fig. 20.5). However, the glands may be asymmetrically enlarged.

Most patients have four parathyroid glands; a right and left superior and a right and left inferior gland. However, patients with as few as two and as many as six parathyroid glands have been reported, with super-

numerary glands most often located in the superior mediastinum [35,36]. The two superior parathyroid glands derive from the fourth branchial cleft pouch. Relatively little migration of the superior glands occurs during embryogenesis, and the superior glands are typically found posterior to the upper third of the

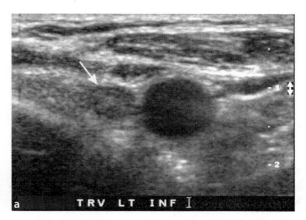

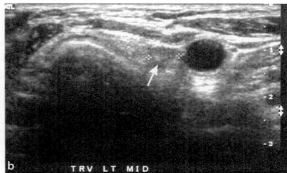

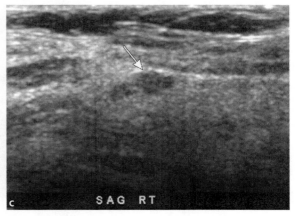

Fig. 20.5 At least three of the four parathyroid glands (*arrows*) are enlarged in this patient with hypercalcemia. All are similar in size and echotexture (**a, b,** and **c**). Although multiple parathyroid adenoma could have a similar appearance, the ultrasound findings are most consistent with the diagnosis of parathyroid hyperplasia

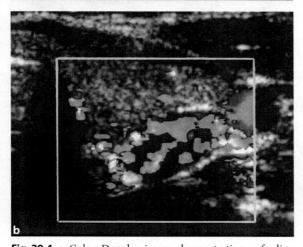

Fig. 20.4 a Color Doppler image demonstrating a feeding vessel (*arrow*) entering the hypoechoic parathyroid adenoma (same patient as in Fig. 20.3). **b** Parathyroid adenoma posterior to the left lobe of the thyroid in a 65-year-old woman with hypercalcemia. Note the prominent peripheral rim of vascularity in an arc-like configuration

thyroid gland. The superior glands are less commonly ectopic in location, but if so, they are most commonly found posteriorly, in the tracheoesophageal groove. The inferior parathyroid glands arise from the third branchial cleft pouch and typically migrate more than the superior glands both inferiorly and anteriorly. Hence, the location of the inferior glands is more variable, with approximately 60% located within 1–2 cm inferior and posterior to the lower pole of the thyroid gland. The most common location for an ectopic inferior gland is in the lower neck or superior mediastinum in association with the thymus gland. However, ectopic inferior glands can also be found high in the neck near the carotid bifurcation or carotid sheath [37–40]. Often they may be seen just anterior to the carotid artery in a location more typical for cervical adenopathy (Fig. 20.6). Rarely a parathyroid gland will be intrathyroidal in location (Fig. 20.7). Hence, full evaluation for a parathyroid adenoma by US will include evaluation of the neck from the angle of the jaw to as deep below the sternal notch as one can visu-

alize, with particular attention to the posterior aspect of the upper third of the thyroid gland, the posterior aspect of the lower pole of the thyroid gland and up and down the carotid artery.

US examination should be performed using a high-resolution, high-frequency, linear-array transducer (at least 7.5–15 MHz) with both gray-scale and color Doppler imaging. If the patient's neck is thick, the use of a lower-frequency 5 MHz transducer may be required to effect adequate penetration. The patient is examined supine with the neck extended. A pillow or rolled towel placed between the shoulders will help to extend the neck in a comfortable fashion. Imaging should begin in a transverse plane concentrating behind the upper third of the thyroid gland, the lower pole of the thyroid gland and any area of abnormality noted on prior imaging study such as nuclear medicine or MRI. Longitudinal images are also obtained. If no lesion is identified, scanning should be extended superiorly along the carotid sheath and internal jugular vein to the angle of the jaw and inferiorly to the

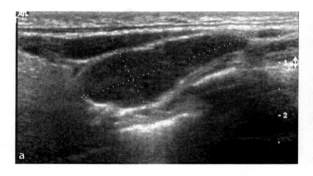

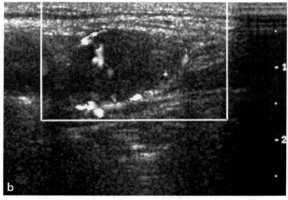

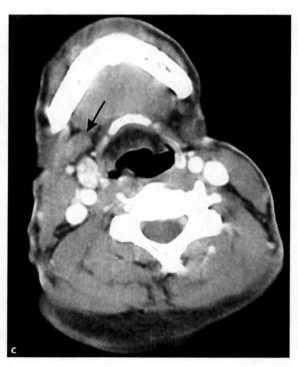

Fig. 20.6 High cervical ectopic parathyroid adenoma. Grey scale (**a**) and Doppler image (**b**) of the superior right neck reveal a hypoechoic vascular mass medial to the right submandibular gland (*calipers* in **a**) in a postsurgical patient with persistent hypercalcemia. Although lymph nodes may occur in this location, this lesion is more vascular than a normal lymph node and lacks the morphologic characteristics of corticomedullary differentiation that is typical of a normal lymph node. Diagnosis was confirmed by fine-needle aspiration and parathyroid hormone (PTH) assay. Computed tomography (CT; **c**) confirms the ultrasound findings; parathyroid adenoma (*arrow*)

clavicle/sternal notch in both transverse and longitudinal planes. At the level of the clavicle, the transducer should be angled inferiorly to search the upper mediastinum as carefully as possible.

If a hypoechoic, extrathyroidal mass is identified, color Doppler imaging should then be used to demonstrate the typical rim pattern of peripheral vascularity [33] and a feeding vessel that enters at the upper or lower pole of the gland [32]. If no lesion is identified, color Doppler imaging may still be helpful by identifying an extrathyroidal feeding artery, which can then be followed to the parathyroid adenoma [3,32]. Lane et al. [32] reported that use of color Doppler to identify a feeding vessel increased the sensitivity of US examination for the detection of parathyroid adenomas from 73 to 88% in their series. In addition, the thyroid gland should then be surveyed with color or power Doppler imaging searching for asymmetry in vascularity as the thyroid gland maybe more vascular in the region of an adenoma [3]. If gray-scale and color or power Doppler imaging still do not identify an adenoma, gray-scale imaging should be repeated using gradually applied graded compression to reevaluate the areas previously described where adenomas are most common [3]. The graded compression technique has been reported to be particularly helpful in visualizing small deep ectopic adenomas (Fig. 20.8). Reeder et al. [3] have reported in their series that the graded compression technique was helpful in visualizing 27% of small adenomas, but was not necessary for identifying adenomas >1 cm in diameter.

Despite careful attention to scanning technique and focused use of color Doppler imaging and graded compression, it may still be difficult to identify retrotracheal or retroesophageal, mediastinal, and intrathyroidal parathyroid adenomas or adenomas located within the carotid sheath. To search the retrotracheal region, a helpful maneuver is to angle the transducer medially while the patient's head is turned to the contralateral side. Repeating this approach on the opposite side of the neck may make the adenoma "pop out" into view (Fig. 20.9). If one can see the esophagus from both sides of the neck, one can confirm that the retrotracheal area has been adequately evaluated [34]. While it is impossible to fully evaluate the mediastinum by US, the superior mediastinum can be partially evaluated by angling the transducer inferior- and posterior-medially around the clavicle with the neck hyperextended. Asking the patient to swallow can sometimes be helpful by causing the parathyroid adenoma to transiently elevate into the field of view. A lower-frequency probe may be required. Intrathyroidal

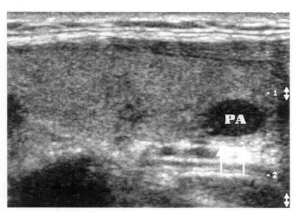

Fig. 20.7 Intrathyroidal parathyroid adenoma (PA). Note that thyroid tissue surrounds the entire periphery of the gland (*arrows*)

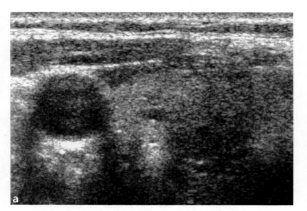
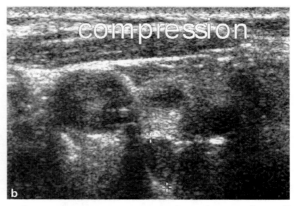

Fig. 20.8 Transverse images without (**a**) and with (**b**) compression, showing dramatic improvement of visualization of a small adenoma (calipers) with compression. (Reprinted with permission from the Journal of Ultrasound in Medicine, the American Institute of Ultrasound in Medicine, and R. Brooke Jeffrey MD (senior author): Reeder et al. (2002) [3]

parathyroid adenomas can be difficult to differentiate from a hypoechoic thyroid nodule, and percutaneous FNA to assess for parathyroid hormone (PTH) may be necessary to confirm the diagnosis. Adenomas within the carotid sheath may be found anywhere along the carotid artery, but are often located superior and anterior to the carotid artery or between the carotid artery and internal jugular vein [34], and can therefore be difficult to distinguish from cervical lymphadenopathy. The Doppler flow pattern may be helpful in discriminating between these two entities (see below).

Cervical lymph nodes, the collapsed esophagus, and the longus colli muscle can occasionally be mistaken for parathyroid adenomas on US examination [3,34,41]. Cervical lymph nodes can most often be distinguished from parathyroid adenomas by their internal architecture and typical vascular pattern. A normal cervical node should demonstrate a central echogenic hilum and surrounding hypoechoic cortex. Normal cervical lymph nodes are kidney-bean in

shape rather than oval. The feeding vessel to a lymph node enters the echogenic hilum centrally rather than peripherally in the polar region, which is more typical for an adenoma. However, inflammatory or malignant lymph nodes may lose their normal corticomedullary differentiation and become more uniformly hypoechoic with a round or oval shape, and therefore be quite difficult to distinguish from parathyroid adenomas on gray-scale imaging. Percutaneous FNA may be required for diagnosis (see below). The esophagus can be recognized on high-resolution US images by the striated appearance of its wall, its position medial to the lower pole of the left lobe of the thyroid, and the fact that it will elongate on coronal or sagittal imaging. The longus colli muscle also lies posterior to the thyroid gland. On transverse images it has a triangular configuration, and although hypoechoic, will contain echogenic striations typical of skeletal muscle. Longitudinal images will reveal elongation of the structure. Dynamic imaging while the patient swallows may also be helpful. The thyroid gland will move, but the longus colli muscle is attached to the spine, and is therefore more stationary [34].

False-negative US examinations in the setting of primary HPTH occur primarily when a parathyroid adenoma is ectopic in location or only minimally enlarged. Mediastinal and retrotracheal adenomas can be extremely difficult to visualize on US despite meticulous imaging techniques. In addition, enlargement of the thyroid gland will displace a deeper adenoma such that it is difficult to visualize and if the surface of the thyroid gland is nodular or lobular, differentiation of an extrathyroidal hypoechoic parathyroid adenoma from an exophytic thyroid nodule will become extremely difficult.

Preoperative imaging is even more important in patients with recurrent HPTH, as the surgical morbidity is higher due to scarring and fibrosis. The risk of recurrent laryngeal nerve damage is substantially higher and the surgical cure rate is lower by approximately 10–30% [42–49]. A combined imaging approach is generally necessary using nuclear medicine, US, MRI, and angiographic venous sampling as there is a much higher incidence of ectopic adenomas in this clinical setting. This multipronged imaging approach has been reported to increase the reoperative surgical success rate to nearly 90% from a surgical success rate of only 62% for the nonimaged patient [49,50].

Preoperative US-guided percutaneous FNA of a suspected parathyroid adenoma is often recommended in patients with recurrent HPTH due to the increased surgical risk. In addition, cervical lymph nodes are commonly identified in the postoperative

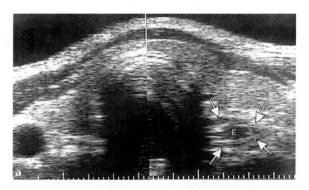

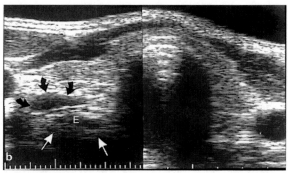

Fig. 20.9 Retroesophageal parathyroid adenoma. **a** Composite split image if the thyroid gland with the patient's head turned to the right. The esophagus (*E* and *arrows*) protrudes to the left of the trachea. The thyroid gland is normal and no parathyroid adenoma is seen. When the patient turns their head to the left (**b**), the esophagus (*E* and *straight arrows*) and the parathyroid adenoma (*curved arrows*) pop out on the right from behind the trachea (courtesy of Dr. Carl Reading)

neck and are a significant cause of false-positive US examinations. To perform an US-guided FNA, the patient's neck is prepped with betadine and local anesthesia is achieved using 1% lidocaine. A 25-gauge beveled needle is then placed into the suspected adenoma under real time US observation. The needle is advanced up and down within the lesion under continuous US visualization approximately 5–10 times with an excursion of at least 0.5 cm. Material is drawn up into the core of the needle by direct capillary action without a syringe. Following aspiration, the sample is aspirated into a syringe containing 0.5 ml of sterile saline and immediately assayed for PTH. This can be accomplished using portable assay equipment in the US suite and takes approximately 7–10 min. If there is inadequate tissue, the aspiration procedure can be repeated using suction with a 5- to 10-ml syringe. Overall accuracy of FNA for diagnosis of parathyroid tissue has been reported to be as high as 87% in a series of 52 patients [51].

In patients at significant surgical risk, US-guided alcohol ablation of adenomas can be performed. Following local anesthesia (this technique is more painful), a 22- to 25-gauge beveled needle is inserted into the adenoma under direct US visualization. The mass is then injected with 95% ethanol. A volume equal to approximately one half of the mass is used and should be injected into multiple areas. The injected area will become markedly echogenic for approximately 1 min and the vascularity of the adenoma should decrease. The injections are repeated every other day until serum calcium or PTH levels normalize. Up to three to five injections may be required and long-term follow up is required to detect the subsequent hypoparathyroidism or recurrent HPTH [34]. Long-term results have been mixed, but cure rates are reported to be less than for surgery [52–55]. Partial responses have been reported in 89–90% of patients. However, a durable complete response over 3–16 months has been reported in only 56–33% of patients, respectively [52,53]. Failures have been hypothesized to be caused by either incomplete ablation or because the correct abnormal gland was not identified. It should be noted that ethanol ablation is not as effective in patients with multiglandular disease, which may be difficult to accurately diagnose. In addition, ethanol ablation can cause severe periglandular fibrosis, which may make subsequent ablation and or surgery extremely difficult. Furthermore, this technique has been associated with injuries to the recurrent laryngeal nerve, which is often in direct apposition to the parathyroid gland. Accordingly, this technique is rarely employed.

20.4 Tomographic Imaging

20.4.1 Computed Tomography

CT is an effective method for the detection of ectopic lower parathyroid adenomas, especially in the anterior mediastinum, with a sensitivity of up to 92% [56]. These glands usually lie within the fat-replaced thymus, and even small adenomas may readily be visualized (Fig. 20.10). Ectopic higher parathyroid adenomas may be localized within the tracheoesophageal

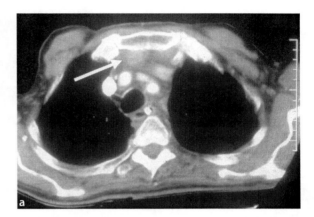

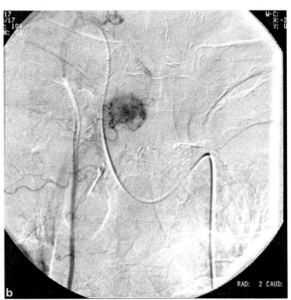

Fig. 20.10 Imaging of ectopic mediastinal parathyroid adenoma: **a** Contrast-enhanced CT scan of the upper mediastinum shows a hyperdense lesion surrounded by the mediastinal fat during arterial contrast dye phase (*arrow*). **b** Further confirmatory evaluation of this adenoma using superselective angiography of the right internal mammary artery reveals the typical blood supply of an anterior mediastinal parathyroid adenoma

groove in the posterosuperior mediastinum. On CT these adenomas are identified as solid masses adjacent to the air-filled esophagus and trachea. Undescended adenomas near the carotid bifurcation at the level of the hyoid bone are also depicted on CT (Fig. 20.6c), proved that the examination includes the entire neck to the level of the mandible [57]. CT correctly identifies the adenoma of initial and reoperative cases in about 70% and 60%, respectively [58–60]. Recently, the possibility of CT-MIBI image fusion has been reported. This appears to be superior to MIBI-SPECT in preoperative parathyroid imaging with improved sensitivity and specificity. CT-MIBI image fusion can be performed on existing CT- and MIBI-SPECT units [61].

20.4.2.   Magnetic Resonance Imaging

MRI provides a higher sensitivity at identifying ectopic parathyroid adenomas than does CT scan [62,63]. MRI resolution with T1-weighted images (Fig. 20.11) of parathyroid adenomas is comparable to that of CT scans, with a low to intermediate signal intensity similar to that of muscle on T1-weighted images. On the other hand, T2-weighted images (Fig. 20.12) or short-tau inversion recovery-pulse sequences produces a bright signal [64]. It must be noted that a minor proportion of abnormal parathyroid glands demonstrate different signal characteristics (i.e., isointense on both T2- and T1-weighted images or hyperintense on both sequences), which may lead to false-negative results [65]. The potential advantage of MRI contrast dye application in this minor proportion of patients with

isointense lesions still remains to be assessed [66]. Reported sensitivities for parathyroid gland localization by MRI are 71–83% [60,67–69]. Sensitivity is superior for the adenomas (87%) but less for parathyroid hyperplasia (75%) [66,70]. Recent studies demonstrate that MRI with surface coils provides exquisite anatomy of the neck and enhanced resolution. Results indicate that approximately 90% of abnormal parathyroid glands can correctly be depicted in patients undergoing reoperations.

20.5   Invasive Localization Tests

Invasive localization tests are almost exclusively indicated in the preoperative work-up for repeat surgery and then only if the advanced noninvasive tests as sonography, scintigraphy, CT, and/or MRI have been negative or inconclusive. These two facts – previous surgery and negative advanced diagnostics – inherently represent an enormous selection bias. Despite these difficulties, cases invasive localization tests can add important pieces to the puzzle.

20.5.1   Selective Parathyroid Venous Sampling

Selective parathyroid venous sampling (SVS) was first described by Reitz and colleagues [71]. If positive, it can indicate the side and the cervical or thoracic location of a PTH-producing lesion. It can not give the exact height and location of an adenoma or hyperplasia, distinguish between the two, or directly

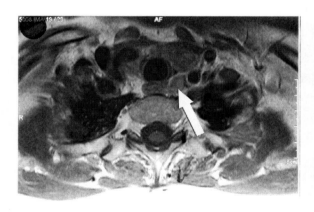

Fig. 20.11 T1-weighted magnetic resonance (MR) image of a left paraesophageal parathyroid adenoma (*arrow*) showing a low- to intermediate-intense lesion that is similar to the MR intensity of muscle tissue

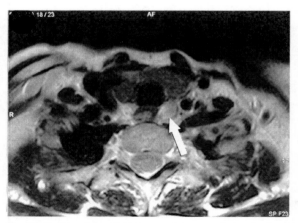

Fig. 20.12 T2-weighted MR image of the same lesion depicted in Fig. 20.11 showing a lesion with a bright, hyperintense signal (*arrow*)

"show" the offending lesion. Unlike imaging tests, its accuracy is not dependent on lesion size, but rather PTH output.

20.5.1.1 Parathyroid Venous Anatomy

The normal venous return of an orthotopic parathyroid gland takes place via the superior, medial, and inferior thyroid veins. The superior and medial thyroid veins in turn drain into the internal jugular veins bilaterally, whereas the inferior thyroid veins normally empty into the left brachiocephalic vein. Ectopic glands may drain via the superior thymic vein or the twin internal thoracic veins given a corresponding location in the thymus or the mediastinum.

Doppman and colleagues postulated that the majority of the parathyroid venous blood flows along the inferior thyroid vein and that there is little if any crossflow from one side to the other [72]. After previous cervical surgery the flow may proceed along the middle and superior thyroid as well as the vertebral and thymic veins. Ectopic mediastinal and thymic parathyroid tissue usually drains via the thymic or internal thoracic veins.

20.5.1.2 Technique of SVS

SVS is a sophisticated technique (Fig. 20.13) that is best performed by an experienced interventional radiologist. It can principally be done from any sufficiently large venous access site. We normally use a transfemoral access and place a 6-F sheath. We then advance a 5-F multipurpose catheter with an additional side hole close to its tip into the superior caval vein and selectively draw blood samples from the locations given on the scheme in Fig. 20.14. Each superselective location is confirmed with digital subtraction venography after sampling. The samples are immediately put on ice and sent to a specialized laboratory. The PTH levels reported are then noted on this scheme as percentages of the value in the superior caval vein. Values above 150–200% are considered positive in the literature [73,74]. A gradient that is continuously decreasing in sequential samples from a peripheral peak to the superior caval vein is another strong indicator for a close location of a PTH-producing lesion. The resulting location is classified as either right or left or bilaterally cervical or mediastinal or thymic, respectively.

Chaffanjon and coworkers report that an elevated PTH value drawn from a vertebral vein in their experience points to "a diseased superior parathyroid

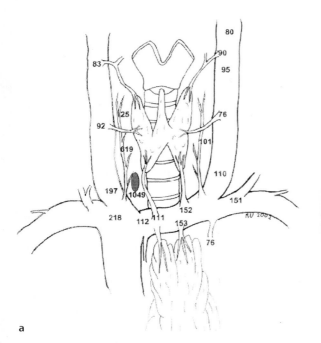

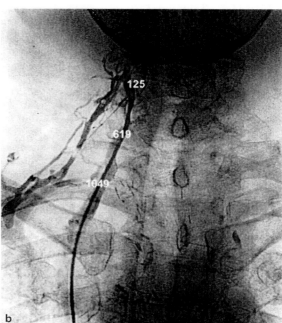

Fig. 20.13 a Venous PTH levels (pg/ml) obtained in the interventional suite in a patient with persistent hyperparathyroidism. A gradient was demonstrated in the right vertebral vein. **b** Highly selective catheterization of this vein and the superimposed PTH values (pg/ml)

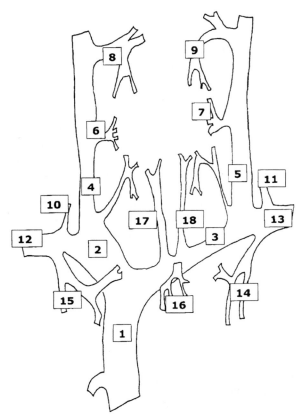

Fig. 20.14 Relevant anatomy for selective parathyroid venous sampling (from [75]). Cervical and mediastinal venous sites selected for blood sampling. *1* superior vena cava, *2* right brachiocephalic vein, *3* left brachiocephalic vein, *4* right internal jugular vein, *5* left internal jugular vein, *6* right middle thyroid vein, *7* left middle thyroid vein, *8* right superior thyroid vein, *9* left superior thyroid vein, *10* right vertebral vein, *11* left vertebral vein, *12* right subclavian vein, *13* left subclavian vein, *14* left internal thoracic vein, *15* right internal thoracic vein, *16* superior thymic vein, *17* right inferior thyroid vein, *18* left inferior thyroid vein

of 71% and a proportion of 9% of false-positives. Compared with sestamibi scanning, SVS provides a higher number of true-positive and false-positive results in 69% and 7% of cases, respectively. In an associated study, the sensitivity of SVS was even reported as at least 90% with no false-positives in 21 patients. The authors conclude that SVS is the gold standard in patients being evaluated for reoperation in whom the noninvasive localization techniques have been negative, equivocal, or inconsistent [73]. It is reasonable to expect that in about three-quarters of this difficult group of patients the pathology can be correctly localized with SVS. This group in itself represents about a quarter of all patients evaluated for repeat surgery.

False-positive localization with SVS studies is probably at least partially due to the fact that during previous surgery the normal venous anatomy has been substantially disturbed, for example by ligation of the inferior thyroid veins. This will lead to collateral flow phenomena that are difficult to factor into the interpretation of an SVS. Arteriography has been recommended to study the venous drainage prior to sampling, but there is no evidence yet that this will lead to a higher accuracy of sampling.

Complications of SVS are rarely reported and where they are, they are mostly without clinical consequences. The possible adverse effects of contrast media application, especially in secondary HPTH, however, must certainly be taken into account.

20.5.2 Parathyroid Arteriography

Parathyroid arteriography can be performed for diagnostic and therapeutic purposes.

20.5.2.1 Diagnostic Parathyroid Angiography

Angiographic localization of parathyroid adenomas goes back to Ivar Seldinger in 1953 [79]. Contrary to SVS angiography can directly demonstrate parathyroid tissue as a hypervascular area (Fig. 20.10b) with a dense contrast media staining that may persist longer than in the thyroid gland. The problem is that this sign is completely unspecific, as are displacement or enlargement of the inferior thyroid artery and an early venous return. The diagnostic arteriography of the parathyroid gland is therefore mostly unnecessary. As said above, it may be helpful in selected cases to elucidate a venous flow altered by surgery.

gland in a homolateral retroesophageal position" whereas an equally elevated value in the internal thoracic vein suggests a location in the thymic tongue [75]. This observation has not been confirmed by other groups, so far.

20.5.1.3 Results of SVS

Results of SVS for localization prior to reoperation have been reported consistently as being both sensitive and specific [74–78]. A recent meta-analysis on localization techniques in persistent or recurrent renal HPTH reports an overall rate of true-positives

20.5.2.2 Parathyroid Transcatheter Ablation

The methods reported in the literature are contrast media staining, embolization [80], and alcohol ablation [81]. Contrast media staining avoids the risk of malembolization and has been reported as being effective in more than 80% of cases [82]. Almost all cases concerned mediastinal adenomas. The same is true for transcatheter alcohol ablation, which is considered to be too risky to cervical application. Mediastinal location is therefore the best indication for any form of transcatheter therapy as it can be performed safely and is much less invasive than open surgery.

20.5.3 Percutaneous Parathyroid Puncture

The role of percutaneous parathyroid biopsy with PTH sampling, pecutaneous ablation using alcohol, or laser techniques has yet to be defined. Direct proof of parathyroid tissue or an elevated PTH level in a hitherto unclassified cervical tumor may certainly be beneficial, but normally the clinical diagnosis of recurrent or persistent HPTH is already established. The therapeutic margin of percutaneous ablation in the neck appears to be rather small regarding complications and recurrences. In the mediastinum, where surgery is most invasive, these techniques are unfortunately not applicable.

20.5.4 Indications for Invasive Localization Tests

In our view, every algorithm for the preoperative evaluation of recurrent or persistent hyperparathyroidism should include SVS as the definitive test if the combined results of the noninvasive tests are equivocal or conflicting with each other or the clinical history.

Acknowledgements

This chapter was shared and the authors contributed as follows: Introduction part and Ultrasound (Dr. Leslie Scoutt); Nuclear Imaging (Dr. David Cheng); and Invasive Localization Tests (Dr. Ludwig Jacob).

References

1. Howe JR (2000) Minimally invasive parathyroid surgery. Surg Clin North Am 80:1399–1426

2. Doppman JL (1968) Reoperative parathyroid surgery: localization procedures, parathyroid surgery. Prog Surg 18:1171–1175

3. Reeder SB, Desser TS, Weigel RJ, Jeffrey RB (2002) Sonography in primary hyperparathyroidism. J Ultrasound Med 21:539–552

4. Udelsman R (2001) Primary hyper parathyroidism. Curr Treat Options Oncol 2:365–372

5. Loevner LA (1996) Imaging of the parathyroid glands. Semin Ultrasound CT MR 17:563–575

6. Sanders LR (1998) Hyperparathyroidism. In: McDermott MT (ed) Endocrine Secrets. Hanley & Belfus, Philadelphia, PA, pp 91–98

7. Van Heerden JA, Beahrs OH, Woolner LB (1977) The pathology and surgical management of primary hyperparathyroidism. Surg Clin North Am 57:557–563

8. Sandrock D, Merino MJ, Norton JA, Neumann RD (1990) Parathyroid imaging by Tc/Tl scintigraphy. Eur J Nucl Med 16:607–613

9. Goris ML, Basso LV, Keeling C (1991) Parathyroid imaging. J Nucl Med 32:887–889

10. Gimlett TM, Brownless SM, Taylor WH, Shields R, Simkin EP (1986) Limits to parathyroid imaging with thallium-201 confirmed by tissue uptake and phantom studies. J Nucl Med 27:1262–1265

11. Young AE, Gaunt JI, Croft DN, et al (1983) Location of parathyroid adenomas by thallium-201 and technetium-9m subtraction scanning. Br Med J 286:1384–1386

12. Intenzo C, Park CH (1985) Co-existent parathyroid adenoma and thyroid carcinoma. Clin Nucl Med 10:560–561

13. Punt JA, De Hooge P, Hoekstra JBL (1985) False positive subtraction scintigram of the parathyroid glands due to metastatic tumour. J Nucl Med 26:155–156

14. Chiu ML, Kronange JF, Piwnica-Worms D (1990) Effect of mitochondrial and plasma-membrane potentials on accumulation of hexakis (2-methoxyisobutylisonitrile) technetium in cultured mouse fibroblasts. J Nucl Med 31:1646–1653

15. Sandrock D, Merino MJ, Norton JA, Neumann RD (1993) Ultrastructural histology correlates of thallium-201/technetium-99m parathyroid subtraction scintigraphy. J Nucl Med 34:24–29

16. Dotzenrath C, Goretzki PE, Sarbia M, Cupisti K, Feldkamp J, Roher H-D (2001) Parathyroid carcinoma: problems in diagnosis and the need for radical surgery even in recurrent disease. Eur J Surg Oncol 27:383–389

17. Pappu S, Donovan P, Cheng D, Udelsman R (2005) Sestamibi scans are not all created equally. Arch Surg 140:383–386

18. Cance WG, Otsuka FL, Dilley WG, et al (1988) A potential new radiopharmaceutical for parathyroid imaging: radiolabeled parathyroid-specific monoclonal antibody. I. Evaluation of 125I-labeled antibody in a nude mouse model system. Int J Radiat Appl Instrum 15:299–303

19. Otsuka FL, Cance WG, Dilley WG, et al (1988) A potential new radiopharmaceutical for parathyroid imaging: radiolabeled parathyroid-specific monoclonal antibody. II. Comparison of 125I and 111In-labeled antibodies. Int J Radiat Appl Instrum 15:305–311

20. Zwas ST, Czerniak A, Boruchowsky S, Itamar A, Wolfstein I (1987) Preoperative parathyroid localization by superimposed iodine-131 toluidine blue and technetium-99m pertechnetate imaging. J Nucl Med 28:298–307

21. Neumann DR, Esselstyn CB Jr, MacIntyre WJ, et al (1996) Comparison of FDG-PET and sestamibi SPECT in primary hyperparathyroidism. J Nucl Med 37:1809–1815

22. Melon P, Luxen A, Hamoir E, et al (1995) Fluorine-18-fluorodeoxyglucose positron emission tomography for pre-operative parathyroid imaging in primary hyperparathyroidism. Eur J Nucl Med 22:556–558

23. Sundin A, Johansson C, Hellman P, et al (1996) PET and parathyroid L-[carbon-11]methionine accumulation in hyperparathyroidism. J Nucl Med 37:1766–1770

24. Price DC (1993) Radioisotopic evaluation of the thyroid and parathyroids. Radiol Clin North Am 31:991–1015

25. Gooding GAW, Okerlund MD, Stark DD (1986) Parathyroid imaging: comparison of double tracer (T1-201, Tc-99m) scintigraphy and high-resolution US. Radiology 161:57–64

26. Krusback AJ, Wilson SD, Lawson TL (1989) Prospective comparison of radionuclide, computer tomographic, sonographic, and magnetic resonance localization of parathyroid tumors. Surgery 106:639–644

27. Mazzeo S, Caramella D, Lencioni R, et al (1996) Comparison among sonography, double tracer subtraction scintigraphy, and double phase scintigraphy in the detection of parathyroid lesions. AJR Am J Roentgenol 166:1465–1470

28. Lloyd MN, Lees WR, Milroy EJ (1990) Pre-operative localization in primary hyperparathyroidism. Clin Radiol 41:239–243

29. Simeone HJ, Mueller PR, Fernucci JT, et al (1981) High-resolution real-time sonography of the parathyroid. Radiology 141:745–751

30. Giron J, Ouhayoun E, Dahan M, et al (1996) Imaging of hyperparathyroidism: US, CT, MRI and MIBI scintigraphy. Eur J Radiol 21:167–173

31. Stein BL, Wexler MJ (1990) Preoperative parathyroid localization: a prospective evaluation of ultrasonography and thallium technetium scintigraphy in hyperparathyroidism. Can Assoc Gen Surg 33:175–180

32. Lane MJ, Desser TS, Weigel RJ, Jeffrey RB Jr (1998) Use of color and power Doppler sonography to identify feeding associated with parathyroid adenomas. AJR Am J Roentgenol 171:819–823

33. Wolf RJ, Cronan JJ, Monchik JM (1994) Color Doppler sonography: an adjunctive technique in assessment of parathyroid adenomas. J Ultrasound Med 13:303–308

34. Huppert BJ, Reading CC (2005) The parathyroid glands. In: Rumack CM, Wilson SR, Charboneau JW (eds) Diagnostic Ultrasound. Elsevier-Mosby, St. Louis, pp 771–794

35. Cotran RS, Kumar V, Robbins SL, Schoen FJ (1994) The endocrine system. In: Cotran RS, Kumar V, Robbins SL, Schoen FJ (eds) Robbins Pathological Basis of Disease. WB Saunders, Philadelphia, PA, pp 1143–1148

36. Russell CF, Grant CS, Van Heerden JA (1982) Hyperfunctioning supernumerary parathyroid glands: an occasional cause of hyperparathyroidism. Mayo Clin Proc 57:121–124

37. Edis AJ, Purnell DC, Van Heerden JA (1979) The undescended "parathymus." An occasional cause of failed neck exploration for hyperparathyroidism. Ann Surg 190:64–68

38. Mansberger AR, Wei JP (1993) Surgical embryology and anatomy of the thyroid and parathyroid glands. Surg Clin North Am 73:727–746

39. Akerstrom G, Malmaeus J, Bergstrom R (1984) Surgical anatomy of human parathyroid glands. Surgery 95:14–21

40. Wang C-A (1976) The anatomic basis of parathyroid surgery. Ann Surg 183:271–275

41. Khati N, Adamson T, Johnson KS, Hill MC (2003) Ultrasound of the thyroid and parathyroid glands. Ultrasound Q 19:162–176

42. Levin KE, Clark OH (1989) The reasons for failure in parathyroid operations. Arch Surg 124:911–914

43. Cheung PSY, Borgstrom A, Thompson NW (1989) Strategy in re-operative surgery for hyperparathyroidism. Arch Surg 124:676–680

44. Palmer JA, Rosen IB (1982) Re-operative surgery for hyperparathyroidism. Am J Surg 144:406–410

45. Prinz RA, Gamvros OI, Allison DJ, et al (1981) Re-operations for hyperparathyroidism. Surg Gynecol Obstet 152:760–764

46. Grant CS, Charboneau JW, James EM, et al (1988) Re-operative parathyroid surgery. Wien Klin Wochenschr 100:360–363

47. Wells SA (1991) Advances in the operative management of persistent hyperparathyroidism. Mayo Clin Proc 66:1175–1177

48. Brennan MF, Marx SJ, Doppman J, et al (1981) Results of re-operation for persistent and recurrent hyperparathyroidism. Ann Surg 194:671–676

49. Thompson GB, Grant CS, Perrier ND, et al (1999) Reoperative parathyroid surgery in the era of sestamibi scanning and intraoperative parathyroid hormone monitoring. Arch Surg 134:699–705

50. Grant CS, Van Heerden JA, Charboneau JW, et al (1986) Clinical management of persistent and/or recurrent primary hyperparathyroidism. World J Surg 10:555–565

51. Solbiati L, Montali G, Croce F, et al (1983) Parathyroid tumors detected by fine-needle aspiration biopsy under ultrasonic guidance. Radiology 148:793–797

52. Harman CR, Grant CS, Hay ID, et al (1998) Indications, technique, and efficacy of alcohol injection of enlarged parathyroid glands in patients with primary hyperparathyroidism. Surgery 124:1011–1020

53. Cercueil JP, Jacob D, Verges B, et al (1998) Percutaneous ethanol injection into parathyroid adenomas: Mid- and long-term results. Eur Radiol 8:1565–1569

54. Karstup S, Hegedus L, Holm HH (1993) Ultrasonically guided chemical parathyroidectomy in patients with primary hyperparathyroidism. A follow-up study: Clin Endocrinol 38:523–530

55. Bennendbaek FN, Karstrup S, Hegedus L (1997) Percutaneous ethanol injection therapy in the treatment of thyroid and parathyroid lesions. Eur J Endocrinol 136:240–247

56. Nwariaku FE, Snyder WH, Burkey SH, Watumull L, Mathews D (2005) Inframanubrial parathyroid glands in patients with primary hyperparathyroidism: alternatives to sternotomy. World J Surg 29:491–494

57. Krudy AG, et al (1981) The detection of mediastinal parathyroid glands by computed tomography, selective arteriography, and venous sampling: an analysis of 17 cases. Radiology 140:739–744

58. Clark P, et al (2004) Providing optimal preoperative localization for recurrent parathyroid carcinoma: a combined parathyroid scintigraphy and computed tomography approach. Clin Nucl Med 29:681–684

59. Sekiyama K, et al (2003) Usefulness of diagnostic imaging in primary hyperparathyroidism. Int J Urol 10:7–11

60. van der HE, et al (1994) [Preoperative noninvasive tests for localization of enlarged parathyroid glands in 115 patients with hyperparathyroidism]. Ned Tijdschr Geneeskd 138:1660–1664

61. Profanter C, et al (2004) CT-MIBI image fusion: a new preoperative localization technique for primary, recurrent, and persistent hyperparathyroidism. Surgery 135:157–162

62. Tziakouri C, et al (1996) Value of ultrasonography, CT and MR imaging in the diagnosis of primary hyperparathyroidism. Acta Radiol 37:720–726

63. Ishibashi M, et al (1997) Localization of ectopic parathyroid glands using technetium-99m sestamibi imaging: comparison with magnetic resonance and computed tomographic imaging. Eur J Nucl Med 24:197–201

64. Wright AR, et al (1992) Fat-suppression magnetic resonance imaging in the preoperative localization of parathyroid adenomas. Clin Radiol 46:324–328

65. Lee VS, et al (1996) The complementary roles of fast spin-echo MR imaging and double-phase 99m Tc-sestamibi scintigraphy for localization of hyperfunctioning parathyroid glands. AJR Am J Roentgenol 167:1555–1562

66. Lopez HE, et al (2000) Preoperative contrast-enhanced MRI of the parathyroid glands in hyperparathyroidism. Invest Radiol 35:426–430

67. Catargi B, et al (1999) Localization of parathyroid tumors using endoscopic ultrasonography in primary hyperparathyroidism. J Endocrinol Invest 22:688–692

68. McDermott VG, et al (1996) Preoperative MR imaging in hyperparathyroidism: results and factors affecting parathyroid detection. AJR Am J Roentgenol 166:705–710

69. Gotway MB, et al (2001) Comparison between MR imaging and 99mTc MIBI scintigraphy in the evaluation of recurrent or persistent hyperparathyroidism. Radiology 218:783–790

70. Wakamatsu H, et al (2001) Technetium-99m tetrofosmin for parathyroid scintigraphy: a direct comparison with (99m)Tc-MIBI, (201)Tl, MRI and US. Eur J Nucl Med 28:1817–1827

71. Reitz RE, Pollard JJ, Wang CA, et al (1969) Localization of parathyroid adenomas by selective venous catheterization and radioimmunoassay. N Engl J Med 281:348–351

72. Doppman JL, Hammond WG (1970) The anatomic basis of parathyroid venous sampling. Radiology 95:603–610

73. Seehofer D, Steinmuller T, Rayes N, et al (2004) Parathyroid hormone venous sampling before reoperative surgery in renal hyperparathyroidism: comparison with noninvasive localization procedures and review of the literature. Arch Surg 139:1331–1338

74. Jones JJ, Brunaud L, Dowd CF, Duh QY, Morita E, Clark OH (2002) Accuracy of selective venous sampling for intact parathyroid hormone in difficult patients with recurrent or persistent hyperparathyroidism. Surgery 132:944–950; discussion 950–941

75. Chaffanjon PC, Voirin D, Vasdev A, Chabre O, Kenyon NM, Brichon PY (2004) Selective venous sampling in recurrent and persistent hyperparathyroidism: indication, technique, and results. World J Surg 28:958–961

76. Eisenberg H, Pallotta J, Sherwood LM (1974) Selective arteriography, venography and venous hormone assay in diagnosis and localization of parathyroid lesions. Am J Med 56:810–820

77. Sugg SL, Fraker DL, Alexander R, et al (1993) Prospective evaluation of selective venous sampling for parathyroid hormone concentration in patients undergoing reoperations for primary hyperparathyroidism. Surgery 114:1004–1009; discussion 1009–1010

78. Jaskowiak N, Norton JA, Alexander HR, et al (1996) A prospective trial evaluating a standard approach to reoperation for missed parathyroid adenoma. Ann Surg 224:308–320; discussion 320–301

79. Gunther R, Georgi M, Diethelm L, Rothmund M (1976) Current status of preoperative localization in primary hyperparathyroidism. Radiologe 16:175–187

80. Doppman JL, Brown EM, Brennan MF, Spiegel A, Marx SJ, Aurbach GD (1979) Angiographic ablation of parathyroid adenomas. Radiology 130:577–582

81. Gunther R, Beyer J, Hesch H, Reinwein D (1984) Percutaneous transcatheter ablation of parathyroid gland tumors by alcohol injection and contrast media infusion. Rofo 140:27–30

82. Miller DL, Doppman JL, Chang R, et al (1987) Angiographic ablation of parathyroid adenomas: lessons from a 10-year experience. Radiology 165:601–607

21 Conventional Surgical Management of Primary Hyperparathyroidism

Heather Yeo, Paola Uranga, and Sanziana Roman

CONTENTS

21.1   Introduction

The first successful parathyroidectomy for primary hyperparathyroidism (HPTH) was performed in Vienna in 1925 by Felix Mandl who performed a neck exploration identifying all four parathyroids. The bilateral neck exploration has remained the conventional treatment of choice for primary HPTH for many decades, until more recently, when minimally invasive parathyroidectomy has been popularized. This time-tested dissection by an experienced endocrine surgeon continues too be the "gold" standard to which all other procedures are compared [1].

The incidence of primary HPTH has been on the rise since the 1960s. With the development of autoanalyzers, serum calcium became routinely screened. Hence, asymptomatic calcium elevations are now readily identified. Approximately 100,000 new cases of primary HPTH are diagnosed each year in the United States. Incidence estimates are as high as 1/1,000 in postmenopausal women [2]. While the advent of many new localization modalities is changing the face of parathyroid surgery, an understanding of the conventional surgical management for parathyroid surgery remains paramount for the successful treatment of primary HPTH.

21.2   Embryology

The embryology of the parathyroid glands is of particular importance for intraoperative determination of their location. The parathyroid glands form during the fifth week of gestation, and develop from the endoderm of the third and fourth branchial pouches. The inferior parathyroid glands arise from the third branchial pouch and, during development, descend along with the thymus. They can be found from the base of the skull to the anterior mediastinum [3]. The superior parathyroid glands develop from the fourth branchial pouch, and do not migrate as far. Their final position is usually superior and posterior to the thyroid gland, although they originated from a lower branchial pouch (for further details please refer to Chapter 2).

Knowledge of the gland arch derivatives and an understanding of their developmental course are very important, as accessory or aberrant tissue from the third and fourth pouches occurs in up to 15–20% of patients [4]. Hyperfunctioning parathyroid glands have been found as high as the internal carotid artery and as low as the aortopulmonary window, both anterior and posterior to the aortic arch. The majority of individuals have four parathyroid glands, but six or more may be found. A fifth supernumerary parathyroid gland located in the thymus is the most common variant.

21.3   Surgical Anatomy

A thorough knowledge of neck anatomy is essential for successful completion of parathyroid surgery. The surgeon must have a complete understanding of the anatomy and embryology of the neck in order to minimize hemorrhagic complications or injury to the recurrent laryngeal nerve, which may course through the bifurcation of the inferior thyroid artery. It is imperative to maintain a dry operative field, as the planes of dissection must be carefully considered throughout the procedure.

Normal parathyroid glands weigh between 30 and 40 mg, are a dark yellow/orange color, and are nestled in a rim of fat. Normal glands appear flat and ovoid, whereas pathological glands tend to more globular and enlarged. In a recent single surgeon retrospective review, adenomas were clearly distinguished from normal glands by cellularity, stromal fat, and intracellular fat in chief cells on intraoperative pathological frozen section. The authors found that the weight of normal parathyroid glands removed at surgery in patients with primary HPTH may be greater than that reported in autopsy studies. Histological features are better measures than weight alone in determining whether a gland is normal, and intraoperative identification of slightly enlarged glands should not lead to immediate subtotal parathyroidectomy [5]. If the viability of a normal gland is in question and the gland appears dusky in color, it is likely to be devascularized and autotransplantation should be considered [4].

The superior parathyroid glands tend to be more constant in their position. They are located in the posterior aspect of the thyroid lobe, near the point where the recurrent laryngeal nerve enters the cricothyroid muscle, or just posterior to this, and where the inferior constrictor muscle fibers are found. They are located in this position in 75% of the population. Other locations include inside the capsule of the posterior upper pole of the thyroid gland, retroesophageal, or retropharyngeal. In order to reach the superior parathyroid glands, the upper pole of the thyroid needs to be medially rotated, preferably without disruption of the main trunk of the superior thyroid artery.

The location of the inferior parathyroid glands is more variable; approximately 40% are located in the tissue immediately adjacent to the lower pole of the thyroid (both anteriorly and posteriorly), 40% are located in the tongue of thymic tissue between the inferior border of the thyroid gland and the clavicle (thyrothymic tract), 15% may be located juxtathyroidal, 1% are located in the lower mediastinum, and 2% are ectopic, at any location along the migration path from the base of tongue to the mediastinum. Approximately 2–5% of all parathyroid glands may be intrathyroidal [6].

The main blood supply to all parathyroid glands is from the inferior thyroid artery. The superior para-

thyroid artery usually arises from a branch of the inferior thyroid artery, but can also arise from the superior thyroid artery. To avoid devascularizing normal parathyroid tissue, the inferior thyroid artery should be preserved. If the decision is made to ligate the vessel, it should be done at the point where it enters the gland.

21.4 Indications for Parathyroidectomy in Primary HPTH

Primary HPTH is a generalized disorder of calcium, phosphate, and bone metabolism due to increased secretion of parathyroid hormone (PTH). The excessive levels of circulating PTH lead to hypercalcemia and hypophosphatemia. The incidence of primary HPTH is 0.2% in patients over age 60, and has an estimated prevalence of 2%. Peak incidence is between the fourth and sixth decades, but may also occur in children. Women are affected at least twice as often as men.

Patients with symptomatic primary HPTH may suffer from nephrolithiasis, bone fractures, osteopenia, muscle weakness, pancreatitis, gastritis, and severe neurocognitive problems such as psychosis, depressed mental status, and coma in extreme cases. These patients are usually treated with parathyroidectomy. In the hands of experienced endocrine surgeons, the conventional operation offers 95–99% cure rates, with minimal morbidity and mortality [7].

Treatment options for "asymptomatic" or "minimally symptomatic" patients with primary HPTH are controversial. The National Institutes of Health (NIH) convened meetings in 1990 and 2001 for experts in the field to develop guidelines for parathyroidectomy [8,9]. Their recommendations are summarized in Table 21.1. This group of experts also recommends that there is a potentially large group of patients with neurocognitive findings who may also benefit from parathyroidectomy.

21.5 Operative Goals and Preoperative Planning

The goal of parathyroidectomy is to achieve long-term postoperative normocalcemia by removing the hyperfunctioning parathyroid tissue. This may require removal of a single adenomatous gland, multiple adenomatous glands, or most of the hyperplastic glands/tissue. The cosmetic result of the surgery needs to be

Table 21.1 Recommendation for parathyroidectomy in primary hyperparathyroidism

1. Significant hypercalcemia defined as serum calcium 1 mg/dl above the upper limit of the normal reference range

2. Significant hypercalciuria defined as 24-hour urinary calcium excretion ≥400 mg

3. Creatinine clearance reduced by 30% compared to age-matched subjects

4. Decreased bone density at the lumbar spine, hip, or distal radius (as determined by dual-energy X-ray absorptiometry) that is more than 2.5 standard deviations below peak bone mass (t-score <-2.5)

5. Age younger than 50 years

6. Patients for whom medical surveillance is neither desirable, nor possible

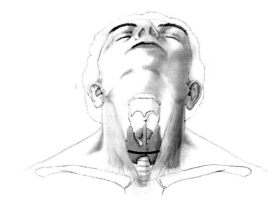

Fig. 21.1 Placement of the collar incision for open parathyroidectomy

kept in mind. Every effort should be made to make the skin incision short and along the natural creases of the neck. Maintaining and defining tissue planes is important in avoiding injury to key structures, such as the recurrent and superior laryngeal nerves. These nerves are in close association with the thyroid gland and aberrant anatomy may make dissection of the parathyroids difficult.

The capsule of the parathyroid glands needs to be kept intact to avoid spilling parathyroid cells, with subsequent risk of implantation and development of ectopic parathyroid proliferation. All glands should be identified during a conventional neck exploration. Preoperative localization studies are not necessary in the conventional neck exploration, but are helpful in reoperations or patients with acute hypercalcemic crisis. Preoperative localization can be achieved by parathyroid ultrasound, with an accuracy of 65–80%, or sestamibi scanning with or without single-photon emission computed tomography (SPECT), with an accuracy of 60–85% [2,7].

21.6   Operative Technique

21.6.1   Anesthesia

The procedure is generally carried out under general anesthesia, although locoregional anesthesia, such as anterior cervical block with sedation, may be used in selected patients.

21.6.2   Positioning

Patients should be placed in the semi-Fowler, neck extension position, with a roll underneath the shoulders, in the "sniffing position." Care should be taken not to hyperextend the neck, but to allow good exposure for the operation (Fig. 21.1).

21.6.3   Procedure

An approximately 5-cm transverse cervical incision is made and extended through the subcutaneous tissue and platysma muscle to the areolar plane just below the platysma muscle, where an avascular plane will be found. The incision should be done carefully, avoiding injury the anterior jugular veins that lie just deep to the areolar tissue plane. Active bleeding and danger of air embolus may occur from accidental openings made into the anterior jugular veins [10]. A subplatysmal flap is developed in this plane up to the level of the thyroid cartilage, laterally to the sternocleidomastoid muscles and inferiorly to the sternal notch, using either sharp dissection or electrocautery along with blunt gauze dissection. Once these flaps are developed, a self-retaining retractor can be placed to give appropriate exposure.

Because statistically parathyroid adenomas arise more commonly in the right lower parathyroid gland, we prefer to start the dissection on the right side of the neck. The strap muscles should be separated in the median raphe and dissected laterally off the thyroid capsule from the thyroid cartilage to the sternal notch. The middle thyroid veins can be ligated and divided to allow full mobilization of the thyroid lobes anteromedially, although in many cases it is not necessary to ligate the middle thyroid veins. Hemostasis is crucial at all times.

The recurrent laryngeal nerve and inferior thyroid artery should be identified. In most patients the recurrent laryngeal nerve lies in the tracheoesophageal groove; less commonly it is lateral to the trachea. Finger retraction using dry gauze is gentle on the thyroid tissue and leads to less trauma and bleeding than clamps. The right thyroid lobe is freed by blunt dissection in order to find the recurrent laryngeal nerve. The lower parathyroid gland is normally found in the thyrothymic tract, inferior to the thyroid lobe and anterior to the recurrent laryngeal nerve. This area is gently dissected. Inferior thyroid veins may be ligated. The parathyroid gland may lie within the capsule of the lower thyroid pole.

A common location for the superior parathyroid gland is within 1 cm of the recurrent laryngeal nerve as it pierces the cricothyroid membrane, posterior to the superior pole of the thyroid (Fig. 21.2). The extent of the operation should not be limited to the excision of one obviously enlarged gland. The remaining glands should be identified and their locations recorded [10]. Some surgeons recommend biopsy of each gland with frozen section identification. However, this practice appears unnecessary, and is associated with an increased incidence of postoperative hypoparathyroidism. If the intraoperative PTH assay is available, fine-needle aspiration of the in situ parathyroid gland with a 25-gauge needle, with washing of the aspirate in 3 cc 0.9% saline, should yield significantly high parathormone levels, thus confirming parathyroid tissue. This maybe used in lieu of biopsy of the gland for identification. In situ biopsy or aspiration of enlarged glands is not recommended, as these techniques are potentially associated with parathyromatosis.

The dissection of the superior gland is carried out in a superior direction on the thyroid capsule toward the upper pole of the thyroid, preserving the branches of the inferior thyroid artery. The thyroid gland should be rotated medially, and the recurrent laryngeal nerve followed. At this point, the branches of the superior thyroid artery may be ligated for better exposure of the posterior aspect of the superior thyroid pole. The posterior branches to the thyroid should be preserved until the parathyroid is identified, or a branch from the inferior thyroid artery to the parathyroid gland is detected.

Because of the possibility of multiple parathyroid gland involvement, every effort must be made to identify all parathyroids. Parathyroid glands will often be located in a mirror image to the contralateral side, therefore knowing where one superior gland lies, may guide the surgeon to the position of the contralateral superior parathyroid gland.

The left neck is explored in a similar fashion. A complete neck exploration requires patience, meticulous hemostasis, and surgical skill.

21.7 Considerations

21.7.1 Single Adenoma

Primary HPTH is the result of a single parathyroid adenoma in 65–85% of patients, and, rarely, parathyroid carcinoma is present in less than 1% of patients [11–13]. Multigland hyperplasia occurs in approximately 15% of patients, and is more common in large endocrine centers due to selective referral of patients with familial forms of primary HPTH. The success rate of the conventional bilateral neck exploration in curing patients with primary HPTH is greater than 95% in the hands of experienced endocrine surgeons [14]. Surgical failures occur due to the inability to locate an ectopic parathyroid adenoma, unrecognized multiple gland hyperplasia, or supernumerary glands.

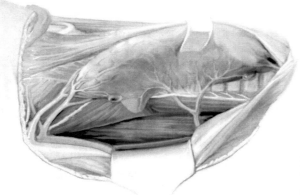

Fig. 21.2 Conventional surgical technique for parathyroidectomy: exposure of the dorsal aspect of the thyroid gland after mobilization of the thyroid lobe

If an enlarged parathyroid gland appears fibrotic, elicits a desmoplastic reaction, and is adherent to other neck structures or the thyroid gland, clinical suspicion should be raised of parathyroid malignancy, and the gland should be resected en bloc with a hemithyroidectomy. If lymphadenopathy is noted, a central lymph node dissection on the ipsilateral side should be undertaken. Frozen section of the parathyroid gland is rarely helpful in confirming a clinical suspicion of malignancy. At no time should the surgeon cut across a suspicious gland in order to obtain a frozen section to confirm parathyroid carcinoma.

21.7.2 Multiglandular Disease

Multigland hyperplasia occurs in 10–30% of patients with primary HPTH [11,12]. The incidence of recurrent or persistent hypercalcemia is highest for patients with multiglandular hyperplasia, either sporadic or in association with multiple endocrine neoplasia (MEN) syndromes. In patients with multiglandular parathyroid hyperplasia, recurrent or persistent HPTH may be found in 5–10% of sporadic cases and in up to 20–40% of familial cases [15,16]. Both familial and sporadic multigland disease exhibit asymmetric parathyroid gland enlargement [17]. If the glands demonstrate hyperplasia, a subtotal parathyroidectomy, whereby three and a half glands are removed, should be performed. Cryopreservation of one gland, which can be stored indefinitely, should be planned, if this modality is available, as this will reduce the potential for permanent hypoparathyroidism, allowing transplantation at a later date [18].

21.7.3 Double Adenomas

Multiple adenomas occur in 5–15% of patients, and was first described as an entity in 1947 by Felix Mandl [19,20]. It remains controversial whether the presence of double adenomas represents a distinct entity or merely asymmetrical diffuse hyperplasia. Many surgeons consider double adenomas as a unique clinical entity of primary HPTH. Double adenomas are found in at least 2% of patients with primary HPTH. A review from the Cleveland Clinic explored anatomical patterns and implications for surgical management in two-gland disease. They found that double adenomas have non-uniform anatomical distribution, with predilection for abnormal growth in bilateral superior parathyroid glands, the embryologic remnants of the fourth branchial pouch. Their conclusions were that

unilateral parathyroidectomy may predispose to recurrent or persistent disease [21].

As with multiglandular hyperplasia, the surgical approach to patients with double adenomas is also controversial. Different operative strategies have been advocated in the event that two enlarged parathyroid glands are found during the initial neck exploration. Supporters of the "hyperplasia theory" recommend subtotal parathyroidectomy (resection of three and a half glands) or total parathyroidectomy with autotransplantation. Surgeons who consider the double adenomas to be a separate disease entity, remove only the clinically enlarged glands. All of these procedures require four-gland exploration [22]. Incomplete resection of diseased parathyroid tissue causes persistence of hypercalcemia and primary HPTH, while unnecessary resection of normal parathyroid glands may cause permanent hypoparathyroidism. The use of intraoperative PTH assays may aid in guiding the extent of parathyroidectomy.

21.7.4 Ectopic Parathyroid Glands

Parathyroid glands are often found in ectopic locations along their embryologic migration path. Aberrant parathyroid tissue has been noted in 15–20% of autopsy studies. The vast majority of patients with primary HPTH who have aberrant parathyroid glands in the neck can be treated successfully through a standard neck exploration (Fig. 21.3).

Depending upon which gland is deemed to be missing, the search for the parathyroid adenoma is undertaken in an organized fashion. Missing superior glands are searched for in the retropharyngeal, retroesophageal planes, posterior mediastinum, inside the thyroid capsule or gland, and the carotid sheath. Inferior glands are found inside the thyroid capsule or lower pole thyroid parenchyma, carotid sheath, and the thymus/mediastinum. If a gland is not found, ipsilateral ligation of the inferior thyroid artery can be performed, thus devascularizing the parathyroid adenoma, or performing a hemithyroidectomy. Obtaining an intraoperative ultrasonographic examination of the neck and thyroid gland may be helpful if an intrathyroidal parathyroid gland is suspected.

Although up to 20% of patients may have parathyroid glands extending into the mediastinum, most of these can be extracted through the neck by performing a cervical thymectomy. Direct mediastinal exploration is required in only 1–2% of cases. Subcarinal parathyroid adenomas may be accessed via a partial or complete median sternotomy while posterior me-

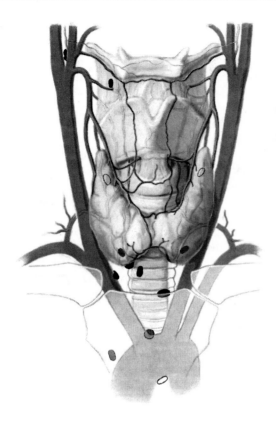

Fig. 21.3 Possible localizations of ectopic parathyroid adenomas. Most of them are surgically accessible by a regular cervicotomy

Step 1
Open and inspect the thyroid capsule, palpate the gland
⊓
Step 2
Dissect the superior thymic/paratracheal tissue, complete a cervical thymectomy
⊓
Step 3
Mobilize the pharynx and esophagus to look in the para- and retro-pharyngeal and esophageal spaces
⊓
Step 4
Open the carotid sheath, and expose the common carotid throughout its course in the neck
⊓
Step 5
Ligate the ipsilateral inferior thyroid artery or perform a thyroid lobectomy, Record location of all confirmed glands identified
⊓
Step 6
Terminate procedure, follow the patient for evidence of persistent hypercalcemia, Image the patient for evidence of parathyroid adenomas outside the neck

Fig. 21.4 Algorithm for identification of the missing parathyroid gland

diastinal parathyroid adenomas may require a thoracotomy, although successful resection of these adenomas using video-assisted thoracoscopic surgery (VATS) is becoming more popular [23]. These procedures are not generally performed at the same time as the primary neck exploration. If the adenoma cannot be identified at the time of the neck exploration and the patient has persistent HPTH, additional imaging techniques, such as thorough neck ultrasonography with the primary potential fine-needle aspiration identification of parathyroid glands, neck and chest MRI or CT scan, sestamibi with SPECT, or selective jugular venous sampling for a PTH differential gradient may need to be employed in order to localize the ectopic glands.

21.7.5   Algorithm for Identification of Missing Glands

When a parathyroid gland cannot be found, it is critical to reflect on the patient's specific anatomy in relation to parathyroid embryologic development. One must identify correctly whether one is missing a superior or an inferior gland. Because the recurrent laryngeal nerve obliquely bisects the lateral aspect of the trachea and esophagus, the inferior glands should generally be located anterior and caudal along this plane and the superior parathyroid glands should be posterior and cranial [3]. However, upper glands are not uncommonly found posterior to the esophagus and inferior to the thyroid gland. Mediastinal adenomas within the thymus are managed by resecting the cranial portion of the thymus by gentle traction on the thyrothymic ligament or by a complete transcervical thymectomy using a substernal retractor [2]. A superior gland may be undescended and found above the level of the thyroid cartilage (Fig. 21.4) [6].

21.8   Conclusions

The incidence of primary HPTH is increasing. While new technologies are enabling preoperative localization of parathyroid gland pathology and the removal of solitary adenomas with minimally invasive approaches, the success of parathyroidectomy remains dependent upon a thorough understanding of the embryology and anatomy of the neck. This is achievable only by the surgeons' experience and intimate knowledge of the traditional bilateral neck exploration.

References

1. Mandl F (1926) Therapeutisher versuch bein falls von ostitis fibrosa generalisata mittles. Exterpation eines epithelkorperchen tumors. Wien Klin Wochenshr Zentral 143:245–284

2. Lowney JK, Lairmore TC (2002) Endocrine surgery. In: Doherty GM (ed) The Washington manual of surgery, 3rd edn. Lippincott Williams & Wilkins, Philadelphia

3. Gauger P, Doherty G (eds) (2004) Parathyroid gland. In: Sabiston textbook of surgery, 17th edn. Elsevier and Saunders, Philadelphia, pp 985–999

4. Petti JG (2001) Parathyroid disease and surgery. In: Calhoun KH, Friedman N, Derkay CS, Gluckman J (eds) Head and neck surgery: otolaryngology, 3rd edn. Lippincott Williams & Wilkins, Philadelphia, p 115

5. Yao K, Singer FR, Roth SI, Sassoon A, Ye C, Giuliano AE (2004) Weight of normal parathyroid glands in patients with parathyroid adenomas. J Clin Endocrinol Metab 89:3208–3213

6. Krempl G, Medina JE, Bouknight AL (2003) Surgical management of the parathyroids. Otolaryngol Clin North Am 36:217–228

7. Van Heerden J, Smith S (1997) Parathyroidectomy for primary hyperparathyroidism (adenoma and carcinoma). Mastery of Surgery 1:508–515

8. Potts JT Jr, Fradkin JE, Aurbach GD, Bilezikian JP, Raisz LG (eds) (1991) Proceedings of the NIH consensus development conference on diagnosis and management of asymptomatic primary hyperparathyroidism, Bethesda, Maryland, 29–31 October 1990. J Bone Miner Res 6(suppl 2):S1–S166

9. Bilezikian JP, Potts JT Jr, Fuleihan GE, Kleerekoper M, Neer R, Peacock M, Rastad J, Silverberg SJ, Udelsman R, Wells SA (2002) Summary statement from a workshop on asymptomatic primary hyperparathyroidism: a perspective for the 21st century. J Clin Endocrinol Metab 87:5353–5361 (reprinted from J Bone Miner Res 17(suppl 2):N2–N11)

10. Zollinger RM Jr, Zollinger R Sr (2003) Parathyroidectomy. In: Zollinger's atlas of surgical operations, 8th edn. Mc-Graw-Hill, New York, pp 364–373

11. Wei J, Burke GJ (1995) Analysis of savings in operative time for primary hyperparathyroidism using localization with technetium 99m sestamibi scan. Am J Surg 170:488–491

12. Wells S, Leight GF, Ross A (1980) Primary hyperparathyroidism. Curr Probl Surg 17:1187–1209

13. Ashley S, Wells SA Jr (1993) Parathyroid glands. In: Editor LG (ed) Surgery: scientific principles and practice. Lippincott, Philadelphia, pp 1187–1209

14. Clark O (1995) Surgical treatment of primary hyperparathyroidism. Adv Endocrinol Metab 6:1–16

15. Oertli D, Richter M, et al (1995) Parathyroidectomy in primary hyperparathyroidism: preoperative localization and routine biopsy of unaltered glands are not necessary. Surgery 117:392–396

16. Burgess J, David R, Parameswaran V, et al (1998) The outcome of subtotal parathyroidectomy for the treatment of hyperparathyroidism in multiple endocrine neoplasia type 1. Arch Surg 133:126–129

17. Thompson N (1995) The surgical management of hyperparathyroidism and endocrine disease of the pancreas in the multiple endocrine neoplasia type 1 patient. J Int Med 238:269–280

18. Berger A, Libutt SK, Bartlett DL, et al (1999) Heterogeneous gland size in sporadic multiple gland parathyroid hyperplasia. J Am Coll Surg 188:382–389

19. Fahey T, Hibbert E, Brady P, et al (1995) Giant double parathyroid adenoma presenting as a hypercalcemic crisis. Aust N Z J Surg 65:292–294

20. Teze A, Shen W, Shaver JK, et al (1993) Double parathyroid adenomas: clinical and biochemical characteristics before and after parathyroidectomy. Ann Surg 218:300–309

21. Milas M, Wagner K, Easley KA, Siperstein A, Weber CJ (2003) Double adenomas revisited: nonuniform distribution favors enlarged superior parathyroids (fourth pouch disease). Surgery 134:995–1004

22. Bartsch D, Nies C, Hasse C, Willuhn J, Rothmund M (1995) Clinical and surgical aspects of double adenoma in patients with primary hyperparathyroidism. Br J Surg 82:926–929

23. Kumar A, Kumar S, Aggarwal S, Kumar R, Tandon N (2002) Thoracoscopy: the preferred method for excision of mediastinal parathyroids. Surg Laparosc Endosc Percutan Tech 12:295–300

24. Carling T, Udelsman R (2005) Parathyroid surgery in familial hyperparathyroid disorders. J Int Med 257:27–37

22 Minimally Invasive Parathyroidectomy

Tobias Carling and Robert Udelsman

22.1   Background

Eighty-five percent of patients with primary hyperparathyroidism (HPTH) harbor a single adenoma and are cured by excision of the incident gland. Thus, with accurate preoperative localization, targeted surgery using unilateral neck exploration under regional or local anesthesia has been developed and evaluated since 1995 and has become the standard of care in an ever-increasing number of specialized centers. Unilateral surgery for primary HPTH was advocated in 1975, and the side to be explored was chosen based on palpation, esophagram, venography, or angiography [1]. If both an enlarged and normal gland were found on the initial side, then contralateral exploration was aborted. Other authors advocated a similar approach, arguing that bilateral exploration increased the risk, cost, and morbidity of surgery for primary hyperparathyroidism [2]. The Lund University surgeons advocated unilateral parathyroidectomy, which they defined as removal of both an adenoma and normal gland from one side [3]. The excised tissue was studied microscopically during surgery with oil-red-O, and the decision to stop the operation at this stage was based on demonstration of a reduction in intracytoplasmic fat droplets in the excised adenomatous parathyroid tissue. Both techniques would fail, however, in the setting of a double adenoma on the contralateral side and if the essentially "random" choice of which side to explore was incorrect. Today, minimally invasive parathyroidectomy (MIP) is performed after preoperative parathyroid localization usually with high-quality sestamibi scans, often under cervical block anesthesia during which a limited exploration is performed, and the rapid intraoperative parathyroid hormone (PTH) assay is employed to confirm an adequate resection [4].

22.2   Indications

The indications for MIP are the same as those for traditional cervical exploration, i.e., symptomatic patients or those with asymptomatic primary HPTH fulfilling the criteria established by the recent NIH consensus meeting [5]. In addition, we believe that there is a large population of patients with subtle neurocognitive impairment who also benefit from parathyroidectomy [6,7]. Preoperative parathyroid localization, generally performed with a high-quality sestamibi scan is performed to localize the parathyroid abnormality. Other imaging techniques including ultrasound as well as computed tomography (CT) or magnetic resonance imaging (MRI) can also be performed, but are less sensitive. Minimally invasive techniques are rarely employed when preoperative localization of the parathyroid tumor has not been performed, is negative, or is consistent with multiglandular enlargement. A standard cervical bilateral exploration is advisable in patients with familial HPTH or secondary HPTH because they almost invariably display multiple parathyroid enlargements [8]. Rare cases when parathyroid carcinoma is diagnosed or suspected preoperatively should undergo radical resection at the initial operation [9].

The role of MIP in the setting of familial HPTH [i.e., multiple endocrine neoplasia type 1 (MEN1), MEN2A, the hyperparathyroidism–jaw tumor syndrome (HPTH-JT), familial isolated HPTH, and HPTH occurring in patients with an underlying mutation in the calcium-sensing receptor (CaSR) gene] is evolving [8]. A conventional cervical exploration should be performed in the vast majority of cases, although MIP may prove to have a limited role in specific instances of familial HPTH. For instance, in HPTH associated with MEN2A, HPTH-JT, and familial isolated HPTH where uniglandular uptake is noted on preoperative imaging, MIP may be considered [8]. Although it is likely that persistence and recurrence rates will be as high or higher compared with the standard cervical exploration, MIP has the advantage of causing minimal tissue trauma facilitating reoperations. MIP may also have a significant role in the familial setting when remedial cervical exploration is required. In those cases when preoperative imaging suggests a single focus of recurrent disease, it is reasonable and probably advantageous to employ MIP techniques and use an adequate decrement in the intraoperative PTH levels to confirm adequateness of resection [10]. In a situation when multiglandular parathyroid enlargements or suspicion of parathyroid carcinoma is encountered peroperatively, the MIP technique can be converted to a standard cervical exploration and general anesthesia can be administered if necessary [11].

22.3   Preoperative Requirements

The development and refinement of parathyroid imaging has been essential for the development of MIP techniques. Several non-invasive preoperative localization methods are available, including sestamibi–technetium 99m (Tc^{99m}) scintigraphy, ultrasonography, CT, MRI, and thallium-201–Tc^{99m} pertechnetate scanning. There is general consensus that the single best study is sestamibi, especially when sestamibi scans are imaged with single-photon emission computed tomography (SPECT), which generates three-dimensional localization [11]. In 1989, it was first reported that the new agent Tc^{99m} used for cardiac imaging was also taken up avidly by parathyroid tissue [12]. Parathyroid cells have a large number of mitochondria, which take up sestamibi/Tc^{99m} [13]. Sestamibi, a monovalent lipophilic cation diffuses passively across cell membranes, concentrates in mitochondria, and accumulates in adenomatous parathyroid tissue because of increased blood supply, higher metabolic activity, and an absence of p-glycoprotein on the cell membrane [14]. Sestamibi imaging can be performed preoperatively to plan a MIP or on the morning of operation in combination with the use of a gamma probe in the operating room to guide the surgeon during the operation. A meta-analysis of the sensitivity and specificity of sestamibi scanning in 6,331 cases gave values of 90.7%

and 98.8%, respectively, and suggested that 87% of the patients with sporadic primary hyperparathyroidism would be candidates for unilateral exploration [15]. The sensitivity of sestamibi is limited in multiglandular disease. In a large study, scintigraphy localized at least one gland in all patients, but only 62% of the total number of hyperplastic glands [16]. SPECT, which allows localization of structures in the anterior/posterior plane, is particularly helpful in detecting smaller lesions and adenomas located behind the thyroid gland. The overall sensitivity for localizing adenomas smaller than 500 mg varies significantly from 52.9% to 92% [17,18]. A major limitation of sestamibi scans is related to the coexistence of thyroid nodules or other metabolically active tissues (e.g., lymph nodes, thyroid nodules, multigland parathyroid hyperplasia, and metastatic thyroid cancer) that can mimic parathyroid adenomas by causing false-positive results on sestamibi scans. This limitation can be overcome in part by using the double-tracer subtraction technique of sestamibi, in which both thyroid and parathyroid nodular abnormalities can be diagnosed simultaneously, or in combination with a neck ultrasound to preoperatively distinguish between thyroid lesions and parathyroid enlargements [19]. Sestamibi scans are now being performed with simultaneous CT imaging, yielding correlative functional and anatomic localization.

Other methods of preoperative localization include ultrasound, CT, and MRI. Ultrasound is effective, non-invasive, and inexpensive, but its limitations include both operator dependency and being limited to application in the neck because it cannot image mediastinal adenomas. By itself, ultrasound has an approximately 50–75% true-positive rate. However, when combined with sestamibi, the true-positive rate approaches 90%, with few false-positives [20]. CT and MRI both provide cross-sectional imaging, and are useful for imaging of parathyroid tumors in the mediastinum, tracheoesophageal groove, and behind the esophagus. MRI does not involve the use of radiation, and parathyroid adenomas may appear very intense on T_2-weighted images. CT is less expensive, and many studies have shown the two techniques to be of equivalent sensitivity. CT has a sensitivity of 70% and a specificity of nearly 100%. In contrast to unexplored patients, those that require remedial cervical exploration often require extensive preoperative imaging. A subset of patients who require re-exploration will have negative, discordant, or non-convincing non-invasive localization studies. Current guidelines recommend that these patients undergo invasive localization procedures in the form of selective arteriography in conjunction with venous sampling for PTH. Rapid PTH measurement is now being used in the angiography suite. Because results are rapidly available on site, interventional radiologists can obtain additional samples from a region in which a subtle but potentially significant PTH gradient is detected [21].

22.4 Technique

All patients undergo a detailed history and physical examination including direct or indirect laryngoscopy. The biochemical data are confirmed and imaging studies are reviewed. Patients with positive or suggestive localization studies are offered MIP.

The awake patient is placed in the semi-Fowler position, and a fan is used to blow room air gently toward his or her face to minimize the sensation of claustrophobia (Fig. 22.1). The skin incision is typically limited to 2–4 cm. A superficial cervical block is administered posterior and deep to the sternal head of the sternocleidomastoid muscle on the ipsilateral side of the preoperatively localized adenoma

(Fig. 22.2). In most patients, 1% lidocaine containing 1:100,000 epinephrine is used and supplemented during the operation as required. Care always is taken to aspirate before delivering the anesthetic to avoid intravascular administration. We have found that by also infiltrating along the anterior border of the sternocleidomastoid muscle, as well as a local field block, excellent analgesia is obtained in virtually every case (Fig. 22.2). The total cumulative volume of lidocaine administered is typically 18–25 ml. Regional anesthesia avoids complications associated with general anesthesia, including endotracheal intubation, which has been reported to cause vocal cord changes in up to 5% of patients [22]. Furthermore, exploring a conscious patients permits intraoperative assessment of the superior and recurrent laryngeal nerve functions because the patient can vocalize throughout the procedure.

The regional block is performed by the surgeon in the operating room, and intravenous supplementation is administered by the anesthesia staff. Propofol may interfere with the PTH assay, but a recent randomized trial has shown that the PTH assay can be employed during propofol sedation [23]. Sedation is used to

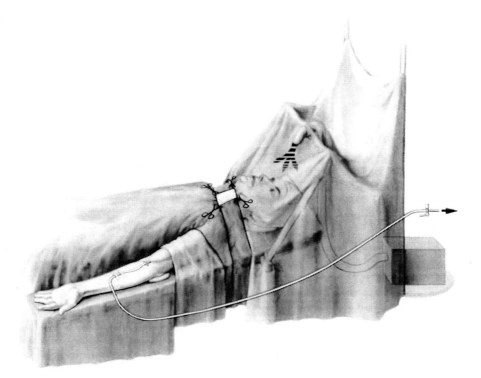

Fig. 22.1 The patient has a large-bore peripheral intravenous line inserted, which is used for medication and fluid administration as well as sampling for parathyroid hormone (PTH) levels. The patient is awake, and a fan is used to blow room air gently toward his or her face to minimize the sensation of claustrophobia. From [32], with permission. (Copyright © 2002, Lippincott Williams & Wilkins)

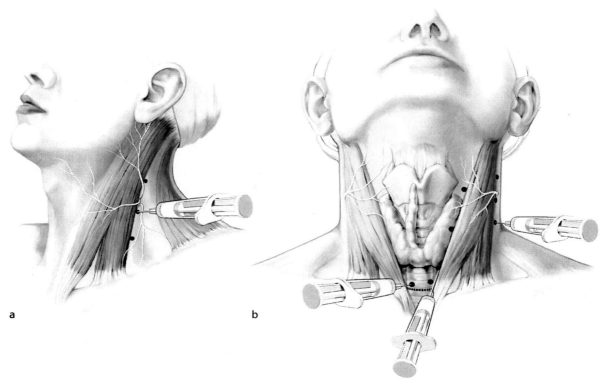

Fig. 22.2 Cervical block anesthesia. **a** A superficial cervical block is administered posteriorly and deep to the sternocleidomastoid muscle (SCM) (*1*). **b** Local infiltration is also performed along the anterior border of the SCM (*2*), and a local field block (*3*) is performed. From [32], with permission. (Copyright © 2002, Lippincott Williams & Wilkins)

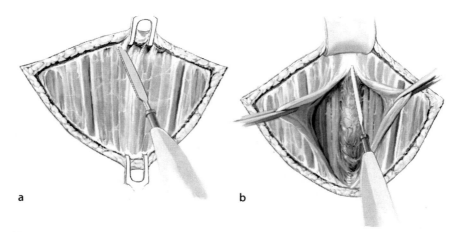

Fig. 22.3 **a** An abbreviated Kocher incision is made and the platysma is divided. **b** The strap muscles are separated. From [32], with permission. (Copyright © 2002, Lippincott Williams & Wilkins)

minimize patient anxiety while maintaining an awake, conscious patient who can phonate. Lo Gerfo and colleagues have shown that bilateral neck exploration under regional anesthesia can be performed safely and effectively in patients with coexisting thyroid disease and a non-localized adenoma. In a series of 236 patients undergoing MIP, 62% had a non-localizing sestamibi scan preoperatively or no scan at all, but only 4 required conversion to general anesthesia. Twenty-three percent had a simultaneous procedure performed for thyroid disease, and 85% underwent a bilateral neck exploration [24]. A focused exploration

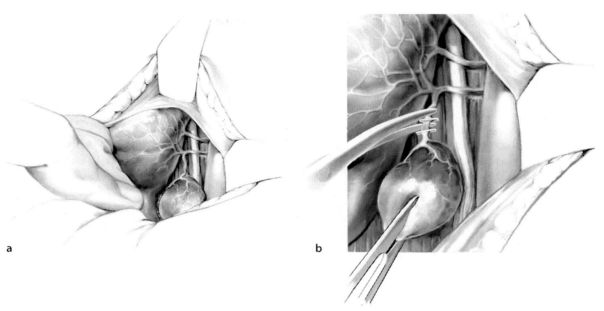

a   b

Fig. 22.4 The parathyroid adenoma is identified, its blood supply is ligated, the recurrent laryngeal nerve is protected, and the adenoma is removed. From [32], with permission. (Copyright © 2002, Lippincott Williams & Wilkins)

is then performed based on the preoperative localization study, and the intraoperative PTH assay is used to confirm the adequacy of parathyroid gland excision in the operating room (Figs. 22.3, 22.4).

The vast majority of patients undergoing MIP are discharged from the same-day surgery unit. They are followed carefully as outpatients, and total serum calcium and PTH levels are measured within the first week of follow-up.

22.5   Intraoperative Parathyroid Hormone Measurements

The rapid intraoperative PTH assay can be used to confirm adequate removal of hypersecreting parathyroid glands and predict a curative procedure. Its use is associated with reduced operating time. The first reported employment of the assay was in 1988, but it has been refined significantly since then, largely because of the work of George Irvin [25]. The rapid PTH immunometric assay utilizes chemiluminescence acridinium esters as a label in the presence of hydrogen peroxide and sodium hydroxide triggers (Nichols Institute Diagnostics, San Juan Capistrano, CA). In their presence, the acridinium esters are oxidized to an excited state, and it is the subsequent return to the ground state that causes an emission of light that is quantified. The amount of bound labeled antibody is directly proportional to the concentration of PTH in

the sample. A certified clinical laboratory technician with training in conducting the complex tests ideally performs each assay either inside the operating room or in direct proximity; results of the assay are available within 12 minutes.

Blood specimens should be obtained in the operating room (Fig. 22.1). Repeated blood specimens from a peripheral intravenous line (best), ipsilateral internal jugular vein, or (rarely) arterial catheter should be drawn before exploration, intraoperatively immediately after resection of the enlarged gland (to capture a potential spike compared with the preoperative baseline caused by manipulation of the gland during exploration) [26], and 5 and 10 minutes after the excision of the incident adenoma. These protocols have been designed to account for the half-life of PTH, which is 2–4 minutes, and to avoid misleading results caused by a spike in PTH that may occur during mobilization of the adenoma. A 50% reduction in the quick PTH value from the baseline level is used as an indication that the exploration has been successful, and this is predictive of cure in 96% of cases [27]. Ex vivo intraoperative needle aspiration of suspected parathyroid tissue for a quick measurement of intraoperative PTH is a useful alternative to frozen section for parathyroid gland identification [10].

The rapid assay is also especially helpful when the surgeon or pathologist has difficulty distinguishing between thyroid tissue, lymph nodes, or a parathyroid adenoma. Aspiration of parathyroid tissue yields substantially higher hormone values than the upper limit of the standard curve; values greater than 1,500 pg/ml secure the tissue diagnosis, and there is minimal incremental cost in cases where the intraoperative PTH assay is being utilized already [10]. Although the assay has not been designated for use with tissue aspirates, samples can be collected by aspiration of the tissue in question with a syringe containing 1 ml saline solution and then injection of the saline into ethylenediaminetetraacetic acid (EDTA) tubes for analysis.

Operative failure rates for initial and reoperative parathyroidectomy appear to have decreased significantly with this intraoperative adjunct. Irvin demonstrated that operative failure rates from initial parathyroidectomy have significantly decreased with the advent of the rapid PTH assay, from 6% to 1.5% [28]. Although experience seems to be variable, even in the more difficult field of reoperation for failed parathyroidectomy, the use of intraoperative PTH testing has been reported to increase success rates from 76% to 94%.

22.6   Results

The success of MIP has been confirmed by evidence of cure and complication rates that are at least as good as those achieved by conventional bilateral exploration. Specifically, in a series of 656 consecutive parathyroidectomies (of which 401 were performed in the standard fashion and 255 were performed with MIP) between 1990 and 2001, there were no significant differences in complication (3.0% and 1.2%, respectively) or cure rates (97% and 99%, respectively) [29]. MIP was associated with an approximately 50% reduction in operating time (1.3 hours for MIP versus 2.4 hours for standard operation), a sevenfold reduction in length of hospital stay (0.24 days versus 1.64 days, respectively), and a mean savings in terms of charges of $2,693 per procedure, which represents a reduction by nearly one half in total hospital charges. A prospective randomized controlled trial comparing unilateral to bilateral neck exploration was recently published [30]. In this study of 91 patients, comparison was made between patients assigned to preoperative sestamibi localization and unilateral neck exploration with the rapid PTH assay *versus* patients assigned to bilateral neck exploration. Patients who underwent unilateral neck exploration had a lower incidence of early postoperative hypocalcemia necessitating calcium supplementation. There were no statistical differences between complication rates, costs, and oper-

ative time between the two groups. The study, which was not blinded, was encumbered by a high-crossover rate; only 62% of patients assigned to unilateral exploration actually underwent this operation. The balance had bilateral neck exploration, probably because sestamibi in the study had a sensitivity of only 71%.

22.7   Variations of Minimally Invasive Parathyroidectomy

There are variations of MIP procedures. One technique uses an endoscopic video-assisted approach (see Chapter 23 "Endoscopic Parathyroidectomy"). Another variation is the use of a handheld intraoperative gamma probe, which uses the same concept as preoperative sestamibi localization. The radionucleotide is administered 2 hours prior to the procedure to enable sestamibi retention within the parathyroid adenoma but to enhance clearance from the thyroid. Once the parathyroid adenoma is extracted residual counts are compared with the surrounding tissue to ensure adequate resection [31]. Results, thus far, seems comparable with that of MIP, but tend to be associated with an increased operative time, and hospitalization.

References

1. Roth SI, Wang CA, Potts JT Jr (1975) The team approach to primary hyperparathyroidism. Hum Pathol 6:645–648
2. Wang CA (1985) Surgical management of primary hyperparathyroidism. Curr Probl Surg 22:1–50
3. Tibblin S, Bondeson AG, Ljungberg O (1982) Unilateral parathyroidectomy in hyperparathyroidism due to single adenoma. Ann Surg 195:245–252
4. Udelsman R, Donovan PI, Sokoll LJ (2000) One hundred consecutive minimally invasive parathyroid explorations. Ann Surg 232:331–339
5. Bilezikian J, Potts JJ, Fuleihan G-H, Kleerekoper M, Neer R, Peacock M, Rastad J, Silverberg S, Udelsman R, Wells S (2002) Summary statement from a workshop on asymptomatic primary hyperparathyroidism: a perspective for the 21st century. J Clin Endocrinol Metab 87:5353–5361
6. Rastad J, Joborn C, Akerstrom G, Ljunghall S (1992) Incidence, type and severity of psychic symptoms in patients with sporadic primary hyperparathyroidism. J Endocrinol Invest 15:149–156
7. Silverberg SJ (2002) Non-classical target organs in primary hyperparathyroidism. J Bone Miner Res 17(suppl 2): N117–N125

8. Carling T, Udelsman R (2005) Parathyroid surgery in familial hyperparathyroid disorders. J Intern Med 257:27–37

9. Carling T, Udelsman R (2003) Parathyroid tumors. Curr Treat Options Oncol 4:319–328

10. Carling T, Donovan P, Santos F, Donabedian R, Udelsman R (2004) The use of intraoperative rapid PTH measurement from parathyroid fine needle aspirates in patients undergoing parathyroidectomy. The Annual Meeting of the International Association of Endocrine Surgeons, Uppsala, Sweden 2004

11. Carling T, Udelsman R (2003) Advancements in the surgical treatment of primary hyperparathyroidism. Probl Gen Surg 20:31–37

12. Coakley AJ, Kettle AG, Wells CP, O'Doherty MJ, Collins RE (1989) 99Tcm sestamibi: a new agent for parathyroid imaging. Nucl Med Commun 10:791–794

13. Hetrakul N, Civelek AC, Stagg CA, Udelsman R (2001) In vitro accumulation of technetium-99m–sestamibi in human parathyroid mitochondria. Surgery 130:1011–1018

14. Mitchell BK, Cornelius EA, Zoghbi S, Murren JR, Ghoussoub R, Flynn SD, Kinder BK (1996) Mechanism of technetium 99m sestamibi parathyroid imaging and the possible role of p-glycoprotein. Surgery 120:1039–1045

15. Denham DW, Norman J (1998) Cost-effectiveness of preoperative sestamibi scan for primary hyperparathyroidism is dependent solely upon the surgeon's choice of operative procedure. J Am Coll Surg 186:293–305

16. Blanco I, Carril JM, Banzo I, Quirce R, Gutierrez C, Uriarte I, Montero A, Vallina NK (1998) Double-phase Tc-99m sestamibi scintigraphy in the preoperative location of lesions causing hyperparathyroidism. Clin Nucl Med 23:291–297

17. Johnston LB, Carroll MJ, Britton KE, Lowe DG, Shand W, Besser GM, Grossman AB (1996) The accuracy of parathyroid gland localization in primary hyperparathyroidism using sestamibi radionuclide imaging. J Clin Endocrinol Metab 81:346–352

18. Jones JM, Russell CF, Ferguson WR, Laird JD (2001) Preoperative sestamibi-technetium subtraction scintigraphy in primary hyperparathyroidism: experience with 156 consecutive patients. Clin Radiol 56:556–559

19. Casara D, Rubello D, Cauzzo C, Pelizzo MR (2002) 99mTc-MIBI radio-guided minimally invasive parathyroidectomy: experience with patients with normal thyroids and nodular goiters. Thyroid 12:53–61

20. Geatti O, Shapiro B, Orsolon PG, Proto G, Guerra UP, Antonucci F, Gasparini D (1994) Localization of parathyroid enlargement: experience with technetium-99m methoxyisobutylisonitrile and thallium-201 scintigraphy, ultrasonography and computed tomography. Eur J Nucl Med 21:17–22

21. Udelsman R, Aruny JE, Donovan PI, Sokoll LJ, Santos F, Donabedian R, Venbrux AC (2003) Rapid parathyroid hormone analysis during venous localization. Ann Surg 237:714–719; discussion 719–721

22. Stojadinovic A, Shaha A, Orlikoff R, Nissan A, Kornak M, Singh B, Boyle J, Shah J, Brennan M, Kraus D (2002) Prospective functional voice assessment in patients undergoing thyroid surgery. Ann Surg 236:823–832

23. Sippel RS, Becker YT, Odorico JS, Springman SR, Chen H (2004) Does propofol anesthesia affect intraoperative parathyroid hormone levels? A randomized, prospective trial. Surgery 136:1138–1142

24. Lo Gerfo P (1999) Bilateral neck exploration for parathyroidectomy under local anesthesia: a viable technique for patients with coexisting thyroid disease with or without sestamibi scanning. Surgery 126:1011–1014; discussion 1014–1015

25. Irvin GL 3rd, Sfakianakis G, Yeung L, Deriso GT, Fishman LM, Molinari AS, Foss JN (1996) Ambulatory parathyroidectomy for primary hyperparathyroidism. Arch Surg 131:1074–1078

26. Yang GP, Levine S, Weigel RJ (2001) A spike in parathyroid hormone during neck exploration may cause a false-negative intraoperative assay result. Arch Surg 136:945–949

27. Garner SC, Leight GS Jr (1999) Initial experience with intraoperative PTH determinations in the surgical management of 130 consecutive cases of primary hyperparathyroidism. Surgery 126:1132–1137; discussion 1137–1138

28. Irvin GL 3rd, Molinari AS, Figueroa C, Carneiro DM (1999) Improved success rate in reoperative parathyroidectomy with intraoperative PTH assay. Ann Surg 229:874–878; discussion 878–879

29. Udelsman R (2002) Six hundred and fifty-six consecutive explorations for primary hyperparathyroidism. Ann Surg 235:665–670

30. Bergenfelz A, Lindblom P, Tibblin S, Westerdahl J (2002) Unilateral versus bilateral neck exploration for primary hyperparathyroidism: a prospective randomized controlled trial. Ann Surg 236:543–551

31. Chen H, Mack E, Starling JR (2003) Radioguided parathyroidectomy is equally effective for both adenomatous and hyperplastic glands. Ann Surg 238:332–337; discussion 337–338

32. Udelsman R (2002) Unilateral neck exploration under local or regional anesthesia. In: Gagner M, Inabnet WB III (eds) Minimally invasive endocrine surgery. Lippincott Williams & Wilkins, Philadelphia

23 Endoscopic Parathyroidectomy

Paolo Miccoli and Gabriele Materazzi

CONTENTS

23.1 Introduction

The first endoscopic parathyroidectomy was performed by M. Gagner who operated on a patient presenting with a primary hyperparathyroidism (HPTH) caused by a hyperplasia of four glands [1]. The operation, although successful, raised a certain degree of scepticism, in particular among endocrine surgeons, probably because the indication was not adequate for such a procedure. In fact, primary HPTH appears to be an ideal disease to be approached endoscopically for several reasons: (1) the tumor giving rise to the hyperfunction is almost always benign, (2) it rarely exceeds 2–3 cm in size, and (3) there is no need for any surgical reconstruction after the small mass removal.

This stimulated several surgeons to search for other minimally invasive approaches to the parathyroid glands either totally [2–5] or partly endoscopic [6]. At present we consider endoscopic or video-assisted parathyroidectomy is to be a valid option [7] for most of the cases of primary HPTH and it is widely performed in several centers as the first option [8,9].

23.2 Indications and Contraindications

As in any other minimally invasive operation for primary HPTH, a proper selection of the patients undergoing these procedures is crucial for their success: without doubt this surgery is mostly indicated for sporadic disease characterized by the presence of a single, well-localized adenoma harbored in a virgin neck. This should imply a positive imaging that, according to some authors [7], should be concordant for both ultrasonography and sestamibi scintiscan. In our experience this concordance proved not to be strictly necessary because the central access allows good exposure of both sides, with the possibility of unveiling an adenoma whose preoperative localization was not perfect. Likewise in cases where the patient had previously undergone surgery on one side of the neck, a lateral access is always possible and the operation can still be performed endoscopically (8 cases in our series). For this reason our selection criteria have been modified as our experience increased according to our learning curve (Fig. 23.10). In spite of the subsequent reduction of patients undergoing open operation for primary HPTH, some contraindications must still be regarded as absolute, and these are mainly represented Table 23.1. Finally, very large adenomas (more than 3 cm in diameter) must be carefully evaluated because of the suspicion that large masses are more at risk of being carcinomas (in particular when associated with very high values of PTH and calcium).

Table 23.1 Contraindications for endoscopic parathyroidectomy

Large goiters
Recurrent disease
Extensive previous neck surgery
MEN and familial primary HPTH
Parathyroid carcinomas

The difference in the interpretation of these inclusion criteria clearly explains the wide differences in the percentage of eligibility of patients for this surgery ranging from values as little as 25% [10] to values as high as 66% [9].

23.3   Surgical Technique

In the majority of cases minimally invasive video-assisted parathyroidectomy (MIVAP) is performed under general anesthesia. Our technique requires neither trocars nor gas insufflation. The patient's neck does not have to be hyperextended (Fig. 23.1) to allow a sufficient operative space under the strap muscles. After conventional neck preparation and draping, a further steri-drape (Bioclusive 2003; Johnson & Johnson, Skipton, UK) is put on the skin to avoid any heating from the electrocautery. A 15-mm transverse incision is made 2 cm above the sternal notch (Fig. 23.2). Subcutaneous fat and platysma are carefully dissected to avoid bleeding. The surgeon should use the electrocautery with its blade, except for the tip, protected with a thin film of sterile drape.

In case of redo surgery, a lateral access instead of the standard midline access is possible. This avoids entering fibrous tissue where recognition of anatomical planes and structures such as the recurrent laryngeal nerve may be difficult. The incision is made just medially to the sternocleidomastoid muscle and blunt dissection is performed until the thyroid space is well exposed.

The strap muscles are then divided in the midline longitudinally for not more than 3 cm. One retractor gently retracts the strap muscles laterally on the side of the suspected adenoma to include the carotid artery while another one retracts the thyroid lobe medially (this retraction can be more easily carried out with the modified conventional Army-Navy retractors shown in Fig. 23.3). The thyrotracheal groove is then exposed after cutting the middle thyroid vein between clips. The lobe is mobilized from the strap muscles only using small spatulas under direct vision.

A 30° endoscope, 5 mm in diameter, is then introduced through the incision and from this moment on the procedure is performed endoscopically using small reusable surgical instruments (spatulas, forceps, scissor, and vascular clips; Fig. 23.4).

Three surgeons are generally involved in this video-assisted procedure: the operator, the first assistant (holding the endoscope and a spatula-aspi-

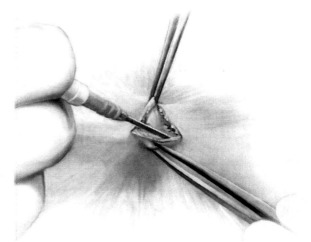

Fig. 23.2 Incision: a 15-mm transverse incision is made 2 cm above the sternal notch

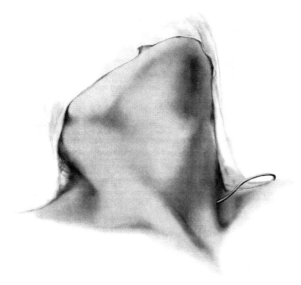

Fig. 23.1 Position of the patient during minimally invasive parathyroidectomy. The patient's neck does not have to be hyperextended to allow a sufficient operative space under the strap muscles

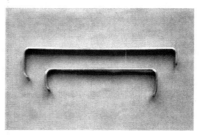

Fig. 23.3 Operative space is continuously maintained by small retractors (modified Army-Navy)

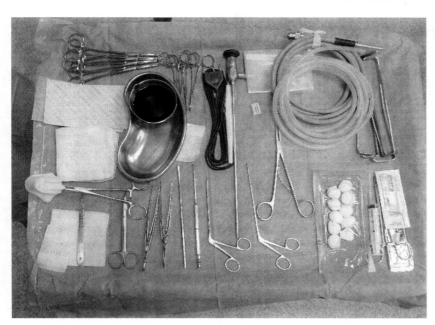

Fig. 23.4 Table instruments for MIVAP

rator), and a second assistant holding the retractors (Fig. 23.5). Usually only one side of the neck is explored but the opposite side can be explored through the same incision if necessary. It is important to stress that the exploration first starts on the side in which the adenoma is supposed to be on the basis of the preoperative imaging, but bilateral exploration can be achieved through the central incisionby just changing the position of the small retractors. The endoscopic magnification allows very easy identification of the relevant neck structures, particularly the recurrent laryngeal nerve, which should be clearly under vision throughout the procedure. Once the adenoma is located it is dissected without disrupting the capsule by cautious blunt dissection using the above-described spatulas. The pedicle of the gland (Fig. 23.6), which is readily visible under optical magnification, is then clipped: the use of small disposable vascular clips is strongly suggested (2 mm) because of the relatively small operative field. Washing and cleaning of the operative field can be simply achieved in the absence of trocars. Water can be injected directly with a syringe; its aspiration is facilitated by the use of the spatula-shaped aspirator (Fig. 23.7). Smoke and fluids can be sucked without introducing extra instruments into the incision.

The adenoma is then retrieved through the skin incision. No drainage is necessary but we strongly advocate not to close the midline tightly in order to enable early detection of postoperative bleeding. The skin is generally closed only by means of a skin

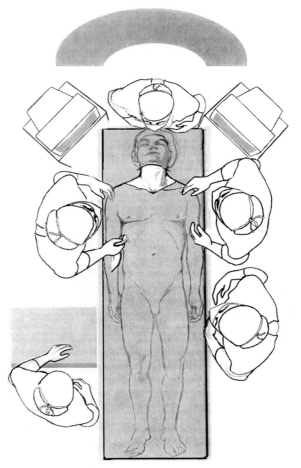

Fig. 23.5 MIVAP: operating room

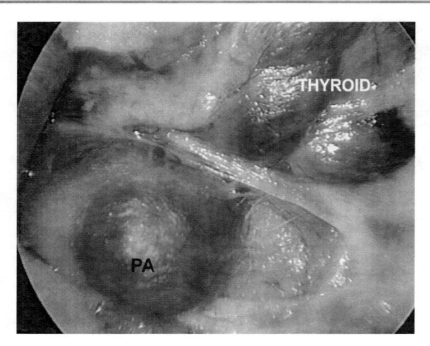

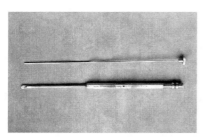

Fig. 23.7 Smoke and fluids can be sucked by introducing the spatula-aspirator

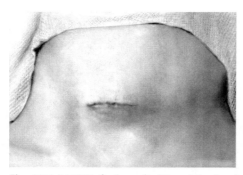

Fig. 23.8 MIVAP final result. Wound is closed by sealant (Dermabond)

sealant (Dermabond) after a subcuticular running suture has been performed in order to approximate the two edges of the incision (Fig. 23.8). Meanwhile the surgeon waits for the result of the Quick intraopera-

tive intact parathyroid hormone assay (qPTHa). The completeness of the surgical resection of all hyperfunctioning parathyroid tissue is confirmed by a decrease of more than 50% in qPTHa values compared to the highest pre-excision level. Measurements are obtained when anesthesia is induced, when the adenoma is visualized, and 5 and 10 minutes after the adenoma is removed (Fig. 23.9).

23.4   Our Experience with Endoscopic Parathyroidectomy

Our experience consists of 463 patients who underwent MIVAP from February 1997 to February 2005. The mean age of the patients was 55.7±13 years (range 20–87 years), with 379 women and 84 men. The mean operative time of the procedure was 33.6±20.1 minutes (range 10–180 minutes). Twenty patients had a concurrent video-assisted thyroid resection for associated diseases (microfollicular nodule, small papillary cancer): 13 thyroid lobectomies (10 ipsilateral and 3 contralateral) and 7 total thyroidectomies. MIVAP was performed under general and local anesthesia in 423 and 40 cases, respectively.

The mean size of the removed adenoma was 1.8 cm in its largest diameter. There were three permanent laryngeal nerve palsies (0.7%). There was one case of postoperative bleeding from a displaced clip

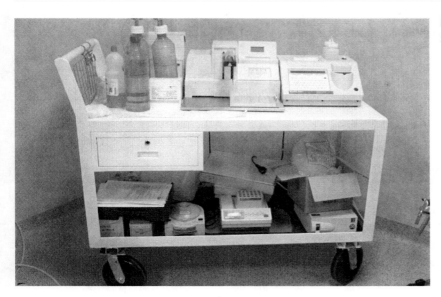

Fig. 23.9 Chemoluminometer for intraoperative PTH measurement

on a middle thyroid vein that required a reoperation 2 hours after surgery. Transient hypocalcemia occurred in 15 patients. Six patients had persistent hyperparathyroidism. In 4 patients the adenoma was not found at exploration even after conversion. These patients are being re-evaluated. In two patients the persistence was due to false-positive qPTHa. A second exploration revealed a second adenoma missed at the time of the first operation. Both missed second adenomas were on the opposite side to the first operation and they were successfully treated again by the minimally invasive video-assisted approach.

In this series 6 patients had previously undergone thyroid surgery and 2 patients had a prior exploration for primary HPTH. We successfully used a lateral approach in these patients to avoid adhesions in the midline. We started to perform this procedure in 1997 [6] and our mean follow-up is now considerable, accounting for an average of 3 years (range 9–91 months): a surgical cure was obtained in 98.7% of the cases who had undergone MIVAT and no case of recurrent primary HPTH was present in the series [11]. Our learning curve with MIVAP is depicted in Fig. 23.10.

23.5   Conversion to Open Surgery: When and How

During MIVAP the necessity for conversion can be due either to a technical difficulty the surgeon encounters when trying to remove the involved adenoma or to the problems or lack of correspondence between the preoperative localization by imaging and the real anatomical situation. Difficulty in controlling bleeding or the impossibility of visualizing correctly the recurrent laryngeal nerve because of a difficult dissection should call for an immediate conversion: the latter situation generally occurs in the presence of bulging thyroids which have been underestimated at preoperative ultrasonography and which are quite common in endemic goiter countries. Suspicion of malignancy or the presence of an intrathyroidal adenoma can represent rarely the reason for a conversion. In case the supposed adenoma does not come into vision, a decision must be made by the surgeon: at least an extensive unilateral exploration should be carried out before shifting to an open procedure. In fact, the endoscopic view should quite easily allow exploration of all the possible sites from the upper neck to the superior mediastinum where an adenoma can be found. If two normal parathyroid glands have been found, it is necessary to explore the opposite side immediately. If the patient is undergoing an operation involving a central access, such as the one we are describing and we currently use, the possibility of a contralateral endoscopic exploration must be taken into account before converting to a different procedure, in particular in all the cases where preoperative localization was undetermined or sestamibi scan and ultrasonography were not concordant. Of course a reasonable period of time should be spent for endoscopic exploration: we suggest that when four glands are present or, in absence of their visualization, more than one hour has gone by, a wide open exploration must be performed. This attitude is not in contrast

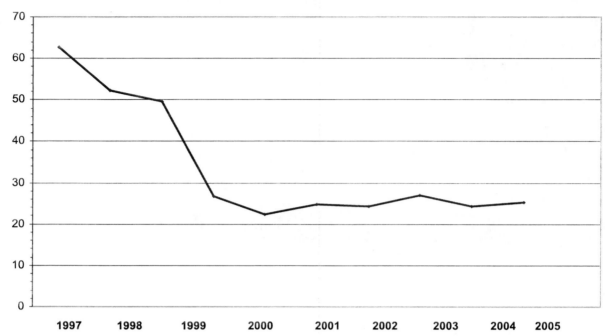

learning curve MIVAP (operative time) 1997-2005

Fig. 23.10 MIVAP operating time learning curve in 463 patients operated on between 1997 and 2005. (*y*-axis: operating time (minutes); *x*-axis: period)

with the fact that these procedures are generally regarded as targeted or focused parathyroidectomies, all of them receiving a validation through the use of qPTHa [12]. Bilateral exploration in fact remains the keystone of the surgical treatment of primary HPTH in all difficult cases [13]: the choice of performing an endoscopic operation through a central access allowing a bilateral exploration was in our case strongly influenced by this concept.

In our experience, conversion to open surgery did not guarantee a successful operation in all the patients: in 4 cases out of 13 in our series the adenoma was not found even after an extensive open exploration. The reasons for conversion in all the other cases were: multiglandular disease in 4 (double adenoma), intrathyroid adenoma in 3, difficult dissection in 8, intraoperative suspicion of parathyroid carcinoma in 1 (confirmed by frozen section and thus treated with synchronous thyroid lobectomy), and inadequate intraoperative PTH assay in 1. The overall incidence of conversions was less than 6.5%. A further advantage of central access is that when shifting to a standard cervicotomy the incision is easier to perform starting from the midline and gives a better aesthetic result.

23.6   Advantages of Video-assisted Parathyroidectomy

The main advantage by far of MIVAP is the cosmetic benefit. This is generally considered obvious because a scar of 1–2 cm tends to be better accepted than a 6-cm one in this region. This particular advantage though is not simple to demonstrate and to measure in an objective way: there are only a few papers dealing with this subject. A single prospective study evaluating patients' satisfaction by means of a visual analog scale score proved that it was significantly higher in MIVAP versus conventional procedures [14]. The same paper demonstrated a less painful course following MIVAP.

It was said that focused approaches would not allow the treatment of concomitant thyroid diseases: this is certainly true in most of these procedures but it is no longer true when considering endoscopic procedures based on a central access, such as described here. In fact, as long as the thyroid mass does not exceed the size established as cut-off for the indications for video-assisted thyroidectomy, it can be easily removed using the same access no matter on which side of the gland it is located. This happened in 5.6% of the cases in our series. Finally there is a wide consensus about the lower incidence of postoperative hypoparathyroidism after any focused operation in comparison to bilateral neck exploration: this aspect is not peculiar to MIVAP but is shared by all minimally invasive or targeted operations for primary HPTH.

References

1. Gagner M (1996) Endoscopic parathyroidectomy (letter). Br J Surg 83:87

2. Henry JF, Defechereux T, Gramatica L, de Boissezon C (1999) Minimally invasive videoscopic parathyroidectomy by lateral approach. Langenbecks Arch Surg 384:298–301

3. Shimizu K, Akira S, Jasmi AY, Kitamura Y, Kitagawa W, Akasu H, Tanaka S (1999) Video-assisted neck surgery: endoscopic resection of thyroid tumors with a very minimal neck wound. J Am Coll Surg 188:697–703

4. Ohgami M, Ishii S, Ohmori T, Noga K, Furukawa T, Kitajima M (2000) Scarless endoscopic thyroidectomy: breast approach better cosmesis. Surg Laparosc Endosc Percutan Tech 10:1–4

5. Ikeda Y, Ikeda Y, Takami H, Sasaki Y, Kan S, Niimi M (2000) Endoscopic neck surgery by the axillary approach. J Am Coll Surg 191:336–340

6. Miccoli P, Cecchini G, Conte M, Bendinelli C, Vignali E, Picone A, Marcocci C (1997) Minimally invasive, video-assisted parathyroid surgery for primary hyperparathyroidism. J Endocrinol Invest 20:429–430

7. Duh QY (2003) Presidential address. Minimally invasive endocrine surgery: standard of treatment or hype? Surgery 134:849–857

8. Henry JF, Jacobone M, Mirallie M, Deveze A, Pili S et al (2001) Indications and results of video assisted parathyroidectomy by a lateral approach in patients with a primary hyperparathyroidism. Surgery 130:999–1004

9. Berti P, Materazzi G, Picone A, Miccoli P (2003) Limits and drawbacks of video-assisted parathyroidectomy. Br J Surg 90:743–747

10. Gauger PG, Reeve TS, Delbridge LW (1999) Endoscopically assisted, minimally invasive parathyroidectomy. Br J Surg 86:1563–1566

11. Vignali E, Picone A, Materazzi G, Steffè S, Berti P, Cianferotti L, Cetani F, Ambrogini E, Miccoli P, Pinchera A, Marcocci C (2002) A quick intraoperative parathyroid hormone assay in the surgical management of patients with primary hyperparathyroidism: a study of 206 consecutive cases. Eur J Endocrinol 146:783–788

12. Udelsman R (2002) Six hundred fifty-six consecutive explorations for primary hyperparathyroidism. Ann Surg 235:665–672

13. Clark OH (2005) Editorial. J Endocrinol Invest (in press)

14. Miccoli P, Bendinelli C, Berti P, et al (1999) Video-assisted versus conventional parathyroidectomy in primary hyperparathyroidism: a prospective randomized study. Surgery 126:1117–1122

24 Multiglandular Parathyroid Disease and MEN Syndromes

Peter Langer, Detlef K. Bartsch, and Matthias Rothmund

24.1   Introduction

Primary hyperparathyroidism (HPTH) is a common endocrine disease with an estimated annual incidence of about 30 per 100,000 inhabitants [1]. The disease is mostly sporadic and caused by a single adenoma in about 80–95% of cases [1]. However primary HPTH has also been associated with hereditary syndromes (Table 24.1). One of the major characteristics of the hereditary syndromes is multiglandular disease. The hereditary variants of primary HPTH require special diagnostic workup and therapeutic consequences. Hereditary forms of primary HPTH may present in different clinical settings.

Hyperparathyroidism is the most common manifestation of multiple endocrine neoplasia type 1 (MEN1) [2–5]. It can also occur in 20–30% of patients as part of MEN2A and very rarely in MEN2B

[6]. The MEN syndromes are familial disorders affecting more than one endocrine gland and are also transmitted as an autosomal dominant trait. They are characterized by high penetrance and synchronously or metachronously developing tumors or hyperplasia of different glands such as thyroid, parathyroid, endocrine pancreas, adrenal, and pituitary glands. MEN1, or Wermer's syndrome, includes lesions of the parathyroids, the endocrine pancreas, and the anterior pituitary [5]. Tumors of the adrenal cortex, lipoma, and foregut carcinoids have also been reported, but are less common [3,4,7,8]. Mutations of the *MEN1-(menin)* gene, located on chromosome 11q13 are responsible for the development of MEN1 and were identified in 1997 [9]. MEN2 is characterized by medullary thyroid carcinoma (MTC) affecting nearly 100% of subjects and unilateral or often bilateral pheochromocytoma. Primary HPTH is a part of MEN2A. Marfanoid habitus and ganglioneuromatosis belong to MEN2B. All subtypes of MEN2 are caused by germline-activating mutations of the *RET* proto-oncogene, which has been mapped to chromosome 10q11.2 [10]. In 1936 Goldman and Smyth reported on siblings with familial HPTH without any other manifestation of MEN [11]. Many other reports about this, later called familial isolated HPTH, appeared in the meantime, although some authors speculate that familial cases of HPTH are a specific allelic variant of MEN1-related HPTH [12–15]. Nevertheless, recent studies showed that a fraction of familial HPTH must have unrecognized causes, since evaluated kindreds did not show any evidence of *MEN1*, calcium-sensing receptor gene (*CaSR*), or *HRPT2* gene mutations [16]. *HRPT2* gene mutations have been identified to cause the hyperparathyroidism–jaw tumor syndrome (HPTH-JT), which is another hereditary entity with primary HPTH, although the clinical presentation of the syndrome with respect to HPTH is often characterized by single parathyroid adenomas [10,17,18]. The incidence of parathyroid carcinoma is higher among patients with HPTH-JT.

Familial hypocalciuric hypercalcemia (FHH) is a very rare disorder. It is characterized by increased/ normal levels of serum calcium, moderate hypophosphoremia, and increased/normal circulating parathormone levels [19]. Patients with FHH are heterozygous for mutations of the *CaSR* gene, whereas children with neonatal severe primary HPTH suffer from the homozygous form of the disease [10,20]. The clinical symptoms of FHH, which is transmitted in an autosomal dominant order, are usually vague and mild and patients do not benefit from parathyroidectomy [21]. Nevertheless, the neonatal variant of the disease requires total parathyroidectomy, autotransplantation, and cryopreservation of parathyroid tissue [19].

The clinical characteristics and responsible genetic defects of the syndromes mentioned above are summarized in Table 24.1. Knowledge of the causing genetic defect makes molecular-genetic screening in affected families possible and therefore early intervention can be achieved in mutation carriers, if indicated.

24.2 Primary Hyperparathyroidism as Part of Multiple Endocrine Neoplasia Type 1 (MEN1)

Multiple endocrine neoplasia type 1 or Wermer's syndrome is classically characterized by the presence of neoplastic lesions in the parathyroid glands, the anterior pituitary gland, and the endocrine pancreas and duodenum [5]. Primary HPTH is the initial feature of the syndrome in the vast majority of patients [2, 4]. The penetrance of HPTH in MEN1 reaches nearly 100% by the age of 50 years [22–25].

24.2.1 Clinical Presentation

Multiple endocrine neoplasia type 1-HPTH may show the same symptoms as in sporadic cases, although it has been stated that MEN1-HPTH has a milder course of the disease. Nevertheless, it has been shown that bone mass in women with HPTH and MEN1 is already low at the age of 35 years due to longstanding HPTH [26]. The authors recently published their own experience with 34 patients with MEN1-HPTH in a German endocrine referral center [27]. In this series 10 patients had renal calculi, one patient had bone pain, another one suffered from headache, and another one had gastrointestinal symptoms that led to the diagnosis. Twenty-one patients were asymptomatic and screening examinations in *MEN1* mutation carriers revealed the diagnosis of HPTH. The average age at the time of diagnosis in this group was 39.2 (17–78) years [27].

24.2.2 Indication for Surgery

Parathyroidectomy should be performed before any treatment of a suspected Zollinger-Ellison syndrome (ZES) due to gastrinoma, because hypercalcemia enhances gastrin secretion and may mimic ZES [28]. After parathyroidectomy hypergastrinemia often disappears. The time and extent of surgery was a matter of debate for a long time. Nevertheless it is nowadays accepted by most groups that surgical intervention is needed when hypercalcemia is noted to prevent renal

Table 24.1 Hereditary syndromes[a] associated with HPTH and multiglandular disease. (*MEN1* Multiple endocrine neoplasia type 1, *MEN2* multiple endocrine neoplasia type 2, *HPTH* hyperparathyroidism, *HPTH-JT* hyperparathyroidism–jaw tumor syndrome, *FHH* familial hypocalciuric hypercalcemia, *PTX* parathyroidectomy, *MTC* medullary thyroid carcinoma)

Syndrome	Genetic defect	Incidence of HPTH	Classical clinical features	Therapy of HPTH
MEN1	*MEN1-(menin)*	80–100%	Parathyroid hyperplasia, gastroenteropancreatic endocrine tumors, pituitary tumors	Total PTX + parathyroid autotransplantation, or subtotal PTX
MEN2A	*RET*	20–30%	MTC, parathyroid hyperplasia/adenoma, pheochromocytoma	Extirpation of enlarged glands, total or subtotal PTX
Familial isolated HPTH	*MEN1, HRPT2, CaSR, ?*	100%	Parathyroid hyperplasia/adenoma	Total or subtotal PTX, extirpation of enlarged glands
HPTH-JT	*HRPT2*	80%	Parathyroid adenoma/carcinoma, fibro-osseous jaw tumors	Extirpation of enlarged glands, total or subtotal PTX
FHH	*CaSR*		Hypercalcemia, hypocalciuria	No surgery
Neonatal severe HPTH	*CaSR*		Severe hypercalcemia	Total PTX + autotransplantation

[a] For a comprehensive review, refer to Marx and Simonds (2005) [61]

calculi, osteopenia, and cardiovascular problems. The authors operate on MEN1 patients fulfilling the diagnostic criteria of primary HPTH (hypercalcemia in combination with elevated or inadequately high parathormone serum levels) irrespective of symptoms. Screening in MEN1 mutation carriers starts at the age of 16 years in our institution.

24.2.3 Surgical Procedure

The main difference of MEN1-HPTH compared to sporadic HPTH is the potential of every parathyroid gland of neoplastic growth. Due to this genetically determined potential the surgical approach to MEN1-primary HPTH should be similar to the approach to secondary HPTH. Patients with MEN1-HPTH usually have three or four enlarged glands and the tumors are typically asymmetric in size. This has been documented by several reports comparing gland volume and gland weights [29–31]. Some authors state that these tumors should be regarded as independent polyclonal adenomas [29], whereas an early hyperplastic phase has been suggested but not proven.

Minimally invasive parathyroidectomy is therefore not recommended because it does not allow the routine examination and extirpation of all parathyroid glands. Adequate surgery for MEN1-HPTH therefore requires subtotal parathyroidectomy (PTX) with transcervical thymectomy, leaving a parathyroid remnant in the neck, or total PTX and transcervical thymectomy with a fresh parathyroid autograft to the forearm. Subtotal PTX has been favored by some authors due to the low incidence of postoperative hypocalcemia [32]. Recurrence rates after subtotal PTX are high especially in older series and can reach 44% if transcervical thymectomy is not performed [33–35]. Additional parathyroid glands located in the thymus can be a source of postoperative parathormone excess and be responsible for recurrences. In the authors series two additional glands have been found in 34 patients and seven parathyroid glands have been found in the thymic horns [27]. Therefore transcervical thymectomy has to be performed routinely. Thompson (1995) reported longtime recurrence rates of 12.5% after subtotal PTX including transcervical thymectomy without postoperative hypocalcemia [30]. Similar results have been published by the French groups [36,37]. These groups left parathyroid remnants of about 60–80 mg in the neck. Another important argument for routine transcervical thymectomy is to prevent the development of thymic carcinoid tumors, which may occur in MEN1 patients. These tumors are malignant in 82% and can be a cause of death related to the syndrome

[38,39]. The most important argument against subtotal PTX with or without transcervical thymectomy compared to total PTX and autotransplantation is the leaving of parathyroid tissue in the neck, mostly in young patients. In case of recurrence and a probably necessary revision of the neck the rates of recurrent laryngeal nerve palsies rise up to 10% even in experienced centers. Low recurrence and persistence rates have been published after total PTX and autotransplantation. Tonelli et al. found no recurrence or persistence after a mean follow-up of 35.5 months [40]. Hellmann et al. described a 20% recurrence rate after a mean follow-up of 5.5 years [34]. In the authors series no recurrence occurred after a median follow-up of 36 months. In cases of recurrence after total PTX and autotransplantation the easy-to-perform "Casanova test" can distinguish between recurrence from the transplant site or a missed additional gland in the neck [41]. Revision of the transplant in the forearm can be performed under local anesthesia in an outpatient setting. However, in our own experience and from literature data recurrences are rare after total PTX and autotransplantation. It is anticipated that all patients who undergo total cervical PTX with immediate autotransplantation of parathyroid tissue experience immediate postoperative hypocalcemia. Also, hypocalcemia has been reported to be a longstanding problem after total PTX and autotransplantation, although transplant function can become evident even after a long postoperative time [34]. From the authors experience it is important that autotransplantation is performed meticulously. The parathyroid tissue must be carefully minced into small, about 1-mm³-large, pieces and then placed into individual muscle pockets of the non-dominant forearm. The pockets are closed and marked by a clip. In cases of postoperative hypocalcemia, oral substitution of calcium and vitamin D is possible and retransplantation of parathyroid tissue can also be performed in an outpatient setting.

Nevertheless, data from prospective randomized trials are lacking to compare the longtime results of subtotal PTX versus total PTX and autotransplantation. Therefore subtotal or total PTX and autotransplantation are the procedures of choice, if performed including transcervical thymectomy with cryopreservation of parathyroid tissue and if performed in experienced centers. Meticulous documentation of the operative site and the number of removed glands including the histological confirmation of every single removed gland is imperative to make reintervention easier, if necessary. It is likely that intraoperative parathyroid hormone (PTH) assays will be helpful in confirming the adequacy of resection in patients with familial forms of primary HPTH.

24.3 Persistence and Recurrences in MEN1-HPTH

In cases of persistence or recurrence the diagnostic workup must begin with confirming the diagnosis of recurrent primary HPTH and reevaluation of previous surgery including operative notes and histology reports. This is followed by localization procedures, starting with ultrasonography of the neck and sestamibi scintigraphy. Magnetic resonance imaging of the neck and mediastinum as well as catheterized venous sampling for serum parathormone are optional and may complete the diagnostic workup. A focused approach to a missed single gland should then be possible in most cases. This focused approach might reduce the risk of recurrent laryngeal nerve palsies. Intraoperative parathormone measurement ("Quick-PTH") is a helpful tool for all redo cases.

In case of recurrence after total PTX and autotransplantation, the first diagnostic procedure has to be the Casanova test to localize the source of parathormone excess in the neck or forearm [41]. Revision of the neck, if necessary, then follows the same workup as mentioned above. Revision of the forearm can be performed under local anesthesia.

24.4 Primary Hyperparathyroidism as Part of Multiple Endocrine Neoplasia Type 2 (MEN2)

The incidence of primary HPTH in MEN2 is not comparable to HPTH in MEN1. HPTH occurs in approximately 20–30% of patients with MEN2A and only very rarely in MEN2B [42–44]. HPTH is the least common endocrinopathy in MEN2. The disease mostly develops after the third decade of life and rarely after thyroidectomy for MTC [45]. Germline mutations of the *RET* proto-oncogene are responsible for MEN2. While a lot of different mutations of the *RET* gene have been described so far, especially mutations of codon 634 in exon 11 predispose patients to HPTH [46]. As in MEN1 and other hereditary syndromes with HPTH the incidence of multiglandular disease is high.

24.4.1 Clinical Presentation

Hyperparathyroidism in MEN2 patients is often asymptomatic, but nevertheless hypercalciuria and renal calculi may occur. The course of the disease has been reported to be milder than MEN1-HPTH [10].

24.4.2 Indication for Surgery

The surgical management of MTC generally dominates the clinical course in patients with MEN2A (refer also to Chapter 11 "Surgery for Medullary Thyroid Cancer"). The diagnostic criteria and the indications for surgical intervention are similar to those in MEN1-HPTH and sporadic HPTH [10,47].

24.4.3 Surgical Procedure

First it is important to rule out a possibly coexisting pheochromocytoma in a patient with MEN2-HPTH to prevent a dangerous hypertensive crisis during the operation. Urine catecholamine measurement is therefore mandatory and in the case of pheochromocytoma adrenalectomy has to be performed prior to neck surgery for HPTH. As for MEN1-HPTH data from randomized prospective trials are not available. The situation is even more difficult due to the rarity of the disease. Only a very few endocrine centers have longtime experience. Some groups recommend a similar surgical approach as to MEN1-HPTH and favor subtotal or total parathyroidectomy with autotransplantation [48,49]. Herfarth et al. found a high rate of recurrent or persistent hyperparathyroidism as a result of either missed glands or development of neoplasia in previously normal parathyroid glands left in situ. This group therefore recommended total parathyroidectomy with routine transcervical thymectomy and autotransplantation. In contrast to this point of view other groups advocated only selective resection of enlarged parathyroid glands [44,47]. This conservative attitude was supported by a retrospective study of the French Calcitonin Tumors Study Group, published in 1996. In this study the authors found that the disease was often mild with moderate asymptomatic hypercalcemia. The recurrence rate in this study was 9% but hypocalcemia occurred in 12 of 56 patients [44]. The consensus guidelines for the diagnosis and treatment of MEN1 and 2, published in 2001, recommended for MEN2-HPTH, that "operation (resection of only enlarged glands, subtotal parathyroidectomy, parathyroidectomy with autotransplantation) should be similar to those in other patients with potential for multiple parathyroid tumors" [50].

Generally, as for MEN1-HPTH, surgery should be performed in experienced centers. The disease tends to be more mild and the parathyroid gland enlargement much more asymmetric and unpredictable. Most surgeons recommend removing enlarged glands and are not as aggressive in MEN2A patients as in MEN1 patients. From our point of view, however, surgical approach should be similar as to MEN1-HPTH. We recommend subtotal PTX or total PTX with immediate autotransplantation and, for both methods, a transcervical thymectomy. Cryopreservation of parathyroid tissue is also mandatory, to have options to treat a possible postoperative hypoparathyroidism. Nevertheless the clinical situation may be even more difficult compared to MEN1-HPTH, due to the association with MTC in MEN2. During neck surgery for MTC in a eucalcemic patient, enlarged parathyroid glands should be removed [51]. In cases where neck surgery has already been performed for MTC, the surgical approach to MEN2A-HPTH should be more tailored to the individual patient. For example in an older patient after thyroidectomy for MTC with mild asymptomatic hypercalcemia, localization procedures and a targeted approach with intraoperative parathormone measurement may then be worthwhile, if possible.

24.5 Familial Isolated Primary Hyperparathyroidism

Other patients with so-called familial HPTH without evidence of MEN syndromes have subsequently been reported [52–55] following the publication of Goldman and Smyth about siblings with HPTH in 1936 [11]. Nevertheless, due to the rarity of the syndrome patients were frequently included in series with MEN-HPTH. Although recently some publications appeared stating that familial isolated HPTH is a distinct entity [16,56], other authors still believe that the syndrome might be a specific allelic variant of MEN1 or HPTH-JTS [13–15,57,58]. To date, the question whether familial isolated HPTH is a distinct entity or not remains unclear.

Carneiro et al. concluded from their study on familial isolated HPTH families that limited parathyroidectomy performed with intraoperative measurement of parathormone is a successful surgical approach in these patients [56]. Long-term follow-up must prove these observations and combined clinical and genetic studies on the background of familial hyperparathyroidism have to answer these questions.

The consequences for the daily work of the endocrine surgeon dealing with these problems are evident. In every case of a family history of hypercalcemia without clinical evidence of MEN syndromes, first FHH has to be ruled out. Then every effort including molecular-genetic analysis has to be made to

screen for MEN or HPTH-JTS. During neck exploration every parathyroid gland should be identified and enlarged glands be removed. In cases of macroscopic multiglandular disease subtotal or total PTX with autotransplantation should be performed. An alternative could be to perform localization procedures and, if positive, perform a unilateral approach with intraoperative parathormone measurement to control surgical success. All patients with familial HPTH have to be followed and screened for possible development of full-blown MEN1 or HPTH-JTS.

24.6 Hyperparathyroidism–Jaw Tumor Syndrome

The HPTH-JTS is an extremely rare syndrome with about 30 kindreds reported in the literature so far. The causative genetic defect, mutations of the *HRPT2* gene, has recently been described [17]. The syndrome is characterized by HPTH, fibro-osseous tumors of the jaw, and rarely kidney tumors. HPTH is the most common feature of the disease, accounting for about 80%. The syndrome is also characterized by a high incidence of parathyroid cancer and may often be uniglandular for HPTH [59–61]. Large series do not exist due to the low incidence, but resection of grossly enlarged parathyroid glands seems to be adequate surgery. However, all parathyroid glands should be seen during neck exploration and subtotal or total PTX and autotransplantation are the alternatives of choice in cases of macroscopic multiglandular disease. In cases of parathyroid carcinoma en bloc resection combined with ipsilateral thyroid lobectomy and lymph node dissection of the medial compartment should be performed.

24.7 Familial Hypocalciuric Hypercalcemia

Familial hypocalciuric hypercalcemia is transmitted in an autosomal dominant fashion and usually a symptomless non-progressive lifelong hypercalcemic disorder with 100% penetration [10,19]. Hypercalcemia is mild and hypocalciuria due to increased renal tubular reabsorbtion is an important feature. The incidence of gallstones, diabetes mellitus, relapsing pancreatitis, and myocardial infarction is slightly increased; the incidence of nephrolithiasis is normal. The urinary calcium level of less than 0.01 for urinary calcium-to-creatinine clearance ratio (C_{ca}/C_{cr}) is the most reliable diagnostic criterion for FHH to distinguish it from HPTH. Patients generally do not benefit from PTX because hypercalcemia persists after operation [21]. Therefore FHH is only a possible differential diagnosis in the focus of the endocrine surgeon.

24.8 Neonatal Severe Primary Hyperparathyroidism

Neonatal severe primary HPTH is a rare disease. Although it has been speculated that some documented cases of neonatal HPTH have been sporadic, it is now accepted that most cases represent the homozygous form of FHH resulting in severe hypercalcemia requiring urgent intervention [10]. The clinical manifestations occur in the first week of life or within the first 6 months. The newborns are usually normal in terms of size and weight. HPTH-associated skeletal manifestations are frequent and pathologic fractures have been reported. Medical therapy, including hydration may be administered to children with a mild course of the disease, but urgent parathyroidectomy is necessary in most patients. Total parathyroidectomy with immediate or later autotransplantation of cryopreserved tissue is the surgical therapy of choice [19].

24.9 Summary

Parathyroid surgery in the setting of familial disorders resulting in multiglandular disease is challenging for the endocrine surgeon. The aim of surgery is to gain eucalcemia for a long time without producing hypocalcemia. Since the syndromes are rare, sufficient data are lacking in most diseases. MEN1-HPTH should be treated with subtotal or total PTX with autotransplantation. Surgery in MEN2A has to be more tailored to the individual patient and subtotal PTX, total PTX and autotransplantation as well as excision of grossly enlarged glands might be alternatives depending on the patient's history of the disease. The surgical approach to patients with HPTH-JTS is the same as to MEN2A-HPTH. Nevertheless radical surgery may be required in this special setting, since the incidence of parathyroid carcinoma is comparably high in these patients.

Cryopreservation of parathyroid tissue is mandatory in all cases of familial HPTH. The role of minimally invasive parathyroid surgery in familial HPTH is limited and should only be performed in redo cases combined with intraoperative PTH measurements.

Patients with FHH do not benefit from parathyroid surgery whereas infants with neonatal severe HPTH need to be operated on and total parathyroidectomy performed.

References

1. Heath H 3rd, Hodgson SF, Kennedy MA (1980) Primary hyperparathyroidism. Incidence, morbidity, and potential economic impact in a community. N Engl J Med 302:189–193
2. Benson L, Ljunghall S, Akerstrom G (1987) Hyperparathyroidism presenting as the first lesion in multiple endocrine neoplasia type 1. Am J Med 82:731–737
3. Carty SE, Helm AK, Amico JA, Clarke MR, Foley TP, Watson CG, Mulvihill JJ (1998) The variable penetrance and spectrum of manifestations of multiple endocrine neoplasia type 1. Surgery 124:1106–1114
4. Vasen HFA, Lamers CB, Lips CJM (1989) Screening for the multiple endocrine neoplasia syndrome type 1: a study of 11 kindreds in the Netherlands. Arch Intern Med 149:2717–2722
5. Wermer P (1954) Genetic aspects of adenomatosis of endocrine glands. Am J Med 16:363–371
6. Kraimps JL, Duh QY, Demeure M, et al (1992) Hyperparathyroidism in multiple endocrine neoplasia syndrome. Surgery 112:1080–1086
7. Langer P, Cupisti K, Bartsch DK, Nies C, Goretzki PE, Rothmund M, Röher HD (2002) Adrenal involvement in multiple endocrine neoplasia type 1. World J Surg 26:891–896
8. Skogseid B, Rastad J, Gobl A, Larsson C, Backlin K, Juhlin C, Akerstrom G, Öberg K (1995) Adrenal lesion in multiple endocrine neoplasia type 1. Surgery 118:1077–1082
9. Chandrasekharappa SC, Guru SC, Manickam P, et al. (1997) Positional cloning of the gene for multiple endocrine neoplasia type 1. Science 276:404–407
10. Brandi ML, Falchetti A (2004) Genetics of primary hyperparathyroidism. Urol Int 72:11–16
11. Goldman L, Smyth FS (1936) Hyperparathyroidism in siblings. Ann Surg 104:971–981
12. Cetani F, Pardi E, Giovannetti A, et al (2002) Genetic analysis of the MEN1 gene and HPRT2 locus in two Italian kindreds with familial isolated hyperparathyroidism. Clin Endocrinol (Oxf) 56:457–464
13. Kassem M, Kruse TA, Wong, FK, Larssun C, Teh BT (2000) Familial isolated hyperparathyroidism as a variant of multiple endocrine neoplasia type 1 in a large Danish pedigree. J Clin Endocrinol Metab 85:165–167
14. Miedlich A, Lohmann T, Schneyer U, Lamesch P, Paschke R (2001) Familial isolated primary hyperparathyroidism: a multiple endocrine neoplasia type 1 variant? Eur J Endocrinol 145:155–160

15. Pannett AA, Kennedy AM, Turner JJ, et al (2003) Multiple endocrine neoplasia type 1 (MEN1) germline mutations in familial isolated primary hyperparathyroidism. Clin Endocrinol (Oxf) 58:639–646

16. Simonds WF, Robbins CM, Agarwal SK, Hendy GN, Carpten JD, Marx SJ (2004) Familial isolated hyperparathyroidism is rarely caused by germline mutation in *HRPT2*, the gene for the hyperparathyroidism-jaw tumor syndrome. J Clin Endocrinol Metab 89:96–102

17. Carpten JD, Robbins CM, Villablanca A, et al (2002) *HRPT2*, encoding parafibromin, is mutated in hyperparathyroidism-jaw tumor syndrome. Nat Genet 32:676–680

18. Cavaco BM, Guerra L, Bradley KJ (2004) Hyperparathyroidism-jaw tumor syndrome in Roma families from Portugal is due to a founder mutation of the HRPT2 gene. J Clin Endocrinol Metab 89:1747–1752

19. Huang SH (1996) Familial hyperparathyroidism. In: Clark OH, Duh QY (eds) Textbook of endocrine surgery, 1st edn. Saunders, Philadelphia, pp 385–393

20. Pollak MR, Brown EM, Chou YH, Hebert SC, Marx SJ, Steinmann B, Levi T, Seidman CE, Seidman JG (1993) Mutations in the human Ca(2+)-sensing receptor gene cause familial hypocalciuric hypercalcemia and neonatal severe hyperparathyroidism. Cell 75:1297–1303

21. Marx SJ, Attie MF, Levine MA, et al (1981) The hypocalciuric or benign variant of familial hypercalcemia: clinical and biochemical features in fifteen kindreds. Medicine 60:397–412

22. Langer P, Wild A, Nies C, Rothmund M, Bartsch DK (2001) Variable expression of multiple endocrine neoplasia type 1: implications for screening strategies. Int J Surg Invest 3:473–481

23. Marx SJ (2001) Multiple endocrine neoplasia type 1. In: Scriver CR, Beaudet AL, Sly WS, Valle D (eds) The metabolic and molecular bases of inherited disease, 8th edn. McGraw-Hill, New York, pp 943–966

24. Skarulis MC (1998) Clinical expressions of multiple endocrine neoplasia type 1 at the National Institutes of Health. Ann Int Med 129:484–494

25. Trump D, Farren B, Wooding C, Pang JT, Besser GM, Buchanan KD, et al (1996) Clinical studies of multiple endocrine neoplasia type 1 (MEN1). QJM 89:653–659

26. Burgess JR, David R, Greenaway TM, Parameswaran V, Shepherd JJ (1999) Osteoporosis in multiple endocrine neoplasia type 1. Arch Surg 134:1119–1123

27. Langer P, Wild A, Schilling T, Nies C, Rothmund M, Bartsch DK (2004) Multiple endocrine neoplasia type 1: surgical therapy of primary hyperparathyroidism. Chirurg 75:900–906

28. Norton JA, Cornelius MJ, Doppmann JL, Maton PN, Garner JD, Jensen RT (1987) Effect of parathyroidectomy in patients with hyperparathyroidism, Zolllinger-Ellison syndrome and multiple endocrine neoplasia type 1: a prospective study. Surgery 102:958–966

29. Marx SJ, Menczel J, Campbell G, Aurbach GD, Spiegel AM, Norton JA (1991) Heterogeneous size of the parathyroid glands in familial multiple endocrine neoplasia type 1. Clin Endocrinol (Oxf) 35:521–526

30. Thompson NW (1995) The surgical management of hyperparathyroidism and endocrine disease of the pancreas in the multiple endocrine neoplasia type 1 patient. J Int Med 238:269–280

31. Grimelius L, Akerstrom G, Bondeson L, Juhlin C, Johansson H, Ljunghall S, Rastad J (1991) The role of the pathologist in diagnosis and surgical decision making in hyperparathyroidism. World J Surg 15:698–705

32. Kraimps JL, Duh QY, Demeure M, Clark OH (1992) Hyperparathyroidism in multiple endocrine neoplasia syndrome. Surgery 112:1080–1088

33. Burgess JR, David R, Parameswaran V, Greenaway TM, Shepherd JJ (1998) The outcome of subtotal parathyroidectomy for the treatment of hyperparathyroidism in multiple endocrine neoplasia type 1. Arch Surg 133:126–129

34. Hellman P, Skogseid B, Öberg K, Juhlin C, Akerström G, Rastad J (1998) Primary and reoperative parathyroid operations in hyperparathyroidism of multiple endocrine neoplasia type 1. Surgery 124:993–999

35. Malmaeus J, Benson L, Johansson H, Ljunghall S, Rastad J, Akerström G, et al (1986) Parathyroid surgery in the multiple endocrine neoplasia type 1 syndrome: choice of surgical procedure. World J Surg 10:668–672

36. Hubbard JG, Sebag F, Majewa S, Henry JF (2002) Primary hyperparathyroidism in MEN1: how radical should surgery be? Langenbecks Arch Surg 386:553–557

37. Goudet P, Cougard P, Vergès B, Murat A, Carnaille B, Calender A, Faivre J, Proye C (2001) Hyperparathyroidism in multiple endocrine neoplasia type 1: surgical trends and results of a 256-patient series from Groupe d'Etude des Néoplasies Endocriniennes Multiples Study Group. World J Surg 25:886–890

38. Duh QY, Hybarger CP, Geist R, et al (1987) Carcinoids associated with multiple endocrine neoplasia syndromes. Am J Surg 154:142–148

39. Teh BT, Zedenius J, Kytölä S, et al (1998) Thymic carcinoids in multiple endocrine neoplasia type 1. Ann Surg 228:99–105

40. Tonelli F, Spini S, Tommasi M, Gabrielli G, Amorosi A, Brocchi A, Brandi ML (2000) Intraoperative parathormone measurement in patients with multiple endocrine neoplasia type 1 syndrome and hyperparathyroidism. World J Surg 24:556–562

41. Casanova D, Sarfati E, De Francisco A, Amado JA, Arias M, Dubost C (1991) Secondary hyperparathyroidism: diagnosis of site of recurrence. World J Surg 15:546–549

42. Howe JR, Norton JA, Wells SA (1993) Prevalence of pheochromocytoma and hyperparathyroidism in multiple endocrine neoplasia type 2A: results of long-term follow-up. Surgery 114:1070–1077

43. O'Riordan DS, O'Brien T, Grant CS, et al (1993) Surgical management of primary hyperparathyroidism in multiple endocrine neoplasia types 1 and 2. Surgery 114:1031–1037

44. Kraimps JL, Denizot A, Carnaille B, et al (French Calcitonin Tumors Study Group), French Association of Endocrine Surgeons (1996) Primary hyperparathyroidism in multiple endocrine neoplasia type IIa: retrospective French multicentric study. World J Surg 20:808–813

45. Gagel RF, Tashjian AH Jr, Cummings T, Papathanasopoulos N, Kaplan MM, DeLellis RA, Wolfe HJ, Reichlin S (1988) The clinical outcome of prospective screening for multiple endocrine neoplasia type 2A: an 18-year experience. N Engl J Med 318:478

46. Schuffeneker I, Virally-Monod M, Brohet R, le Groupe D'Etude des Tumeurs a Calcitonine (1998) Risk and penetrance of primary hyperparathyroidism in multiple endocrine neoplasia type 2A families with mutations at codon 634 of the *RET* proto-oncogene. J Clin Endorinol Metab 83:487–491

47. van Heerden JA, Kent III RB, Sizemore GW, et al (1983) Primary hyperparathyroidism in patients with multiple endocrine neoplasia syndromes. Surgical experience. Arch Surg 118:533–536

48. Herfarth KK, Bartsch D, Doherty GM, Wells SA Jr, Lairmore TC (1996) Surgical management of hyperparathyroidism in patients with multiple endocrine neoplasia type 2A. Surgery 120:966–973

49. Mallette LE (1994) Management of hyperparathyroidism in the multiple endocrine neoplasia syndromes and other familial endocrinopathies. Endocrinol Metab Clin North Am 23:19–36

50. Brandi ML, Gagel RF, Angeli A, et al (2001) Guidelines for diagnosis and therapy of MEN type 1 and type 2. J Clin Endocrinol Metab 86:5658–5671

51. Marx SJ, Agarwal SK, Simonds WF, et al (2002) Hyperparathyroidism in hereditary syndromes: special expressions and special managements. J Bone Miner Res 17(suppl 2):N37–N43

52. Clark OH, Way LW, Hunt TK (1976) Recurrent hyperparathyroidism. Ann Surg 184:391–402

53. Allo M, Thompson NW (1982) Familial hyperparathyroidism caused by solitary adenomas. Surgery 92:486–490

54. Law WM, Hodgson SF, Heath H III (1983) Autosomal inheritance of familial hyperparathyroidism. N Engl J Med 309:650–653

55. Doury P, Eulry F, Pattin S, Fromantin M, Gautier D, Bernard J, Tabaraud F, Masson C, Dano P (1983) Recurrent familial hyperparathyroidism: a propos of seven adenomas in three members of the same family and a review of the literature. Sem Hop Paris 59:3427–3430

56. Carneiro D, Irvin GL, Inabnet WB (2002) Limited versus radical parathyroidectomy in familial isolated primary hyperparathyroidism. Surgery 132:1050–1055

57. Perrier ND, Villablanca A, Larsson C, Wong M, Ituarte P, Teh BT, Clark OH (2002) Genetic screening for *MEN1* mutations in families presenting with familial primary hyperparathyroidism. World J Surg 26:907–913

58. Carrasco CA, Gonzalez AA, Carvajal CA, Campusano C, Oestreicher E, Arteaga E, Wohllk N, Fardella CE (2004) Novel intronic mutation of MEN1 gene causing familial isolated hyperparathyroidism. J Clin Endocrinol Metab 89:4124–4129

59. Szabo J, Heath B, Hill VM, et al (1995) Hereditary hyperparathyroidism-jaw tumor syndrome: the endocrine tumor gene HRPT2 maps to chromosome 1q21-q31. Am J Hum Genet 56:944–950

60. Haven CJ, Wong FK, van Dam EW, et al (2000) A genotypic and histopathologic study of a large Dutch kindred with hyperparathyroidism-jaw tumor syndrome. J Clin Endocrinol Metab 85:1449–1454

61. Marx SJ, Simonds WF (2005) Hereditary hormone excess: genes, molecular pathways, and syndromes. Endocr Rev 26:615–661

25 Pathophysiology and Treatment of Secondary and Tertiary Hyperparathyroidism

Ulrich Güller and Michael Mayr

CONTENTS

25.1   Introduction

Secondary hyperparathyroidism (HPTH) is a disorder of mineral homeostasis occurring predominantly in patients with chronic kidney disease (CKD). As a consequence of renal insufficiency, phosphate retention, vitamin D deficiency, and hypocalcemia develop and result in a pathological increase in parathyroid hormone (PTH) secretion [1]. The pathogenesis of parathyroid disease is not yet fully understood. Already in the early course of the disease, polyclonal hyperplasia of parathyroid cells occurs. In the further course of HPTH, neoplastic transformation of pre-existing polyclonal hyperplasia to monoclonal areas is common and likely to play a major role in disease development [2]. However, histopathological categories that discriminate nodular versus generalized hyperplasia are not useful predictors of clonal status [2]. Polyclonal hyperplasia and areas of monoclonal proliferation often coexist and alter response to endogenous regulatory mechanisms and medical therapy. In areas of monoclonal expansion, the morphological substrate of tertiary HPTH, parathyroid cells escape regulatory control of serum calcium concentration and vitamin D.

25.2   Clinical Aspects of Secondary Hyperparathyroidism

From the large list of detrimental effects associated with secondary HPTH (Table 25.1), both renal osteodystrophy and progressive vascular calcifications have a major impact on patients' health [3–14]. These disorders begin in the early course of CKD. For the clinical management of secondary HPTH, both diagnosis and therapy, it is necessary to adequately judge the underlying renal function. The stages of CKD are defined by the National Kidney Foundation - Kidney Disease Outcomes Quality Initiative (NKF-K/DOQI) (Table 25.2) [15]. CKD is defined as either kidney damage (abnormalities in blood or urine tests or imaging studies) independent of glomerular filtration

Table 25.1 Detrimental effects of uremic refractory hyperparathyroidism

Sequels of hyperparathyroidism	References
Pruritus	[9]
Impaired T cell proliferation	[14]
Impaired humoral immunology	[13]
Hypertension	[12]
Anemia	[8]
Cardiopathy	[12]
Renal osteodystrophy	[5–7]
Increased mortality	[10,11,24]

Table 25.2 Stages of chronic kidney disease [15]. (*GFR* Glomerular filtration rate)

Stage	Description	GFR (ml/min per 1.73 m²)
1	Kidney damage[a] with normal or increased GFR	≥90
2	Kidney damage[a] with mild decrease in GFR	60–89
3	Moderate decrease in GFR	30–59
4	Severe decrease in GFR	15–29
5	Kidney failure	<15

[a] Kidney damage is defined as pathological abnormalities or markers of damage, including abnormalities in blood or urine tests or imaging studies

rate (GFR) or GFR <60 ml/min per 1.73 m² for more than 3 months [15].

25.2.1   Renal Osteodystrophy

Changes in bone structure due to secondary HPTH are common and begin in the early stages of CKD [16]. The term renal bone disease or renal osteodystrophy includes two major pathologies: osteitis fibrosa cystica and adynamic bone disease. In mixed osteodystrophy features of both osteitis fibrosa and decreased mineralization coexist [17].

Osteitis fibrosa cystica is a disease of high bone turnover. The disease is a consequence of increased PTH secretion. There is a correlation between the serum level of PTH and the rate of bone formation. The probability of high-turnover bone disease increases with rising serum PTH concentrations [7]. Serum values of PTH greater than 450 pg/ml (44 pmol/l)

are closely related to high-turnover bone disease in hemodialysis and peritoneal dialysis patients [6]. Osteitis fibrosa cystica is characterized by increases in osteoclasts, osteoblasts, osteocytes, and fibroblasts. These cells produce a peritrabecular fibrosis that is the hallmark of osteitis fibrosa cystica [5]. Since it has become possible to suppress PTH secretion with the administration of calcium and vitamin D, the frequency of osteitis fibrosa cystica and mixed forms is decreasing, while the frequency of adynamic bone disease is increasing [4,18].

Adynamic bone disease is typically associated with low levels of serum PTH. Histologically, this disease is characterized by unequal decreased numbers of both osteoclasts and osteoblasts, whereas the deficiency of osteoblasts is overbalanced. Low bone formation rates lead to decreased bone mass [5]. A special form of adynamic bone disease, osteomalacia, is related to aluminum exposition. Aluminum-based phosphate binders were commonly used to treat hyperphosphatemia in CKD. Its use decreased rapidly in the 1990s after the serious side effects became known (microcytic anemia, encephalopathy, osteomalacia). This led to a low prevalence of aluminum-induced adynamic bone disease. The disease is histologically characterized by stainable bone aluminum, increased osteoid formation, and defective mineralization [4].

Renal osteodystrophy is associated with high morbidity and mortality. The incidence of hip fractures in patients undergoing dialysis is reported to be up to 17 times higher than in the general population. Additionally, dialysis patients sustain hip fractures at a median age 11–15 years younger than their counterparts in the general population. The 1-year mortality related to hip fracture is 64% and thus 2.4 times higher than found in the general population [19]. In middle-aged Japanese men on dialysis the rate of vertebral fractures is reported to be three times higher than that in healthy men [20]. Patients with low levels of PTH seem to be at greatest risk for fractures [19,20]. It may be assumed that these populations represent predominantly patients with low-turnover bone disease, however, strict evidence correlating PTH levels, fractures, and biopsy-proven patterns of bone disease is still lacking. In addition to an increased risk of fractures, both high- and low-turnover bone disease seem to be involved in cardiovascular-related mortality. This may be due either to an increased release of calcium and phosphate from bone or to a low calcium-buffering capacity of bone, thus promoting vascular and soft tissue calcifications [4].

With respect to the pathophysiology of renal bone disease it becomes clear that the most important step in preventing renal osteodystrophy and its detrimen-

Table 25.3 Target range of intact PTH, phosphorus, calcium, and Ca × P product by stage of chronic kidney disease [21]

Stage	Intact PTH	Phosphorus	Calcium	Ca × P product
3	35–70 pg/ml (3.85–7.7 pmol/l)	2.7–4.6 mg/dl (0.87–1.48 mmol/l)	Within the normal range	<55 mg²/dl² (4.44 mmol²/l²)
4	70–110 pg/ml (7.7–12.1 pmol/l)	2.7–4.6 mg/dl (0.87–1.48 mmol/l)	Within the normal range	See stage 3
5	150–300 pg/ml (16.5–33.0 pmol/l)	3.3–5.5 mg/dl (1.13–1.78 mmol/l)	8.4-9.5 mg/dl (2.1-2.37 mmol/l)	See stage 3

tal effects is well-balanced PTH secretion. As recommended in the guidelines of the NKF-K/DOQI, the target levels of serum intact PTH should be based on the stage of CKD. In stage 4 serum intact PTH levels of 70–110 pg/ml (7.7–12.1 pmol/l) and in stage 5 of 150–300 pg/ml (16.5–33.0 pmol/l) should be the goal (Table 25.3) [21]. To reach these targets restriction of dietary phosphate intake is mandatory. Dependent on the serum levels of intact PTH as well as serum calcium and phosphorus, the attributable use of phosphate binders and/or calcitriol or one of its analogs may be necessary. The use of aluminum-based phosphate binders should be avoided whenever possible.

25.2.2 Vascular Calcifications

Despite deepened insights into the pathogenesis of renal disease, advances in medical interventions, and improvements in dialysis, mortality rates exceed 20% per year in patients suffering from end-stage renal disease (ESRD) [22]. Cardiovascular illness is an important factor of morbidity and mortality in CKD. The pathophysiological processes contributing to cardiovascular disease start early in the course of renal disease [23]. Classic risk factors and factors associated with renal insufficiency contribute to the occurrence and progression of cardiovascular disease. A growing body of evidence indicates that disorders of mineral metabolism in the context of secondary HPTH, i.e., high concentrations of serum phosphorus, serum calcium, calcium-phosphorus product as well as the degree of secondary HPTH itself are associated with increased risk of death [24]. It remains speculative as to why disturbances in mineral metabolism are associated with high mortality and morbidity rates. However, there are increasing data indicating that the dysregulation of mineral metabolism in CKD may influence vascular calcification [25–27] and may, in turn, at least partly contribute to the extremely high cardiovascular mortality rates in CKD [27]. Consequently, the treatment of secondary HPTH should not exclusively aim for ideal levels of serum PTH but should also focus on serum phosphorus, calcium, and calcium-phosphorus product.

25.3 Management of Secondary Hyperparathyroidism

25.3.1 Dietary Phosphate Intake

Phosphate retention represents one of the major factors in the development of secondary HPTH. Therefore, control of serum phosphorus is crucial in the prevention and treatment of secondary HPTH. The first step to control serum phosphorus is to reduce phosphate intake (Table 25.4). Experimental data from animals and humans show that a low phosphate diet can both prevent and ameliorate secondary HPTH [28–30]. Patients should be instructed to begin controlling dietary phosphate as soon as GFR is reduced. Dietary phosphate should be restricted to 800–1,000 mg/day to keep serum phosphorus levels below 4.6 mg/dl (1.49 mmol/l) in stage 3 and 4 CKD and 5.5 mg/dl (1.78 mmol/l) in stage 5 (Table 25.3) [21].

25.3.2 Phosphate Binders

The extent of dietary phosphate restriction is limited by malnutrition associated with inadequate protein intake and poor patient compliance. Therefore, the use of phosphate binders is required in almost all patients, at least in those who are on dialysis (Table 25.4). There are three types of phosphate binders: calcium-based, aluminum-based, and neither calcium- nor aluminum-based phosphate binders.

In spite of the effective phosphate binding by orally administered aluminum hydroxide, its use should be avoided because of the potential danger of aluminum intoxication. Coadministration of citrate is contraindicated in all patients ingesting aluminum-containing

Table 25.4 Consequences of medical and surgical therapy of secondary hyperparathyroidism and mineral metabolism in chronic kidney disease

Therapy	Phosphorus	Calcium	Ca × P product	PTH
Dietary phosphate restriction	↓	↔	↓	↓
Calcium-based phosphate binders	↓	↑	↓	↓
Calcium-free phosphate binders	↓	↔	↓	↓
Vitamin D sterols	↑	↑	↑	↓↓
Calcimimetics	↓	↓	↓	↓↓↓
Dialysis	↓	↔	↓	↓↓
Parathyroidectomy	↔	↓↓	↓	↓↓↓↓

compounds. Citrate enhances, even in low doses, intestinal aluminum absorption and, hence, intoxication [31].

Calcium carbonate and calcium acetate have been the favorite agents for controlling phosphate over the past 20 years. They are effective in lowering serum phosphorus and in preventing secondary HPTH [32,33]. Either drug should be given midway between meals to achieve maximal phosphate binding. In order to avoid undesirable calcium absorption, no more than 6 g per day (corresponding to approximately 1,200 mg elemental calcium) should be administered [34]. Studies demonstrated an independent association between dose of calcium-containing phosphate binders and vascular calcifications [35,36].

In patients with serum calcium levels greater than 10.2 mg/dl (2.54 mmol/l) (Table 25.3) calcium-based phosphate binders should be reduced or discontinued [21]. In patients with hypercalcemia and uncontrolled hyperphosphatemia a combination with calcium-free phosphate binders should be considered (Table 25.4). There are several calcium-free phosphate binders. One of them is sevelamer, a polyallamine hydrochloride. It can control serum phosphorus and reduce the levels of PTH without inducing hypercalcemia [37,38]. There is some evidence that effective lowering of phosphorus levels with sevelamer is less likely to cause progressive coronary and aortic calcification in hemodialysis patients than with calcium-based phosphate binders [39]. The daily amount of sevelamer equivalent to calcium-containing phosphate binders is approximately 6.5 g per day [38,40]. Currently, treating hypercalcemia with a combination of reduced doses of calcium-based phosphate binders and sevelamer should be preferred to monotherapy: sevelamer in monotherapy can lead to relevant hypocalcemia [37] and it is roughly ten times more expensive than calcium-based phosphate binders [41].

Another non-calcium-based phosphate binder currently under investigation is lanthanum carbonate, a rare earth element. Preliminary studies on end-stage renal disease are promising [42,43]. Although a study with bone biopsies performed at one year showed no signs of osteomalacia [42], concerns remain about potential long-term toxic side effects of absorption and accumulation.

25.3.3 Vitamin D Sterols

After achieving the desired serum phosphorus levels with phosphate restriction and the use of phosphate binders, secondary HPTH may often persist due to vitamin D deficiency. In this case vitamin D should be substituted. $1,25-(OH)_2D_3$, the most active metabolite of vitamin D, is important in controlling PTH synthesis and secretion (Table 25.4) [44]. However, in the setting of CKD there are potential adverse effects: calcitriol also promotes the intestinal absorption of calcium and phosphate leading to hypercalcemia and hyperphosphatemia followed by a rise in calcium-phosphorus product [45], a known risk factor of mortality in CDK [24]. Furthermore, oversuppression of PTH secretion leads to adynamic bone disease and may, in turn, aggravate hypercalcemia and hyperphosphatemia [45]. Therefore, vitamin D should not be administered until the serum phosphorus is under adequate control.

These undesired side effects have led to the development of vitamin D analogs that should retain the suppressive action on PTH and parathyroid gland growth with concomitantly less calcemic and phosphatemic activity [44]. Currently, three vitamin D analogs are available: paricalcitol (19-nor-1,25-dihydroxyvitamin D_2) and doxercalciferol (1α-hydroxyvitamin D_2) in the United States, and maxacalcitol

(22-oxacalcitriol) in Japan. Data comparing vitamin D analogs and calcitriol are sparse. One prospective study suggested that paricalcitol corrects secondary HPTH more rapidly than calcitriol, with fewer prolonged episodes of hypercalcemia [46]. Additional studies are needed to clarify the long-term benefits of newer vitamin D sterols over calcitriol.

The recommended initial dosing in patients with stages 3 and 4 CKD is calcitriol 0.25 μg/day or alfacalcidol 0.25 μg/day or doxercalciferol 2.5 μg three times per week. In patients on hemodialysis it is advisable to administer vitamin D sterols orally or intravenously three times per week after each hemodialysis session: calcitriol 0.5–1.5 μg, paricalcitol 2.5–5 μg, or doxercalciferol 5 μg oral or 2 μg i.v. Higher doses may be necessary depending on PTH serum levels [21]. However, it should be reemphasized that good control of phosphorus is a mandatory prerequisite for initiating high-dose active vitamin D therapy. Initially, at least monthly monitoring of serum calcium and phosphorus levels is advisable to avoid hypercalcemia and/or hyperphosphatemia. Serum intact PTH should be measured every 3–6 months.

25.3.4   Calcimimetics

The parathyroid calcium-sensing receptor (CaR), first cloned by Brown and his colleagues in 1995, regulates parathyroid secretion [47]. A key step in the development of secondary HPTH is the partial loss of calcium-regulated PTH suppression due to the underexpression of the CaR. Calcimimetics allosterically modulate the CaR, thereby sensitizing it to extracellular calcium ions [48]. The reestablished sensitivity to calcium ions leads to suppression of PTH secretion. In contrast to vitamin D sterols, which show an effect on PTH levels in hours or days by inhibition of PTH synthesis, the modification of the CaR and the resulting inhibition of PTH secretion leads to changes in serum PTH in minutes to a few hours [49]. Until now, medical therapy of HPTH was limited by hypercalcemia induced by vitamin D sterols and calcium-containing phosphate binders. The advantage of calcimimetics is their capacity to suppress PTH secretion without concomitant rise in serum calcium and phosphorus (Table 25.4).

The first clinically approved calcimimetic was cinacalcet hydrochloride. In two randomized clinical trials cinacalcet effectively reduced PTH levels in secondary HPTH with favorable influence on serum calcium and phosphorus [50]. Cinacalcet was well tolerated; only nausea and vomiting occurred more often

in the patients treated with cinacalcet [50]. Based on the published studies and with regard to limited long-term clinical experiences, the appropriate patients to start with cinacalcet are those on hemodialysis with inadequately controlled secondary HPTH despite adequate therapy. It is recommended to start with 30 mg once daily and increase the dose by 30 mg every 2–4 weeks until the target PTH is reached. During the titration phase, serum calcium should be controlled every week to twice weekly, whereas, during the maintenance period monitoring should be monthly to avoid hypocalcemia. Further studies will show what the role of cinacalcet is in the early phase of HPTH, in first-line therapy of established HPTH, and in patients with predominant autonomous areas in parathyreoidea.

25.3.5   Indications for Parathyroidectomy

Parathyroidectomy (PTX) is recommended in patients with therapy refractory HPTH. Analysis of the United States Renal Data System (USRDS) including patients on chronic dialysis and kidney transplant patients showed a clear-cut decline in the use of PTX from 1994 (0.8%) to 1998 (0.5%) [51]. The cause of this drop may be due to better medical management of HPTH, in consequence of better removal of phosphorus by dialysis and the use of better and less toxic phosphate binders. However, it is noteworthy that the indications for PTX are not well described and there are no studies that unequivocally define biochemical parameters indicating that medical therapy is not effective and surgery is required to control HPTH. The classic indication for surgical PTX is therapy-resistant hypercalcemia and hyperphosphatemia in the presence of severe HPTH (i.e., PTH levels approximately eight times over the normal range). Calciphylaxis with PTH levels greater than 500 pg/ml (55 pmol/l) is still an absolute indication [21,52].

25.4   Hyperparathyroidism after Renal Transplantation

25.4.1   Clinical Aspects of Hyperparathyroidism after Renal Transplantation

Successful renal transplantation should have beneficial effects on HPTH by reversal of abnormalities in mineral and bone metabolism. The functioning renal graft leads to a decrease of the plasma phosphate concentration by increasing urinary phosphate excretion and by renewing the synthesis of 1,25-dihydroxyvitamin D_3 [53]. PTH levels tend to fall rapidly during the first 3 months after transplantation and remain substantially stable thereafter [54]. However, complete resolution of secondary HPTH is an inconsistent finding after renal transplantation. In 20–50% of patients, PTH levels remain elevated, sometimes even years after transplantation [54–57]. Besides a non-optimal functioning graft [57,58], long duration of dialysis and high levels of PTH prior to kidney transplantation are associated with persistent HPTH after transplantation [54,56–59]. This supports the concept that the degree of HPTH after transplantation is largely dependent on the glandular volume, the degree of hyperplasia (number of parathyroid cells), and of monoclonal proliferation during the course of CKD and uremia. The mean lifespan of parathyroids cells is about 20 years [60], thus the involution of the parathyroid gland after transplantation is a very slow act, if it does indeed occur [61]. Therefore, it is plausible that spontaneous resolution of HPTH after renal transplantation does not necessarily occur. The importance of the vitamin D receptor genotype on the persistence of HPTH by influencing the sensitivity of the parathyroidea to calcitriol activity is still controversial. Fernandez [62] and Messa [54] noted lower PTH levels post-transplantation in patients with BB genotype whereas Torres [63] found lower PTH levels in patients with bb genotype.

Persistent post-transplant HPTH is associated with some deleterious effects. PTH represents an important regulator of renal phosphate handling as it increases renal phosphate excretion. The phosphaturic action of PTH results from inhibition of proximal tubular brush border membrane Na/Pi co-transporter by decreased expression of type IIa Na/Pi cotransport protein activity [64]. In consequence, high post-transplant PTH levels may induce hyperphosphaturia and hypophosphatemia [65,66]. During the first months after transplantation up to 90% of the graft recipients develop hypophosphatemia [67]. In the early post-transplant period muscle phosphate concentration was found to be decreased by 25%; however, the correlation with the serum phosphorus concentration was poor [67]. Patients with low serum phosphate concentrations may suffer from muscle weakness [68], and severe hypophosphatemia below 1.0 mg/dl (0.30 mmol/l), although rare, may lead to rhabdomyolysis [69], impaired cardiac contractility [70], respiratory failure [71,72], hemolytic anemia [73], leukocyte dysfunction [74], and neurological dysfunction [75].

Hypophosphatemia and, even more so, preexisting and persistent HPTH are considered to be important cofactors in disturbances of post-transplant bone remodeling [63,76]. Prospective studies have demonstrated that rapid bone loss occurs in the first 6–12 months after transplantation [77–79]. The location and rate of bone loss varies between men and women, with women losing bone mainly from the lumbar spine and men from the femoral neck. Bone loss rates of 1.7% per year to 1.6% per month at the lumbar spine and 3.6% per 3 months at the proximal femur have been reported [77,78,80]. The decrease of bone mineral density places the renal transplant recipient at a high risk for spontaneous fractures. The fracture rate which exceeds 10% is much higher in this population than in the general population, with vertebral bodies, hips, feet, and ankles being the sites most often affected [81–83].

Scarce data exist about the histological patterns and the dynamics of bone disease after kidney transplantation. In a study with bone biopsies before and 6 months after kidney transplantation, Cruz and colleagues found that bone histology changed: whereas high-turnover bone disease improved in all cases, low-turnover bone disease emerged and was the predominant form in most of them. No correlation between PTH and histomorphometric parameters could be detected [84]. Further, a decrease in trabecular bone volume and sometimes even osteomalacia were found in histomorphological analysis [85,86]. Impaired osteoblastogenesis and early osteoblast apoptosis seem to play an important role in the pathogenesis of post-transplant osteoporosis and appear to correlate with low serum phosphorus levels, whereas PTH is thought to have a protective effect by preserving osteoblast survival [87].

The effect of increased PTH concentrations on different target tissues leads to the common problem of post-transplant hypercalcemia. Hypercalcemia is seen in up to 50% of patients after transplantation [88]. High PTH concentrations stimulate the renal synthesis of 1,25-dihydroxycholecalciferol which, in turn, increases intestinal calcium absorption and improves the skeletal mobilization of calcium. Furthermore, the resolution of the skeletal resistance to PTH by correction of uremia and normalization of serum phosphorus levels facilitate release of calcium due to osteoclastic bone resorption [89]. Hypercalcemia after transplantation may become manifest in one of three forms: subacute hypercalcemia, transient self-limited hypercalcemia, and persistent hypercalcemia [56]. Subacute hypercalcemia develops within the first 3 months with calcium levels up to 15 mg/dl

(3.75 mmol/l) and presents a serious adverse event with potential graft dysfunction and calciphylaxis requiring rapid PTX. However, due to the improved pretransplantation management of secondary HPTH subacute hypercalcemia is nowadays a rare event [56]. Transient hypercalcemia is the most common form of post-transplant hypercalcemia and resolves in most cases within the first year. In 4–10% of kidney graft recipients mild hypercalcemia continues beyond the first year and gradually resolves within 2–5 additional years. Such persistent mild hypercalcemia (serum calcium concentration 10.5–11.5 mg/dl; 2.63–3.00 mmol/l) is generally well tolerated and not associated with severe side effects. However, a small group of recipients (<5%) maintain persistent hypercalcemia above 12 mg/dl (3.0 mmol/l) with the risk of renal dysfunction, nephrocalcinosis, pancreatitis, and vascular calcifications. In these cases elective PTX should be considered [56,89].

25.4.2 Management of Hyperparathyroidism after Transplantation and Indications for Parathyroidectomy

In general, treatment of disturbances in PTH, mineral, and bone metabolism is determined by the level of graft function in the transplant recipient and analog the guidelines for CKD (NFK-K/DOQI) (see paragraph 25.3). In the next paragraphs management of HPTH is focused on disorders emerging characteristically after kidney transplantation.

25.4.2.1 Hypercalcemia

In the rare cases of subacute post-transplant hypercalcemia (occurring within the first 3 months after transplantation) with serum calcium concentrations as high as 15 mg/dl (3.75 mmol/l) early PTX is required. Graft dysfunction and vascular calcifications of the small vessels with ischemic necrosis (calciphylaxis) can thereby be prevented. In cases (1–5% of the recipients) of persistent serum calcium concentrations above 12 mg/dl (3.0 mmol/l) elective PTX is recommended to avoid the complications of graft dysfunction, nephrolithiasis, pancreatitis, and vascular calcifications [21,56,89]. The place of calcimimetics, a new class of drugs introduced in the therapy of secondary HPTH, in the management of post-transplant HPTH with hypercalcemia is not yet clarified and represents a challenge for further investigations.

25.4.2.2 Hypophosphatemia

Besides primary tubular dysfunction of the allograft, persistent HPTH is the main cause of hyperphosphaturia and hypophosphatemia. In most cases relevant hypophosphatemia is transient and resolves within 1 month due to normalization of PTH levels and tubular function [61]. It has been shown that oral phosphate supplements are able to increase serum phosphate concentration and muscle phosphate content after transplantation [67]. However, it is not yet fully clear at which serum phosphorus levels phosphate supplementation should be started after kidney transplantation. Most authors agree that all recipients with severe hypophosphatemia [serum phosphorus levels less than 1.0 mg/dl (0.32 mmol/l)] or less severe hypophosphatemia in cases of cardiac dysfunction, respiratory failure, muscle weakness, or impaired tissue oxygenation should be treated, when coexisting hypercalcemia is excluded [90,91]. Otherwise, it should be kept in mind that phosphate stimulates PTH synthesis and secretion. Therefore, supplementation of phosphate bears the risk of worsening HPTH. Whereas in the early course after transplantation serum calcium and PTH concentrations seem not to be affected by oral phosphate supplements, a significant increase in PTH levels was found in patients receiving oral phosphate supplements in the late course of transplantation [58,67].

25.5 Different Surgical Approaches in the Treatment of Secondary and Tertiary Hyperparathyroidism

The objective of the surgical management of secondary and tertiary HPTH is to eliminate the symptoms due to the overproduction of parathormone (PTH) while avoiding postoperative hypocalcemia due to the complete lack of parathyroid glands. It is thus cardinal that vital parathyroid tissue remains in the patient. There are two commonly used surgical strategies in the treatment of secondary and tertiary HPTH which will be described here:
1. Subtotal PTX
2. Total PTX and autotransplantation

Total PTX without autotransplantation results in a complete lack of PTH, requires a lifelong substitution therapy with calcium and vitamin D, and may have grave implications on the bone mineralization. Therefore, this technique has been abandoned by the vast majority of surgeons in the treatment of secondary and tertiary HPTH.

25.5.1   Technique of Subtotal Parathyroidectomy

Ideally, the operation should be planned 1 day after the patient has been on dialysis. The access to the parathyroid glands resembles that for thyroidectomy which has been described in detail in Chapter 7. Briefly, conventional PTX is performed through a standard collar incision. Strap muscles are separated in the midline. The anterior part of the thyroid gland is exposed by predominantly blunt dissection. To access the posterior part of the thyroid where the parathyroid glands are located, meticulous, "bloodless" dissection is necessary. After careful identification of the recurrent laryngeal nerve and the inferior thyroid artery, it is critically important to visualize all parathyroid glands. The parathyroid glands are commonly located near the junction of the recurrent laryngeal nerve and inferior thyroid artery [92,93]. The superior parathyroid glands are usually found after mobilizing the superior pole of the thyroid gland while the inferior parathyroid glands are in close proximity to the lower thyroid pole [93]. It is of the utmost importance to identify at least four parathyroid glands as well as all supernumerary glands [94,95]. If less than four parathyroid glands can be identified, it is critically important to search for ectopic upper parathyroid glands in the para- and retroesophageal area [96], in the area of the upper thyroid pole, as well as in the posterosuperior mediastinum [92,97]. If the lower parathyroid glands can not be visualized, one must actively look for them in the thyrothymic ligament and a cervical thymectomy should be performed [97]. Some recommend performing a cervical thymectomy for all patients with secondary and tertiary HPTH due to the high probability of supernumerary intrathymic parathyroid glands. Also, if a lower parathyroid gland can not be found, a partial or complete thyroid lobectomy should be performed due to the possible existence of an intrathyroid parathyroid gland. If less than four parathyroid glands can be identified despite thorough examination of the above-mentioned anatomical structures, all identified glands must be removed. We do not recommend a sternotomy during the first surgical intervention to search for parathyroid glands in the mediastinum.

After all parathyroid glands have been identified, the smallest is resected in that approximately 30–50 mg of tissue remain in situ [92]. To avoid post-operative hypocalcemia, it is critically important to preserve the blood supply for the parathyroid tissue remaining in situ. It is often challenging to gauge the amount of tissue remaining in situ. However, thorough preparation of the parathyroid gland prior to resection facilitates this step.

During the resection of the parathyroid glands parathyroid cells may be disseminated [98], a phenomenon called "seeding". Thus, careful handling is cardinal during removal of parathyroid tissue [98].

All removed parathyroid tissue should be verified by frozen section [97,99,100] or by ex vivo aspiration of the parathyroid glands and use of a rapid PTH assay. This enables identifying with certainty the number of removed parathyroid glands and decreases the risk of persistent HPTH.

It is of the utmost importance to have profound knowledge in the anatomy of the location of parathyroid glands [101]. A sound anatomical knowledge combined with vast experience in parathyroid surgery represent the most important factors to achieve excellent postoperative outcomes.

25.5.2   Technique of Total Parathyroidectomy and Autotransplantation

Total PTX is performed similarly to subtotal PTX as described above except that no parathyroid tissue is left in situ (Fig. 25.1). As for subtotal PTX, it is critically important to avoid peroperative "seeding."

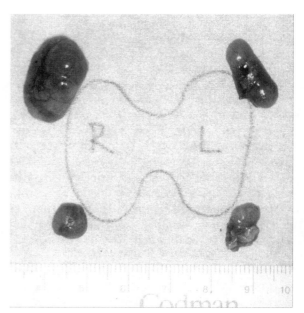

Fig. 25.1 Total parathyroidectomy: ex situ photograph of four hyperplastic parathyroid glands with sketch of their location

Over the past decades, several different techniques of total PTX plus autotransplantation have been described [102–104]. While the complete removal of all parathyroid glands is common to all techniques, the site of replantation varies. The most common site of replantation is in the forearm muscles, but autotransplantation of parathyroid tissue to the sternocleidomastoid muscle [103], subcutaneous abdominal adipose tissue [104], presternal subcutaneous tissue [102], and subcutaneous forearm tissue [105] have been described as well.

The technique of autotransplantation to the forearm was described for the first time by Wells and colleagues [99] and remains the gold standard in current practice. It has proven to work efficiently, is safe, and allows, in case of recurrent HPTH due to graft hyperplasia, removal of the grafted parathyroid tissue under local anesthesia. We thus exclusively describe the technique of autotransplantation to the forearm.

Immediately after removal of the parathyroid glands, one or two are placed in a sterile, physiological solution at 4°C [106]. Due to the low temperature, the parathyroid glands become firm, which facilitates the subsequent slicing and autotransplantation (Fig. 25.2) [106]. The parathyroid glands are sliced into small pieces of about 1×3 mm (Fig. 25.3) [106]. Approximately 50 mg parathyroid tissue should be autotransplanted [92,94,107].

Through a longitudinal incision in the volar surface of the non-dominant forearm, 20–25 slices of parathyroid gland are placed in muscle pouches of the brachioradialis or flexor muscle group (Fig. 25.4). It is cardinal to perform hemostasis as the formation of a postoperative hematoma may compromise the function of the autotransplanted parathyroid tissue [108].

For each piece of parathyroid tissue, a separate muscle pouch is created [92,94,95,99] which, after placing the slice, is closed with a non-resorbable thin suture [106]. Alternatively, metal clips can be used to mark the site of replantation. This is critically important [107] as it enables the identification of the implantation site if reoperation due to recurrent disease becomes necessary [106].

If less than four parathyroid glands are found during the neck exploration, no autotransplantation should be performed [92,109]. If, however, postoperative hypocalcemia persists, autotransplantation of cryopreserved parathyroid tissue should be considered (see below) [110].

25.5.3 Transcervical Thymectomy

It is well known that supernumerary parathyroid glands are commonly located adjacent to the thymus [95,96,111–115]. In an autopsy study by Akerstrom et al. [93] parathyroid glands were dissected in 503 cases. Supernumerary glands, most frequently located in the thymus, were found in 64 cases (13%). Some authors suggest to routinely perform a partial thymectomy (removal of the thymic tongue) [95,96,116]. In fact, Tominaga reported that almost 40% of the supernumerary glands in their series of 519 patients were located in the thymic tongue [95]. We and others concur and advocate to systematically performing a cervical thymectomy [92,93,112–114,117] or at least

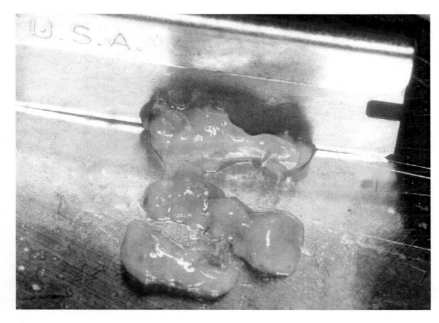

Fig. 25.2 Preparation of parathyroid autotransplantation: the gland with the least hyperplasia is sliced using a sterile blade

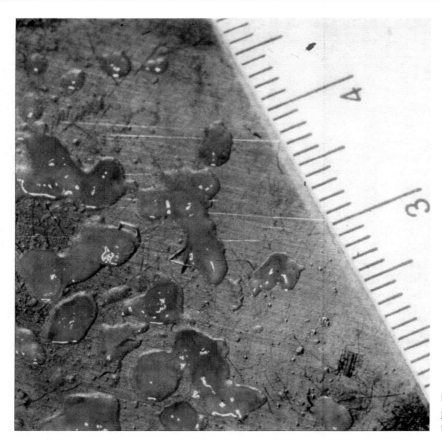

Fig. 25.3 Parathyroid autotransplantation: the gland is minced into tiny cubes

to remove the thymic tongue [108] which enables the removal of supernumerary glands, decreases the risk of recurrent HPTH, and lowers the rate of reoperations to the neck.

25.5.4 Intraoperative PTH Measurement

Intraoperative PTH measurement represents an established tool in determining the successful removal of parathyroid tissue in patients undergoing surgery for primary HPTH [118–123]. Recent reports have provided suggestive evidence that intraoperative PTH measurement may also be useful during surgery for secondary HPTH [124–126]. The premise is simple. The PTH levels are measured prior to removing the parathyroid glands. Due to chronic renal failure, PTH levels in patients with secondary HPTH are usually high. After removal of the four parathyroid glands, a relevant and rapid decline of PTH is expected [124–126]. A persisting high PTH level can result from non-identified supernumerary parathyroid glands and further identification and removal of additional parathyroid glands are indicated [125].

Although these preliminary reports are promising, the usefulness of routine intraoperative PTH measurement during surgery for secondary and tertiary HPTH must be investigated in larger studies prior to its routine implementation in current practice.

25.5.5 Postoperative Function of the Autografted Parathyroid Tissue

The function of grafted parathyroid tissue after total PTX has been measured and described in numerous studies [95,97,99,114]. In the vast majority of investigations the graft function was very satisfactory [95,97,99,114]. Also, the implantation of cryopreserved parathyroid tissue has proved successful [97].

It should be emphasized that several months are required until the autografted parathyroid tissue starts working properly. Indeed, Rothmund and colleagues reported that it takes, on average, 6 months postsurgery—for some patients longer—until replacement therapy can be discontinued [97]. Therefore, they advocated that persisting hypocalcemia 5–6 months

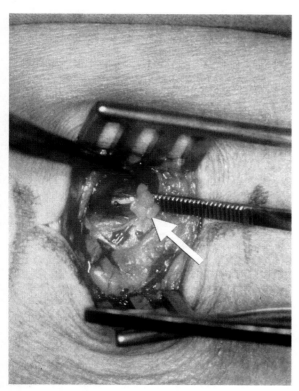

Fig. 25.4 Parathyroid autotransplantation: the minced pieces of one parathyroid gland (*arrow*) are implanted into a small pocket in the brachioradial muscle

after autotransplantation should per se not be considered an indication for regrafting [97].

25.5.6 Postoperative Management after Parathyroidectomy

The decrease of PTH concentration after successful PTX is usually accompanied by a rapid decline of calcium. In particular, patients with high-turnover bone disease carry the risk of severe postoperative hypocalcemia due to eminent uptake of calcium by the skeleton, known as "hungry bone syndrome." Rapid occurrence of severe hypocalcemia leads to tetany with positive Chvostek phenomenon (twitching of the corner of the mouth and the face after tapping of the branch of the facial nerve) and Trousseau sign (maximal flexion of hands). The ECG typically shows a prolongation of the Q–T interval. If a patient develops symptomatic hypocalcemia, calcium gluconate infusion should be administered [dosage: 90 mg (1–2 mg/kg body weight) of elemental calcium per hour] [21]. However, the primary goal is to prevent the occurrence of severe hypocalcemia after PTX.

Therefore, serum calcium levels should be measured closely, at least every 6–12 hours for the first 2 days after surgery. Oral supplementation of elemental calcium should be started early after surgery. In clinical practice, we recommend 1,000 mg twice daily. More than 3,000 mg of calcium in organic salts are not well tolerated by patients due to the common side effect of diarrhea. It is thus advisable to co-administer vitamin D sterols to stimulate active intestinal calcium absorption. A common starting dosage is 0.5 µg calcitriol per day. The appropriate dosage of both calcium and active vitamin must be adjusted according to the measured serum calcium levels.

25.5.7 Cryopreservation of Parathyroid Glands

Cryopreservation of parathyroid glands after total PTX and autotransplantation was introduced by Wells and colleagues almost 30 years ago [99]. The parathyroid tissue is placed in vials containing 10% dimethylsulfoxide, 10% human serum, and 80% tissue culture media. The vials are then frozen and stored in a nitrogen storage freezer at −200°C [106]. It is now ubiquitously accepted that cryopreserving resected parathyroid tissue should be routinely performed [92,101,104–108,127] as it enables further parathyroid grafting if postoperative hypoparathyroidism with consecutive hypocalcemia occurs. As previously mentioned, no autotransplantation should be performed if less than four parathyroid glands were found and removed because it can be assumed that unidentified parathyroid tissue remained in situ. However, it has been emphasized that cryopreservation of parathyroid tissue is particularly important in this scenario as it is possible that all parathyroid glands were removed. Replantation of cryopreserved parathyroid tissue facilitates treatment of permanent hypocalcemia and may prevent lifelong vitamin D and calcium substitution [110].

25.5.8 Advantages and Drawbacks of Subtotal Parathyroidectomy versus Total Parathyroidectomy and Autotransplantation

The respective advantages and drawbacks of subtotal PTX versus total PTX plus autotransplantation are listed in Table 25.5. The most important strength of performing the latter is that, in case of a recurrence, the autotransplanted parathyroid tissue can be removed

Table 25.5 Advantages and drawbacks of subtotal parathyroidectomy versus total parathyroidectomy and autotransplantation

	Advantages	Disadvantages
Total parathyroidectomy plus autotransplantation	Reoperation in case of graft hyperplasia possible under local anesthesia [100,117,129–132] Low risk of seeding [129] Easy functional testing of the grafted parathyroid tissue in vivo [95,129]	Period of postoperative hypocalcemia [95] Graft hyperplasia and infiltration of adjacent structures [137–139]
Subtotal parathyroidectomy	Short or absent postoperative hypocalcemia	Reoperation to the neck may be difficult and associated with increased morbidity [100,117,133] Higher risk of seeding [129]

under local anesthesia and with low associated morbidity [100,117,128–131]. Conversely, a recurrent HPTH after subtotal PTX requires a second exploration of the neck, may be difficult due to fibrosed and scarred tissue, and is associated with an increased incidence of postoperative complications [132].

The critical analysis of the literature reveals that compelling data supporting one or the other approach are scarce. Most investigations comparing the two procedures are non-randomized case series [112,113,117,130,133] and have the associated limitations and drawbacks of these study types. There is only one randomized clinical trial comparing the two procedures [100,101]. Forty patients with secondary HPTH were randomized to subtotal PTX versus total PTX plus autotransplantation to the forearm muscles. The latter operation was associated with more frequent normalization of serum-calcium product, higher regression of radiological alterations, and significantly better improvement of clinical symptoms such as pruritus and muscular weakness compared with subtotal PTX. Moreover, while 2 patients after subtotal PTX required re-exploration of the neck due to recurrences, no reoperations were necessary in the group of total PTX plus autotransplantation. Based on these results and the fact that reoperation of the autograft is less challenging compared with reoperation to the neck, the authors recommended total PTX plus autotransplantation as the procedure of choice in the treatment of secondary HPTH [100,101]. We as well as others concur that total PTX plus autotransplantation is advantageous compared with subtotal PTX [95,108,128,129].

25.6 Problem of Supernumerary Glands and Graft Hyperplasia

The variability of the number of parathyroid glands is well known [93,95–97,113]. In a report on 519 patients undergoing total PTX plus forearm autotransplantation, supernumerary glands were found in 75 patients (14.5%) [95]. The most frequent location of supernumerary glands (39%) was the thymic tongue.

It is of the utmost importance to remove at least four parathyroid glands during total PTX and to leave no more than 30–40 mg of a well-vascularized parathyroid gland in situ during subtotal PTX. Also, all supernumerary glands must be identified and removed. If parathyroid glands remain undetected, persistent or recurrent disease will occur and require reoperation. Indeed, missing or supernumerary glands represent a frequent cause of persistent HPTH after parathyroid surgery [101,109,112,117,134,135].

Several reports have described the phenomenon of graft hyperplasia [136–138]. Frei et al. [137] reported on 41 patients with secondary HPTH in whom total PTX and autotransplantation to the forearm muscles were performed. Five patients developed recurrent HPTH due to graft hyperplasia requiring reoperation. The weight of the removed grafts was between 0.9 and 3.1 g, a multiple of the initially implanted parathyroid tissue. Some grafts showed signs of infiltration of adjacent structures and even invasion of blood vessels, and required extensive and repeated surgery for complete removal. Based on these findings the authors recommended abandoning total PTX and autotransplantation as the treatment of choice of secondary HPTH [137]. There are several other reports that advocate against the autotransplantation of parathyroid tissue [136,138] particularly if atypical cellular features or frequent mitoses are found in the intraoperative frozen sections, a factor that may lead to graft hyperplasia and reoperation [139].

It has been emphasized that graft hyperplasia is relevantly higher when a *nodular* gland is implanted compared with a *diffusely hyperplastic* gland [95,133]. Therefore, Tominaga et al. emphasized avoiding autografting nodular hyperplastic parathyroid tissue [95]. Neyer and colleagues [128] pointed out, however, that discriminating between nodular versus diffuse hyperplasia is insufficient. They proposed to use a stereomagnifier to select parathyroid tissue with low proliferative potential for autotransplantation. Interestingly, of 37 patients who underwent total PTX plus concomitant autotransplantation only one recurred, a rate which compares very favorably to others [103,109,136,140,141].

Although we recognize the fact that tumor-like infiltration of the autograft in adjacent structures does occur, it represents a rare phenomenon and should not be considered as a reason against performing total PTX plus autotransplantation.

25.7   Summary

The surgical indications for patients with secondary or tertiary HPTH are not clearly defined. In general patients who develop PTH autonomy and do not respond to medical management will require PTX. It is also critical to screen all patients who are potential renal transplant recipients for secondary HPTH and to treat severe HPTH prior to transplantation. Both subtotal PTX and total cervical PTX with immediate heterotopic parathyroid transplantation are accepted surgical techniques. Cryopreservation is extremely useful and should always be employed during surgery. The intraoperative PTH assay appears to be a useful adjunct in early studies.

References

1. Moe SM, Drueke TB (2003) Management of secondary hyperparathyroidism: the importance and the challenge of controlling parathyroid hormone levels without elevating calcium, phosphorus, and calcium-phosphorus product. Am J Nephrol 23:369–379

2. Arnold A, Brown MF, Urena P, Gaz RD, Sarfati E, Drueke TB (1995) Monoclonality of parathyroid tumors in chronic renal failure and in primary parathyroid hyperplasia. J Clin Invest 95:2047–2053

3. Block GA (2000) Prevalence and clinical consequences of elevated Ca x P product in hemodialysis patients. Clin Nephrol 54:318–324

4. Malluche HH, Mawad H, Monier-Faugere MC (2004) The importance of bone health in end-stage renal disease: out of the frying pan, into the fire? Nephrol Dial Transplant 19(suppl 1):i9–13

5. Hruska K (2000) Pathophysiology of renal osteodystrophy. Pediatr Nephrol 14:636–640

6. Qi Q, Monier-Faugere MC, Geng Z, Malluche HH (1995) Predictive value of serum parathyroid hormone levels for bone turnover in patients on chronic maintenance dialysis. Am J Kidney Dis 26:622–631

7. Wang M, Hercz G, Sherrard DJ, Maloney NA, Segre GV, Pei Y (1995) Relationship between intact 1-84 parathyroid hormone and bone histomorphometric parameters in dialysis patients without aluminum toxicity. Am J Kidney Dis 26:836–844

8. Brancaccio D, Cozzolino M, Gallieni M (2004) Hyperparathyroidism and anemia in uremic subjects: a combined therapeutic approach. J Am Soc Nephrol 15(suppl 1):S21–S24

9. Chou FF, Ho JC, Huang SC, Sheen-Chen SM (2000) A study on pruritus after parathyroidectomy for secondary hyperparathyroidism. J Am Coll Surg 190:65–70

10. Ganesh SK, Stack AG, Levin NW, Hulbert-Shearon T, Port FK (2001) Association of elevated serum PO(4), Ca x PO(4) product, and parathyroid hormone with cardiac mortality risk in chronic hemodialysis patients. J Am Soc Nephrol 12:2131–2138

11. Marco MP, Craver L, Betriu A, Belart M, Fibla J, Fernandez E (2003) Higher impact of mineral metabolism on cardiovascular mortality in a European hemodialysis population. Kidney Int Suppl 2003:S111–S114

12. Rostand SG, Drueke TB (1999) Parathyroid hormone, vitamin D, and cardiovascular disease in chronic renal failure. Kidney Int 56:383–392

13. Tzanno-Martins C, Futata E, Jorgetti V, Duarte AJ (2000) Restoration of impaired T-cell proliferation after parathyroidectomy in hemodialysis patients. Nephron 84:224–227

14. Yasunaga C, Nakamoto M, Matsuo K, Nishihara G, Yoshida T, Goya T (1999) Effects of a parathyroidectomy on the immune system and nutritional condition in chronic dialysis patients with secondary hyperparathyroidism. Am J Surg 178:332–336

15. National Kidney Foundation (2002) K/DOQI clinical practice guidelines for chronic kidney disease: evaluation, classification, and stratification. Am J Kidney Dis 39: S1–S266

16. Rix M, Andreassen H, Eskildsen P, Langdahl B, Olgaard K (1999) Bone mineral density and biochemical markers of bone turnover in patients with predialysis chronic renal failure. Kidney Int 56:1084–1093

17. Coen G, Ballanti P, Bonucci E, Calabria S, Costantini S, Ferrannini M, Giustini M, Giordano R, Nicolai G, Manni M, Sardella D, Taggi F (2002) Renal osteodystrophy in predialysis and hemodialysis patients: comparison of histologic patterns and diagnostic predictivity of intact PTH. Nephron 91:103–111

18. Gal-Moscovici A, Popovtzer MM (2002) Parathyroid hormone-independent osteoclastic resorptive bone disease: a new variant of adynamic bone disease in haemodialysis patients. Nephrol Dial Transplant 17:620–624

19. Coco M, Rush H (2000) Increased incidence of hip fractures in dialysis patients with low serum parathyroid hormone. Am J Kidney Dis 36:1115–1121

20. Atsumi K, Kushida K, Yamazaki K, Shimizu S, Ohmura A, Inoue T (1999) Risk factors for vertebral fractures in renal osteodystrophy. Am J Kidney Dis 33:287–293

21. National Kidney Foundation (2003) K/DOQI clinical practice guidelines for bone metabolism and disease in chronic kidney disease. Am J Kidney Dis 42:S1–S201

22. US Renal Data System (2003) USRDS 2003 Annual Report, Bethesda, MD, National Institutes of Health, National Institute of Diabetes and Digestive and Kidney Diseases

23. Levin A, Foley RN (2000) Cardiovascular disease in chronic renal insufficiency. Am J Kidney Dis 36:S24–S30

24. Block GA, Klassen PS, Lazarus JM, Ofsthun N, Lowrie EG, Chertow GM (2004) Mineral metabolism, mortality, and morbidity in maintenance hemodialysis. J Am Soc Nephrol 15:2208–2218

25. Guerin AP, London GM, Marchais SJ, Metivier F (2000) Arterial stiffening and vascular calcifications in end-stage renal disease. Nephrol Dial Transplant 15:1014–1021

26. Raggi P, Boulay A, Chasan-Taber S, Amin N, Dillon M, Burke SK, Chertow GM (2002) Cardiac calcification in adult hemodialysis patients. A link between end-stage renal disease and cardiovascular disease? J Am Coll Cardiol 39:695–701

27. Salgueira M, del Toro N, Moreno-Alba R, Jimenez E, Areste N, Palma A (2003) Vascular calcification in the uremic patient: a cardiovascular risk? Kidney Int Suppl 2003: S119–S121

28. Aparicio M, Combe C, Lafage MH, de P, V, Potaux L, Bouchet JL (1993) In advanced renal failure, dietary phosphorus restriction reverses hyperparathyroidism independent of changes in the levels of calcitriol. Nephron 63:122–123

29. Martinez I, Saracho R, Montenegro J, Llach F (1997) The importance of dietary calcium and phosphorous in the secondary hyperparathyroidism of patients with early renal failure. Am J Kidney Dis 29:496–502

30. Slatopolsky E, Caglar S, Pennell JP, Taggart DD, Canterbury JM, Reiss E, Bricker NS (1971) On the pathogenesis of hyperparathyroidism in chronic experimental renal insufficiency in the dog. J Clin Invest 50:492–499

31. Nestel AW, Meyers AM, Paiker J, Rollin HB (1994) Effect of calcium supplement preparation containing small amounts of citrate on the absorption of aluminium in normal subjects and in renal failure patients. Nephron 68:197–201

32. Emmett M, Sirmon MD, Kirkpatrick WG, Nolan CR, Schmitt GW, Cleveland MB (1991) Calcium acetate control of serum phosphorus in hemodialysis patients. Am J Kidney Dis 17:544–550

33. Slatopolsky E, Weerts C, Lopez-Hilker S, Norwood K, Zink M, Windus D, Delmez J (1986) Calcium carbonate as a phosphate binder in patients with chronic renal failure undergoing dialysis. N Engl J Med 315:157–161

34. Drueke TB (2000) Renal osteodystrophy: management of hyperphosphataemia. Nephrol Dial Transplant 15(suppl 5):32–33

35. Goodman WG, Goldin J, Kuizon BD, Yoon C, Gales B, Sider D, Wang Y, Chung J, Emerick A, Greaser L, Elashoff RM, Salusky IB (2000) Coronary-artery calcification in young adults with end-stage renal disease who are undergoing dialysis. N Engl J Med 342:1478–1483

36. Guerin AP, London GM, Marchais SJ, Metivier F (2000) Arterial stiffening and vascular calcifications in end-stage renal disease. Nephrol Dial Transplant 15:1014–1021

37. Bleyer AJ, Burke SK, Dillon M, Garrett B, Kant KS, Lynch D, Rahman SN, Schoenfeld P, Teitelbaum I, Zeig S, Slatopolsky E (1999) A comparison of the calcium-free phosphate binder sevelamer hydrochloride with calcium acetate in the treatment of hyperphosphatemia in hemodialysis patients. Am J Kidney Dis 33:694–701

38. Slatopolsky EA, Burke SK, Dillon MA (1999) RenaGel, a nonabsorbed calcium- and aluminum-free phosphate binder, lowers serum phosphorus and parathyroid hormone. The RenaGel Study Group. Kidney Int 55:299–307

39. Chertow GM, Burke SK, Raggi P (2002) Sevelamer attenuates the progression of coronary and aortic calcification in hemodialysis patients. Kidney Int 62:245–252

40. Qunibi WY, Hootkins RE, McDowell LL, Meyer MS, Simon M, Garza RO, Pelham RW, Cleveland MV, Muenz LR, He DY, Nolan CR (2004) Treatment of hyperphosphatemia in hemodialysis patients: The Calcium Acetate Renagel Evaluation (CARE Study). Kidney Int 65:1914–1926

41. Hergesell O, Ritz E (2002) Phosphate binders in uraemia: pharmacodynamics, pharmacoeconomics, pharmacoethics. Nephrol Dial Transplant 17:14–17

42. D'Haese PC, Spasovski GB, Sikole A, Hutchison A, Freemont TJ, Sulkova S, Swanepoel C, Pejanovic S, Djukanovic L, Balducci A, Coen G, Sulowicz W, Ferreira A, Torres A, Curic S, Popovic M, Dimkovic N, De Broe ME (2003) A multicenter study on the effects of lanthanum carbonate (Fosrenol) and calcium carbonate on renal bone disease in dialysis patients. Kidney Int Suppl S73–S78

43. Finn WF, Joy MS, Hladik G (2004) Efficacy and safety of lanthanum carbonate for reduction of serum phosphorus in patients with chronic renal failure receiving hemodialysis. Clin Nephrol 62:193–201

44. Slatopolsky E, Finch J, Brown A (2003) New vitamin D analogs. Kidney Int Suppl 2003:S83–S87

45. Malluche HH, Mawad H, Koszewski NJ (2002) Update on vitamin D and its newer analogues: actions and rationale for treatment in chronic renal failure. Kidney Int 62:367–374

46. Sprague SM, Llach F, Amdahl M, Taccetta C, Batlle D (2003) Paricalcitol versus calcitriol in the treatment of secondary hyperparathyroidism. Kidney Int 63:1483–1490

47. Brown EM, Gamba G, Riccardi D, Lombardi M, Butters R, Kifor O, Sun A, Hediger MA, Lytton J, Hebert SC (1993) Cloning and characterization of an extracellular Ca(2+)-sensing receptor from bovine parathyroid. Nature 366:575–580

48. Nemeth EF, Steffey ME, Hammerland LG, Hung BC, Van Wagenen BC, DelMar EG, Balandrin MF (1998) Calcimimetics with potent and selective activity on the parathyroid calcium receptor. Proc Natl Acad Sci U S A 95:4040–4045

49. Goodman WG, Hladik GA, Turner SA, Blaisdell PW, Goodkin DA, Liu W, Barri YM, Cohen RM, Coburn JW (2002) The calcimimetic agent AMG 073 lowers plasma parathyroid hormone levels in hemodialysis patients with secondary hyperparathyroidism. J Am Soc Nephrol 13:1017–1024

50. Block GA, Martin KJ, de Francisco AL, Turner SA, Avram MM, Suranyi MG, Hercz G, Cunningham J, Abu-Alfa AK, Messa P, Coyne DW, Locatelli F, Cohen RM, Evenepoel P, Moe SM, Fournier A, Braun J, McCary LC, Zani VJ, Olson KA, Drueke TB, Goodman WG (2004) Cinacalcet for secondary hyperparathyroidism in patients receiving hemodialysis. N Engl J Med 350:1516–1525

51. Cohen EP, Moulder JE (2001) Parathyroidectomy in chronic renal failure: has medical care reduced the need for surgery? Nephron 89:271–273

52. Jorge Cannata-Andia JP-DER (2000) Management of the renal patient: experts' recommendations and clinical algorithms on renal osteodystrophy and cardiovascular risk factors. Nephrol Dial Transplant 15:S1–S154

53. Saha HH, Salmela KT, Ahonen PJ, Pietila KO, Morsky PJ, Mustonen JT, Lalla ML, Pasternack AI (1994) Sequential changes in vitamin D and calcium metabolism after successful renal transplantation. Scand J Urol Nephrol 28:21–27

54. Messa P, Sindici C, Cannella G, Miotti V, Risaliti A, Gropuzzo M, Di Loreto PL, Bresadola F, Mioni G (1998) Persistent secondary hyperparathyroidism after renal transplantation. Kidney Int 54:1704–1713

55. Heaf J, Tvedegaard E, Kanstrup IL, Fogh-Andersen N (2000) Bone loss after renal transplantation: role of hyperparathyroidism, acidosis, cyclosporine and systemic disease. Clin Transplant 14:457–463

56. Julian BA, Quarles LD, Niemann KM (1992) Musculoskeletal complications after renal transplantation: pathogenesis and treatment. Am J Kidney Dis 19:99–120

57. Torres A, Rodriguez AP, Concepcion MT, Garcia S, Rufino M, Martin B, Perez L, Machado M, de Bonis E, Losada M, Hernandez D, Lorenzo V (1998) Parathyroid function in long-term renal transplant patients: importance of pretransplant PTH concentrations. Nephrol Dial Transplant 13(suppl 3):94–97

58. Caravaca F, Fernandez MA, Ruiz-Calero R, Cubero J, Aparicio A, Jimenez F, Garcia MC (1998) Effects of oral phosphorus supplementation on mineral metabolism of renal transplant recipients. Nephrol Dial Transplant 13:2605–2611

59. Koch Nogueira PC, David L, Cochat P (2000) Evolution of secondary hyperparathyroidism after renal transplantation. Pediatr Nephrol 14:342–346

60. Parfitt AM (1997) The hyperparathyroidism of chronic renal failure: a disorder of growth. Kidney Int 52:3–9

61. Bonarek H, Merville P, Bonarek M, Moreau K, Morel D, Aparicio M, Potaux L (1999) Reduced parathyroid functional mass after successful kidney transplantation. Kidney Int 56:642–649

62. Fernandez E, Fibla J, Betriu A, Piulats JM, Almirall J, Montoliu J (1997) Association between vitamin D receptor gene polymorphism and relative hypoparathyroidism in patients with chronic renal failure. J Am Soc Nephrol 8:1546–1552

63. Torres A, Machado M, Concepcion MT, Martin N, Lorenzo V, Hernandez D, Rodriguez AP, Rodriguez A, de Bonis E, Gonzalez-Posada JM, Hernandez A, Salido E (1996) Influence of vitamin D receptor genotype on bone mass changes after renal transplantation. Kidney Int 50:1726–1733

64. Lotscher M, Scarpetta Y, Levi M, Halaihel N, Wang H, Zajicek HK, Biber J, Murer H, Kaissling B (1999) Rapid downregulation of rat renal Na/P(i) cotransporter in response to parathyroid hormone involves microtubule rearrangement. J Clin Invest 104:483–494

65. Pabico RC, McKenna BA (1988) Metabolic problems in renal transplant patients. Persistent hyperparathyroidism and hypophosphatemia: effects of intravenous calcium infusion. Transplant Proc 20:438–442

66. Steiner RW, Ziegler M, Halasz NA, Catherwood BD, Manolagas S, Deftos LJ (1993) Effect of daily oral vitamin D and calcium therapy, hypophosphatemia, and endogenous 1-25 dihydroxycholecalciferol on parathyroid hormone and phosphate wasting in renal transplant recipients. Transplantation 56:843–846

67. Ambuhl PM, Meier D, Wolf B, Dydak U, Boesiger P, Binswanger U (1999) Metabolic aspects of phosphate replacement therapy for hypophosphatemia after renal transplantation: impact on muscular phosphate content, mineral metabolism, and acid/base homeostasis. Am J Kidney Dis 34:875–883

68. Ravid M, Robson M (1976) Proximal myopathy caused by iatrogenic phosphate depletion. JAMA 236:1380–1381

69. Knochel JP (1992) Hypophosphatemia and rhabdomyolysis. Am J Med 92:455–457

70. O'Connor LR, Wheeler WS, Bethune JE (1977) Effect of hypophosphatemia on myocardial performance in man. N Engl J Med 297:901–903

71. Newman JH, Neff TA, Ziporin P (1977) Acute respiratory failure associated with hypophosphatemia. N Engl J Med 296:1101–1103

72. Planas RF, McBrayer RH, Koen PA (1982) Effects of hypophosphatemia on pulmonary muscle performance. Adv Exp Med Biol 151:283–290

73. Klock JC, Williams HE, Mentzer WC (1974) Hemolytic anemia and somatic cell dysfunction in severe hypophosphatemia. Arch Intern Med 134:360–364

74. Craddock PR, Yawata Y, VanSanten L, Gilberstadt S, Silvis S, Jacob HS (1974) Acquired phagocyte dysfunction. A complication of the hypophosphatemia of parenteral hyperalimentation. N Engl J Med 290:1403–1407

75. Subramanian R, Khardori R (2000) Severe hypophosphatemia. Pathophysiologic implications, clinical presentations, and treatment. Medicine (Baltimore) 79:1–8

76. Bellorin-Font E, Rojas E, Carlini RG, Suniaga O, Weisinger JR (2003) Bone remodeling after renal transplantation. Kidney Int Suppl 2003:S125–S128

77. Almond MK, Kwan JT, Evans K, Cunningham J (1994) Loss of regional bone mineral density in the first 12 months following renal transplantation. Nephron 66:52–57

78. Horber FF, Casez JP, Steiger U, Czerniak A, Montandon A, Jaeger P (1994) Changes in bone mass early after kidney transplantation. J Bone Miner Res 9:1–9

79. Julian BA, Laskow DA, Dubovsky J, Dubovsky EV, Curtis JJ, Quarles LD (1991) Rapid loss of vertebral mineral density after renal transplantation. N Engl J Med 325:544–550

80. Pichette V, Bonnardeaux A, Prudhomme L, Gagne M, Cardinal J, Ouimet D (1996) Long-term bone loss in kidney transplant recipients: a cross-sectional and longitudinal study. Am J Kidney Dis 28:105–114

81. Grotz WH, Mundinger FA, Gugel B, Exner V, Kirste G, Schollmeyer PJ (1994) Bone fracture and osteodensitometry with dual energy X-ray absorptiometry in kidney transplant recipients. Transplantation 58:912–915

82. Nisbeth U, Lindh E, Ljunghall S, Backman U, Fellstrom B (1999) Increased fracture rate in diabetes mellitus and females after renal transplantation. Transplantation 67:1218–1222

83. Ramsey-Goldman R, Dunn JE, Dunlop DD, Stuart FP, Abecassis MM, Kaufman DB, Langman CB, Salinger MH, Sprague SM (1999) Increased risk of fracture in patients receiving solid organ transplants. J Bone Miner Res 14:456–463

84. Cruz EA, Lugon JR, Jorgetti V, Draibe SA, Carvalho AB (2004) Histologic evolution of bone disease 6 months after successful kidney transplantation. Am J Kidney Dis 44:747–756

85. Felsenfeld AJ, Gutman RA, Drezner M, Llach F (1986) Hypophosphatemia in long-term renal transplant recipients: effects on bone histology and 1,25-dihydroxycholecalciferol. Miner Electrolyte Metab 12:333–341

86. Monier-Faugere MC, Mawad H, Qi Q, Friedler RM, Malluche HH (2000) High prevalence of low bone turnover and occurrence of osteomalacia after kidney transplantation. J Am Soc Nephrol 11:1093–1099

87. Rojas E, Carlini RG, Clesca P, Arminio A, Suniaga O, De Elguezabal K, Weisinger JR, Hruska KA, Bellorin-Font E (2003) The pathogenesis of osteodystrophy after renal transplantation as detected by early alterations in bone remodeling. Kidney Int 63:1915–1923

88. Reinhardt W, Bartelworth H, Jockenhovel F, Schmidt-Gayk H, Witzke O, Wagner K, Heemann UW, Reinwein D, Philipp T, Mann K (1998) Sequential changes of biochemical bone parameters after kidney transplantation. Nephrol Dial Transplant 13:436–442

89. Torres A, Lorenzo V, Salido E (2002) Calcium metabolism and skeletal problems after transplantation. J Am Soc Nephrol 13:551–558

90. Peppers MP, Geheb M, Desai T (1991) Endocrine crises. Hypophosphatemia and hyperphosphatemia. Crit Care Clin 7:201–214

91. Lentz RD, Brown DM, Kjellstrand CM (1978) Treatment of severe hypophosphatemia. Ann Intern Med 89:941–944

92. Niederle B (2000) Sekundärer Hyperparathyreoidismus: Operative Therapie. In: Siewert JR, Harder F, Rothmund M (eds) Praxis der Viszeralchirurgie. Endokrine Chirurgie. Springer, Berlin, Heidelberg, New York, pp 309–315

93. Akerstrom G, Malmaeus J, Bergstrom R (1984) Surgical anatomy of human parathyroid glands. Surgery 95:14–21

94. Sitges-Serra A, Caralps-Riera A (1987) Hyperparathyroidism associated with renal disease. Pathogenesis, natural history, and surgical treatment. Surg Clin North Am 67:359–377

95. Tominaga Y, Numano M, Tanaka Y, et al (1997) Surgical treatment of renal hyperparathyroidism. Semin Surg Oncol 13:87–96

96. Numano M, Tominaga Y, Uchida K, et al (1998) Surgical significance of supernumerary parathyroid glands in renal hyperparathyroidism. World J Surg 22:1098–1102; discussion 1103

97. Rothmund M, Wagner PK (1983) Total parathyroidectomy and autotransplantation of parathyroid tissue for renal hyperparathyroidism. A one- to six-year follow-up. Ann Surg 197:7–16

98. Akerstrom G, Rudberg C, Grimelius L, Rastad J (1988) Recurrent hyperparathyroidism due to peroperative seeding of neoplastic or hyperplastic parathyroid tissue. Case report. Acta Chir Scand 154:549–552

99. Wells SA Jr, Gunnells JC, Shelburne JD, et al (1975) Transplantation of the parathyroid glands in man: clinical indications and results. Surgery 78:34–44

100. Rothmund M, Wagner PK, Schark C (1991) Subtotal parathyroidectomy versus total parathyroidectomy and autotransplantation in secondary hyperparathyroidism: a randomized trial. World J Surg 15:745–750

101. Wagner PK, Eckhardt J, Rothmund M (1991) [Subtotal parathyroidectomy versus total parathyroidectomy with autotransplantation in secondary hyperparathyroidism. A randomized study]. Chirurg 62:189–194

102. Kinnaert P, Salmon I, Decoster-Gervy C, et al (1993) Total parathyroidectomy and presternal subcutaneous implantation of parathyroid tissue for renal hyperparathyroidism. Surg Gynecol Obstet 176:135–138

103. Skinner KA, Zuckerbraun L (1996) Recurrent secondary hyperparathyroidism. An argument for total parathyroidectomy. Arch Surg 131:724–727

104. Jansson S, Tisell LE (1987) Autotransplantation of diseased parathyroid glands into subcutaneous abdominal adipose tissue. Surgery 101:549–556

105. Chou FF, Chan HM, Huang TJ, et al (1998) Autotransplantation of parathyroid glands into subcutaneous forearm tissue for renal hyperparathyroidism. Surgery 124:1–5

106. Wells SA Jr, Ross AJ 3rd, Dale JK, Gray RS (1979) Transplantation of the parathyroid glands: current status. Surg Clin North Am 59:167–177

107. D'Avanzo A, Parangi S, Morita E, et al (2000) Hyperparathyroidism after thyroid surgery and autotransplantation of histologically normal parathyroid glands. J Am Coll Surg 190:546–552

108. Rothmund M (1986) Surgical treatment of secondary hyperparathyroidism: indication, operative management and results. Karger, Basel

109. Edis AJ, Levitt MD (1987) Supernumerary parathyroid glands: implications for the surgical treatment of secondary hyperparathyroidism. World J Surg 11:398–401

110. Donckier V, Decoster-Gervy C, Kinnaert P (1997) Long-term results after surgical treatment of renal hyperparathyroidism when fewer than four glands are identified at operation. J Am Coll Surg 184:70–74

111. Freeman JB, Sherman BM, Mason EE (1976) Transcervical thymectomy: an integral part of neck exploration for hyperparathyroidism. Arch Surg 111:359–364

112. Dotzenrath C, Cupisti K, Goretzki E, et al (2003) Operative treatment of renal autonomous hyperparathyroidism: cause of persistent or recurrent disease in 304 patients. Langenbecks Arch Surg 387:348–354

113. Proye C, Carnaille B, Sautier M (1990) [Hyperparathyroidism in patients with chronic renal failure: subtotal parathyroidectomy or total parathyroidectomy with autotransplantation? Experience with 121 cases]. J Chir (Paris) 127:136–140

114. Malmaeus J, Akerstrom G, Johansson H, et al (1982) Parathyroid surgery in chronic renal insufficiency. Subtotal parathyroidectomy versus total parathyroidectomy with autotransplantation to the forearm. Acta Chir Scand 148:229–238

115. Ahlers J, Rothmund M (1980) [Cervical thymectomy as an expanded surgical method in primary and secondary hyperparathyroidism]. Chirurg 51:629–633

116. Hibi Y, Tominaga Y, Sato T, et al (2002) Reoperation for renal hyperparathyroidism. World J Surg 26:1301–1307

117. Dotzenrath C, Goretzki PE, Roher HD (1996) [Results of surgical therapy in renal hyperparathyroidism. Follow-up of 143 patients]. Langenbecks Arch Chir 381:46–50

118. Maier GW, Kreis ME, Renn W, et al (1998) Parathyroid hormone after adenectomy for primary hyperparathyroidism. A study of peptide hormone elimination kinetics in humans. J Clin Endocrinol Metab 83:3852–3856

119. Mandell DL, Genden EM, Mechanick JI, et al (2001) The influence of intraoperative parathyroid hormone monitoring on the surgical management of hyperparathyroidism. Arch Otolaryngol Head Neck Surg 127:821–827

120. Maweja S, Sebag F, Hubbard J, et al (2004) Immediate and medium-term results of intraoperative parathyroid hormone monitoring during video-assisted parathyroidectomy. Arch Surg 139:1301–1303

121. Chapuis Y, Fulla Y, Bonnichon P, et al (1996) Values of ultrasonography, sestamibi scintigraphy, and intraoperative measurement of 1-84 PTH for unilateral neck exploration of primary hyperparathyroidism. World J Surg 20:835–839; discussion 839–840

122. Westerdahl J, Lindblom P, Bergenfelz A (2002) Measurement of intraoperative parathyroid hormone predicts long-term operative success. Arch Surg 137:186–190

123. Beck TM, Huber PR, Oertli D (2003) Intraoperative parathormone measurement in patients with primary hyperparathyroidism: a prospective clinical study. Swiss Med Wkly 133:206–209

124. Clary BM, Garner SC, Leight GS Jr (1997) Intraoperative parathyroid hormone monitoring during parathyroidectomy for secondary hyperparathyroidism. Surgery 122:1034–1038; discussion 1038–1039

125. Chou FF, Lee CH, Chen JB, et al (2002) Intraoperative parathyroid hormone measurement in patients with secondary hyperparathyroidism. Arch Surg 137:341–344

126. Seehofer D, Rayes N, Ulrich F, et al (2001) Intraoperative measurement of intact parathyroid hormone in renal hyperparathyroidism by an inexpensive routine assay. Langenbecks Arch Surg 386:440–443

127. Niederle B, Roka R, Brennan MF (1982) The transplantation of parathyroid tissue in man: development, indications, technique, and results. Endocr Rev 3:245–279

128. Neyer U, Hoerandner H, Haid A, et al (2002) Total parathyroidectomy with autotransplantation in renal hyperparathyroidism: low recurrence after intra-operative tissue selection. Nephrol Dial Transplant 17:625–629

129. Brunt LM, Wells SA Jr (1983) Surgical treatment of secondary hyperparathyroidism. Ann Chir Gynaecol 72:139–145

130. Welsh CL, Taylor GW, Cattell WR, Baker LR (1984) Parathyroid surgery in chronic renal failure: subtotal parathyroidectomy or autotransplantation? Br J Surg 71:591–592

131. Takagi H, Tominaga Y, Uchida K, et al (1984) Subtotal versus total parathyroidectomy with forearm autograft for secondary hyperparathyroidism in chronic renal failure. Ann Surg 200:18–23

132. Patow CA, Norton JA, Brennan MF (1986) Vocal cord paralysis and reoperative parathyroidectomy. A prospective study. Ann Surg 203:282–285

133. Gagne ER, Urena P, Leite-Silva S, et al (1992) Short- and long-term efficacy of total parathyroidectomy with immediate autografting compared with subtotal parathyroidectomy in hemodialysis patients. J Am Soc Nephrol 3:1008–1017

134. Alexander PT, Schuman ES, Vetto RM, et al (1988) Repeat parathyroid operation associated with renal disease. Am J Surg 155:686–689

135. Kaye M, D'Amour P, Henderson J (1989) Elective total parathyroidectomy without autotransplant in end-stage renal disease. Kidney Int 35:1390–1399

136. Hampl H, Steinmuller T, Stabell U, et al (1991) Recurrent hyperparathyroidism after total parathyroidectomy and autotransplantation in patients with long-term hemodialysis. Miner Electrolyte Metab 17:256–260

137. Frei U, Klempa I, Schneider M, et al (1981) Tumour-like growth of parathyroid autografts in uraemic patients. Proc Eur Dial Transplant Assoc 18:548–555

138. Korzets Z, Magen H, Kraus L, Bernheim J (1987) Total parathyroidectomy with autotransplantation in haemodialysed patients with secondary hyperparathyroidism: should it be abandoned? Nephrol Dial Transplant 2:341–346

139. Ellis HA (1988) Fate of long-term parathyroid autografts in patients with chronic renal failure treated by parathyroidectomy: a histopathological study of autografts, parathyroid glands and bone. Histopathology 13:289–309

140. Max MH, Flint LM, Richardson JD, et al (1981) Total parathyroidectomy and parathyroid autotransplantation in patients with chronic renal failure. Surg Gynecol Obstet 153:177–180

141. Mozes MF, Soper WD, Jonasson O, Lang GR (1980) Total parathyroidectomy and autotransplantation in secondary hyperparathyroidism. Arch Surg 115:378–385

26 Parathyroid Carcinoma

Janice L. Pasieka and Moosa Khalil

26.1   Introduction

Parathyroid carcinoma is a rare malignant neoplasm derived from the parenchymal cells of the parathyroid gland. The first description of this malignant tumor was by de Quervain in 1904 [1]. Making up only a small percentage of parathyroid carcinomas seen today, the first tumor described was non-functioning. It was not until 1933 when Sainton and Millot first described a case of metastatic parathyroid carcinoma causing manifestations of Recklinghausen's disease, commonly known today as hyperparathyroidism (HPTH) [2]. Parathyroid carcinoma is an uncommon cause of parathyroid hormone (PTH)-dependant hypercalcemia accounting for only 1–3% of cases of primary HPTH [3–9]. Since de Quervain's initial article, there have been over 700 cases reported in the literature [3–5,7–28]. From these reports, it is apparent that parathyroid cancer characteristically presents with more profound manifestations of HPTH than parathyroid adenomas and benign hyperplasia. Unfortunately, the histological diagnosis is not straightforward unless there is evidence of tumor invasiveness. For the pathologist, diagnostic difficulties arise in distinguishing hyperplasia, adenoma, and recurrent disease following inadequate surgery from carcinoma [13,29]. Recent advances in the molecular pathogenesis of parathyroid carcinoma will hopefully aid in the diagnosis of this disease. It has been shown that both familial and sporadic forms of parathyroid carcinoma are associated with mutations of the tumor-suppressor gene *HRPT2* [30–32]. These findings suggest that *HRPT2* mutation may be an early event in the pathogenesis of parathyroid carcinoma. A better understanding of this rare tumor will have valuable impact in the diagnosis and the treatment of these patients in the years to come.

Although parathyroid carcinoma is a rare disease, every surgeon who treats primary HPTH must be aware of its clinical presentation and unique operative findings, as early recognition and complete resection is the only means of cure. Unlike other malignancies, parathyroid carcinoma rarely causes death by tumor spread; instead, death is usually a result of the complications arising from excessive PTH secretion [4,5]. This chapter will discuss the current understanding of the pathogenesis, its clinical presentation, and treatment options for both the primary tumor and metastatic disease.

26.2   Incidence

Parathyroid carcinoma is a rare cause of primary HPTH. In 1999 the National Cancer Data Base (NCDB) reported 286 cases of parathyroid carcinoma, the largest single series published to date spanning a 10-year period [33]. They found that parathyroid carcinoma accounted for 0.005% of NCDB cancer cases. More recently, Beus and Stack reviewed all reports of parathyroid carcinoma in the literature since 1904 and found a total of 711 cases [10]. Many of these cases are likely reported multiple times, highlighting the rarity of this unique tumor. In most series, parathyroid carcinoma accounts for less than 1% of patients presenting with primary HPTH [3,4,6,13]. Interestingly, there appears to be a higher incidence of this disease in the Japanese and Italian populations, reporting an incidence of 5% [5,34,35]. The discrepancy likely arises from either the diagnostic difficulties that face the pathologist in the absence of tumor invasiveness and distant disease, or an absolute increase in the disease due to genetic and environmental factors.

26.3   Etiology and Molecular Pathogenesis

The etiology of parathyroid carcinoma remains to be fully elucidated. Until recently, clinical associations with predisposing factors such as head and neck radiation, chronic stimulation from renal failure, and familial syndromes were the only clues. Recent advances in molecular genetics, however, have increased our understanding of the pathogenesis of this disease. Several clinical associations that may predispose to the development of parathyroid carcinoma have been reported. Parathyroid carcinoma following head and neck radiation has been reported in a few patients [5,18,36–39]. Three out of these patients developed parathyroid carcinoma 25, 49, and 53 years following radiation and a further patient also had chronic renal failure, another possible stimulus. Therefore, the etiological significance of head and neck radiation is not clearly understood.

Parathyroid carcinoma has also been described in several patients with chronic renal failure (CRF) on hemodialysis. In a recent review of the literature, Miki et al. found 12 patients with CRF in whom parathyroid carcinoma developed [14]. They outline the difficulty in distinguishing, clinically, parathyroid carcinoma from progressive secondary HPTH in patients with CRF. In none of the reported cases was the diagnosis of carcinoma made preoperatively because of the biochemical and clinical similarities that both of these conditions present. With an increase in the number of patients on hemodialysis worldwide, it is interesting that the prevalence of the carcinoma has remained fairly constant [33]. Contributing to this may be the pathological difficulty in distinguishing hyperplasia from carcinoma. Therefore, the relationship between CRF and parathyroid carcinoma has yet to be clearly defined.

Familial HPTH, first reported in 1936, is now known to be a separate entity from multiple endocrine neoplasia type 1 syndrome (MEN1) [40]. Familial HPTH has an autosomal dominate mode of inheritance. This syndrome is characterized by hypercalcemia, elevated PTH levels, and isolated para-

thyroid tumors, with no evidence of hyperfunction of any other endocrine tissue. Although multigland hyperplasia is the most common finding, solitary adenomas have been reported in up to 25% of patients [41,42]. Parathyroid carcinoma was reported in five of the affected families, leading the authors to conclude that these patients are at increased risk of this rare malignancy [15,43]. This clinical syndrome of isolated familial HPTH appeared to be distinct from another hereditary HPTH syndrome called hyperparathyroidism–jaw tumor syndrome (HPTH-JT) [15,43,44]. HPTH-JT syndrome is a rare autosomal dominate condition associated with ossifying fibromas of the mandible and maxilla, renal cyst, renal hamartomas, and Wilms' tumors (Fig. 26.1) [45–49]. The incidence of parathyroid carcinoma is approximately 10% in HPTH-JT syndrome patients compared to 1% in patients with sporadic HPTH [15,30,43,44,50].

Since 1995, evidence for the role of both a tumor-suppressor gene and/or an oncogene in the pathogenesis of parathyroid tumors have been reported. The identification of the gene, *HRPT2*, responsible for HPTH-JT syndrome was recently mapped to the 1q25-q32 region [34]. Carpten et al. identified 13 different mutations of *HRPT2* in 14 families with HPTH-JT syndrome. Their study supported the previously held belief that this is a tumor-suppressor gene that encodes for the protein parafibromin. The role of parafibromin is presently unknown. Inactivating germline mutations of this gene were identified in the majority of kindreds with HPTH-JT syndrome, in which parathyroid carcinoma is overrepresented, therefore, Shattuck et al. investigated if *HRPT2* mutations could be responsible for the development of sporadic parathyroid carcinoma. Ten of the 15 parathyroid cancers studied demonstrated *HRPT2* mutations, all of which inactivated the encoded parafibromin protein [32]. Therefore, *HRPT2* mutation leading to an inactiva-

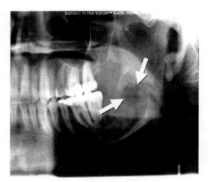

Fig. 26.1 An ossifying fibroma (*arrows*) of the mandible in a young patient with hereditary jaw tumor syndrome

tion of parafibromin is likely an important contributor to the pathogenesis of parathyroid carcinoma. In support of this thesis, Howell et al. also demonstrated *HRPT2* somatic mutations in four of four parathyroid carcinomas, and germline mutations in five HPTH-JT tumors and two additional tumors from a familial HPTH kindred [31]. These data provided further evidence for *HRPT2* as the causative gene in HPTH-JT and a subset of familial HPTH. Both these studies support the hypothesis that *HRPT2* mutation is an early event that may lead to the development of parathyroid carcinoma.

Unexpectedly, three patients in Shattuck et al.'s study of sporadic parathyroid carcinoma were found to have germline mutations [32]. This finding suggests that some of the sporadic carcinomas may be a phenotypic variant of HPTH-JT syndrome. The clinical implications of this finding are significant. Patients, especially the young, should be considered for DNA testing looking for germline mutations of the *HRPT2* gene. If mutations are found, then family members can be tested and, if positive, appropriate surveillance can be implemented [32,51].

Further evidence to support the important role that *HRPT2* gene plays in the pathogenesis of parathyroid carcinoma is the finding of an increased loss of heterozygosity (LOH) at chromosome 1q in sporadic carcinomas. In Haven et al.'s study that included 22 parathyroid carcinomas, 12 (55%) showed LOH of chromosome 1q whereas, LOH is only found in 8% of parathyroid adenomas [50,52]. This is not the entire story, however, as this group also found 50% of parathyroid carcinomas that demonstrated LOH of chromosome 11q13, the location of the *MENIN* gene. This gene is responsible for MEN1 syndrome, an autosomal dominate disorder characterized by parathyroid hyperplasia, pituitary, pancreatic, carcinoid, and adrenal cortical tumors. It has been previously reported that 30% of cases of parathyroid adenomas demonstrate LOH in chromosome 11q13 [53,54] and, therefore, suggest that the *MENIN* gene may play a role in tumorigenesis. Of interest was that 36% of the parathyroid carcinomas in Haven et al.'s study demonstrated LOH in both chromosomes 1q and 11q13. This finding suggests that inactivation of the *HRPT2* gene may function both independently and in concert with the *MENIN* gene inactivation to promote parathyroid carcinogenesis [50].

PRAD1/Cyclin D1 has also been implicated in the development of parathyroid tumors [55–58]. *PRAD1/Cyclin D1* is an oncogene located at chromosome 11q13; its protein product is thought to play a significant role in transition of cells from the G1-phase of the cell cycle into the S-phase [55]. The *PRAD1/Cyclin D1* oncoprotein is overexpressed in 18–40% of parathyroid adenomas [50,55,57,58]. Overexpression of this protein was found at a significantly higher frequency in parathyroid carcinomas (57–91%) [50,57]. Although these data suggest an important role of this protein in parathyroid carcinomas, the genetic effect of *PRAD1/Cyclin D1* activation in the context of the development of parathyroid carcinoma remains to be determined.

One possible mechanism for the oncogenic activity of *PRAD1/Cyclin D1* is via the inactivation of the growth inhibitory effects of the protein product of the retinoblastoma (*Rb*) gene [59]. *Rb* is a tumor-suppressor gene that has been implicated in parathyroid carcinomas. Several investigators have demonstrated an LOH on chromosome 13q, a region known to include both the *Rb* and the *BRCA2* genes [60–62]. However, recently Shattuck's group was unable to demonstrate tumor-specific somatic mutations in either *Rb* or *BRCA2* in six parathyroid carcinomas that demonstrated LOH at chromosome 13q [59]. While decreased expression of these genes may contribute to the pathogenesis of parathyroid carcinomas, their role in tumorigenesis needs further investigation.

26.4 Clinical Presentation

The distinction between benign primary HPTH and malignant disease can be difficult. Frequently, the diagnosis is only made when hypercalcemia reoccurs years later [13]. Consideration of carcinoma in the differential diagnosis of PTH-dependant hypercalcemia has been shown to lead to optimal outcomes, as completeness of resection offers the best chance for cure [3,5,51,61,63,64]. Clinical and laboratory findings may suggest parathyroid carcinoma, however these findings are non-specific (Table 26.1). Several clinical features should, however, alert the surgeon to the possibility for this diagnosis and cause him/her to plan appropriately for an en bloc resection. In contrast to benign HPTH where there is a predominance of females to males (4:1), parathyroid carcinoma affects both males and females equally [3,65]. In a recent review of the literature, Koea and Shaw found that the average age of presentation was 49 years (13–80) [65]. This is approximately 10 years younger than the average age for benign primary HPTH. Biochemically, the degree of hypercalcemia is more marked in patients with carcinoma than in benign HPTH. The average calcium level in benign HPTH is 2.7 mmol/l as compared to 3.75–3.97 mmol/l reported in the literature

Table 26.1 The clinical and biochemical features of parathyroid carcinoma compared to benign primary hyperparathyroidism (*HPTH*)

	Benign HPTH	Parathyroid carcinoma
Female to male	4 to 1	1 to 1
Average calcium (mmol/l)	2.7–2.9	3.75–4.0
Average PTH (ng/l)	<2× normal	>3–10× normal
Average age	Sixth decade	Fifth decade
Palpable mass	<2%	30–76%
Osteitis fibrosa cystica	5%	40–75%
Nephrolithiasis	10–15%	40%
Renal and bone disease	Rare	40–50%
Asymptomatic	80%	2%

for parathyroid carcinoma [65]. The PTH levels are also significantly higher, reported to be greater than five to ten times the normal range [3–5,13]. In a review of reported cases between 1974 and 1998, the mean increase in PTH values was 512% above normal [65]. Although such high levels of PTH are seen in progressive secondary and tertiary HPTH, primary HPTH rarely has such marked elevation.

In contrast to benign primary HPTH, where the majority of patients that present today are "asymptomatic" and lacking in significant manifestations of renal or bone disease [66,67], parathyroid carcinoma patients usually present with clinical manifestations of end-organ disease (Table 26.1) [3–5,65]. The prevalence of renal involvement including nephrolithiasis and impaired glomerular filtration is less than 20% in benign primary HPTH [67,68]. In contrast, nephrolithiasis was found in 56% of patients and renal insufficiency in 84% of patients with parathyroid carcinoma [4]. Overt radiographic manifestation of HPTH, such as osteitis fibrosa cystica, Brown's tumors, diffuse osteopenia, and subperiosteal bone resorption, is seen in 45–91% of carcinoma patients in contrast to benign HPTH where they are seen in only 5% of the population (Figs. 26.2, 26.3) [3,4,65,67,68]. An additional clinical clue to the diagnosis of parathyroid carcinoma is the presence of both renal and bone disease found in up to 50% of patients. Concomitant renal and bone disease is rarely seen today in benign disease [3,65]. There are rare cases of non-functioning parathyroid carcinoma reported [1,26,69,70]. Because of the lack of an endocrinopathy, these tumors tend to present late with diffuse metastatic disease. In a review by Klink et al., only 14 cases in the literature were found, making up less than 2% of all parathyroid carcinomas reported [69].

On physical examination, parathyroid cancer patients may display constitutional signs of malignancy, such as weight loss, significant fatigue, anorexia, and muscle wasting. The vague non-specific manifestations of HPTH are markedly pronounced and unlike benign HPTH usually have a rapid onset in patients with carcinoma. Recurrent laryngeal nerve (RLN) palsy in a patient with HPTH and no previous neck surgery should be suspicious for invasive disease. A palpable neck mass is found in 36–52% of patients with carcinoma, something that is found in less than 5% of benign HPTH patients [65].

26.5   Preoperative Investigations

Since 1995, there has been a paradigm shift in the surgical treatment of HPTH. With better imaging modalities and the development of intraoperative PTH, minimal, image-directed surgery has become standard practice in selected patients over a four-gland exploration [71]. It is important, therefore, that the surgeon continue to utilize appropriate patient selection, as preoperative suspicion of carcinoma would necessitate the need for a non-minimal approach to the patient. As a result, when carcinoma is suggested on clinical presentation, preoperative investigation may help not only make the diagnosis, but also help with surgical planning. Ultrasound (U/S) of the neck can raise the suspicion of invasive disease. Malignancy should be considered when the U/S demonstrates signs of gross invasion, marked tumor irregularity, and evidence of metastatic nodal disease [5,72,73]. Other non-invasive imaging has been the use of computed tomography (CT) and magnetic resonance imaging (MRI). Both of these imaging

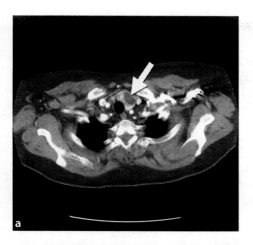

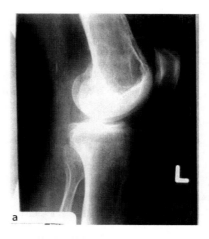

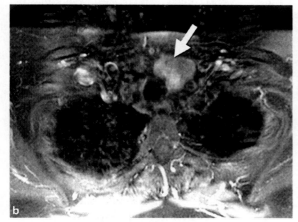

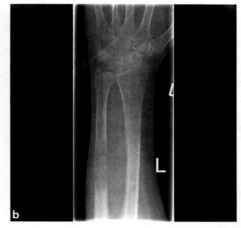

Fig. 26.2 a A CT scan of the neck demonstrating a large parathyroid carcinoma in the left lobe of the thyroid (*arrow*). **b** An MRI scan of the same patient illustrating the large carcinoma on the left side of the neck (*arrow*)

Fig. 26.3 Plain radiographs of the femur (**a**) and the radius (**b**) demonstrating lytic bony lesion initially thought to be consistent with metastatic disease. On further investigations, the patient was found to have parathyroid carcinoma and these lesions proved to be Brown's tumors consistent with osteitis fibrosa cystica

modalities can demonstrate the extent of the tumor, its involvement in adjacent structures, and evidence of regional and distant metastases (Figs. 26.2, 26.4). Recently, positive emission tomography (PET) has been described in the detection of parathyroid malignancies [27]. The role of PET in the future will continue to evolve as we gain more experience with this modality.

Tc-99m pertechnetate/Tc-99m sestamibi (MIBI) imaging has become the standard preoperative image modality in primary HPTH. MIBI scans have been helpful in the diagnosis of parathyroid carcinoma for they not only localize the primary tumor even in the face of non-function, but have also been shown to display distant metastases [69,74]. It is, therefore, important to obtain a whole-body MIBI scan when the diagnosis of parathyroid carcinoma is considered as it will help differentiate Brown's tumors from meta-static bone disease (Fig. 26.5). Bone scans have also been shown to be helpful in the preoperative diagnosis of parathyroid carcinoma. The classical features of a nuclear bone scan would consist of evidence of increased bone turnover consistent with metabolic bone disease as well as demonstrating both Brown's tumors and metastatic deposits (Fig. 26.6) [64].

The use of fine-needle aspiration in a suspected case of carcinoma is not recommended for two reasons. First, the diagnosis of parathyroid carcinoma can be extremely difficult histologically and sampling error may lead to false-negatives thus misleading the surgeon preoperatively [75]. Second, by violating the capsule of the tumor there is a risk of seeding parathyroid cells, which has been previously reported [76].

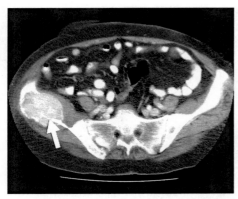

Fig. 26.4 A large destructive bony metastasis (*arrow*) of the right pelvis in a patient with parathyroid carcinoma

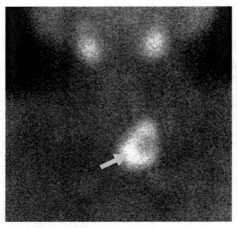

Fig. 26.5 A sestamibi scan demonstrating a large parathyroid lesion (*arrow*) that histologically proved to be parathyroid carcinoma

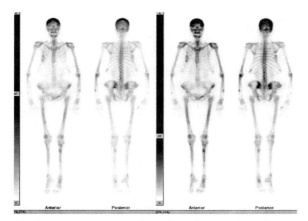

Fig. 26.6 The bone scan of a patient with parathyroid carcinoma. Note the increased uptake in the tibial region consistent with increased bone turnover. The Brown's tumors from Fig. 26.2 are also highlighted on this scan

26.6   Surgical Management

The single most effective treatment of parathyroid carcinoma is complete surgical resection of the primary and regional disease [5,6,20,64,65,77]. Preoperative suspicion and intraoperative recognition are paramount in the treatment of these patients. When preoperative clinical features are suspicious for carcinoma, appropriate investigation as outlined above should be undertaken and a planned en bloc resection should be carried out. Intraoperative findings suggestive of a carcinoma include a large, firm, white or gray parathyroid lesion and adherence or invasion into adjacent structures (the strap muscles, thyroid, trachea, RLN, esophagus, and sternocleidomastoid muscle). In a review of 358 reported cases of parathyroid carcinoma, the diagnosis was made or suspected intraoperatively because of evidence of invasion in 178 patients, and in an additional 46 cases the diagnosis was based on the appearance of the gland [65].

The surgical approach is through a collar incision exposing the strap muscles. The contralateral side should be explored to rule out hyperplasia of the parathyroid glands, since some patients will have four-gland disease associated with the carcinoma [15,19]. If hyperplasia is encountered, in addition to an en bloc resection of the involved side, the remaining parathyroid glands should also be removed and autotransplanted into the forearm away from the neck. If both contralateral parathyroid glands are normal in appearance, they should be left in situ, undisturbed. The en bloc resection involves division of the strap muscles, leaving them on the thyroid and the tumor. Identification of the remaining normal parathyroid gland on the affected side should be attempted. This gland should be included in the specimen to ensure all parathyroid tissue is removed from the affected side to aid in follow-up. The tumor is removed en bloc along with the thyroid lobe, the cervical thymus, and the contents of the central compartment (level VI) (Fig. 26.7) [64]. Great care must be taken not to rupture the capsule of the gland to avoid tumor spillage which will lead to an increase in recurrence. If the RLN is involved, it should be resected with the specimen. This illustrates the importance of performing a direct laryngoscopy preoperatively on all these patients. Comprehensive lateral lymphadenectomy (levels I, II, III, IV, or V) is usually not indicated unless grossly involved. In the NCDB report, lymph node status was documented in 105 cases; in 15% of these patients the lymph nodes were pathologically involved [33]. Currently, the use of intraoperative

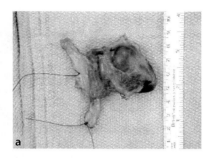

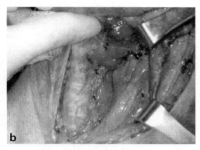

Fig. 26.7 a The en bloc surgical specimen. One suture is on the isthmus of the ipsilateral thyroid lobe. Two sutures mark the thymus and central compartment. **b** The residual tumor bed upon completion of the en bloc resection including the central compartment, ipsilateral thyroid lobe, and both the parathyroid carcinoma and normal ipsilateral gland

PTH will help guide the extent of surgery. A significant reduction in PTH with the objective to return to a normal level at 30 minutes postresection, should be attempted [77].

The more difficult scenario is when the diagnosis is made in the early postoperative period. If gross characteristics of the lesion are typical for carcinoma and if the pathology demonstrates an aggressive tumor with extensive invasion, or the patient remains hypercalcemic, then re-exploration of the neck excising the surgical bed and the structures adjacent to the tumor bed is indicated, once distant disease has been ruled out. If, however, none of those features are present, and the diagnosis is made solely on histopathology, reoperation may not be necessary. Such a patient should be observed for evidence of recurrence by measuring their PTH and calcium levels.

The postoperative management of these patients requires special attention to calcium homeostasis. These patients usually present with hungry bone syndrome and, as calcium and phosphorus are deposited into the skeleton, a significant drop in calcium will occur. The hypocalcemia following successful surgical intervention may be severe and protracted, requiring both oral and intravenous calcium. Pa-

tients should be given both oral elemental calcium and vitamin D supplements immediately following surgery and titrated to maintain serum calcium at the lower end of normal to aid in the recovery of the normal parathyroid glands. As the bones heal and the remaining parathyroid glands start to function, the required dosage of calcium will decline. Depending on the degree of hungry bone disease, the PTH levels following surgery may remain elevated as part of the normal physiological response of the bones. The clue that this elevation in PTH is not persistent disease but rather hungry bone disease is that the calcium level is not elevated in the latter.

26.7 Adjuvant Therapy

Historically, adjuvant radiotherapy had not been considered effective in the treatment of parathyroid carcinoma [3,7–9,78]. External beam radiation proved to be ineffective in reducing tumor size and/or correcting the hypocalcemia when given to treat bulky, unresectable disease. Similarly, disappointing results have been obtained in the treatment of bony metastases. However, recent reports have questioned the role of adjuvant radiotherapy postoperatively when given for histological close or positive margins. Munson et al. reported on 65 patients, four of whom had adjuvant therapy and four of whom were treated for locoregional disease control [79]. Overall locoregional recurrence occurred in 44% of patients, however, all four patients treated with adjuvant therapy were alive without disease. Similarly, both MD Anderson and the Princess Margaret Cancer Centers have reported a lower locoregional recurrence if adjuvant radiation of 40–50 Gy is applied postoperatively [17,77]. It therefore appears that, although the numbers are small, adjuvant radiation may play an important role in locoregional control of the disease.

Chemotherapy has been disappointing in the treatment of this disease. Because of the rarity of this disease, there are no large scale trials to evaluate its role as an adjuvant or therapeutic regimen. Most of the time, chemotherapy is given to patients with extensive local and/or regional disease that is considered unresectable. Several regimens including vincristine, adriamycin, cyclophosphamide, and 5-fluorouracil have been used as single agents or in combination, yet have proved to be ineffective [4,80,81]. Currently, there appears to be no role for the use of chemotherapy in the treatment of patients with parathyroid carcinoma.

26.8   Pathology

26.8.1   Histological Features

Without evidence of metastatic disease or invasion, the diagnosis of parathyroid carcinoma can be a challenge for the pathologist. The classic histological features of parathyroid carcinoma described by Schantz and Castleman [82] and used by other investigators [4–6,37,83,84] include trabecular architecture, mitotic figures, thick fibrous bands, and capsular and blood vessel invasion. In a recent review of 27 parathyroid carcinoma patients, Clayman et al. found that fibrous bands, mitosis, and vascular invasion were observed individually in 37% of patients [77]. Capsule invasion was found in only 26% of cases and trabeculae and lymphatic invasion in only 11% of cases. This study illustrates the fact that the "classic" pathological features of carcinoma are not always present in parathyroid carcinoma, nor are they specific for malignant disease. In addition to the trabecular architecture (Fig. 26.8), solid sheets of homogeneous cells resembling the histological appearance of many adenomas may be encountered (Fig. 26.9). The fibrous bands seen in carcinoma tend to be of dense hyaline fibrous tissue similar to that seen in many thymomas (Fig. 26.10). If the fibrous tissue is associated with evidence of old hemorrhage or previous surgery, however, it may be a feature of adenoma [37].

The presence of mitoses in tumor cells has been used by some authors as the most useful indication of carcinoma [6,82]. However, others have observed mitotic figures in adenomas [37,85]. The triad of high mitotic rate (>5 per 50 high-power fields), macronucleoli, and necrosis was associated with tumors that were more aggressive in terms of recurrent or metastatic disease (Fig. 26.11) [86].

The capsules of most parathyroid carcinomas are thicker than those of adenomas of similar size (Fig. 26.12). Capsular invasion is characterized by the extension of the neoplastic tissue in a tongue-like protrusion through the collagenous fibers of the cap-

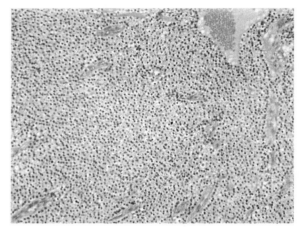

Fig. 26.9 Photomicrograph of a histological section of parathyroid carcinoma. Solid (sheet-like) proliferation of monotonous cells with bland nuclei and clear cytoplasm resembling the histological appearance of a chief cell adenoma. (H&E; 10×)

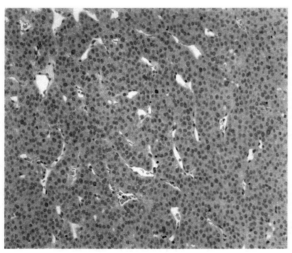

Fig. 26.8 Photomicrograph of a histological section of parathyroid carcinoma demonstrating a trabecular growth pattern. (H&E stain; 10×)

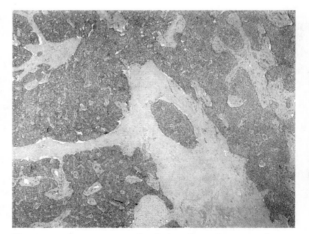

Fig. 26.10 Photomicrograph of a histological section of parathyroid carcinoma demonstrating thick hyalinized fibrous bands within the tumor. (H&E; 4×)

sule. Infiltrative growth through the capsule into the adjacent tissues allows a definitive diagnosis of carcinoma. The most common sites of local invasion are adipose tissue and muscle, esophagus, thyroid gland, RLN, and trachea [87].

Vascular invasion is seen in approximately 10–15% of parathyroid carcinomas and is considered to be virtually diagnostic of malignancy. To qualify as a bona fide feature, the tumor must not only be present within a vascular channel but must also be at least partially attached to its wall (Fig. 26.13) [28].

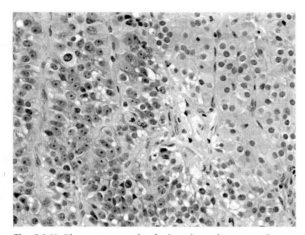

Fig. 26.11 Photomicrograph of a histological section of parathyroid carcinoma showing variable cytomorphology (cells with clear, amphophilic, and oxyphilic cytoplasm). Notice the nuclear enlargement, high N/C ratio, and prominent nucleoli (*left*). Two mitotic figures are seen near the *center*. (H&E; 40×)

26.8.2 Electron Microscopy

Under the electron microscope the cells from parathyroid carcinomas are large with tortuous, interdigitating plasma membranes. They have very active cytoplasm frequently with a partially dilated ergastoplasm that does not show any polarity or juxtanuclear distribution. Desmosomes are difficult to find. Lipid and glycogen are reduced, but many electron-dense secretory granules are usually seen. The nucleus varies considerably in size and shape. A loss of the nuclear membrane, as seen in prophase, can be observed even though mitosis may not be evident in light microscope sections. The nucleolus is enlarged and dense and the chromatin is clumped and dispersed through the karyoplasm giving rise to the "angry nucleus" appearance [37,88]. The latter feature is considered by some authors to be suggestive of malignancy as it has not been described in adenomas while others find electron microscopic investigation is of limited diagnostic value [5].

26.8.3 Flow Cytometric DNA Analysis

Some studies have shown that aneuploidy is significantly associated with malignancy in parathyroid tumors [5,89]. However, because of the overlap of results with adenomas, ploidy is not regarded as a useful tool in the differential diagnosis of carcinoma and adenoma [90]. In contrast the S-phase fraction may be helpful. One study suggests that a diagnosis of carcinoma should be considered in the presence of

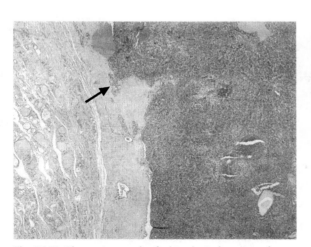

Fig. 26.12 Photomicrograph of a histological section of parathyroid carcinoma. The tumor (*right*) has a thick fibrous capsule that separates it from the thyroid gland (*left*). A tongue of neoplastic cells protrudes into the capsule (*arrow*) but complete capsular penetration is not evident. (H&E; 4×)

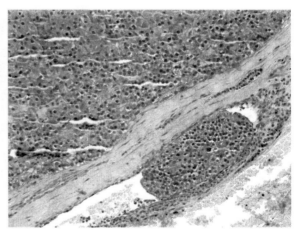

Fig. 26.13 Photomicrograph of a histological section of parathyroid carcinoma. Vascular invasion is seen outside the tumor capsule. The tumor embolus is partially attached to the vessel wall. (Musto stain; 20×)

an S-phase fraction greater than 4% and DNA index greater than 1.2% [91].

26.8.4 Immunohistochemistry

Immunohistochemical staining with the monoclonal MIB-1 antibody that detects the cell cycle-associated marker, *Ki-67* antigen, in paraffin sections can be used to evaluate the tumor-proliferative fraction (TPF). The latter is expressed as the number of *Ki-67*-positive nuclei per 1,000 parenchymal cells [85]. One study has shown that the mean TPF is significantly greater in parathyroid carcinomas in comparison to hyperplastic glands and adenomas. The authors concluded that a TPF exceeding 60 in 1000 cells is consistent with the diagnosis of parathyroid carcinoma and is an indication of malignant behavior both in terms of locally aggressive disease and distant spread [92]. Other investigators found the results of *Ki-67* staining inconclusive for the distinction between benign and malignant parathyroid lesions [93]. It would appear that less than 30% of parathyroid carcinomas have *Ki-67* positivity compared to 2% of adenomas [84]. Therefore, when present in the appropriate clinical scenario it can aid in the diagnosis, but its absence does not rule out malignancy.

Immunohistochemical staining for the protein product of the tumor-suppressor gene retinoblastoma (Rb) may be of diagnostic value. Parathyroid carcinomas are reported to lack staining for Rb protein while there is positive staining in adenomas [77]. This finding correlates with the allelic loss of *Rb* gene found in carcinomas [61]. One study, however, found that staining for Rb protein is not reliable for the distinction between benign and malignant tumors [93].

It has been shown that *PRAD1/Cyclin D1* is frequently overexpressed in parathyroid carcinoma [50,57]. This overexpression can be detected by immunohistochemistry, however to date it has not been useful in distinguishing carcinomas from adenomas [57]. With the recent evidence that mutations in the *HRPT2* gene are found in parathyroid carcinoma, loss of the parafibromin in parathyroid tumor may help distinguish carcinoma from benign tissue [32,58]. Utilizing a novel anti-parafibromin monoclonal antibody, Tan et al. found that loss of parafibromin immunoreactivity had a 96% sensitivity and 99% specificity in diagnosing carcinoma [94]. This molecular marker shows promise in aiding the pathologist in the diagnosis of parathyroid carcinoma.

26.9 Natural History and Prognosis

Although the biological behavior of parathyroid carcinoma can be aggressive in a few patients, the majority of patients display an indolent course. The 5-year survival rate varies in the literature from 44% to 85%, likely reflecting the difficultly in confirming the histological diagnosis in all cases [4,6,13]. In the recent NCDB study, the overall 5-year and 10-year relative survival rates were 85.5% and 49%, respectively [33]. Neither tumor size nor lymph node status predicted survival in this cohort.

Recurrence following initial surgery is common with rates ranging from 33% to 78% [4,13,20,22,65]. In their review of the literature, Koea and Shaw were able to analysis 301 patients with adequate treatment and follow-up data [65]. They found that a total of 179 patients were treated with parathyroidectomy only. Of these 92 (51%) recurred locally in a mean time of 41 months. Ninety percent of patients who developed recurrence died of their disease at a mean time of 62 months. In contrast, 104 patients underwent an en bloc resection with curative intent. Eight percent recurred locally and an additional 3 patients developed distant metastases, demonstrating the important of clinical recognition and extensive initial surgery.

Persistent hypercalcemia following initial surgery has been shown to be a poor prognostic indicator [4]. Sixty percent of patients with persistent disease were dead from their disease within 3 years. Surgical resection and/or debulking of locoregional or metastatic disease has been shown to result in periods of normocalcemia ranging from months to years [3,65]. Survival benefit has also been demonstrated in patients that underwent metastasectomy compared to similar patients treated symptomatically [65].

26.10 Palliative Therapies

When parathyroid carcinoma becomes widely disseminated, patients usually die from the metabolic complications of hypercalcemia [5,63]. The management of hypercalcemia involves rehydration, and promotion of calciuresis with a loop diuretic [95]. However, unlike other cause of hypercalcemia, parathyroid carcinoma rarely responds solely to these measures. Bisphosphonates are a class of drugs that inhibit osteoclast-mediated bone resorption. Pamidronate when infused over 2–24 hours in doses of 30–90 mg/day have been effective in lowering serum calcium levels in patients with parathyroid carcinoma, at least transiently [5,19,96]. New and more potent bisphosphonates, such as zoledronate, will likely replace pamidronate in these patients in the future [97].

A new class of drugs, the calcimimetics, show promise in the long-term treatment of parathyroid carcinoma-induced hypercalcemia [98,99]. These drugs are an allosteric modulator of the calcium-sensing receptors (CaRs) that are responsible for the regulation of PTH secretion. In a multicenter study, cinacalcet, a second-generation calcimimetic, safely normalized calcium levels and lowered PTH concentrations in patients with hypercalcemia seen in HPTH [100]. The authors concluded that this drug had great potential for the palliative treatment of parathyroid carcinoma patients.

Most recently, a novel treatment of parathyroid carcinoma was reported utilizing anti-parathyroid hormone immunotherapy [101]. In their report of a patient with refractory hypercalcemia from pulmonary metastases, the Betea et al. found that after the fourth immunization both PTH and serum calcium levels decreased. They also found a reduction in the sizes of the pulmonary metastases, demonstrating promise for this type of therapy in the future.

Finally, the somatostatin analog, octreotide, has been reported to inhibit PTH secretion [102]. Recent reports have demonstrated palliative benefit from the use of indium-labeled octreotide therapy for metastatic neuroendocrine tumors [103]. It is therefore possible that, in the future, utilization of radionuclide therapy may provide therapeutic benefit to patients with metastatic parathyroid carcinoma.

26.11   Summary

Although parathyroid carcinoma is a rare disease, every surgeon who treats HPTH must have a comprehensive understanding of the clinical presentation, operative findings, and the pathological pitfalls of this disease. Surgical en bloc resection remains the treatment of choice and provides the only means of cure. The addition of external beam radiation therapy may provide better locoregional control in selected patients. Recent advances have increased our understanding of the molecular pathogenesis of this disease. It would appear that the *HRPT2* gene plays an important role in the development of carcinoma, and provides a genetic marker for those patients at risk. Unlike other malignancies, parathyroid carcinoma rarely causes death by tumor spread; instead, death is usually a result of the complications arising from excessive PTH secretion. Therefore, palliative therapies directed at reducing the hypercalcemia and PTH se-

cretion have been shown to benefit the patient suffering from this disease.

References

1. de Quervain F (1904) Parastruma maligna aberrata. Dtsch Z Chir 100:334–352
2. Sainton P, Millot J (1933) Malegne d'un adenome parathyroidiene eosinophile. Au cours d'une de Recklinghausen. Ann Anat Pathol 10:813–814
3. Shane E (2001) Clinical review 122: parathyroid carcinoma. J Clin Endocrinol Metab 86:485–493
4. Wynne AG, van Heerden J, Carney JA, Fitzpatrick LA (1992) Parathyroid carcinoma: clinical and pathologic features in 43 patients. Medicine 71:197–205
5. Obara T, Fujimoto Y (1991) Diagnosis and treatment of patients with parathyroid carcinoma: an update and review. World J Surg 15:738–744
6. Wang CA, Gaz RD (1985) Natural history of parathyroid carcinoma. Diagnosis, treatment, and results. Am J Surg 149:522–527
7. Cohn K, Silverman M, Corrado J, Sedgewick C (1985) Parathyroid carcinoma: the Lahey Clinic experience. Surgery 98:1095–1100
8. Hakaim AG, Esselstyn CB (1993) Parathyroid carcinoma: 50-year experience at the Cleveland Clinic Foundation. Cleve Clin J Med 60:331–335
9. Fujimota Y, Obara T (1987) How to recognize and treat parathyroid carcinoma. Surg Clin North Am 67:343–357
10. Beus KS, Stack BC Jr (2004) Parathyroid carcinoma. Otolaryngol Clin North Am 37:845–854
11. Shane E (1994) Parathyroid carcinoma. Curr Ther Endocrinol Metab 5:565–568
12. Salusky IB, Goodman WG, Kuizon BD (2000) Implications of intermittent calcitriol therapy on growth and secondary hyperparathyroidism. Pediatr Nephrol 14:641–645
13. Sandelin K, Auer G, Bondeson L, Grimelius L, Farnebo L-O (1992) Prognostic factors in parathyroid cancer: a review of 95 cases. World J Surg 16:724–731
14. Miki H, Sumitomo M, Inoue H, Kita S, Monden Y (1996) Parathyroid carcinoma in patients with chronic renal failure on maintenance hemodialysis. Surgery 120:897–901
15. Streeten EA, Weinstein LS, Norton JA, Mulvihill JJ, White BJ, Friedman E, Jaffe G, Brandi ML, Stewart K, Zimering MB (1992) Studies in a kindred with parathyroid carcinoma. J Clin Endocrinol Metab 75:362–366
16. Cordeiro AC, Montenegro FL, Kulcsar MA, Dellanegra LA, Tavares MR, Michaluart P Jr, Ferraz AR (1998) Parathyroid carcinoma. Am J Surg 175:52–55
17. Chow E, Tsang RW, Brierley JD, Filice S (1998) Parathyroid carcinoma: the Princess Margaret Hospital experience. Int J Radiat Oncol Biol Phys 41:569–572

18. Mashburn MA, Chonkich GD, Chase DR, Petti GH Jr (1987) Parathyroid carcinoma. Two new cases: diagnosis, therapy, and treatment. Laryngoscope 97:215–218

19. de Papp AE, Kinder B, LiVolsi V, Gupta SM, Stewart AF (1994) Parathyroid carcinoma arising from parathyroid hyperplasia: autoinfarction following intravenous treatment with pamidronate. Am J Med 97:399–400

20. Favia G, Lumachi F, Polistina F, D'Amico DF (1998) Parathyroid carcinoma: sixteen new cases and suggestions for correct management. World J Surg 22:1225–1230

21. Hauptman JB, Modlinger RS, Ertel NH (1983) Pheochromocytoma resistant to alpha adrenergic blockade. Arch Intern Med 143:2321–2323

22. Kebebew E, Arici C, Duh QY, Clark OH (2001) Localization and reoperation results for persistent and recurrent parathyroid carcinoma. Arch Surg 136:878–885

23. Dionisi S, Minisola S, Pepe J, De Geronimo S, Paglia F, Memeo L, Fitzpatrick LA (2002) Concurrent parathyroid adenomas and carcinoma in the setting of multiple endocrine neoplasia type 1: presentation as hypercalcemic crisis. Mayo Clin Proc 77:866–869

24. Schmidt JL, Perry RC, Philippsen LP, Wu HH (2002) Intrathyroidal parathyroid carcinoma presenting with only hypercalcemia. Otolaryngol Head Neck Surg 127:352–353

25. Chandran M, Deftos L, Stuenkel C, Haghihi P, Orloff L (2003) Thymic parathyroid carcinoma and postoperative hungry bone syndrome. Am Surg 9:152–156

26. Aldinger KA, Hickey RC, Ibanez ML, Samaan NA (1982) Parathyroid carcinoma: a clinical study of seven cases of functioning and two cases of nonfunctioning parathyroid cancer. Cancer 49:388–397

27. Snell SB, Gaar EE, Stevens SP, Flynn MB (2003) Parathyroid cancer, a continued diagnostic and therapeutic dilemma: report of four cases and review of the literature. Am Surg 69:711–716

28. Iacobone M, Lumachi F, Favia G (2004) Up-to-date on parathyroid carcinoma: analysis of an experience of 19 cases. J Surg Oncol 88:223–228

29. Morrison C, Farrar W, Kneile J, Williams N, Liu-Stratton Y, Bakaletz A, Aldred MA, Eng C (2004) Molecular classification of parathyroid neoplasia by gene expression profiling. Am J Pathol 165:565–576

30. Szabo J, Heath B, Hill VM, Jackson CE, Zarbo RJ, Mallette LE, Chew SL, Besser GM, Thakker RV, Huff V (1995) Hereditary hyperparathyroidism-jaw tumor syndrome: the endocrine tumor gene HRPT2 maps to chromosome 1q21-q31. Am J Hum Genet 56:944–950

31. Howell VM, Haven CJ, Kahnoski K, Khoo SK, Petillo D, Chen J, Fleuren GJ, Robinson BG, Delbridge LW, Philips J, Nelson AE, Krause U, Hammje K, Dralle H, Hoang-Vu C, Gimm O, Marsh DJ, Morreau H, Teh BT (2003) HRPT2 mutations are associated with malignancy in sporadic parathyroid tumours. J Med Genet 40:657–663

32. Shattuck TM, Valimaki S, Obara T, Gaz RD, Clark OH, Shoback D, Wierman ME, Tojo K, Robbins CM, Carpten JD, Farnebo LO, Larsson C, Arnold A (2003) Somatic and germ-line mutations of the HRPT2 gene in sporadic parathyroid carcinoma. N Engl J Med 349:1722–1729

33. Hundahl SA, Fleming ID, Fremgen AM, Menck HR (1999) Two hundred eighty-six cases of parathyroid carcinoma treated in the U.S. between 1985–1995: a National Cancer Data Base Report. The American College of Surgeons Commission on Cancer and the American Cancer Society. Cancer 86:538–544

34. Carpten JD, Robbins CM, Villablanca A, Forsberg L, Presciuttini S, Bailey-Wilson J, Simonds WF, Gillanders EM, Kennedy AM, Chen JD, Agarwal SK, Sood R, Jones MP, Moses TY, Haven C, Petillo D, Leotlela PD, Harding B, Cameron D, Pannett AA, Hoog A, Heath H III, James-Newton LA, Robinson B, Zarbo RJ, Cavaco BM, Wassif W, Perrier ND, Rosen IB, Kristoffersson U, Turnpenny PD, Farnebo LO, Besser GM, Jackson CE, Morreau H, Trent JM, Thakker RV, Marx SJ, Teh BT, Larsson C, Hobbs MR (2002) HRPT2, encoding parafibromin, is mutated in hyperparathyroidism-jaw tumor syndrome. Nat Genet 32:676–680

35. Ishida T, Yokoe T, Izuo M (1991) Nationwide survey of parathyroid operations in Japan 1980–1989. Endocr Surg 8:37–45

36. Ireland JP, Fleming SJ, Levison DA, Cattell WR, Baker LR (1985) Parathyroid carcinoma associated with chronic renal failure and previous radiotherapy to the neck. J Clin Pathol 38:1114–1118

37. Smith JF (1993) The pathological diagnosis of carcinoma of the parathyroid. Clin Endocrinol (Oxf) 38:662

38. Christmas TJ, Chapple CR, Noble JG, Milroy EJ, Cowie AG (1988) Hyperparathyroidism after neck irradiation. Br J Surg 75:873–874

39. Tisell LE, Hansson G, Lindberg S, Ragnhult I (1977) Hyperparathyroidism in persons treated with X-rays for tuberculous cervical adenitis. Cancer 40:846–854

40. Goldman L, Smyth FS (1936) Hyperparathyroidism in siblings. Ann Surg 104:971–981

41. Huang S-M, Duh Q-Y, Shaver J, Siperstein AE, Kraimps J-L, Clark OH (1997) Familial hyperparathyroidism without multiple endocrine neoplasia. World J Surg 21:22–29

42. Barry MK, van Heerden JA, Grant CS, Thompson GB, Khosla S (1997) Is familial hyperparathyroidism a unique disease. Surgery 122:1028–1033

43. Wassif WS, Moniz CF, Friedman E, Wong S, Weber G, Nordenskjold M, Peters TJ, Larsson C (1993) Familial isolated hyperparathyroidism: a distinct genetic entity with an increased risk of parathyroid cancer. J Clin Endocrinol Metab 77:1485–1489

44. Jackson CE, Norum RA, Boyd SB, Talpos GB, Wilson SD, Taggart T, Mallette LE (1990) Hereditary hyperparathyroidism and multiple ossifying jaw fibromas: A clinically and genetically distinct syndrome. Surg 108:1006–1013

45. Haven CJ, Wong FK, van Dam EW, van der JR, van Asperen C, Jansen J, Rosenberg C, de Wit M, Roijers J, Hoppener J, Lips CJ, Larsson C, Teh BT, Morreau H (2000) A genotypic and histopathological study of a large Dutch kindred with hyperparathyroidism-jaw tumor syndrome. J Clin Endocrinol Metab 85:1449–1454

46. Cavaco BM, Guerra L, Bradley KJ, Carvalho D, Harding B, Oliveira A, Santos MA, Sobrinho LG, Thakker RV, Leite V (2004) Hyperparathyroidism-jaw tumor syndrome in Roma families from Portugal is due to a founder mutation of the HRPT2 gene. J Clin Endocrinol Metab 89:1747–1752

47. Teh BT, Farnebo F, Kristoffersson U, Sundelin B, Cardinal J, Axelson R, Yap A, Epstein M, Heath H III, Cameron D, Larsson C (1996) Autosomal dominant primary hyperparathyroidism and jaw tumor syndrome associated with renal hamartomas and cystic kidney disease: linkage to 1q21-q32 and loss of the wild type allele in renal hamartomas. J Clin Endocrinol Metab 81:4204–4211

48. Cavaco BM, Barros L, Pannett AA, Ruas L, Carvalheiro M, Ruas MM, Krausz T, Santos MA, Sobrinho LG, Leite V, Thakker RV (2001) The hyperparathyroidism-jaw tumour syndrome in a Portuguese kindred. QJM 94:213–222

49. Wassif WS, Farnebo F, Teh BT, Moniz CF, Li FY, Harrison JD, Peters TJ, Larsson C, Harris P (1999) Genetic studies of a family with hereditary hyperparathyroidism-jaw tumour syndrome. Clin Endocrinol 50:191–196

50. Haven CJ, Howell VM, Eilers PH, Dunne R, Takahashi M, van Puijenbroek M, Furge K, Kievit J, Tan MH, Fleuren GJ, Robinson BG, Delbridge LW, Philips J, Nelson AE, Krause U, Dralle H, Hoang-Vu C, Gimm O, Morreau H, Marsh DJ, Teh BT (2004) Gene expression of parathyroid tumors: molecular subclassification and identification of the potential malignant phenotype. Cancer Res 64:7405–7411

51. Weinstein LS, Simonds WF (2003) HRPT2, a marker of parathyroid cancer. N Engl J Med 349:1691–1692

52. Farnebo F, Teh BT, Dotzenrath C, Wassif WS, Svensson A, White I, Betz R, Goretzki P, Sandelin K, Farnebo LO, Larsson C (1997) Differential loss of heterozygosity in familial, sporadic, and uremic hyperparathyroidism. Hum Genet 99:342–349

53. Farnebo F, Teh BT, Kytola S, Svensson A, Phelan C, Sandelin K, Thompson NW, Hoog A, Weber G, Farnebo LO, Larsson C (1998) Alterations of the MEN1 gene in sporadic parathyroid tumors. J Clin Endocrinol Metab 83:2627–2630

54. Dwight T, Twigg S, Delbridge L, Wong FK, Farnebo F, Richardson AL, Nelson A, Zedenius J, Philips J, Larsson C, Teh BT, Robinson B (2000) Loss of heterozygosity in sporadic parathyroid tumours: involvement of chromosome 1 and the MEN1 gene locus in 11q13. Clin Endocrinol (Oxf) 53:85–92

55. Mallya SM, Arnold A (2000) Cyclin D1 in parathyroid disease. Front Biosci 5:D367–D371

56. Hemmer S, Wasenius VM, Haglund C, Zhu Y, Knuutila S, Franssila K, Joensuu H (2001) Deletion of 11q23 and cyclin D1 overexpression are frequent aberrations in parathyroid adenomas. Am J Pathol 158:1355–1362

57. Vasef MA, Brynes RK, Sturm M, Bromley C, Robinson RA (1999) Expression of cyclin D1 in parathyroid carcinomas, adenomas, and hyperplasias: a paraffin immunohistochemical study. Mod Pathol 12:412–416

58. Hsi ED, Zukerberg LR, Yang WI, Arnold A (1996) Cyclin D1/PRAD1 expression in parathyroid adenomas: an immunohistochemical study. J Clin Endocrinol Metab 81:1736–1739

59. Shattuck TM, Kim TS, Costa J, Yandell DW, Imanishi Y, Palanisamy N, Gaz RD, Shoback D, Clark OH, Monchik JM, Wierman ME, Hollenberg A, Tojo K, Chaganti RS, Arnold A (2003) Mutational analyses of RB and BRCA2 as candidate tumour suppressor genes in parathyroid carcinoma. Clin Endocrinol 59:180–189

60. Pearce SH, Trump D, Wooding C, Sheppard MN, Clayton RN, Thakker RV (1996) Loss of heterozygosity studies at the retinoblastoma and breast cancer susceptibility (BRCA2) loci in pituitary, parathyroid, pancreatic and carcinoid tumours. Clin Endocrinol 45:195–200

61. Cryns VL, Thor A, Xu HJ, Hu SX, Wierman ME, Vickery AL Jr, Benedict WF, Arnold A (1994) Loss of the retinoblastoma tumor-suppressor gene in parathyroid carcinoma. N Engl J Med 330:757–761

62. Venkitaraman AR (2001) Chromosome stability, DNA recombination and the BRCA2 tumour suppressor. Curr Opin Cell Biol 13:338–343

63. Mittendorf E, McHenry CR (2005) Parathyroid carcinoma. J Surg Oncol 89:137–142

64. Pasieka JL (1999) Parathyroid carcinoma. Operative Tech Gen Surg 1:71–84

65. Koea JB, Shaw JH (1999) Parathyroid cancer: biology and management. Surg Oncol 8:155–165

66. Silverberg SJ, Bilezikian JP (1997) Primary hyperparathyroidism: still evolving? J Bone Miner Res 12:856–862

67. Silverberg SJ, Bilezikian JP (1996) Evaluation and management of primary hyperparathyroidism. J Clin Endocrinol Metab 81:2036–2040

68. Heath H III, Hodgson SF, Kennedy MA (1980) Primary hyperparathyroidism. Incidence, morbidity, and potential economic impact in a community. N Engl J Med 302:189–193

69. Klink BK, Karulf RE, Maimon WN, Peoples JB (1991) Nonfunctioning parathyroid carcinoma. Am Surg 57:463–467

70. Murphy MN, Glennon PG, Diocee MS, Wick MR, Cavers DJ (1986) Nonsecretory parathyroid carcinoma of the mediastinum. Light microscopic, immunocytochemical, and ultrastructural features of a case, and review of the literature. Cancer 58:2468–2476

71. Palazzo F, Delbridge LW (2004) Minimal-access/minimally invasive parathyroidectomy for primary hyperparathyroidism. Surg Clin of North Am 84:717–734

72. Edmonson GR, Charboneau JW, James EM, Reading CC, Grant CS (1986) Parathyroid carcinoma: high-frequency sonographic features. Radiology 161:65–67

73. Kinoshita Y, Fukase M, Uchihashi M, Takenaka M, Hishikawa R, Nakada M, Nonaka H, Kondo T, Fujita T (1985) Significance of preoperative use of ultrasonography in parathyroid neoplasms: comparison of sonographic textures with histologic findings. J Clin Ultrasound 13:457–460

74. Johnston LB, Carroll MJ, Britton KE, Lowe DG, Shand W, Besser GM, Grossman AB (1996) The accuracy of parathyroid gland localization in primary hyperparathyroidism using sestamibi radionuclide imaging. J Clin Endocrinol Metab 81:346–352

75. Thompson SD, Prichard AJ (2004) The management of parathyroid carcinoma. Curr Opin Otolaryngol Head Neck Surg 12:93–97

76. Spinelli C, Bonadio AG, Berti P, Materazzi G, Miccoli P (2000) Cutaneous spreading of parathyroid carcinoma after fine needle aspiration cytology. J Endocrinol Invest 23:255–257

77. Clayman GL, Gonzalez HE, El Naggar A, Vassilopoulou-Sellin R (2004) Parathyroid carcinoma: evaluation and interdisciplinary management. Cancer 100:900–905

78. Vetto JT, Brennan MF, Woodruf J, Burt M (1993) Parathyroid carcinoma: diagnosis and clinical history. Surgery 114:882–892

79. Munson ND, Foote RL, Northcutt RC, Tiegs RD, Fitzpatrick LA, Grant CS, van Heerden JA, Thompson GB, Lloyd RV (2003) Parathyroid carcinoma: is there a role for adjuvant radiation therapy? Cancer 98:2378–2384

80. Anderson BJ, Samaan NA, Vassilopoulou-Sellin R, Ordonez NG, Hickey RC (1983) Parathyroid carcinoma: features and difficulties in diagnosis and management. Surgery 94:906–915

81. Grammes CF, Eyerly RC (1980) Hyperparathyroidism and parathyroid carcinoma. South Med J 73:814–816

82. Schantz A, Castleman B (1973) Parathyroid carcinoma. A study of 70 cases. Cancer 31:600–605

83. Sandelin K, Tullgren O, Farnebo LO (1994) Clinical course of metastatic parathyroid cancer. World J Surg 18:594–598

84. Stojadinovic A, Hoos A, Nissan A, Dudas ME, Cordon-Cardo C, Shaha AR, Brennan MF, Singh B, Ghossein RA (2003) Parathyroid neoplasms: clinical, histopathological, and tissue microarray-based molecular analysis. Hum Pathol 34:54–64

85. DeLellis RA (1995) Does the evaluation of proliferative activity predict malignancy of prognosis in endocrine tumors? Hum Pathol 26:131–134

86. Bondeson L, Sandelin K, Grimelius L (1993) Histopathological variables and DNA cytometry in parathyroid carcinoma. Am J Surg Pathol 17:820–829

87. Busaidy NL, Jimenez C, Habra MA, Schultz PN, El Naggar AK, Clayman GL, Asper JA, Diaz EM Jr, Evans DB, Gagel RF, Garden A, Hoff AO, Lee JE, Morrison WH, Rosenthal DI, Sherman SI, Sturgis EM, Waguespack SG, Weber RS, Wirfel K, Vassilopoulou-Sellin R (2004) Parathyroid carcinoma: a 22-year experience. Head Neck 26:716–726

88. Faccini JM (1970) The ultrastructure of parathyroid glands removed from patients with primary hyperparathyroidism: a report of 40 cases, including four carcinomata. J Pathol 102:189–199

89. Levin KE, Chew KL, Ljung B, Mayall BH, Siperstein AE, Clark OH (1988) Deoxyribonucleic acid cytometry helps identify parathyroid carcinomas. J Clin Endocrinol Metab 67:779–784

90. Mallette LE (1992) DNA quantitation in the study of parathyroid lesions. Am J Clin Pathol 98:305–311

91. Harlow S, Roth SI, Bauer K, Marshall RB (1991) Flow cytometric DNA analysis of normal and pathologic parathyroid glands. Mod Pathol 4:310–315

92. Abbona GC, Papotti M, Gasparri G, Bussolati G (1995) Proliferative activity in parathyroid tumors as detected by Ki-67 immunostaining. Hum Pathol 26:135–138

93. Farnebo F, Auer G, Farnebo LO, Teh BT, Twigg S, Aspenblad U, Thompson NW, Grimelius L, Larsson C, Sandelin K (1999) Evaluation of retinoblastoma and Ki-67 immunostaining as diagnostic markers of benign and malignant parathyroid disease. World J Surg 23:68–74

94. Tan MH, Morrison C, Wang P, Yang X, Haven CJ, Zhang C, Zhao P, Tretiakova MS, Korpi-Hyovalti E, Burgess JR, Soo KC, Cheah WK, Cao B, Resau J, Morreau H, Teh BT (2004) Loss of parafibromin immunoreactivity is a distinguishing feature of parathyroid carcinoma. Clin Cancer Res 10:6629–6637

95. Bilezikian JP (1992) Management of acute hypercalcemia. N Engl J Med 326:1196–1203

96. Sandelin K, Thompson NW, Bondeson L (1991) Metastatic parathyroid carcinoma: dilemmas in management. Surgery 110:978–988

97. Hurtado J, Esbrit P (2002) Treatment of malignant hypercalcaemia. Expert Opin Pharmacother 3:521–527

98. Collins MT, Skarulis MC, Bilezikian JP, Silverberg SJ, Spiegel AM, Marx SJ (1998) Treatment of hypercalcemia secondary to parathyroid carcinoma with a novel calcimimetic agent. J Clin Endocrinol Metab 83:1083–1088

99. Nemeth EF, Steffey ME, Hammerland LG, Hung BC, Van Wagenen BC, DelMar EG, Balandrin MF (1998) Calcimimetics with potent and selective activity on the parathyroid calcium receptor. Proc Natl Acad Sci U S A 95:4040–4045

100. Shoback DM, Bilezikian JP, Turner SA, McCary LC, Guo MD, Peacock M (2003) The calcimimetic cinacalcet normalizes serum calcium in subjects with primary hyperparathyroidism. J Clin Endocrinol Metab 88:5644–5649

101. Betea D, Bradwell AR, Harvey TC, Mead GP, Schmidt-Gayk H, Ghaye B, Daly AF, Beckers A (2004) Hormonal and biochemical normalization and tumor shrinkage induced by anti-parathyroid hormone immunotherapy in a patient with metastatic parathyroid carcinoma. J Clin Endocrinol Metab 89:3413–3420

102. Koyano H, Shishiba Y, Shimizu T, Suzuki N, Nakazawa H, Tachibana S, Murata H, Furui S (1994) Successful treatment by surgical removal of bone metastasis producing PTH: new approach to the management of metastatic parathyroid carcinoma. Intern Med 33:697–702

103. Pasieka JL, McEwan A, Rorstad O (2004) The palliative role of 131I mIBG and 111In-octreotide in patients with metastatic progressive neuroendocrine tumors. Surgery 136:1218–1226

27 Reoperative Parathyroid Surgery

Cord Sturgeon, Nadine Caron, and Quan-Yang Duh

CONTENTS

27.1   Definition and Introduction

The success of parathyroidectomy for primary hyperparathyroidism (HPTH), with or without preoperative localization, is higher than 95% in the hands of experienced surgeons [1]. In contrast, the success rate for surgeons who perform less than ten parathyroidectomies per year is only approximately 70% [2]. The majority of parathyroid operations in the USA are not, in fact, performed by experienced parathyroid surgeons. Consequently, for some patients disease is not cured and HPTH persists following surgery. Recurrence develops in about 1% of patients with sporadic primary HPTH and one third of patients with familial primary HPTH. Overall, about 5–10% of patients operated on for HPTH will develop recurrent or persistent disease. When hypercalcemia persists immediately following surgery or is diagnosed up to 6 months following surgery, the patient is said to have "persistent" disease. Persistent HPTH is usually due to a missed parathyroid adenoma, and is the most common indication for parathyroid reoperation. Hypercalcemia that develops more than 6 months after apparently curative surgery is called "recurrent". Recurrent HPTH is most frequently due to the biology of the underlying disease process. The most common causes of persistent and recurrent HPTH are listed in Table 27.1.

Persistent and recurrent HPTH has been called the *bête noire* of the endocrine surgeon [3]. This notorious disease has haunted surgeons from the time that Dr Felix Mandl performed the first parathyroidectomy in 1925. Ironically, this operation resulted in recurrence of disease from what may have been parathyroid cancer. In one of the most infamous cases of HPTH from the same era, Captain Charles Martell suffered persistent HPTH following neck exploration and ultimately underwent seven operations before a mediastinal gland was identified and removed. These early failures demonstrate that the biology of this disease has not dramatically changed in the past 80 years; physicians and patients still face the same pitfalls and challenges today.

In some series, the incidence of recurrent or persistent disease has been reported to be as high as 30% [4–6]. The success rate of repeat parathyroidectomy is about 80–90% in experienced hands; however, the optimal time to cure the patient is during the index operation, when the likelihood of cure is greatest and the risks of surgical complications are lowest. This chapter will highlight the causes of persistent and recurrent HPTH, discuss the indications for reoperative surgery, and outline a preoperative strategy for approaching this disease.

Table 27.1 Causes of persistent and recurrent hyperparathyroidism (*HPTH*)

Persistent HPTH:
• Failure to identify or remove the parathyroid adenoma
• Failure to identify or remove all adenomatous or hyperplastic parathyroid tissue
• Inadequate subtotal resection in four-gland hyperplasia
• Subtotal resection of a parathyroid adenoma
• Residual or metastatic parathyroid carcinoma
• Parathyromatosis
• Failed percutaneous ablation techniques
Recurrent HPTH:
• Regrowth of hyperplastic parathyroid tissue (especially in familial HPTH)
• Regrowth of autotransplanted parathyroid tissue
• Recurrent or metastatic parathyroid carcinoma
• Parathyromatosis

27.2 Anatomy and Embryology of the Parathyroid Gland

Approximately 80–85% of cases of primary HPTH are caused by a single parathyroid adenoma. Hyperplasia accounts for about 12%, double or triple adenomas are responsible for 2–3%, and the remaining 1% are due to parathyroid cancer [7]. Most parathyroid glands responsible for primary HPTH are found in the normal anatomic location. Occasionally parathyroid glands are encountered in ectopic sites such as the thyrothymic ligament, thymus, mediastinum, retroesophageal space, thyroid gland, carotid sheath, or undescended at the skull base. Supernumerary parathyroid glands may also be encountered in up to 15% of patients.

The embryology of the parathyroid glands explains the potential anatomic variants of parathyroid location. The inferior glands arise from the third branchial pouches, and the superior from the fourth. Other glands associated with these branchial pouches include the thymus (third) and the thyroid (fourth). During embryologic migration the superior parathyroids migrate with the thyroid gland along a relatively short path. Superior glands are less variable in location, probably because they have less distance to travel during migration. They remain close to the posterior aspect of the midportion of the thyroid gland. In an adult the non-pathologic superior parathyroid glands are usually (85%) found on the posterior aspect of the thyroid, in an area within one centimeter of the crossing of the inferior thyroid artery and recurrent laryngeal nerve. The inferior parathyroids migrate along with the thymus, and have a relatively long migration path. Subsequently, the final location of the inferior parathyroid glands is much more variable. During migration, the thymus and inferior parathyroids are both drawn toward the anterior mediastinum. The inferior parathyroid glands usually halt their migration in the neck at the level of the inferior pole of the thyroid lobe. It is not uncommon to find normal glands in the thyrothymic ligament, or in the cervical thymus.

The superior parathyroid glands usually retain their posterior relationship to the recurrent laryngeal nerve, and the inferior glands are almost always found anterior to the nerve. The inferior parathyroid gland crosses the superior gland during embryologic migration, and consequently the two glands can sometimes be found very closely associated with each other. This usually occurs at the level of the insertion of the inferior thyroid artery into the thyroid gland. Sometimes it may be very difficult to separate or distinguish the two glands; however parathyroid glands always have independent vascular pedicles, regardless of how intimate they are with the other parathyroid gland. In 80% of cases the parathyroid glands are supplied by a single branch of the inferior thyroid artery. In the remaining 20% the arterial supply may be branched. Also, in approximately 20% of cases the blood supply to the superior parathyroid glands is derived from the superior thyroid artery [8].

About 13% of patients have five glands and about 3% have three glands [9]. Superior glands are symmetric in about 80% of cases and inferior glands in about 70% of cases [9].

27.3 Causes of Persistent and Recurrent Hyperparathyroidism

To successfully treat patients for persistent or recurrent HPTH it is essential to understand why treatment failures occur. Treatment failures may be caused by factors associated with the initial surgery, the patient's anatomy, or the biology of the disease. Each of these factors may act independently or in concert. Surgeon inexperience leading to faulty operative technique is a significant contributor to initial treatment failure. Variations in gland number or migration pattern may also contribute to the failure rate. Multigland disease (sporadic or familial), malignancy, and parathyromatosis all create considerable difficulty in the management of HPTH.

27.3.1 Persistent Hyperparathyroidism

The most common cause of persistent HPTH is the failure to identify and/or remove the abnormal parathyroid tissue. This may be due to an ectopic adenoma or failure to identify an adenoma in the normal anatomic position. Failure to identify and remove a second abnormal gland in the case of double adenoma will probably become more common in the age of focused minimally invasive parathyroidectomy. Inadequate or subtotal resection of abnormal parathyroid tissue can occur when an inappropriately large remnant is left during a three and one-half gland parathyroidectomy, or when abnormally shaped adenomas are inadvertently subtotally resected. Parathyromatosis and parathyroid carcinoma with residual or metastatic disease can cause persistence of HPTH, and are quite challenging to treat.

27.3.2 Recurrent Hyperparathyroidism

The etiology of recurrent HPTH is usually distinct from that of persistent disease. The most common cause of recurrent HPTH is the regrowth of abnormal parathyroid tissue. This is most common in inherited syndromes such as familial HPTH and multiple endocrine neoplasia (MEN). Regrowth of autotransplanted parathyroid tissue in MEN and secondary HPTH is commonly seen as well. Parathyromatosis and recurrent or metastatic parathyroid carcinoma may also cause recurrent HPTH.

27.4 Is Reoperation Indicated? Why Reoperate?

The symptoms and metabolic complications associated with HPTH are legion, and their enumeration is beyond the scope of this chapter. The indications for reoperative parathyroidectomy are essentially the same as for initial exploration. There may be a slightly higher threshold for surgery for persistent and recurrent HPTH because the operative risks are slightly higher than at initial operation. There is general agreement that surgery is indicated for all patients with HPTH who are younger than 50 years old, or who have serum calcium greater than 11.5 mg/dl. Furthermore, most physicians also agree that surgery is indicated for all patients who are symptomatic due to their HPTH. Successful surgery can significantly benefit these patients [10]. In fact, parathyroidectomy improves symptoms in approximately 85% of patients

with primary HPTH, including those who are considered asymptomatic [11]. With hypercalcemia alleviated there is improvement in a wide range of symptoms. The greatest improvement is in those patients with the most severe complications, such as osteitis fibrosa cystica, nephrolithiasis, and pancreatitis. Other complications such as osteoporosis and osteopenia are also substantially improved. In some patients bone density can increase by as much as 20% one year following successful parathyroid surgery [12]. Most of the non-specific symptoms of HPTH, such as weakness, fatigue and lethargy, joint and bone pain, and depression, are improved by parathyroidectomy. Several studies have also suggested that surgical cure of HPTH may also decrease the risk of premature death from cardiovascular disease and cancer [13–16].

27.5 Preoperative Strategy

27.5.1 Reconfirm the Diagnosis of Hyperparathyroidism

Prior to reoperation the diagnosis of HPTH must be reconfirmed. The first step is to perform a thorough personal and family history and physical examination. The history should be focused on identifying misdiagnoses such as benign familial hypocalciuric hypercalcemia (BFHH; discussed below), idiopathic hypercalciuria, and malignancy. A review of the biochemical studies that initially established the diagnosis of HPTH is essential. Biochemical studies done following surgery should be reviewed as well to differentiate between persistent and recurrent HPTH. The diagnosis of HPTH is confirmed by elevated serum calcium and intact PTH, without hypocalciuria. Elevated serum calcium with a normal but inappropriately high PTH can be a clinical conundrum. We consider these patients to have primary HPTH. Patients may also present with elevated PTH but total serum calcium levels at the upper limit of normal. Checking an ionized calcium level can help confirm the diagnosis of HPTH in most of these patients. Some patients will have idiopathic hypercalciuria, which is discussed below.

The next step is to repeat a complete set of biochemical tests including concomitant serum calcium and intact PTH, and a 24-hour urinary calcium clearance. Patients with hypocalciuria may have benign familial hypocalciuric hypercalcemia (BFHH), a rare inherited condition characterized by mildly elevated serum calcium and PTH and low urinary calcium (clearance <100 mg/day). The serum magnesium may be high, and the ratio of urinary calcium clearance to creatinine is less than 0.01. These patients do not benefit from parathyroidectomy. A careful family history will often shed light on this diagnosis. Sadly, a history of family members with failed parathyroid operations is commonly found.

Idiopathic hypercalciuria (formerly known as "renal leak" hypercalciuria) can also be mistaken for normocalcemic primary HPTH. These patients are usually normocalcemic, but have elevated PTH, kidney stones, and osteoporosis. These patients should be treated with a thiazide diuretic (e.g., hydrochlorothiazide, 25 mg p.o. b.i.d. for 10 days) to decrease urinary calcium loss. Following this treatment the PTH and urinary calcium transiently return to normal in patients with idiopathic hypercalciuria. The PTH and urinary calcium do not normalize in patients with normocalcemic HPTH. Patients with BFHH or idiopathic hypercalciuria, who were initially operated on due to a misdiagnosis of HPTH, will not benefit from further surgery.

A third possible cause of initial misdiagnosis is hypercalcemia of malignancy. This occurs most commonly in the setting of advanced malignancy with bone metastases and is also known as local osteolytic hypercalcemia. Humoral hypercalcemia of malignancy is more uncommon and is caused by the elaboration of PTH [17] or PTH-related peptide (PTHrP) by the tumor, or $1,25(OH)_2D$ (as is seen in lymphoma) [18]. Hypercalcemia of malignancy should be suspected when there is a history of cancer that frequently metastasizes to bone, such as breast carcinoma. Documentation of an elevated serum intact PTH usually rules out the possibility of hypercalcemia of malignancy, other than the very rare tumor that produces PTH. The diagnosis of hypercalcemia of malignancy is supported biochemically by detection of PTHrP or increased urinary cyclic AMP (cAMP) levels in association with low or normal serum PTH levels.

Following successful parathyroidectomy some patients may have a persistent elevation of the PTH level despite clinical cure of hypercalcemia [19]. This occurs most commonly in patients who have had profound HPTH preoperatively, especially those patients with elevated preoperative alkaline phosphatase who develop "bone hunger" postoperatively, or in patients with renal dysfunction. In patients with severe bone disease, the PTH level may return to normal only after several months, and with oral calcium supplementation.

27.5.2 Review the Old Localization Studies, Operative Notes, and Pathology Reports

Old preoperative localization studies and surgery and pathology reports are critical to help determine the location of potentially normal and abnormal glands. The extent of the parathyroidectomy, the limits of dissection and where scar tissue can be expected to be encountered, the relationship of the glands to the recurrent laryngeal nerve, and the number and position of normal and abnormal glands are all critical to operative planning. The location of a missing parathyroid adenoma can often be predicted based on information from the operative and pathology reports alone. A review of this information should be done before obtaining localization studies because the interpretation of such studies may be impacted by information in the surgical reports that suggests the presence of hyperplasia versus missed adenoma. Needless to say, documentation of prior removal of four normal parathyroid glands is very worrisome for a missed supernumerary parathyroid adenoma. Failure to perform autotransplantation of parathyroid tissue following removal of the remaining parathyroid gland would result in permanent hypoparathyroidism. This underscores the need to thoroughly evaluate the prior operative and pathology reports, and to discuss the case directly with the surgeon(s) involved in the prior operation(s).

27.5.3 Employ Complementary Localization Procedures

Since complication rates are higher and surgical cure rates are lower in reoperative parathyroidectomy, we employ extensive localization studies prior to reoperation. Ideally, localization studies will lead us toward a focused approach to a single missed adenoma if the history, prior surgical and pathologic findings, and new localization studies suggest single gland disease. Single gland disease, such as ectopic glands or missed second adenomas, are common in persistent HPTH. Multiglandular disease and hyperplasia are more common in recurrent HPTH. Approximately 90% of missed parathyroid tumors can be removed through a cervical incision.

We recommend a combination of functional and anatomic localization studies prior to reoperation due to their complementary nature. Our current practice is to start with ^{99}Tc sestamibi radionuclide scanning (Fig. 27.1) and cervical ultrasonography (US;

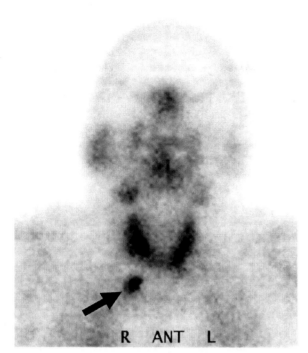

Fig. 27.1 99Tc sestamibi radionuclide scanning of an ectopic retrosternal right lower parathyroid gland (*arrow*) that has been surgically removed from the tongue of the thymus through a collar incision

Fig. 27.2). The best regimen for localizing parathyroid adenomas is a matter of some debate. Preoperative US and sestamibi scanning provide complementary information for localization of parathyroid adenomas in primary HPTH. The combined accuracy when both tests are used is 89–98%. When both tests show abnormalities at the same location the accuracy for single gland disease is about 95% [20]. When preoperative localization tests are discordant or discrepant multiple gland disease is more likely. In double adenoma, the accuracy of combined US and sestamibi was 60% in a report by Haciyanli et al. [21]. Furthermore, in double adenoma the addition of intraoperative PTH (IOPTH) measurement to US and sestamibi scanning resulted in an accuracy of 80%. When US and sestamibi studies were concordant for single gland disease the addition of IOPTH yielded a success rate of 97%.

Ultrasound is non-invasive and is the least expensive of the preoperative imaging modalities. It provides information about the size, depth, and location of the adenoma, but it is very radiologist and/or technician dependent. The typical US appearance is that of a hypoechoic homogenous well-demarcated lesion. It is possible to have a cystic component to the parathyroid adenoma, but it is usually solid. Coexisting thyroid abnormalities and intrathyroidal adenomas are also identified. US is poor for mediastinal, paraesophageal, and some ectopic locations (undescended and lateral). Sensitivity is about 70–80% and specificity is about 90–95%. It can be combined with fine-needle aspiration (FNA) of a lesion suspicious for parathyroid adenoma, and the aspirate sent for PTH assay [22–24].

Sestamibi is concentrated by the thyroid and parathyroids. It is rapidly washed out of the thyroid but is retained by the parathyroid glands; therefore the parathyroids are usually seen on delayed images at 2–4 hours. Sestamibi has a short half-life of 6 hours. It localizes in mitochondria. Parathyroid adenomas

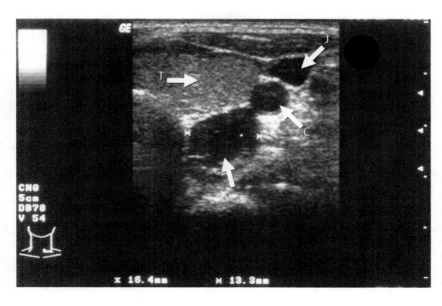

Fig. 27.2 Ultrasonographic view of a 16-mm parathyroid adenoma in the left neck. The sonographic appearance of the adenoma is typically hypoechogenic (*arrow*). The nearby anatomic structures are: *T* thyroid gland, *J* internal jugular vein, *C* carotid artery

are believed to have high metabolic activity and mitochondria-rich oxyphil cell content. The generally accepted sensitivity range for sestamibi scanning is 75–80% for single gland disease and 60% or less for multigland disease; for hyperplasia success is also low at 50–60%. Sestamibi scanning is not as anatomically precise as US, but is not limited by mediastinal gland location. There is minimal operator dependence, and its success depends less on the size of the gland. The causes of false-negative sestamibi scans include small glands (<100 mg), parathyroid hyperplasia, multiple adenomas, and delayed washout from the thyroid (multinodular goiter, Hashimoto's thyroiditis, adenomatous nodules, and thyroid carcinoma). False-positive sestamibi studies may be due to sarcoidosis, carcinoid disease, lymph nodes, adenomatous nodules, and thyroid carcinoma. ^{99}Tc sestamibi single-photon emission computed tomography (MIBI-SPECT) is a method to generate a three-dimensional image of the tracer distribution. It can be helpful in discriminating between anterior mediastinal versus aorticopulmonary window glands.

On magnetic resonance imaging (MRI), parathyroid adenomas show enhancement on T2-weighted images (Fig. 27.3). They are isointense on T1 (Fig. 27.4). Parathyroid glands usually also enhance with gadolinium. Sensitivity is about 80% for glands in the neck and 90% for glands in the mediastinum. For hyperplasia, the sensitivity is about 70%. MRI is particularly useful for ectopic sites such as the mediastinum.

Computed tomography (CT) of the parathyroids should be done with thin (3-5 mm) cuts. Only 25% of adenomas enhance with i.v. contrast (Fig. 27.5). The use of iodinated contrast obviates the use of nuclear imaging or radioiodine treatment for 6–8 weeks which may be important for some patients with concomitant thyroid disease. The sensitivity of CT is about 55%, and specificity is as high as 98% for single gland disease, but only 40% for hyperplasia.

Highly selective venous catheterization (SVC) can be performed by experienced interventionalists by placing catheters in tributaries that drain regions of the neck where parathyroid adenomas are likely to be. The major disadvantage of this invasive localization study is that it merely lateralizes disease. We have limited the use of highly selective venous catheterization for PTH to those cases when US, sestamibi, and MRI are negative, equivocal, or reveal different glands. We employ this study in only about 10% of our reoperative cases.

Selective transarterial angiography is another invasive method for imaging and treatment of parathyroid adenomas (Fig. 27.6). Angiographic ablation, the deliberate injection of large doses of contrast material into the artery that selectively perfuses the adenoma, may be successful in up to 73% of cases [25].

Localization studies fail when there is coexistent disease such as thyroid cancer or adenomatous thyroid nodules which cause false-positive US or sestamibi studies. Also, sarcoid and carcinoid disease may take up sestamibi and give a false-positive result. Prior

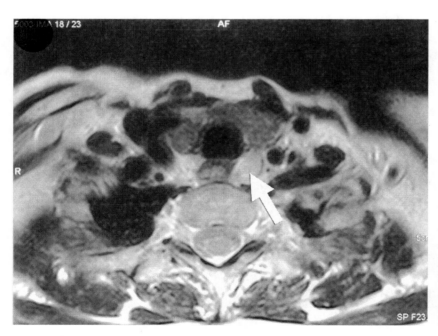

Fig. 27.3 MR image of an upper left parathyroid adenoma (*arrow*) in the neck in a paraesophageal location. Note the gadolinium enhancement in the T2-weighted scan

thyroid or parathyroid operations are also associated with a lower accuracy for US and SVC studies. Multiglandular disease, whether sporadic or associated with MEN or familial HPTH, is associated with lower sensitivity for US and sestamibi studies.

27.5.4 Discuss Risks with Patient

The risks of reoperative parathyroidectomy are higher than at initial neck exploration. Vocal cord paralysis can occur in up to 4–10% of reoperative cases [26–28]. An evaluation of vocal cord function prior to reoperation by direct or indirect laryngoscopy is important because some patients with unilateral vocal cord paralysis are difficult to diagnose clinically. Inadvertent damage to the contralateral recurrent laryngeal nerve would necessitate potentially permanent tracheostomy. Patients should understand their individual risk of nerve injury and tracheostomy before surgery.

Transient postoperative hypocalcemia is common following parathyroid surgery. Approximately 10–20%

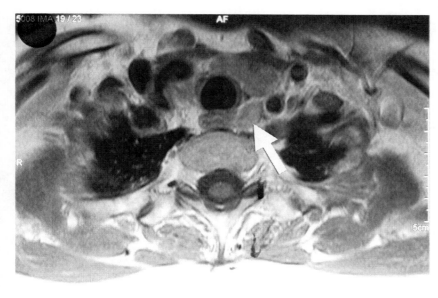

Fig. 27.4 MR image of the same gland (*arrow*) as depicted in Fig. 27.3. The T1-weighted scan shows an isointense signal of the adenoma compared with the thyroid parenchyma

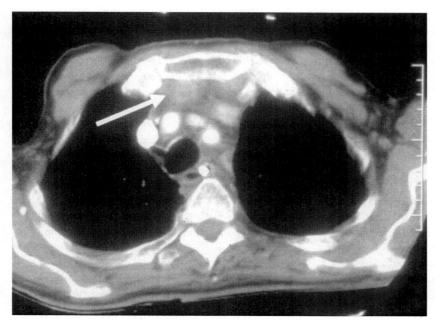

Fig. 27.5 CT scan of an ectopic retrosternal adenoma (*arrow*) in the arterial phase after i.v. contrast dye administration

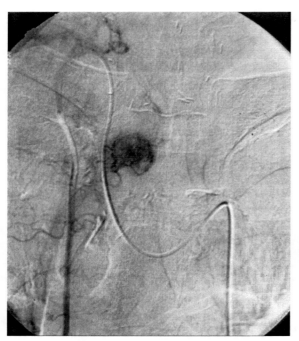

Fig. 27.6 Super-selective angiography of the right internal mammary artery shows the contrast flush of the ectopic gland that is also depicted in Fig. 27.5

of patients may have permanent hypoparathyroidism following reoperation, but there are reports of up to a 35% incidence of permanent hypoparathyroidism [29–31]. Knowledge of the remaining parathyroid anatomy will hopefully prevent the removal of all remaining parathyroid tissue in these patients.

Persistent hypercalcemia may occur in 5–10% of patients reoperated for persistent or recurrent HPTH [30]. Patients with familial HPTH, parathyroid carcinoma, parathyromatosis, or who have unlocalized ectopic adenomas are more likely to have a failed reoperation.

27.6   Operative Strategy

27.6.1   Choose an Appropriate Time and Operative Approach

Reoperative surgery is easiest within the first week or after 3 months because of scar formation. The optimal strategy is a focused exploration, avoiding the need for placing both recurrent laryngeal nerves and any contralateral remaining parathyroid tissue at risk. This type of focused exploration reduces the risk of permanent hypoparathyroidism and nerve injury. When entering the reoperative neck it is beneficial to

use the lateral or "back door" approach to the central neck (Fig. 27.7). This is done by dissecting medial to the sternocleidomastoid muscle but lateral to the strap muscles and thyroid. Dissection is carried down medial to the carotid sheath, and the thyroid and strap muscles are retracted anteromedially to reveal the central neck. This usually allows dissection through a relatively undisturbed field posterior to the plane used during the standard anterior approach. Great care must be taken to avoid injuring the recurrent laryngeal nerve during this dissection technique.

The operative approach should also be tailored to the identity of the missing parathyroid gland(s). You can usually determine if a missed adenoma is a superior or inferior gland based on review of the operative and pathology reports. The lateral approach is most beneficial in the case of a missing superior parathyroid gland. Even in an ectopic location, the superior glands usually maintain their posterior relationship to the recurrent laryngeal nerve. The search for missing inferior glands is best accomplished through an anterior approach. These tumors are almost always located anterior to the recurrent laryngeal nerve, and there should be no need to dissect in the region of the recurrent laryngeal nerve through a previously operated field.

27.6.2   Consider Ectopic or Unusual Locations (Know Where to Look)

Most missed glands (approximately 40%) are located in the normal location. The thymus (approximately 10%), and the anterior mediastinum (approximately 13%) are also common locations for missed single adenomas. Other less common sites include paraesophageal (approximately 6%), intrathyroidal (approximately 5%), the carotid sheath (approximately 2%), and undescended (approximately 1%) [30]. When a superior gland is suspected it is most likely located low in the neck in the tracheoesophageal groove, or in the posterior superior mediastinum. A superior gland may also be found in the carotid sheath. As discussed above, superior glands have a shorter migration path during embryogenesis and are, therefore, less likely to be in ectopic locations than inferior glands. When an inferior gland is suspected it can usually be found in the thyrothymic ligament or in the thymus itself in the anterior superior mediastinum. Most mediastinal adenomas (80%) are located close to or within the thymus. Because the blood supply to these glands is from the inferior thyroid artery, most can safely be removed through a cervical approach without risking uncontrollable hemorrhage. Parathyroid tumors

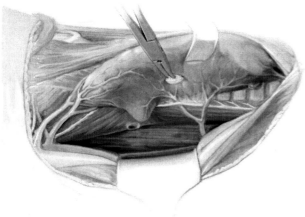

Fig. 27.7 The so-called "back door" approach to the thyroid and parathyroid glands on the right side

located in the aortopulmonary window are not amenable to cervical resection and should be an indication for transthoracic removal.

27.6.3 Consider Using IOPTH or Other Intraoperative Localization Techniques

Intraoperative PTH measurement was made feasible by the development of an assay for intact PTH in 1987. Intact PTH is rapidly cleared by the kidneys and has a half-life of about 5 minutes. Blood is drawn from the patient during surgery either from a peripheral vein by the anesthesiologist or one of the internal jugular veins by the surgeon. Post-parathyroidectomy PTH values are compared to baseline values. A drop of PTH greater than 50% from the highest pre-incision or pre-excision value is considered predictive of success by some surgeons [20, 32–35]. At some centers they also require that the PTH fall into the normal range. PTH in the serum is measured by microbeads coated with goat anti-human PTH antibody specific for one end of the molecule. A second antibody binds to the other end of the molecule, and in doing so creates a luminescent reaction that can be measured by colorimeter. Accuracy of intraoperative PTH is being examined by our group and others. Some studies have revealed that an appropriate fall in IOPTH predicts cure approximately 95% of the time or better [32,36,37], but other studies show that the accuracy in primary HPTH may only be as high as about 80% [20,34].

Intraoperative ultrasound (IOUS) is especially helpful for identifying intrathyroidal parathyroid adenomas, and should reduce the need for blind hemithyroidectomy. The US can also be combined with needle aspiration for PTH to interrogate hypo-echoic structures identified in the thyroid or neck intraoperatively.

The hand-held gamma probe can also be used intraoperatively to identify parathyroid glands. The patient is given an intravenous dose of radiolabeled sestamibi approximately 2 hours before surgery. The probe is then used to scan areas of the neck and mark out areas of high isotope concentration to guide the surgery. In our hands it is not a consistently reliable tool, and it does not appear to be cost-effective when compared to preoperative imaging. Other investigators have also reported a high false-negative rate with this technique [36].

27.6.4 Employ Cryopreservation

The use of cryopreservation is important in cases where several parathyroid glands have already been removed, or if prior surgery has placed the parathyroid glands at risk for inadvertent resection or ischemic necrosis. The removal of all remaining parathyroid tissue would result in permanent hypoparathyroidism requiring the lifelong administration of calcium and vitamin D. Patients who have had a subtotal parathyroid resection but who still suffer from persistent or recurrent HPTH may require cryopreservation.

27.7 Results of Surgery for Recurrent or Persistent Hyperparathyroidism

The results of reoperative parathyroid surgery are usually not as good as a first-time operation for HPTH. Cure rates have been reported to be as high as 95% [27,38], however most authors report that the success rate for reoperative surgery is approximately 90% [26,30,31,39–42]. Furthermore, there appears to be a much greater risk of complications, such as temporary or permanent nerve injury (4–10%) or hypoparathyroidism (10–20%), after reoperative surgery [31,39,42,43]. Hopefully, by employing the methods and caveats highlighted in this chapter, success will be maximized, while minimizing the rate of complications such as failed exploration, nerve injury, and permanent hypoparathyroidism.

27.8   Summary

Overall, about 5–10% of patients operated on for primary HPTH develop persistent or recurrent disease. Persistent HPTH is usually due to a missed parathyroid adenoma, whereas recurrence is most often a function of the underlying disease process. Treatment failures may be caused by factors associated with the index operation, aberrant anatomy, or the biology of disease. Each of these factors may act independently or in concert to thwart the efforts of experienced endocrine surgeons.

The most common cause of persistent HPTH is the failure to identify or remove abnormal parathyroid tissue. This may be from failure to identify an adenoma in the normal anatomic position or in predictable ectopic locations. The most common cause of recurrent HPTH is the regrowth of abnormal parathyroid tissue. This is most often seen in multiglandular or inherited syndromes such as familial HPTH and MEN.

A sound preoperative strategy is central to successful management of persistent or recurrent disease. After confirming the diagnosis a thorough review of all old localization studies, operative notes, and pathology reports is necessary. Complementary localization studies should be repeated to localize or at least lateralize the disease process. An evaluation of vocal cord function should also be done. The patient should be aware of the increased risk of complications and failure to cure HPTH that accompanies reoperation. An operative approach should be chosen based on data from the prior surgery and new preoperative studies, and knowledge of parathyroid ectopias. The use of adjunctive measures such as IOPTH or intraoperative localization tools should be strongly considered. A low threshold for cryopreservation and/or autotransplantation of resected parathyroid tissue is wise in many cases.

References

1. Clark OH (1998) Symposium: parathyroid disease, part 1. Contemp Surg 52:137–152
2. Malmaeus J, Granberg PO, et al (1988) Parathyroid surgery in Scandinavia. Acta Chir Scand 154:409–413
3. Caron N, Sturgeon C, et al (2004) Persistent and recurrent hyperparathyroidism. Curr Treat Options Oncol 5:335–345
4. Wadstrom C, Zedenius J, et al (1998) Re-operative surgery for recurrent or persistent primary hyperparathyroidism. Aust N Z J Surg 68:103–107
5. Mundschenk J, Klose S, et al (1999) Diagnostic strategies and surgical procedures in persistent or recurrent primary hyperparathyroidism. Exp Clin Endocrinol Diabetes 107:331–336
6. al-Fehaily M, Clark OH (2003) Persistent or recurrent primary hyperparathyroidism. Ann Ital Chir 74:423–434
7. Kebebew E (2001) Parathyroid carcinoma. Curr Treat Options Oncol 2:347–354
8. Bliss RD, Gauger PG, et al (2000) Surgeon's approach to the thyroid gland: surgical anatomy and the importance of technique. World J Surg 24:891–897
9. Akerstrom G, Malmaeus J, et al (1984) Surgical anatomy of human parathyroid glands. Surgery 95:14–21
10. Eigelberger MS, Cheah WK, et al (2004) The NIH criteria for parathyroidectomy in asymptomatic primary hyperparathyroidism: are they too limited? Ann Surg 239:1–8
11. Sywak MS, Knowlton ST, et al (2002) Do the National Institutes of Health consensus guidelines for parathyroidectomy predict symptom severity and surgical outcome in patients with primary hyperparathyroidism? Surgery 132:1013–1019; discussion 1019–1020
12. Abdelhadi M, Nordenstrom J (1998) Bone mineral recovery after parathyroidectomy in patients with primary and renal hyperparathyroidism. J Clin Endocrinol Metab 83:3845–3851
13. Palmer M, Adami HO, et al (1987) Survival and renal function in untreated hypercalcaemia. Population-based cohort study with 14 years of follow-up. Lancet 1:59–62
14. Hedback G, Tisell LE, et al (1990) Premature death in patients operated on for primary hyperparathyroidism. World J Surg 14:829–835; discussion 836
15. Hedback G, Oden A (1998) Increased risk of death from primary hyperparathyroidism: an update. Eur J Clin Invest 28:271–276
16. Hedback G, Oden A (1998) Death risk factor analysis in primary hyperparathyroidism. Eur J Clin Invest 28:1011–1018
17. Strewler GJ, Budayr AA, et al (1993) Production of parathyroid hormone by a malignant nonparathyroid tumor in a hypercalcemic patient. J Clin Endocrinol Metab 76:1373–1375

18. Spiegel AM (2003) The parathyroid glands, hypercalcemia, and hypocalcemia. In: Goldman L, Bennett JC (eds) Cecil textbook of medicine. Saunders, Philadelphia, pp 1398–1406

19. Mittendorf EA, McHenry CR (2002) Persistent parathyroid hormone elevation following curative parathyroidectomy for primary hyperparathyroidism. Arch Otolaryngol Head Neck Surg 128:275–279

20. Miura D, Wada N, et al (2002) Does intraoperative quick parathyroid hormone assay improve the results of parathyroidectomy? World J Surg 26:926–930

21. Haciyanli M, Lal G, et al (2003) Accuracy of preoperative localization studies and intraoperative parathyroid hormone assay in patients with primary hyperparathyroidism and double adenoma. J Am Coll Surg 197:739–746

22. Doppman JL, Krudy AG, et al (1983) Aspiration of enlarged parathyroid glands for parathyroid hormone assay. Radiology 148:31–35

23. Abati A, Skarulis MC, et al (1995) Ultrasound-guided fine-needle aspiration of parathyroid lesions: a morphological and immunocytochemical approach. Hum Pathol 26:338–343

24. Tseng FY, Hsiao YL, et al (2002) Ultrasound-guided fine needle aspiration cytology of parathyroid lesions. A review of 72 cases. Acta Cytol 46:1029–1036

25. Doherty GM, Doppman JL, Miller DL, Gee MS, Marx SJ, Spiegel AM, Aurbach GC, Pass, HI, Brennan MF, Nortno JA (1992) Results of a multidisciplinary strategy for management of mediastinal parathyroid adenomas as a cause of persistent primary hyperparathyroidism. Ann Surg 215:101–106

26. Brennan MF, Norton JA (1985) Reoperation for persistent and recurrent hyperparathyroidism. Ann Surg 201:40–44

27. Shen W, Duren M, et al (1996) Reoperation for persistent or recurrent primary hyperparathyroidism. Arch Surg 131:861–867; discussion 867–869

28. Mariette C, Pellissier L, et al (1998) Reoperation for persistent or recurrent primary hyperparathyroidism. Langenbecks Arch Surg 383:174–179

29. Brennan MF, Doppman JL, et al (1982) Assessment of techniques for preoperative parathyroid gland localization in patients undergoing reoperation for hyperparathyroidism. Surgery 91:6–11

30. Lo C-Y, van Heerden JA (1997) Parathyroid reoperations. In: Clark OH, Duh QY (eds) Textbook of endocrine surgery. Saunders, Philadelphia, pp 411–417

31. Gaz RD (2003) Revision parathyroid surgery. In: Randolph GW (ed) Surgery of the thyroid and parathyroid glands. Saunders, Philadelphia, pp 564–570

32. Irvin GL 3rd, Dembrow VD, et al (1993) Clinical usefulness of an intraoperative "quick parathyroid hormone" assay. Surgery 114:1019–1022; discussion 1022–1023

33. Henry JF, Iacobone M, et al (2001) Indications and results of video-assisted parathyroidectomy by a lateral approach in patients with primary hyperparathyroidism. Surgery 130:999–1004

34. Perrier ND, Ituarte PH, et al (2002) Parathyroid surgery: separating promise from reality. J Clin Endocrinol Metab 87:1024–1029

35. Lo CY, Chan WF, et al (2003) Minimally invasive endoscopic-assisted parathyroidectomy for primary hyperparathyroidism. Surg Endosc 17:1932–1936

35. Burkey SH, Van Heerden JA, et al (2002) Will directed parathyroidectomy utilizing the gamma probe or intraoperative parathyroid hormone assay replace bilateral cervical exploration as the preferred operation for primary hyperparathyroidism? World J Surg 26:914–920

37. Westerdahl J, Lindblom P, et al (2002) Measurement of intraoperative parathyroid hormone predicts long-term operative success. Arch Surg 137:186–190

38. Carty SE, Norton JA (1991) Management of patients with persistent or recurrent primary hyperparathyroidism. World J Surg 15:716–723

39. Wang CA (1977) Parathyroid re-exploration. A clinical and pathological study of 112 cases. Ann Surg 186:140–145

40. Grant CS, van Heerden JA, et al (1986) Clinical management of persistent and/or recurrent primary hyperparathyroidism. World J Surg 10:555–565

41. Levin KE, Clark OH (1989) The reasons for failure in parathyroid operations. Arch Surg 124:911–914; discussion 914–915

42. Akerstrom G, Rudberg C, et al (1992) Causes of failed primary exploration and technical aspects of re-operation in primary hyperparathyroidism. World J Surg 16:562–568; discussion 568–569

43. Jaskowiak N, Norton JA, et al (1996) A prospective trial evaluating a standard approach to reoperation for missed parathyroid adenoma. Ann Surg 224:308–320; discussion 320–321

28 Outcomes Analysis in Parathyroid Surgery

Leon D. Boudourakis and Julie Ann Sosa

28.1 Introduction

Primary hyperparathyroidism (HPTH) is the unregulated overproduction of parathyroid hormone (PTH) resulting in abnormal calcium homeostasis. Epidemiologic data suggest that the prevalence of this disease is 4 cases per 100,000 persons in the USA [1]. As the third most prevalent endocrine disorder after diabetes mellitus and thyroid disease, primary HPTH is an important public health concern. It is a disorder which affects women at least twice as frequently as men, and the elderly much more than the young. Parathyroidectomy, the only potential cure for primary HPTH, was estimated to cost $282 million annually in the USA in 1998 [2]. Overall expenditures (including direct and indirect costs) attributed to this disease can be presumed to be much greater today, although no reliable estimate has been published to date [3].

With advancements in laboratory medicine and the development of automated serum screening in the 1970s, the clinical profile of primary HPTH shifted from the classic hypercalcemic symptoms of "bones, moans, stones, and abdominal groans" to asymptomatic or "minimally symptomatic" disease, whereby the diagnosis is established in asymptomatic patients when hypercalcemia is incidentally discovered based on a routine chemistry panel. Likewise, the surgical management of primary HPTH has evolved with the advent of minimally invasive parathyroidectomy (MIP) and the development of the rapid PTH assay. Together, these technologies have revolutionized parathyroidectomy from a procedure performed under general anesthesia with bilateral neck exploration to a safer, less-invasive procedure performed in the ambulatory setting through a smaller incision with unilateral neck exploration. Given this frameshift in the epidemiology of primary HPTH, the advent of new technologies, and a relative paucity of parathyroidectomy outcomes research, there continues to be controversy about the optimal threshold for early surgical referral.

28.2 Early Parathyroid Surgery

The original description of the parathyroid gland was made from the dissection of an Indian rhinoceros in 1850 by Sir Richard Owen [4]. However, it was not until 37 years later that a histologic analysis was performed by the Swedish medical student, Ivar Sandström. His description of the "glandularae parathyreoidae" attracted little, if any, immediate attention [5]. Early insight into the function of the parathyroids was serendipitous. Anton Wolfer described tetany in a patient who underwent thyroidectomy and incidental total parathyroidectomy in 1879 [6]. Ironically, it was a poor outcome following thyroidectomy that led to a better understanding of the parathyroids.

Diseases attributed to the parathyroids were managed with surgery as early as the 1920s. Famous patients include the Viennese tram-car conductor Albert Gahne, who underwent two operations by Felix Mandl, and the Merchant Marine captain Charles Martell, who underwent seven operations by Oliver

Cope and others in New York and Boston; ultimately, a mediastinal parathyroid adenoma was removed [7,8]. Unfortunately, Gahne and Martell succumbed to their disease, and it was not until Issac Olch removed a large parathyroid adenoma from Elva Dawkins in St Louis in 1928 that the first successful parathyroidectomy was documented in the USA. However, this was not without postoperative complications; Dawkins suffered from severe hypocalcemia requiring parathyroid extract and calcium supplementation [9,10]. Thus, early outcomes from parathyroidectomy were dismal, in part because of the relative lack of experience of the surgeons performing the operations (see also Chapter 1 "History of Thyroid and Parathyroid Surgery").

28.3   Obstacles to Performing Parathyroidectomy Outcomes Research

The first efforts to systematically study outcomes in surgery date from 1979, when Luft and colleagues demonstrated lower mortality rates at high-volume centers compared with low-volume centers in high-risk procedures such as coronary artery bypass graft surgery (CABG), vascular surgery, and transurethral prostatectomy. These studies relentlessly demonstrated a statistically significant association between hospital volume and procedure-specific mortality rates. Patient-mix-adjusted mortality rates were lower by 25% to 41% at hospitals performing more than 200 procedures per year [11]. This set the groundwork for outcomes research for a litany of other high-risk, morbid procedures and mortal diseases, where in-hospital and 30-day mortality were meaningful endpoints.

Lower-risk surgical procedures, such as parathyroidectomy, have received less attention among health services researchers, in large part because mortality is not a meaningful outcome. Large administrative databases conventionally used for surgical outcomes research are most reliable for definitive outcomes, such as death, which hospital coders easily capture. In contrast, outcomes from parathyroidectomy are often difficult to establish and are measurable only in a delayed fashion after discharge. Also, many claims databases capture inpatient data only, and thus the assessment of complications potentially occurring after discharge may be inaccurate. For example, cure after parathyroidectomy is defined as a normal serum calcium level six months after surgery. Complications from surgery such as laryngeal nerve injury and permanent hypoparathyroidism also can be hard to cap-

ture. Neurapraxia is transient, while other laryngeal nerve injuries can be permanent. Indirect laryngoscopy is often delayed several months to distinguish between the two and allow temporary changes to resolve. MIP is performed in the ambulatory setting, so symptoms and signs of hypoparathyroidism usually are not apparent until well-after discharge, at which point patients typically are managed in the outpatient setting with calcium and/or vitamin D supplementation. Thus, they are not captured by many databases.

To date, there has not been a prospective, controlled, multi-institutional trial comparing the clinical and economic outcomes for newer surgical techniques, such as MIP or radio-guided parathyroidectomy, with traditional parathyroidectomy or medical strategies in the management of asymptomatic and minimally symptomatic primary HPTH.

28.4   Predictors of Outcomes for Parathyroidectomy

28.4.1   Patient Demographics

There is a substantial body of evidence showing that patients with primary HPTH who are younger than 50 years are at particular risk for going on to develop complications from their disease, such as reduced bone mineral density. As a result, the Consensus Development Conference on Asymptomatic Primary HPTH in 1990 and the Workshop on Asymptomatic Primary HPTH in 2002 held at the National Institutes of Health (NIH) both recommended that all of these patients should be referred for surgical management [12,13]. However, the implication should not be that patients older than 50 years must be treated non-operatively. Recent data suggested that parathyroidectomy is safe in elderly patients and is associated with high cure rates, low morbidity, short lengths of stay (LOS), and high patient satisfaction.

In a prospective study of 211 patients who underwent parathyroidectomy by one surgeon, Chen et al. compared outcome data of elderly patients (>70 years of age, $n = 36$) to younger patients (<70 years of age, $n = 148$) with hyperparathyroidism. Preoperative symptoms of mental impairment, bone disease, and fatigue were more common in elderly patients ($P<0.05$), and nephrolithiasis was more frequent in younger patients ($P<0.03$). Despite the higher preoperative PTH levels among the elderly cohort compared to the younger cohort (301.9±63.3 versus 169.2±14.3 pg/ml, respectively; $P<0.05$), the rates of cure, morbidity, and mortality associated with parathyroidectomy were comparable (94.4%, 5.5%, and 0% for the elderly versus 98%, 1.4%, and 0% for younger patients). The more advanced disease seen in elderly patients suggests that they are referred for surgery with a higher threshold than younger patients. However, the study results suggest that the benefits of parathyroidectomy outweigh the risks and argue for a lower threshold for referral [14].

28.4.2 Hospital Volume and Surgeon Experience

In 2002, Birkmeyer et al. firmly established the association between hospital volume and outcomes for high-risk procedures by examining the experience of 2.5 million patients using data from the Nationwide Inpatient Sample (NIS) and the Medicare claims database [15]. Over a six-year period, operative mortality was shown to decrease as hospital volume increased for 14 types of procedures; absolute differences in adjusted mortality rates between very low and very high volume hospitals ranged from over 12% for pancreatic resection to 0.2% for carotid endarterectomy.

However, there is no evidence that such a relationship exists for relatively low risk parathyroidectomy. There is evidence that outcomes from parathyroidectomy vary widely between individual surgeons and are associated with surgeon experience [16]. Whereas outcomes in high-risk surgery are dependent on hospital volume, outcomes from parathyroidectomy appear to be dependent on individual surgeon skill.

Sosa et al. used a survey of North American members of the American Association of Endocrine Surgeons (AAES) to assess the relationship between physician characteristics, practice patterns, and outcomes [16]. There was a 77% survey response rate. Compared to high-volume surgeons (>50 cases/year), low-volume surgeons (1–15 cases/year) reported significantly higher complication rates after primary operation (1.0% versus 1.9%, respectively; $P<0.01$), higher reoperation rates (1.55 versus 3.8%; $P<0.001$), and higher mortality rates (0.04% versus 1.0%; $P<0.05$) (Table 28.1). The associations between current surgical volume and outcomes were present even when adjustment was made for the number of years surgeons had been in practice. According to the survey, high-volume surgeons also tended to have lower thresholds to operate with respect to abnormalities in preoperative creatinine clearance, bone densitometry changes, and levels of intact PTH and urinary calcium compared with lower-volume surgeons (Fig. 28.1). Even among a group of high-volume endocrine surgeons, practice patterns and thresholds for surgery varied significantly. The results of this survey almost certainly underestimate the practice pattern variation that exists in the broader surgical community, where surgeons generally have less endocrine surgery expertise and less experience performing parathyroidectomies.

It should be noted that a limitation of this study was that survey results were based on self-report, leading to the potential for respondent reporting bias. Ultimately, it is impossible from a cross-sectional study such as this to prove causation, as temporal effects

Table 28.1 Self-reported outcomes of parathyroidectomy and their association with surgeon annual caseload. (*NS* Not significant; $P>0.05$)

Outcome	Primary operation		Reoperation	
	Percent with outcome (mean ± SEM)	Outcome-caseload P value [a]	Percent with outcome (mean ± SEM)	Outcome-caseload P value [a]
Eucalcemia 6 months postoperative	95.2±1.0	<0.01	82.7±2.5	NS
Hypocalcemia 6 months postoperative	2.7±1.1	NS	6.3±1.4	NS
Hypercalcemia 6 months postoperative	3.4±1.0	<0.05	8.4±1.2	NS
Minor complications	2.9±0.6	NS	3.3±0.8	NS
Major complications	1.0±0.1	<0.01	2.0±0.2	<0.01
In-hospital death	0.1±0.03	NS	0.1±0.03	NS

[a] *P* value of linear regression model with specified outcome as dependent variable and surgeon's parathyroidectomy caseload as the independent variable

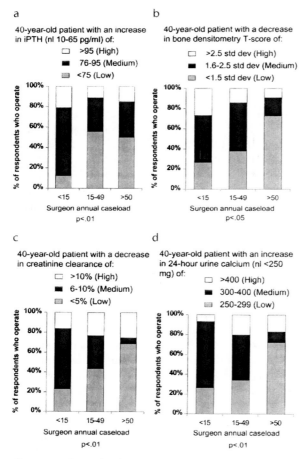

a 40-year-old patient with an increase in iPTH (nl 10-65 pg/ml) of:
- □ >95 (High)
- ■ 76-95 (Medium)
- ▨ <75 (Low)

b 40-year-old patient with a decrease in bone densitometry T-score of:
- □ >2.5 std dev (High)
- ■ 1.6-2.5 std dev (Medium)
- ▨ <1.5 std dev (Low)

c 40-year-old patient with a decrease in creatinine clearance of:
- □ >10% (High)
- ■ 6-10% (Medium)
- ▨ <5% (Low)

d 40-year-old patient with an increase in 24-hour urine calcium (nl <250 mg) of:
- □ >400 (High)
- ■ 300-400 (Medium)
- ▨ 250-299 (Low)

Fig. 28.1 Relationship between surgeon annual case load and low, medium, and high thresholds for surgery using intact parathyroid hormone (*iPTH*; **a**), bone densitometry T-score (**b**), creatinine clearance (**c**), and 24-hour urinary calcium (**d**)

cannot be captured. This is still the rudimentary state of the science of outcomes analysis from parathyroidectomy. Nevertheless, evidence supporting a volume–outcome relationship was deemed sufficient to lead the 2002 NIH Workshop on Asymptomatic Primary HPTH to emphasize that "parathyroidectomy should be performed only by experienced, expert parathyroid surgeons" [12]. The late Dr John Doppman cleverly described this when he said that the best preoperative localization test for hyperparathyroidism is to localize an experienced parathyroid surgeon [17].

Currently, a thorough understanding of the national patterns of endocrine surgery is lacking. Knowledge of clinical practice patterns would allow for a more accurate study of outcomes in the context of surgeon volume and would facilitate the planning of future needs for parathyroid surgery specialists. It is known that the great majority of operations for

endocrine surgery are performed by surgeons whose clinical practice is not focused heavily in endocrine surgery [18]. In addition, the number of surgeons whose practice is focused in endocrine surgery comprises a very small percentage of the total number of surgeons who are performing common operations for endocrine problems.

Based on a 2003 review by Saunders et al. using the International Classification of Disease, 9th revision (ICD-9) and the NIS administrative database, only 1.1% of parathyroidectomies performed in the USA between 1998 and 2000 were performed by surgeons with practices that are focused in endocrine surgery (>75% of practice performing parathyroidectomy, thyroidectomy, and adrenalectomy). The majority of parathyroidectomies were performed by general surgeons [18]. There were 14,232 patients who were identified as having undergone parathyroidectomy by 6,100 unique surgeons during the study period. Surgeons whose practice was focused on endocrine procedures performed 769 parathyroidectomies (5% of total), while general surgeons (<25% of practice dedicated to endocrine surgery) performed 11,071 parathyroidectomies (78% of total). The 242 highest volume parathyroid surgeons (27–182 parathyroidectomies per year) represented only 4% of the surgeons captured in the database, while the 2,995 surgeons who performed only 1–3 parathyroidectomies per year accounted for 49% of the surgeons in the database (Fig. 28.2).

28.4.3 Surgeon Training and Specialty

The development of new technologies such as MIP, the rapid intraoperative PTH assay, and radio-guided parathyroidectomy has made parathyroid surgery more complex. Despite this, the Accreditation Council for Graduate Medical Education (ACGME) sets no minimum number of parathyroid procedures required for completion of a general surgery residency. Moreover, the number of parathyroidectomies performed by graduating chief residents varies widely across the country. Recent evidence regarding the operative experience of general surgery residents in parathyroid disease showed the average number of procedures to be between 4.1 and 5.1, with a standard deviation of 3.44. The maximum cumulative number of parathyroid operations ranged from 25 to 60, and the most common annual caseload was only 2 [19]. With the implementation of the 80-hour resident work week in the USA, it is conceivable that these numbers might decrease even further, raising the question of whether

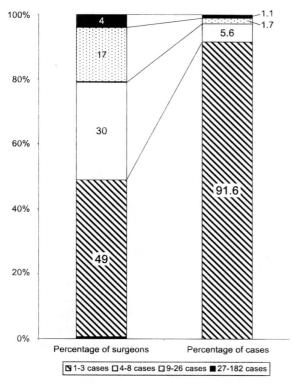

Fig. 28.2 Summary of the distribution of surgeons performing parathyroidectomy and parathyroidectomy cases by four surgeon volume groups

the majority of chief residents in general surgery are competent to perform parathyroidectomy after graduation [20].

Although outcomes from parathyroid surgery appear to be associated with experience based on self-reported data, there also are data which show that when residents perform parathyroidectomy under the supervision of an experienced parathyroid surgeon, clinical outcomes are excellent [21]. Willeke et al. reviewed the outcomes of 230 patients who underwent bilateral neck exploration for primary HPTH at the University of Heidelberg over an eight-year study period and demonstrated that inexperienced surgeons had comparable clinical outcomes to experienced consultants as long as they were under the supervision of an experienced surgeon (defined as having done >40 parathyroidectomies for primary HPTH). Complications were observed in 13.5% of patients, with no statistical difference between the experienced and the inexperienced supervised surgeons. There were 11 complications in 75 operations for the experienced surgeons, versus 25 complications in 155 operations for the supervised trainees ($P = 0.85$; difference 2.2%; 95% CI 7% to 11.4%). However, there were

some important differences between the two groups. Parathyroidectomy was significantly shorter when the operating surgeon was more experienced (median operation time, 85 versus 100 minutes; $P < 0.001$), and experienced surgeons more frequently were able to identify all parathyroid glands (at least four) during exploration than surgeons in training (56 of 75 for a 74.7% success rate, as compared to 80 of 155 for a 51.6% success rate; $P < 0.001$).

28.4.4 New Technologies

In the current era of cost containment, efforts to reduce LOS and associated costs have resulted in the development of a number of new surgical techniques, including MIP and radio-guided parathyroidectomy. MIP, described in 1994 by George Irvin and colleagues at the University of Miami, has dramatically changed the way parathyroidectomy is performed [22]. Unilateral neck exploration is conducted with the rapid PTH assay used as an intraoperative adjunct when patients have had successful preoperative localization. In the first report of the procedure, 16 of 18 study patients had sestamibi results that allowed for successful unilateral exploration with intraoperative confirmation of cure via the rapid PTH assay. Patients in the series who underwent MIP had an operative time that was shortened by an average of 54 minutes (90 versus 36 minutes).

Minimally invasive parathyroidectomy is becoming the standard of care among endocrine surgeons worldwide [23]. Sacket et al. surveyed members of the International Association of Endocrine Surgeons in 2002 and found that 59% of surgeons who are members of the Association perform MIP, and in these surgeons' practices, nearly half of patients with primary HPTH are candidates for the procedure (44%). There are now data showing that patients undergoing a unilateral procedure facilitated by preoperative localization have a lower incidence of biochemical and severe symptomatic hypocalcemia in the early postoperative period compared with patients undergoing traditional bilateral exploration [24]. In a prospective study of 91 patients with primary HPTH who were randomized to unilateral or bilateral neck exploration at Lund University Hospital, Bergenfelz et al. showed that patients in the bilateral neck exploration group consumed more oral calcium (4.20 versus 1.92 g; $P < 0.05$), had lower serum calcium values on postoperative days 1–4 (2.15 versus 2.26 mmol/l; $P < 0.05$), and had a higher incidence of early severe symptomatic hypocalcemia (11% versus 0%; $P < 0.05$) compared to patients in the unilateral group. In addition, for patients undergoing surgery for a solitary parathyroid adenoma, unilateral neck exploration was associated with a shorter operative time (62 versus 84 minutes; $P<0.01$). The cost of the two procedures, however, did not differ significantly.

Using a computer-generated mathematical model and decision tree analysis, Fahy et al. showed that limited parathyroid surgery facilitated by localization technologies (e.g., rapid PTH assay, preoperative sestamibi imaging, and intraoperative radio-guidance) has better clinical and economic outcomes than standard parathyroidectomy with bilateral neck exploration [25]. Specifically, the use of these new technologies reduced total charges, risk of persistent primary HPTH, and risk of recurrent laryngeal nerve injury in the decision analysis. Input variables were based on probabilities and costs culled from the literature. The best outcomes (i.e., greatest cost savings and lowest risk of nerve injury) from limited parathyroidectomy were achieved when sestamibi scanning was performed preoperatively and the gamma probe was used intraoperatively. The lowest incidence of persistent primary HPTH was seen when preoperative sestamibi scanning was combined with intraoperative use of the rapid PTH assay.

28.5   Outcomes from Parathyroidectomy

28.5.1   Clinical Outcomes

While complications from untreated primary HPTH sometimes led to death in the early 1900s, such outcomes are rare today. Instead, rare complications include recurrent laryngeal nerve injury, hemorrhage, wound complications, and postoperative hypocalcemia. Hypocalcemia is generally not severe and is managed successfully in the outpatient setting with calcium and vitamin D supplements. At the Cleveland Clinic, Tarazi et al. examined 70 consecutive patients who underwent parathyroidectomy for primary HPTH [26]. Only 2 developed symptoms of mild tetany after discharge, which responded to an increased dose of oral calcium.

Experienced parathyroid surgeons today achieve cure rates of up to 98% with both minimally invasive and conventional techniques [27]. In the largest published clinical series to date of parathyroid explorations compiled by a single surgeon for patients with primary HPTH ($n=656$), Udelsman demonstrated equivalent cure rates for patients who underwent tra-

ditional parathyroidectomy with bilateral neck exploration and MIP (97% versus 99%, respectively). Four hundred and one patients (61%) underwent standard bilateral cervical exploration under general anesthesia (13 of these had multiple endocrine neoplasia I or IIA), and 255 patients (39%) underwent MIP. There were no perioperative deaths in the series, and complication rates were 3.0% in the conventional group and 1.2% in the MIP group. Patients who underwent MIP were compared to historical controls, so comparisons were imperfect and tests of statistical significance were not performed.

There is still not perfect consensus among endocrinologists and endocrine surgeons about whether patients with minimally symptomatic and asymptomatic primary HPTH should undergo surveillance, non-operative (medical) therapy, or early surgery. The value of parathyroidectomy in asymptomatic patients with mild to moderate hypercalcemia has been debated because the natural history of primary HPTH is still not well understood, and rapid increases in the serum calcium level and/or progression of symptoms or complications is uncommon in patients with borderline hypercalcemia.

The neuromuscular symptoms of primary HPTH vary from series to series in their presentation and response to parathyroidectomy. However, (proximal) muscle weakness detected by examination (i.e., isokinetic strength of knee extension and flexion) appears to have a higher prevalence and to have a good response to parathyroidectomy, as does respiratory muscle capacity [28]. Significant increases in bone mineral density occur in the lumbar spine and hip following successful parathyroidectomy, and these improvements are maintained. The changes in bone remodeling and bone density are apparent within six months of parathyroidectomy [29]. Improvements in gastric ulcer incidence and fracture risk after parathyroidectomy were demonstrated by Vestergaard and Mosekidle, who compared patients with primary HPTH managed with parathyroidectomy versus non-operative strategies [30]. In this Danish nationwide cohort study of 3,213 patients with primary HPTH, 1,934 (60%) underwent surgery and 1,279 (40%) were managed medically. Patients treated with parathyroidectomy subsequently had a reduced risk of fracture (hazards ratio 0.69; 95% CI 0.56–0.84) and gastric ulcers (0.59; 95% CI 0.41–0.84) compared to similar patients without surgery.

No effect of successful surgery has been noted on either blood pressure or renal impairment [31]. Both urinary calcium excretion and the incidence of renal stones are reduced by successful parathyroidectomy

[32]. There are still no data proving that surgical cure increases life expectancy. A Swedish case-control study showed that 23 patients who underwent parathyroidectomy had a hazard ratio for death of 0.89, as compared to matched controls in the normal population. While this difference may be of clinical relevance, the study was clearly underpowered to reach statistical significance [33].

Psychiatric symptoms such as mental dullness, confusion, and loss of consciousness have been shown to improve within days after parathyroidectomy, although to date it has not been possible to predict which patients are most likely to benefit from surgery [34]. There have been reports of neurocognitive impairments associated with this disease, but well-performed, controlled clinical trials examining the effect of parathyroidectomy have not been published to date. However, our group at Yale University has preliminary data suggesting that parathyroidectomy significantly improves these impairments [35]. In this ongoing multidisciplinary, prospective study, we compare patients with primary HPTH with benign, euthyroid disease controls. Neurocognitive function is examined preoperatively and postoperatively using several well-validated and novel tests of memory and concentration, such as the Beck Depression Inventory, the Spielberger State/Trait Inventory, the Brief Symptom Inventory, the Rey Auditory Verbal Learning Test, and the PGRD Maze Learning Test. Compared to preoperative performance, patients with primary HPTH improve in their learning performance after surgery and appear to function at a level equivalent to the patients with thyroid disease after thyroidectomy. Preoperatively, patients with primary HPTH show greater delays in their spatial learning than thyroid controls, as evidenced by fewer correct moves per second across five learning trials and in a delayed response trial. These results suggest that primary HPTH may be associated with a spatial learning deficit and processing that improves with parathyroidectomy. Longer term follow-up is necessary to reach final conclusions, but neurocognitive symptoms might be considered in the future as criteria for parathyroidectomy in the treatment of primary HPTH.

28.5.2 Economic Outcomes

Variation in practice patterns has important implications for healthcare costs and quality of care. This issue was first addressed in 1980, when a break-even analysis suggested that the cost of early operation for primary HPTH would be exceeded by the cost of 5.5 years of medical surveillance [36]. The economic impact of variation in practice patterns is presumably even greater today, given that the costs of American healthcare have increased in the last two decades. A 1998 national survey of endocrine surgeons by Sosa et al. showed that health expenditures on primary HPTH could exceed $70 million in the USA annually, depending on whether management strategies involving low or high use of resources were employed [2]. Survey respondents ($n=109$) performed an average of 33 parathyroidectomies annually. Seventy-five percent of respondents reported using localization techniques before initial exploration. Their choice of localization studies varied significantly; in order of preference, these studies were sestamibi (43%), ultrasonography (28%), and sestamibi with single-photon emission computed tomography (SPECT) (26%). There was significant variation among endocrine surgeons in their patients' average total hospital costs. Even postoperative surveillance of patients with primary HPTH with laboratory tests and clinic visits was characterized by variation in practice patterns. For example, the number of postoperative office visits to the surgeon varied from one to nine, with median of two visits, whereas the number of iPTH tests (each of which cost $62 in 1998) varied from zero to 11. Overall, cost per patient undergoing a parathyroidectomy, assuming average use of resources, was about $7,500, but this cost could be $1,000 lower or higher based on assumptions of alternative use of resources, and 70% of the difference would stem from variation in in-hospital costs.

Given that the vast majority of parathyroidectomies performed in the USA are performed by non-endocrine surgeons and would not be reflected in this survey, variation in practice patterns might well be even higher. The recent introduction of MIP and other new technologies in parathyroid surgery also makes such studies out of date in 2006. According to Udelsman, the economic impact of MIP on average total hospital charges is significant [27]. In his clinical series, the mean LOS for MIP was 0.24 days, which compared favorably with the average LOS of 1.64 days for patients who underwent standard exploration. The mean savings per MIP was calculated as $2,693, which represented 49% of the total hospital charge.

28.5.3 Patient Utilities

As long as there continues to be lack of consensus among clinicians about how to optimize outcomes for patients with primary HPTH, patient preferences should be allowed at least in part to mold clinical decision making, and studies to measure preferences and quality of life in the field of primary HPTH are needed. Quiros et al. in 2003 asked 61 patients who underwent parathyroidectomy for hyperparathyroidism over a 16-month study period to complete a 53-question survey based on the Health Outcomes Institute Health Status Questionnaire 2.0 at three time points: before surgery, and 1 month and 3–24 months after surgery [37]. The survey included questions on overall health, daily activities, mood, and medical conditions. At both postoperative evaluations, patients' perception of general health, muscle strength, energy level, and mood significantly improved ($P<0.05$).

28.6   Policy Implications for Parathyroid Surgery

Given that primary HPTH is more prevalent among the elderly, one could speculate that incidence and prevalence of the disease might increase in the future as the number of Americans over age 65 is projected to grow [36,38]. "Baby boomers" (those born between 1946 and 1964) will begin turning 65 in 2011, when they will number 40.4 million (13% of the population); by 2030, the number of elderly over age 65 is projected to increase to 70.3 million (20% of the population) (http://www.census.gov/Press-Release/www/2000/cb00-05.html). Clearly, primary HPTH will continue to be a pressing public health concern, and outcomes research examining the surgical management of the disease must keep pace.

Surgical outcomes research has led policy makers and payers to practice "evidence-based hospital referral." The most visible of these efforts has been directed by the non-profit Leapfrog Group, which began its initiative in November 2000 in response to a 1999 Institute of Medicine (IOM) report which showed that preventable medical errors in hospitals account for approximately 98,000 deaths per year (http://www.leapfroggroup.org). Leapfrog is an employer-led endeavor whereby a coalition of more than 150 public and private healthcare purchasers representing over 40 million people encourages improvements in the quality of patient outcomes by directing patient referrals to hospitals which meet minimum-volume standards. Leapfrog requires that hospitals maintain certain procedure-specific volume caseloads per year for high-risk surgical procedures such as CABG (500 procedures per year), coronary angioplasty (400 per year), carotid endarterectomy (100 per year), repair of abdominal aortic aneurysm (30 per year), and esophagectomy for cancer (6 per year). There is compelling evidence that higher volumes is correlated with better outcomes for these procedures [15].

Leapfrog has not included parathyroidectomy among its list of procedures, perhaps in part because there is a paucity of outcomes research in the field. However, with time this may change, as outcomes data for endocrine surgery are assembled to inform debate. Existing databases do not lend themselves to this purpose, since parathyroidectomy is increasingly performed in the ambulatory setting. Therefore, multi-institutional prospective primary data collection will be essential.

The creation of clinical practice guidelines intended to standardize the medical and surgical management of primary HPTH could help in reducing variation in practice patterns. In light of the persistent controversy surrounding the optimal management of asymptomatic primary HPTH, the NIH established a consensus panel in 1990 and a Workshop in 2002 to formulate and reformulate recommendations to standardize patient care. However, national surveys of endocrinologists and endocrine surgeons showed that the management of primary HPTH is highly variable among both groups and compliance is poor with many of the practice guidelines outlined in the NIH consensus statements [16,39]. Among surgeons, thresholds were higher than those recommended by the NIH for younger patients and lower than those recommended for older patients. For example, although both NIH consensus statements recommended surgery for *all* patients with primary HPTH below 50 years of age, endocrine surgeons in the survey reported using additional laboratory and clinical criteria to decide whether to operate on younger patients [16]. High-volume endocrinologists, who are likely to be most experienced in managing primary HPTH, were more aware of the NIH guidelines than low-volume physicians in the 1998 national survey of 374 endocrinologists [39].

It is possible that many surgeons are not aware of the NIH guidelines. Alternatively, they could be aware of the guidelines but intentionally do not follow them; for example, surgeons might believe that there is not enough evidence (e.g., prospective randomized trials) supporting the consensus statements. This raises the question of whether the guidelines are obsolete and require yet another reformulation, as third-party payers such as the Leapfrog initiative might use published recommendations to guide their reimbursement strategies. Clearly, guidelines for the (surgical) management of primary HPTH must be more widely disseminated and strongly recommended if practice patterns are to be influenced and clinical outcomes improved.

Clinical pathways are one method healthcare providers and hospital administrators use to standardize care [40]. When a clinical pathway for parathyroidectomy was implemented from July 1998 through July 1999 at the University of Virginia Health System, average LOS decreased from 2.4 to 1.5 days ($P = 0.26$). This, in turn, had economic implications, with per case average cost decreasing from \$5,071 to \$4,291 ($P = 0.50$). Although these differences were not statistically significant due to the relatively small sample size, they can be considered as clinically relevant.

In light of evidence linking surgeon experience with clinical and economic outcomes for parathyroidectomy, there has been a trend toward the creation of centers of excellence in endocrine surgery and parathyroidectomy. There are a growing number of North American fellowship programs in endocrine surgery; however, none are yet certified. Such high-volume parathyroidectomy centers could facilitate the training of young high-volume surgeons in new techniques such as MIP, as well as the creation of evidence-based referral initiatives in parathyroid surgery. However, it also has worrisome implications for access to quality care, especially in rural parts of the country where patients with primary HPTH might be unable to easily access high-volume parathyroid surgeons because of geographic or economic barriers. It will be important for internists, endocrinologists, surgeons, payers, and policymakers to work together in a collaborative fashion. Only then will it be possible to prospectively assemble the primary, up-to-date outcomes data needed to optimize practice patterns and allow for a reasonable balance between cost-effectiveness, quality of care, and access to high-volume providers of parathyroidectomy.

References

1. Wermers RA, Khosla S, et al (1997) The rise and fall of primary hyperparathyroidism: a population-based study in Rochester, Minnesota, 1965–1992. Ann Intern Med 126:433–440

2. Sosa JA, Powe NR, et al (1998) Cost implications of different surgical management strategies for primary hyperparathyroidism. Surgery 124:1028–1035; discussion 1035–1036

3. Melton LJ 3rd (2002) The epidemiology of primary hyperparathyroidism in North America. J Bone Miner Res 17(suppl 2):N12–N17

4. Owen R (1862) On the anatomy of the Indian rhinoceros (*Rh. Unicornis*, L). Trans Zool Soc Lond 4:31–58

5. Carney JA (1996) The glandulae parathyroideae of Ivar Sandström. Contributions from two continents. Am J Surg Pathol 20:1123–1144

6. Organ CH Jr (2000) The history of parathyroid surgery, 1850–1996: the Excelsior Surgical Society 1998 Edward D. Churchill Lecture. J Am Coll Surg 191:284–299

7. Bauer FA, Aub JC (1930) A case of osteitis fibrosa cystica (osteomalacia?) with evidence of hyperactivity of the parathyroid bodies: a metabolic study. J Clin Invest 8:229–248

8. Mandl F (1926) Attempt to treat generalized fibrous osteitis by extirpation of parathyroid tumor. Zentralbl F Chir 53:260–264

9. Barr D, Bulger H, Dixon H (1929) Hyperparathyroidism. JAMA 92:951–952

10. Guy C (1929) Tumors of the parathyroid glands. Surg Gynecol Obstet 48:557–565

11. Luft HS, Bunker JP, Enthoven AC (1979) Should operations be regionalized? The empirical relation between surgical volume and mortality. N Engl J Med 301:1364–1369

12. Bilezikian JP, Potts JT Jr, et al (2002) Summary statement from a workshop on asymptomatic primary hyperparathyroidism: a perspective for the 21st century. J Clin Endocrinol Metab 87:5353–5361

13. National Institutes of Health (1990) Diagnosis and management of asymptomatic primary hyperparathyroidism. National Institutes of Health Consensus Development Conference, 29–31 October 1990. Consens Statement 8:1–18

14. Chen H, Parkerson S, Udelsman R (1998) Parathyroidectomy in the elderly: do the benefits outweigh the risks? World J Surg 22:531–535; discussion 535–536

15. Birkmeyer JD, Siewers AE, et al (2002) Hospital volume and surgical mortality in the United States. N Engl J Med 346:1128–1137

16. Sosa JA, Powe NR, et al (1998) Profile of a clinical practice: thresholds for surgery and surgical outcomes for patients with primary hyperparathyroidism. A national survey of endocrine surgeons. J Clin Endocrinol Metab 83:2658–2665

17. Doppman JL, Miller DL (1991) Localization of parathyroid tumors in patients with asymptomatic hyperparathyroidism and no previous surgery. J Bone Miner Res 6(suppl 2):S153–S158; discussion S159

18. Saunders BD, Wainess RM, et al (2003) Who performs endocrine operations in the United States? Surgery 134:924–931; discussion 931

19. Harness JK, Organ CH Jr, Thompson NW (1995) Operative experience of U.S. general surgery residents in thyroid and parathyroid disease. Surgery 118:1063–1069; discussion 1069–1070

20. Jarman BT, Miller MR, et al (2004) The 80-hour work week: will we have less-experienced graduating surgeons? Curr Surg 61:612–615

21. Willeke F, Willeke M, et al (1998) Effect of surgeon expertise on the outcome in primary hyperparathyroidism. Arch Surg 133:1066–1070; discussion 1071

22. Irvin GL 3rd, Prudhomme DL, et al (1994) A new approach to parathyroidectomy. Ann Surg 219:574–579; discussion 579–581

23. Sackett WR, Barraclough B, et al (2002) Worldwide trends in the surgical treatment of primary hyperparathyroidism in the era of minimally invasive parathyroidectomy. Arch Surg 137:1055–1059

24. Bergenfelz A, Lindblom P, et al (2002) Unilateral versus bilateral neck exploration for primary hyperparathyroidism: a prospective randomized controlled trial. Ann Surg 236:543–551

25. Fahy BN, Bold RJ, et al (2002) Modern parathyroid surgery: a cost-benefit analysis of localizing strategies. Arch Surg 137:917–922; discussion 922–923

26. Tarazi R, Esselstyn CB Jr, Coccia MR (1984) Parathyroidectomy for primary hyperparathyroidism: early discharge. Surgery 96:1158–1162

27. Udelsman R (2002) Six hundred fifty-six consecutive explorations for primary hyperparathyroidism. Ann Surg 235:665–670; discussion 670–672

28. Joborn C, Joborn H, et al (1988) Maximal isokinetic muscle strength in patients with primary hyperparathyroidism before and after parathyroid surgery. Br J Surg 75:77–80

29. Christiansen P, Steiniche T, et al (1999) Primary hyperparathyroidism: effect of parathyroidectomy on regional bone mineral density in Danish patients: a three-year follow-up study. Bone 25:589–595

30. Vestergaard P, Mosekilde L (2003) Cohort study on effects of parathyroid surgery on multiple outcomes in primary hyperparathyroidism. BMJ 327:530–534

31. Salahudeen AK, Thomas TH, et al (1989) Hypertension and renal dysfunction in primary hyperparathyroidism: effect of parathyroidectomy. Clin Sci (Colch) 76:289–296

32. Silverberg SJ, Shane E, et al (1999) A 10-year prospective study of primary hyperparathyroidism with or without parathyroid surgery. N Engl J Med 341:1249–1255

33. Lundgren E, Lind L, et al (2001) Increased cardiovascular mortality and normalized serum calcium in patients with mild hypercalcemia followed up for 25 years. Surgery 130:978–985

34. Joborn C, Hetta J, et al (1989) Self-rated psychiatric symptoms in patients operated on because of primary hyperparathyroidism and in patients with long-standing mild hypercalcemia. Surgery 105:72–78

35. Roman S, Sosa JA, et al (2005) Parathyroidectomy improves neurocognitive deficits in patients with primary hyperparathyroidism. Surgery (in press)

36. Heath H 3rd, Hodgson SF, Kennedy MA (1980) Primary hyperparathyroidism. Incidence, morbidity, and potential economic impact in a community. N Engl J Med 302:189–193

37. Quiros RM, Alef MJ, et al (2003) Health-related quality of life in hyperparathyroidism measurably improves after parathyroidectomy. Surgery 134:675–681; discussion 681–683

38. Tibblin S, Palsson N, Rydberg J (1983) Hyperparathyroidism in the elderly. Ann Surg 197:135–138

39. Mahadevia PJ, Sosa JA, et al (2003) Clinical management of primary hyperparathyroidism and thresholds for surgical referral: a national study examining concordance between practice patterns and consensus panel recommendations. Endocr Pract 9:494–503

40. Markey DW, McGowan J, Hanks JB (2000) The effect of clinical pathway implementation on total hospital costs for thyroidectomy and parathyroidectomy patients. Am Surg 66:533–538; discussion 538–539

Subject Index